Sustainable Development Goals Series

The **Sustainable Development Goals Series** is Springer Nature's inaugural cross-imprint book series that addresses and supports the United Nations' seventeen Sustainable Development Goals. The series fosters comprehensive research focused on these global targets and endeavours to address some of society's greatest grand challenges. The SDGs are inherently multidisciplinary, and they bring people working across different fields together and working towards a common goal. In this spirit, the Sustainable Development Goals series is the first at Springer Nature to publish books under both the Springer and Palgrave Macmillan imprints, bringing the strengths of our imprints together.

The Sustainable Development Goals Series is organized into eighteen subseries: one subseries based around each of the seventeen respective Sustainable Development Goals, and an eighteenth subseries, "Connecting the Goals," which serves as a home for volumes addressing multiple goals or studying the SDGs as a whole. Each subseries is guided by an expert Subseries Advisor with years or decades of experience studying and addressing core components of their respective Goal.

The SDG Series has a remit as broad as the SDGs themselves, and contributions are welcome from scientists, academics, policymakers, and researchers working in fields related to any of the seventeen goals. If you are interested in contributing a monograph or curated volume to the series, please contact the Publishers: Zachary Romano [Springer; zachary.romano@springer.com] and Rachael Ballard [Palgrave Macmillan; rachael.ballard@palgrave.com].

Mario C. B. Raviglione • Fabrizio Tediosi
Simone Villa • Núria Casamitjana
Antoni Plasència
Editors

Global Health Essentials

Springer

Editors
Mario C. B. Raviglione
Centre for Multidisciplinary Research in Health Science (MACH)
University of Milan
Milan, Italy

Fabrizio Tediosi
Department of Epidemiology and Public Health
Swiss Tropical and Public Health Institute
Allschwill, Switzerland

Simone Villa
Centre for Multidisciplinary Research in Health Science (MACH)
University of Milan
Milan, Italy

Núria Casamitjana
Barcelona Institute for Global Health (ISGlobal), Hospital Clínic
University of Barcelona
Barcelona, Spain

Antoni Plasència
Barcelona Institute for Global Health (ISGlobal), Hospital Clínic
University of Barcelona
Barcelona, Spain

ISSN 2523-3084 ISSN 2523-3092 (electronic)
Sustainable Development Goals Series
ISBN 978-3-031-33853-3 ISBN 978-3-031-33851-9 (eBook)
https://doi.org/10.1007/978-3-031-33851-9

This Springer imprint is published by the registered company Springer Nature Switzerland AG
The registered company address is: Gewerbestrasse 11, 6330 Cham, Switzerland

Foreword

Global Health Essentials provides a comprehensive overview of global health, rooted in the principles outlined in the World Health Organization's constitution and the health targets of the Sustainable Development Goals. The book is designed to be accessible to readers from diverse professional backgrounds from both the health and non-health sectors, including students, global health professionals, policy-makers, and others seeking to broaden their knowledge of global health, regardless of their background.

The book embraces a multidisciplinary and cross-sectoral approach, delving into various scientific fields beyond traditional health disciplines, including human development, health economics, social sciences, digital technologies, climate change, and communication sciences, to provide a comprehensive and wide-ranging look at the many factors influencing global health. The book takes into account not only academic perspectives, but also that of implementers, governmental and diplomatic officials, and civil society and community groups. Of the book's 88 chapters, 37 are authored by current or former WHO staff.

The book emphasizes the important role of many of the SDGs in promoting population health across sectors. It highlights the practical implications of assessing the determinants of health, recognizing the interplay between social, economic, commercial, and environmental factors. By comprehensively exploring these determinants, the book provides readers with a nuanced understanding of the multifaceted nature of global health.

The book addresses the need to rethink global health in light of the lessons learned and challenges resulting from the COVID-19 pandemic and other emerging global health threats, including environmental and climate changes, the ecological approach to health and the "One Health" approach, and the health of the planet as a whole.

Finally, the book promotes global solidarity and social justice as critical to positively impacting people's health. It reflects on contemporary social movements that are calling for a re-thinking of global health, and the structural injustices that both make communities more vulnerable to health risks and prevent them from accessing health services. It also considers the need for supporting the training and retention of the health workforce, particularly in low-resource communities and countries. The book considers the impact of a variety of challenges, including poverty, racism, sexism, homophobia, and other inequalities that impact the most vulnerable populations worldwide, including children, adolescents, women, and ageing people.

Global Health Essentials is an important addition to the global health curriculum, offering valuable perspectives from a broad array of disciplines and specialties.

Tedros Adhanom Ghebreyesus
Director-General
World Health Organization
Geneva, Switzerland

Preface

Health is a state of complete physical, mental and social well-being and not merely the absence of disease or infirmity. The enjoyment of the highest attainable standard of health is one of the fundamental rights of every human being without distinction of race, religion, political belief, economic or social condition. The health of all peoples is fundamental to the attainment of peace and security and is dependent on the fullest co-operation of individuals and States. (WHO Constitution, 1946)

These opening statements of the Constitution of the World Health Organization (WHO) were formally adopted by the representatives of 61 States during the International Health Conference held in New York between 19 June and 22 July 1946. They reflected the outcome of discussions by a group of sixteen visionary persons chosen for their expert qualifications that constituted the Technical Preparatory Committee set up during the historical United Nations Conference on International Organization in 1945 at San Francisco. A few months later, the Committee started to work intensively to conceive and design the future WHO. Although the term "global health" is a recent one, dating back a couple of decades during the "era of globalization", the broad philosophy outlined in the first few words of the preamble of the WHO Constitution keeps inspiring those like us who believe in the principles of global health so well captured in the wording of the United Nations (UN) Sustainable Development Goal (SDG) 3: "To ensure healthy lives and promote well-being for all at all ages". These straightforward words promote the fundamental quest for equitable access to health for all without exception.

In this manual we have endeavoured to present the key themes and challenges of global health in a manner that is accessible to readers from diverse professional backgrounds. Whether the reader is a student interested in the well-being of world populations, a global health professional, or simply someone seeking to broaden knowledge of global health and its vast scope, we have carefully designed this book to be user-friendly and concise. The manual serves as an essential introduction to global health, particularly for those pursuing postgraduate studies in disciplines directly or indirectly related to the populations' health. To accomplish this goal, each chapter has been designed to be brief yet informative. Furthermore, we have included an essential bibliographic list of references, enabling interested and knowledgeable readers to delve deeper into the themes described within this compact volume. Finally, the book can be used as a pocket manual by individuals enrolled in specific global health courses. It provides them with convenient and expedient access to fundamental concepts and themes, supporting their studies and enhancing their understanding of this field.

The manual is structured around eight overarching macro-topics, aiming to comprehensively cover the field of global health. These topics include Introduction to Global Health; Global Burden of Disease (divided into four sections: Introduction; Health Throughout the Life Course; Communicable Diseases; Non-communicable Diseases); Social Determinants of Health; Health Systems; Innovations in Global Health; Governance of Global Health; Era of Sustainable Development; Methods in Global Health. Within the "Global Burden of Disease" section, one can find concise and focused chapters dedicated to individual high-burden conditions or diseases of global significance. These chapters are designed to provide essential knowledge on epidemiology, challenges, strategies, and response, particularly for readers who may be less familiar with these specific topics. They serve as short yet informative snapshots, offering a valuable overview of each disease or condition.

In light of the sustainable development context that underpins the foundation of global health, the structure of this manual is inherently multidisciplinary and cross-sectoral. It encompasses a wide range of disciplines and sciences that are fundamental for comprehensive understanding of the field. At its core, the book delves into the fundamental sciences that form the basis of global health in a multi- and interdisciplinary approach. In addition to areas of study such as epidemiology, biostatistics, high-burden diseases and conditions, and health systems, this manual explores various other topics of great significance. These topics encompass areas of study such as human development and cooperation, health economics and financing, social science perspectives with focus on health determinants and challenges, including migrant health and the human rights perspectives. Moreover, the manual explores innovative digital technologies, the agri-food system and its impact on nutrition, veterinarian public health and the "One Health" approach, the impact of climate change on human health, and communication sciences. By incorporating such diverse and interconnected subjects, we aim to provide readers with a comprehensive understanding of global health that transcends traditional disciplinary boundaries. This multidimensional approach allows for a holistic exploration of the complex factors that shape global health outcomes and underscores the interconnectedness of various scientific fields.

Overall, therefore, this manual is centred around the "integrated and indivisible" UN SDGs. There is a specific section devoted to sustainable development, the SDGs and their history, their significance in health and for health. The SDG framework philosophy is transpiring from every chapter of the book. For instance, when the highest burden diseases and conditions are described, references to SDG targets set within the health SDG (SDG-3) are made. Indeed, the book also serves a crucial role in educating readers on the importance of non-health SDGs and their targets in safeguarding population health. It places strong emphasis on the practical implications of assessing the determinants of health, which go beyond the traditional health factors. It involves recognizing the intricated interplay between various social, economic, and environmental dimensions that shape population health outcomes.

By highlighting the importance of non-health SDGs, this book underscores the need to address a wide range of interconnected factors to promote and ensure the well-being of populations. In practical terms, assessing the determinants of health entails recognizing the influence of factors encompassed within the SDGs, such as education, poverty alleviation, gender equality, clean water and sanitation, sustainable cities and communities, climate action, and other relevant factors. By comprehensively exploring these determinants, the book provides readers with a nuanced understanding of the multifaceted nature of global health.

In consideration of emerging discussions, and beyond the more traditional and essential topics, the book also looks at the need to re-think the whole concept of global health in view of the "new normality" expected to result from the COVID-19 pandemic and the upcoming challenges and threats in the context of our world geopolitics. This means addressing environmental and climate changes, the need of an ecological approach to health including "One Health", and, ultimately, the health of our planet as a whole.

Furthermore, there is today a social movement calling for a re-thinking of global health given the structural injustice that still precludes the full contributions of low-resource country professionals to the public good of health. Scholars in global health everywhere need therefore to embark on concrete research, development, and implementation of policies addressing challenges originating from the inequitable and often demeaning world we live in. These challenges include racism, sexism, homophobia, and other discriminating attitudes that impact on the most vulnerable fragments of populations worldwide, including children, adolescents, women, and ageing people. It also means dealing with the uncomfortable, embarrassing issue of "decolonization" and elimination of the "white supremacy", thus pursuing a comprehensive global health agenda and permitting all to contribute to their best and in full respect of their cultures. COVID-19 has clearly unveiled global injustice and unfairness, well exemplified by the COVID-19 vaccine "apartheid" and inequities.

The urgency of promoting global solidarity and social justice to positively impact people's health necessitates the dissemination of information and education. This book strives to address this critical need and fulfil the principles of global health. With a genuine commitment to equity, diversity, and inclusiveness, we aim to advance the agenda in these areas. Our aspiration is for this manual to reach a global audience, transcending boundaries and not solely catering to those in economically privileged settings. We commend Springer for exploring ways of making the book affordable everywhere. Additionally, recognizing the importance of accessibility, the manual will also be available as an e-book. This digital format will facilitate wider dissemination, particularly in low- and middle-income countries, as well as among students enrolled in global health courses around the world. By embracing this inclusive perspective, we aim to ensure that individuals from diverse backgrounds, irrespective of economic circumstances, can benefit from the knowledge and insights presented in this book. We firmly believe that everyone should have the opportunity to engage with and contribute to the field of global health.

This manual is conceived as part of the new Springer Series devoted to the Sustainable Development Goals being focused on SDG-3: "Good health and well-being". While several other books on global health and SDGs have been published in the past few years, most tend to be specific around certain aspects of global health and do not cover the entire field. Different from most, our book is an agile, succinct manual that addresses, as explained above, all fields within global health with the contributions of multiple authors and experts in different disciplines and sectors and with diverse backgrounds and cultures.

The challenges faced in the field of global health are enormous, surpassing the current capacity to address them. Considering this, it becomes crucial to prioritize the education and training of young professionals, equipping them with a "global health mindset". Our ultimate goal is therefore to impart knowledge and promote sound scientific practices in this multifaceted and cross-disciplinary field of global health. We believe that by nurturing a global health mindset, professionals from various disciplines and every citizen of the world can actively contribute to the realization of the fundamental human right of "health for all". This aspiration requires a collective effort and a deep understanding of the interconnectedness and complexities of global health challenges.

Milan, Italy — Mario C. B. Raviglione
Allschwil, Switzerland — Fabrizio Tediosi
Milan, Italy — Simone Villa
Barcelona, Spain — Núria Casamitjana
Barcelona, Spain — Antoni Plasència

Acknowledgements

The Editors are indebted to Dr Beat Stoll of the University of Geneva for his precious suggestions of topics and authors during the conceptual phase of preparation, and to Prof. Richard Skolnik for useful discussions on global health and inspiring input especially in the "Global Burden of Disease" section.

Contents

Part I

Introduction to Global Health

1 Definition, Principles, and Evolution of Global Health

Mario C. B. Raviglione

Abstract

Building on the principles of public health and of the World Health Organization (WHO) definition of health, a definition of global health (GH) was outlined by some as a "cross-discipline" for "study, research, and practice placing a priority on improving health and achieving equity in health for all people worldwide". As such, GH focuses "on transnational health issues, determinants, and solutions; involves many disciplines within and beyond health sciences; promotes interdisciplinary collaboration; and is a synthesis of population-based prevention with individual-level clinical care". Subsequently, systemic and ecological dimensions were added as part of sustainable solutions. The concept of globality emphasizes more than geographical considerations being articulated along several points, including holistic approach, dependence on transnational determinants, awareness that big challenges must be addressed in their totality and through an equity lens that includes one's own community, comprehensive vision of health priorities, and "globality" of disciplines and sectors. The study of global health is rich and vast. It covers its evolution from tropical medicine to public and international health; analysis of global burden of disease, epidemiological transition and progress in health outcomes; assessment of social and economic determinants of health; relationship between health and development; impact of globalization on health; role of the UN Sustainable Development Goals (SDG) in fostering access to health; governance of global health and role of major actors; principles of international cooperation; and assessment of big challenges including pandemic response and preparedness, "One Health" approaches to prevention and management of zoonotic conditions, and impacts of migration and climate change on health.

Keywords

Global health · Public health · International health · Tropical medicine · World Health Organization (WHO) · World Bank · Millennium Development Goals (MDGs) · Sustainable Development Goals (SDGs) · Planetary health

What is Global Health? How do we define it and understand its origins and evolution starting from the definition of "health" in the visionary Constitution of the World Health Organization

M. C. B. Raviglione (✉)
Centre for Multidisciplinary Research in Health Science (MACH), University of Milan, Milan, Italy
e-mail: mario.raviglione@unimi.it

M. C. B. Raviglione et al. (eds.), *Global Health Essentials*, Sustainable Development Goals Series,
https://doi.org/10.1007/978-3-031-33851-9_1

(WHO): "a *state of complete physical, mental and social well-being and not merely the absence of disease*" [1] (see Box 1.1)? How do we recognize its significance today and visualize its future? How do we both distinguish it from, and connect it with, public health and what used to be called "international health"?

Box 1.1 The Constitution of the World Health Organization [1]

The WHO Constitution declares: *"Health is a state of complete physical, mental and social well-being and not merely the absence of disease or infirmity.*

The enjoyment of the highest attainable standard of health is one of the fundamental rights of every human being without distinction of race, religion, political belief, economic or social condition.

The health of all peoples is fundamental to the attainment of peace and security and is dependent upon the fullest cooperation of individuals and States.

The achievement of any State in the promotion and protection of health is of value to all".

Global health (GH), according to an original and early attempt of description proposed by experts in 2009, is "an area for study, research and practice that places a priority on improving health and achieving equity in access to health for people worldwide. Global health emphasizes transnational health issues, determinants, and solutions; involves many disciplines within and beyond the health sciences and promotes interdisciplinary collaboration; and is a synthesis of population-based prevention with individual-level clinical care" [2]. One can indeed consider it as a "cross-discipline" or an area spanning across multiple sectors with a transversal perspective which goes beyond the mere geographical considerations (Box 1.2, freely adapted from [3]).

This chapter introduces the main characteristics and roles of global health, origins and relevance, its links with international health and public health, and the evolution towards "precision global health" and the concept of "planetary health" further emphasizing its ecological dimension (Table 1.1).

Box 1.2 *What is so "global" about Global Health?*

Global aim: Any health issue concerning many countries, affected by transnational determinants (e.g., climate change), and requiring transnational solutions (e.g., a vaccine).

Global scope of problems beyond geographic location. Besides cross-border issues, it can also focus on domestic disparities and inequities among marginalized populations.

Global view: All major health problems, beyond infectious diseases and maternal and child health, embracing the epidemiological transition, and prioritization based on global burden of disease and economic evaluation.

Global in disciplines and sectors: It implies approaches that are both interdisciplinary and multi-sectorial towards both prevention and curative care and are not limited to the health sector alone.

Selected examples of Global Health issues: Emerging and re-emerging infectious diseases; pandemics; antimicrobial resistance; eradication of polio; control of tuberculosis, malaria and HIV; the growing challenge of non-communicable conditions such as cardiovascular diseases, cancer, chronic obstructive lung disease, diabetes, mental health disorders; as well as the impact of climate change and phenomena such as migration.

The most obvious recent example is the pandemic of COVID-19, which emerged in late 2019 and has caused hundreds of millions of cases and millions of deaths worldwide with profound social, economic, and political consequences.

Table 1.1 Differences among global, international, and public health

	Global health	International health	Public health
Geographical reach	Focuses on issues that directly or indirectly affect health but that can transcend national boundaries	Focuses on health issues of countries other than one's own, especially those of low-income and middle-income	Focuses on issues that affect the health of the population of a particular community or country
Level of cooperation	Development and implementation of solutions often requires global cooperation	Development and implementation of solutions usually requires binational cooperation	Development and implementation of solutions does not usually require global cooperation
Individuals or populations	Embraces both prevention in populations and clinical care of individuals	Embraces both prevention in populations and clinical care of individuals	Mainly focused on prevention programmes for populations
Access to health	Health equity among nations and for all people is a major objective	Seeks to help people of other nations	Health equity within a nation or community is a major objective
Range of disciplines	Highly interdisciplinary and multidisciplinary within and beyond health sciences	Embraces a few disciplines but has not emphasized multidisciplinarity	Encourages multidisciplinary approaches, particularly within health sciences and with social sciences

(Reproduced with permission from Koplan et al. 2009)

Public health (PH) emerged as a concept and new discipline in the second half of the 1800s in Great Britain, other European countries, and the USA. It was made possible by the emerging quest for social reforms and increased scientific knowledge of the time. Evidence—from national vital statistics, health surveillance, and medical laboratories—enabled better decision-making by governments and health authorities. After centuries during which "health" was essentially a concept closely linked to "medicine", the focus progressively moved to the health of population besides that of individuals. There was an emphasis on prevention beyond curative care; and the goal of social justice took root.

Ever since, PH has been and remains concerned with the health of the population of a given country. Each country has its own health system and health services and may not need global cooperation. Public health's main focus is on prevention programmes for the population and health equity is a major objective within the nation and its communities. One of the most used and surely visionary definitions is from Winslow in 1920 [4] (Box 1.3).

Box 1.3 Public Health: The Winslow Definition [4]

"Public health is the science and the art of preventing disease, prolonging life, and promoting physical health and efficiency through organized community efforts for the sanitation of the environment, the control of community infections, the education of the individual in principles of personal hygiene, the organization of medical and nursing service for the early diagnosis and preventive treatment of disease, and the development of the social machinery which will ensure to every individual in the community a standard of living adequate for the maintenance of health".

The concept of **international health** emerged after the end of World War II and during the "decolonization" era. It focused on other countries in addition to one's own with an emphasis on low- and middle-income countries. It is an evolution of ideas born during the colonial era with the advent of Colonial Medicine and the discipline of Tropical Medicine. Colonial medicine is linked mainly to the consequences of colonization of tropical countries: it became soon clear that European colonization had enormous effects on the health of both indigenous populations and colonists through the transfer of new diseases, mechanisms of oppression, and the process of urbanization. **Tropical medicine** is the branch of clinical medicine dealing with health problems that occur predominantly, are more widespread, or prove more difficult to contain in tropical and sub-tropical regions. Great Britain was a leader in the establishment of the discipline of tropical medicine in the late nineteenth century, in parallel to the consolidation of its colonial empire. Sir Patrick Manson, a Scottish physician who founded the London School of Hygiene and Tropical Medicine in 1899, is dubbed the "Father of Tropical Medicine". The original main focus of tropical medicine was infections that were, and still are, endemic in tropical zones. However, today, tropical medicine cannot ignore non-communicable conditions, such as malnutrition, cardiovascular and chronic obstructive lung diseases, cancer, and diabetes, and therefore, their social and economic determinants that are common in the tropics.

Based on the experiences from the fields of public health and tropical medicine, the concept of **international health** developed together with a growing humanitarian sentiment whereby higher-income countries felt indebted to poorer, exploited and former colonized countries. The establishment of WHO in 1948 strengthened and further consolidated such powerful sense of humanitarian involvement in the health and development of poorer nations. A new sense of global solidarity prevailed. Box 1.4 illustrates how international health was born and developed during the twentieth century.

Box 1.4 The history of international health before and after the creation of the World Health Organization

1902: Founding of the International Sanitary Office of the American Republics, later Pan American Sanitary Bureau, eventually the Panamerican Health Organization (PAHO) in Washington, DC. PAHO is now the WHO's Regional Office for the Americas.

1907: In Paris, the Office International d'Hygiène Publique (OIHP) is established.

1913: In New York state, the Rockefeller Foundation establishes its International Health Division and goes on to tackle infectious diseases such as yellow fever and malaria.

1920: In Geneva, the League of Nations Health Organization, antecedent of WHO, is set up.

1945: In San Francisco, an international conference approves creation of the United Nations and a new specialized health agency is promoted.

1946: In the Constitution of WHO is written, with 16 member countries (see Box 1.4). A few months later the first International Health Conference is held in New York.

1948, in Geneva, held on 24 June–24 July, the first annual World Health Assembly formally establishes WHO as an international and intergovernmental agency with a global perspective.

Global health (GH) is the further evolution of international health. GH relates to issues that transcend national boundaries, are important to many countries at the same time, and require global cooperation. To fight pandemics such as COVID-19, for example, global cooperation is essential, as is confronting climate change and its health consequences. GH, in seeking equitable access to health care for people in all countries, pursues the concept of primary health care (PHC) and of universal health coverage (UHC). Furthermore, it is multidisciplinary and extends well beyond the health sciences which is, per se, a fascinating challenge in didactic terms. While being strongly rooted within health sciences, GH implementation needs to embrace multiple sciences beyond health and to balance them to pursue concrete outcomes when facing complex issues. Considering its wide range of action, GH is an "umbrella" term that may encompass different sectors and fields as long its global, multidisciplinary core and equitable access principles are preserved [5].

The origins of GH can be traced to the start of the globalization era and the end of the cold war. Globalization represents "a complex and multi-faceted set of processes… that change the nature of human interaction across a wide range of spheres, e.g. economic, political, social, technological and environmental… resulting in the erosion of boundaries of various kind" [6]. Others have compressed the definition: "globalization is about intensifying planetary interconnectivity" [7].

In the era of globalization, novel concepts on how to confront complex global health problems emerged. The World Bank was paramount in reshaping the intellectual and philosophical approach to health through its landmark World Development Report 1993 "Investing in Health". That Report assessed the benefits and costs of health interventions. Its main messages were that evidence-based health expenditures are an investment not only in health, but also in economic prosperity; and that additional resources should be spent on cost-effective interventions to address high-burden diseases. It advocated greater government spending on health, with a package of public health interventions, and fostering an environment to enable households to improve health, promoting pro-poor economic policies, education (especially for girls), and advancing the rights of women. It also promoted diversity and competition, encouraging social or private health insurance. The Report introduced the new concepts of the "global burden of disease" estimates and of measuring cost-effectiveness through indicators including deaths and disability-adjusted life years (DALYs) [8].

Simultaneously, the 1993 WHO World Health Assembly reviewed WHO's role in a rapidly changing global context. It emphasized global health issues and a rethink of WHO's coordinating role. In a sense, global health became "fashionable" with an initial emphasis on global infectious threats. Since the 1970s, in fact, nearly 50 new infectious diseases had been discovered. COVID-19 is the most recent, but others include its closest relative SARS (Severe Acute Respiratory Syndrome) in 2003 and the other Coronavirus epidemic of MERS (Middle Eastern Respiratory Syndrome), as well as avian and swine flu, Ebola, ZIKA, and a multiplicity of antimicrobial resistant bacterial infections such as multidrug-resistant tuberculosis (MDR-TB), or carbapenem-resistant Enterobacterales. The concern for pandemics, certainly a driving force behind the development of the new concept of global health, is well illustrated by the US Centers for Disease Control (CDC) establishment of a new scientific journal "Emerging Infectious Diseases", and the Institute of Medicine's Board of International Health and other important publications in the 1990s that influenced the health of the world for ever [9].

Another fundamental milestone in the development of GH was the inclusion of health within the new United Nations (UN) Millennium Development Goals (MDG) 2000–2015. The well-recognized international health challenges of child and maternal health, and that of combating the three major infectious killers—HIV/AIDS, malaria, and tuberculosis—became prominent in the MDG agenda constituting 3 of 8 MDGs. With the advent of the UN Sustainable Development Goals (SDGs) (https://www.undp.org/sustainable-development-goals), GH evolved towards a more pronounced emphasis on systems thinking, innovations such as digital tools, sustainability and inter-/trans-disciplinarity well expressed by the "One Health" approach integrating interventions across the human, animal, and environmental perspectives in any given socio-ecological context [10].

In the last few years, two new terms have gained currency in international medical and public health journals even causing some controversy: **precision public health and precision global health**. Building on the concept of "precision public health", emphasizing "application and combination of new and existing technologies, and the tailoring of preventive interventions for high-risk populations" [11] and the use of "the best available data to target more effectively and efficiently interventions of all kinds to those most in need" [12], "**precision global health**" (PGH) has been proposed. PGH is, in brief, "an approach that leverages life sciences, social sciences, and data sciences, augmented with artificial intelligence (AI), in order to identify transnational problems and deliver targeted and impactful interventions through integrated and participatory approaches" [13]. Finally, the evolution of the GH concept continues with "**planetary health**". Although ecological perspectives are already intrinsically linked to GH, it emphasizes further the importance of safeguarding both the health of human civilization and the natural systems that underpin it. As well articulated by the Rockefeller Foundation—Lancet Commission on Planetary Health in 2015 [14], human health and the health of the natural environment need to be considered together and indeed protected together in the face of unprecedented environmental challenges such as those linked to climate change that threaten both. Planetary health can thus be described as a field where health sciences converge with ecology and Earth sciences, system theory, ethics, social sciences, One Health, Ecohealth, climatology and other sciences towards the common aim of human and environmental health.

In conclusion, GH is a lively, dynamic, and evolving field addressing ethical dimensions of health, such as the elimination of inequities and inequalities, the impact on well-being and productivity of individuals, its links with economic and social development in countries, and its major implications for global security and open societies. If we accept that in many ways boundaries no longer exist, "the health of anyone, anywhere, is the health of everyone, everywhere".

References

1. World Health Organization. Constitution of the World Health Organization. Official records 2, 100. Geneva: World Health Organization; 1946.
2. Koplan JP, Bond TC, Merson MH, et al. Towards a common definition of global health. Lancet. 2009;373:1993–5.
3. Skolnik R. Global health 101. 3rd ed. Burlington: Jones & Bartlett Learning; 2016.
4. Winslow CEA. The untilled fields of public health. Science. 1920;51(1306):23–33. https://doi.org/10.1126/science.51.1306.23.
5. Havemann M, Bösner S. Global health as "umbrella term"—a qualitative study among global health teachers in German medical education. Glob Health. 2018;14:32. https://doi.org/10.1186/s12992-018-0352-y.
6. Saker L, Lee K, Cannito B, Gilmore A, Campbell-Lendrum Diarmid D, et al. Globalization and infectious diseases: a review of the linkages. Geneva: World Health Organization; 2004. https://apps.who.int/iris/handle/10665/68726
7. Steger MB. Globalization. A very short introduction. 5th ed. Oxford: Oxford University Press; 2020.
8. World Bank. World development report 1993. Investing in health. Oxford: Oxford University Press; 1993.
9. Brown TM, Cueto M, Fee E. The World Health Organization and the transition from "international" to "global" public health. Am J Public Health. 2006;96:62–72.
10. Wernli D, Tanner M, Kickbusch I, Escher G, Paccaud F, Flahault A. Moving global health forward in academic institutions. J Glob Health. 2016;6(1):010409. https://doi.org/10.7189/jogh.06.010409.
11. Weeramanthri TS, Dawkins HJS, Baynam G, Bellgard M, Gudes O, Semmens JB. Editorial: Precision public health. Front Public Health. 2018;6:121. https://doi.org/10.3389/fpubh.2018.00121.
12. Horton R. Offline: In defence of precision public health. Lancet. 2018;392:1504.
13. Sheath DJ, Ruiz de Castañeda R, Bempong NE, Raviglione M, Machalaba C, et al. Precision global health: a roadmap for augmented action. J Public Health Emerg. 2020;4:5. https://doi.org/10.21037/jphe.2020.01.01.
14. Whitmee S, Haines A, Beyrer C, Boltz F, Capon AG, de Souza F, Dias B, et al. The Rockefeller Foundation–Lancet Commission on planetary health safeguarding human health in the Anthropocene epoch: report of The Rockefeller Foundation–Lancet Commission on planetary health. Lancet. 2015;386:1973–2028. https://doi.org/10.1016/S0140-6736(15)60901-1.

2 The Changing World of Global Health

Mario C. B. Raviglione, Ariel Pablos-Méndez, and Simone Villa

Abstract

Global health is a rapidly evolving cross-discipline promoting principles that partly also originated from the HIV/AIDS activism that, in the last decade of the twentieth century spread from high-income countries of the Global North to the Global South. This movement highlighted how health is not a siloed sector but deeply depends on, and interacts with, other sectors of human development. This led to the creation of new international mechanisms to finance country efforts and research to combat AIDS and other major killers. Eventually it resulted in a much higher position of health in the global political agenda, including through the United Nations priority development goals. As more and more actors joined the global stage, the health financing architecture became more complex given the need to address a wider group of health priorities as countries and populations are transitioning demographically, economically, and epidemiologically. Although societies are becoming older and affected by a higher burden of non-communicable diseases, life expectancy and per capita income are increasing across the globe and poverty may still keep decreasing almost everywhere. Middle-income countries are now investing more domestic funds in health services thus graduating from a north-to-south assistance. Overall, therefore, despite all odds linked to the COVID-19 pandemic and other major threats, global health may still progress towards a more equitable access to prevention and care for all.

Keywords

Global health · Millennium development goals (MDGs) · Sustainable development goals (SDGs) · Epidemiological transition · Demographic transition

2.1 Introduction

During the recent three decades, global health evolved to become a recognized cross-discipline with a sound multidisciplinary and academic background. Several traditional educational programmes have been offering integrated approaches from sciences as diverse as anthro-

M. C. B. Raviglione (✉) · S. Villa
Centre for Multidisciplinary Research in Health Science (MACH), University of Milan, Milan, Italy
e-mail: mario.raviglione@unimi.it; simone.villa@unimi.it

A. Pablos-Méndez
Division of General Medicine, Columbia University Medical Centre, New York, NY, USA
e-mail: ap39@cumc.columbia.edu

M. C. B. Raviglione et al. (eds.), *Global Health Essentials*, Sustainable Development Goals Series,
https://doi.org/10.1007/978-3-031-33851-9_2

pology, sociology, psychology, economics, engineering, business management, policy, and law, on top of subjects that are taught in schools of public health and medicine [1]. These advances resulted in a new consolidated field for study, research, and practice aiming at equitable access to health for all people worldwide. Recent challenges, such as the COVID-19 pandemic, economic recession, climate change, and major conflicts are now threatening progress in global health by destabilizing countries, impoverishing people, affecting their well-being, and potentially reducing investments in the health of populations. This chapter, building on progress in global health over the recent decades through effective advocacy, attempts to define the future of global health vis-à-vis current and new threats.

2.2 Global Health Advocacy in the New Millennium

Global health has never been as visible as the time around the turn of the century and the first several years of the new millennium [2]. This has been defined as the "golden era" of global health and has been followed by significant developments that risk being halted by new challenges [2]. Perhaps, we are in front of a new world health era that will result from an equilibrium between macro challenges such as those above and the achievements of the past decades [2]. Visibility was one of such achievements. A powerful advocacy movement for global health originated in large part from HIV/AIDS activism. A phenomenon seen early on in high-income countries (HICs) like the United States of America (USA) and parts of Europe, and later expanding in low- and middle-income settings (LMICs) such as Brazil and South Africa, HIV/AIDS activism had long-lasting social, economic, and political impacts [3].

"AIDS exceptionalism" promoted the idea that such a complex societal problem required a response "above and beyond normal health interventions" and was followed by unprecedented mobilization of disease-specific resources to address the epidemic in an effective manner. The Global Fund to fight AIDS, tuberculosis, and malaria is a clear example of a new and unique institution that since 2002 has been disbursing billions of US dollars (USD) to poorer countries in the effort to alleviate the suffering imposed by HIV/AIDS as well as tuberculosis and malaria[1] [4]. A similarly massive investment has been made by the US Government with the creation of the US President's Emergency Plan for AIDS Relief [5] that has disbursed over USD 100 billion since 2003.[2] Another model to support the global fight against HIV/AIDS was that of Unitaid, launched in 2006 by the governments of Brazil, Chile, France, Norway, and the United Kingdom, with the aim of accelerating access to tools against HIV/AIDS, malaria, and tuberculosis in poor countries through innovative financing mechanisms such as a new tax on air travels [6]. Such "exceptionalism" was built on principles of compassion, social justice, proper funding for research and care, and originated as well new institutions and ways to face regulatory and access issues under emergency conditions. Although disease-specific and, according to some critics, disruptive of health system development, energized advocacy also led to the inclusion of three goals devoted to health within the eight United Nations' (UN) Millennium Development Goals (MDGs) 2000–2015.

[1] See: https://www.theglobalfund.org/en.

[2] See https://www.state.gov/pepfar/.

During the first decade of the new century, development assistance for health (DAH) and new philanthropy emerged as powerful boosts to address major global health issues. DAH grew from annual USD 6–7 billion in the early 1990s to nearly 40 billion in 2015. Meanwhile also emerging economies including the BRICS countries (Brazil, Russia, India, China, and South Africa) started investing more of their own resources in domestic health interventions in what represents a progressive "graduation" from previous reliance mainly on international aid.

However, following the 2007–2008 financial crisis in "western economies", DAH stagnated around USD 40 billion per year despite inflation [7]. The potential adverse effects on health financing caused by the COVID-19 pandemic are not yet clear, but it may well be that investments in global health (outside of COVID-19) could have eroded further. This is obviously a matter of great concern both in aid-recipient LIMCs and HICs that could result in the loss of the progress made in the previous "golden era". Moreover, the shift in political economy towards nationalism and "slowbalization"[3] and conflicts worldwide could further erode international solidarity and cooperation for the most vulnerable and poorest populations.

The question is therefore: what will global health be like in the next decades? Will it regress or continue progressing? Will we enter a "new world health era"? [2]. Several factors will be of critical importance in determining the future of global health and the burden to be faced by humanity: from demographic and epidemiological transitions to the impact of economic and geo-political instabilities.

[3]The term "slowbalization" refers to the significant waning of globalization's previous trend, characterized by a decrease in international trade and investments.

2.3 An Era of Transitions: Potential Headwinds

Demographic pressures are mounting and getting more complex. The size of the world's population doubled three times during the last century and is projected to reach 8 billion by the end of 2022 and 10 billion by the end of this century (Fig. 2.1). In the last 50 years, the largest growth (fivefold increase) has been observed in Sub-Saharan Africa where the population already surpasses 1 billion. At the same time, population is already shrinking in many European and Asian countries, creating labour, social, and immigration challenges.

The demographic transition refers to the historical shift from high birth and death rates in LICs towards lower rates in HICs. This translates into a rapidly ageing of the population, with currently more than 700 million persons aged ≥65 years (10% of the total), a figure bound to double to 1.5 billion in 2050. This will result in greater economic dependency ratios from a shrinking labour pool while increasing the burden of age-related conditions, i.e. mainly non-communicable diseases.

The parallel growing phenomenon of urbanization will likely continue. Four billion people already live in cities, and it is projected that by 2050 more than 2/3 of the human population will dwell in urban areas often in poor living conditions. The health implications include the increase in: (1) non-communicable diseases (including mental conditions) because of increased air, water, and sound pollution, reduced physical activity, easy access to unhealthy food; (2) infectious disease outbreaks because of poorer sanitation and waste management; and (3) injuries because of high risk of abuse and violence—especially among children, women, and older people—and road traffic accidents.

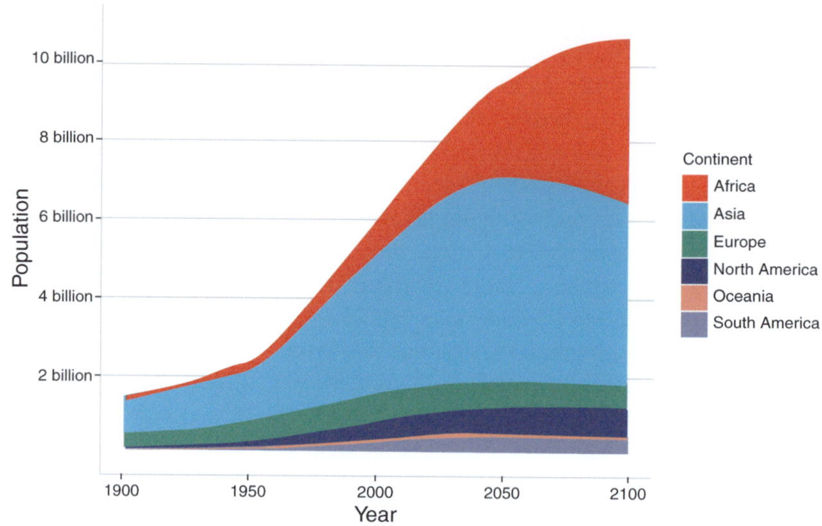

Fig. 2.1 World population by continent, 1950–2100. [Source: Our World in Data (CC BY)]

2.4 An Era of Transitions: Potential Tailwinds

Given the serious headwinds facing us, one could expect a general worsening of the health of populations. However, life expectancy has nearly doubled in the last century and should continue growing after COVID-19, including in continents still ravaged by disease and with poorer health infrastructure, such as Africa. Improved social and economic conditions, sanitation, and tools such as antimicrobials and vaccines play a major role in this historical success (Fig. 2.2).

Furthermore, after centuries of stagnant income per capita, there has been an economic renaissance beyond Europe, USA and other HICs in the last 50 years. The World Bank projects a continued shift from low- to middle-income level and from middle to high income.[4] This is typically accompanied by a growth of total health spending often faster than the GDP [8]. This "first law of health economics" [8] should have a positive impact on the health of people, though it may also lead to impoverishing and out-of-pocket expenditures in the absence of cross-subsidized risk-pooled financing of the population (see **Chapter on Universal Health Coverage**).

As countries get richer, the number of people living in extreme poverty (i.e. USD <2.15 per capita per day) is projected to continue its decrease (persistent inequalities notwithstanding). Poverty had declined most notably in South-East Asia and Pacific by the year 2000, but there are still 700 million people living in extreme poverty, most of them in Africa. The COVID-19 pandemic will likely send millions of families back to poverty, but the pre-pandemic downward trajectory is projected to resume.[5]

Importantly, half a century ago, Preston published an influential article where he showed a clear relationship between life expectancy and per capita income [9]. The "Preston curve" shows that life expectancy grows steeply as gross domestic product (GDP)/capita increases to about USD 3000, plateauing when the USD 20,000-level is reached. It means that the maximum benefit can be seen when investing in health in the poorest settings [10, 11]. Researchers later found that factors other than GDP, such as education (associated with rising income), are also crucially important in determining increase of life expectancy and better health [12].

[4] See https://datatopics.worldbank.org/world-development-indicators/the-world-by-income-and-region.html.

[5] See https://www.worldbank.org/en/topic/poverty/overview.

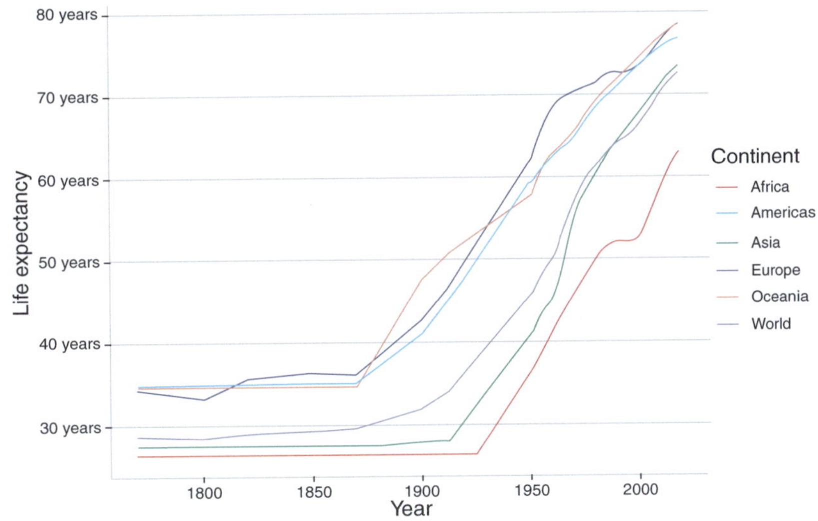

Fig. 2.2 Life expectancy by continent, 1770–2019. [Source: Our World in Data (CC BY)]

2.5 How Will Health Challenges and Opportunities Balance Out in the Next Decades?

That general economic development is a key factor in determining better health of populations has been known for a long time [9]. As long as economic growth reaches the poor and new resources are well spent [13], health of households and populations improves. However, it is well accepted that health shapes socio-economic development of a country as well: health and development are synergistic. This was one of the main conclusions of the historical World Bank World Development Report 1993 "Investing in Health" and reiterated by the WHO Commission on Macroeconomics and Health in the year 2000 [14]. Not by chance, health was the focus of three of the eight MDGs and inspired major financial mechanisms and unprecedented sums of aid money.

The launch of the SDGs for the period 2016–2030 builds on the MDGs and adapts to a new world. Not only do SGDs recognize the demographic and epidemiological changes, but also the economic and political standing of all nations. As traditional aid's footprint shrinks and shifts towards global public goods, peer cooperation replaces assistance and development thrives on domestic resource mobilization. With this approach, the quest for a more equitable world through cross-sectoral and multidisciplinary interventions becomes the priority. Within the SDG framework, health itself has remained visible in the political agenda of leaders as both a pre-requisite to, and an outcome of, sustainable development. The demand for universal health coverage and social protection to guarantee equitable access to prevention and care of diseases in a context of people-centred health system strengthening remains high in the SDGs era. This is seen as the *sine qua non* for political commitment to continue investing in health.

Together with continuously advancing technologies and progress in research—as proven by the extraordinary response to COVID-19—global health may indeed continue being a priority for mobilization of resources and establishment of sustainable and well-funded supportive mechanisms within countries and internationally.

2.6 Conclusions

In this delicate balance between hurdles and pro-health opportunities, there are several fundamental priorities to address as we enter in the "new normal" after the COVID-19 pandemic and the other crises. Among those, the first is to address the epidemiological shifts resulting from the demographic and economic transitions. Ageing and related conditions will be a dominant theme in the future global health. The second is to build proper prevention, preparedness, and response mechanisms to face future public health emergencies, informed by the lessons recently learned. The third is to continuously revisit efforts to alleviate the impact of climate changes on the health of people acting well beyond the ministries of health. A top priority is to pursue financial sustainability of systems guaranteeing access to health for all people: this requires political commitment to reorganized health financing away from out-of-pocket spending and towards universal health coverage. Finally, the movement for "de-colonisation" of global health needs to deliver in such a way that institutions from all countries—in the "Global North" and in the "Global South"—identify the most effective ways to collaborate as peers for furthering promotion of global health and health equity.

References

1. Merson MH. University engagement in global health. N Engl J Med. 2014;370(18):1676–8.
2. Pablos-Méndez A, Raviglione MC. A new world health era. Glob Health Sci Pract. 2018;6(1):8–16.
3. Smith JH, Whiteside A. The history of AIDS exceptionalism. J Int AIDS Soc. 2010;13:47.
4. Brugha R, Donoghue M, Starling M, Ndubani P, Ssengooba F, et al. The global fund: managing great expectations. Lancet. 2004;364(9428):95–100.
5. Fauci AS, Eisinger RW. PEPFAR—15 years and counting the lives saved. N Engl J Med. 2018;378(4):314–6.
6. Samarasekera U. Unitaid at 15. Lancet. 2021;398(10305):1032–3.
7. Global Burden of Disease Health Financing Collaborator Network. Health sector spending and spending on HIV/AIDS, tuberculosis, and malaria, and development assistance for health: progress towards sustainable development goal 3. Lancet. 2020;396(10252):693–724.
8. van der Gaag J, Štimac V. Technical partner paper 3—Toward a new paradigm for health sector development. New York: Rockefeller Foundation; 2008.
9. Preston SH. The changing relation between mortality and level of economic development. Popul Stud. 1975;29:231–48.
10. Lutz W, Kebede Z. Education and health: redrawing the Preston curve. Popul Dev Rev. 2018;44(2):343–61.
11. Jamison DT, Summers LH, Alleyne G, et al. Global health 2035: a world converging within a generation. Lancet. 2013;382:1898–955. https://doi.org/10.1016/S0140-6736(13)62105-4.
12. Lange S, Vollmer S. The effect of economic development on population health: a review of the empirical evidence. Br Med Bull. 2017;121:47–60.
13. World Bank. World Development Report 1993: Investing in Health. New York: Oxford University Press; 1993.
14. World Health Organization. Macroeconomics and health: investing in health for economic development. In: Report of the Commission on Macroeconomics and Health. Geneva: World Health Organization; 2001.

Part II

The Global Burden of Disease: Introduction

3 The Global Burden of Disease and Risk Factors

Emily Briskin

Abstract

In most country income groups and geographic regions worldwide, the burden of disease is primarily noncommunicable, except sub-Saharan Africa and low-income countries where communicable diseases are still the most common causes of death. This pattern represents a shift that has been fueled primarily by a reduction in communicable diseases, linked also to access to antimicrobials and vaccines, as well as the aging of populations. The five leading causes of deaths globally in 2019 were ischemic heart disease; stroke; chronic obstructive pulmonary disease; lower respiratory infections; and tracheal, bronchus, and lung cancer. Globally, the five leading causes of years lived with disability in 2019 were low back pain, depressive disorders, headache disorders, age-related hearing loss, and iron-deficiency anemia. The top five risk factors for the disease globally in 2019 were high blood pressure, particulate matter, smoking, high fasting plasma glucose, and low birth weight and short gestation. Since 2020, COVID-19 has ranked among the five leading causes of deaths and is a substantial source of disability in many countries (World Health Organization, 2022, Nature, 2022).

Keywords

Global burden of disease · Risk factors · The determinants of health · The epidemiological transition · The demographic transition

3.1 Measuring the Burden of Disease

One of the most used indicators in global health is called the disability-adjusted life year or DALY. A DALY is defined as "the sum of years lost due to premature death (YLLs) and years lived with disability (YLDs). DALYs are also defined as years of healthy life lost" [1]. While life expectancy only allows for comparisons of years of life lived, DALYs take into account not only the years lived but also the health status and quality of those years.

The calculation of years lost to premature death is based on the difference between the age at which one dies and one's life expectancy at that age, based on a reference standard that takes into account the highest life expectancy at birth globally. For example, for the 2016 study, this reference standard was set at 86.6 years [2]. To calculate the value for years lived with disability, the number of years lived with disability is multiplied by a weight assigned to that disability [3].

E. Briskin (✉)
Epicentre, Paris, France

M. C. B. Raviglione et al. (eds.), *Global Health Essentials*, Sustainable Development Goals Series,
https://doi.org/10.1007/978-3-031-33851-9_3

Of course, this system is imperfect, as it is difficult to estimate the exact effect of a given illness or disability on any individual's quality of life, but these calculations allow for reasonable comparisons at a population level. The more premature death, illness, and disability that are present in a society equate to more DALYs per person and poorer health.

3.2 Burden of Disease Data

The data that follow on the burden of disease and risk factors are based on the findings of the Global Burden of Disease Study 2019, coordinated by the Institute of Health Metrics and Evaluation (IHME) and published in *The Lancet* in 2020 [4]. Much of the data used in this chapter is drawn from interactive data visualizations available through the IHME website [5]. In this chapter, while some data refer to "deaths" and some data refer to "DALYs," references to the "burden of disease" refer to DALYs. Causes of death and DALYs are generally grouped into three categories:

1. Communicable diseases like HIV, tuberculosis, malaria, and diarrhea, plus maternal, perinatal, and nutritional diseases
2. Noncommunicable diseases like congenital defects, cardiovascular diseases, cancer, or diabetes
3. Injuries like road injuries or interpersonal violence

By examining the tables below, one can see how the types of conditions affecting a population change by income group.

3.3 The Leading Causes of Deaths and DALYs

The burden of deaths and DALYs vary by age, sex, and country income group as shown below.

Table 3.1 shows the five leading causes of death for children aged 0–5 years by country income group.

Examining Table 3.1, one can notice that neonatal disorders, congenital anomalies, and lower respiratory infections are important causes of death among under-five children regardless of country income group. However, as country incomes rise the pattern of young child deaths changes somewhat, with relatively fewer deaths from malaria and diarrhea in wealthier countries.

Table 3.2 examines the five leading causes of deaths and DALYs for the age group 15–49 years by World Bank country income group.

Table 3.2 shows that HIV/AIDS and tuberculosis are leading causes of death and DALYs for all country income groups except for high-income countries. As countries get wealthier, communicable diseases are less common and injuries and chronic diseases rank higher among the causes of death and DALYs.

Table 3.1 Five leading causes of death under 5 years of age by World Bank country income group, 2019

Cause Rank	High-income	Upper middle-income	Lower middle-income	Low-income
1	Neonatal disorders	Neonatal disorders	Neonatal disorders	Neonatal disorders
2	Congenital defects	Congenital defects	Lower respiratory infections	Lower respiratory infections
3	Sudden infant death syndrome (SIDS)	Lower respiratory infections	Diarrheal diseases	Malaria
4	Foreign body	Diarrheal diseases	Congenital defects	Diarrheal diseases
5	Lower respiratory infections	Foreign body	Malaria	Congenital defects

Data from Institute of Health Metrics and Evaluation (IHME). nd GBD. Compare: Viz Hub. Retrieved from https://vizhub.healthdata.org/gbd-compare/

Table 3.2 Five leading causes of deaths and DALYs, 15–49, both sexes, by World Bank country income group, 2019

High-income countries		
Cause		
Rank	Deaths	DALYs
1	Self-harm	Low back pain
2	Road injuries	Drug use disorders
3	Drug use disorders	Headache disorders
4	Ischemic heart disease	Depressive disorders
5	Cirrhosis	Road injuries
Upper middle-income countries		
Cause		
Rank	Deaths	DALYs
1	Road injuries	Road injuries
2	HIV/AIDS	Interpersonal violence
3	Ischemic heart disease	Headache disorders
4	Interpersonal violence	HIV/AIDS
5	Stroke	Low back pain
Lower middle-income countries		
Cause		
Rank	Deaths	DALYs
1	Ischemic heart disease	Road injuries
2	Road injuries	Ischemic heart disease
3	Tuberculosis	Tuberculosis
4	HIV/AIDS	Headache disorders
5	Cirrhosis	HIV/AIDS
Low-income countries		
Cause		
Rank	Deaths	DALYs
1	HIV/AIDS	HIV/AIDS
2	Tuberculosis	Tuberculosis
3	Maternal disorders	Road injuries
4	Road injuries	Maternal disorders
5	Diarrheal diseases	Depressive disorders

Acronym: *AIDS* acquired immunodeficiency syndrome; *HIV* human immunodeficiency virus. Data from Institute of Health Metrics and Evaluation (IHME). nd GBD. Compare: Viz Hub. Retrieved from https://vizhub.healthdata.org/gbd-compare/

3.4 Causes of Deaths and DALYs by Sex

Table 3.3 examines leading causes of DALYs by sex and by country income group in 2019.

Table 3.3 shows that the burden of disease is largely similar across sexes within each country

Table 3.3 Five leading causes of DALYs, males and females, all ages, by World Bank country income group, 2019

High-income countries		
Cause		
Rank	Male	Female
1	Ischemic heart disease	Ischemic heart disease
2	Tracheal, bronchus, and lung cancer	Low back pain
3	Low back pain	Stroke
4	Stroke	Diabetes
5	Diabetes	Alzheimer's disease and other dementias
Upper middle-income countries		
Cause		
Rank	Male	Female
1	Ischemic heart disease	Stroke
2	Stroke	Ischemic heart disease
3	Road injuries	Low back pain
4	Tracheal, bronchus, and lung cancer	Diabetes
5	COPD	COPD
Lower middle-income countries		
Cause		
Rank	Male	Female
1	Neonatal disorders	Neonatal disorders
2	Ischemic heart disease	Ischemic heart disease
3	Lower respiratory infections	Diarrheal diseases
4	Stroke	Lower respiratory infections
5	Diarrheal diseases	Stroke
Low-income countries		
Cause		
Rank	Male	Female
1	Neonatal disorders	Neonatal disorders
2	Diarrheal diseases	Lower respiratory infections
3	Lower respiratory infections	Malaria
4	Malaria	Diarrheal diseases
5	Tuberculosis	HIV/AIDS

Acronym: *AIDS* acquired immunodeficiency syndrome; *COPD* chronic obstructive pulmonary disease; *HIV* human immunodeficiency virus. Data from Institute of Health Metrics and Evaluation (IHME). nd *GBD*. Compare: Viz Hub. Retrieved from https://vizhub.healthdata.org/gbd-compare/

income group. However, certain conditions, such as HIV/AIDS, and Alzheimer's disease and other dementias represent more of the burden of disease in females, while road traffic injuries and tracheal, bronchus, and lung cancer contribute more to the burden of disease more among males.

3.5 The Burden of Deaths and Disease Within Countries

As we consider causes of death and the burden of disease globally and across countries, it is also important to consider how demographic and socioeconomic factors such as ethnicity, income, and education level can affect a person's health within a given country. While not true in all countries or settings, the following trends are often observed:

- Disadvantaged ethnic minorities are less healthy than more privileged populations.
- Females are less healthy than males, in relation to their often disadvantaged social positions and to the risks linked to pregnancy.
- Less educated people are less healthy than more educated people.
- Lower-income people are less healthy than wealthier people.
- Rural populations are less healthy than urban populations.

Conditions relating to smoking and alcohol use are generally more common in people of lower socioeconomic status than among wealthier people. People in lower socioeconomic groups often face a higher burden of communicable diseases, malnutrition, and maternal deaths than people of higher socioeconomic status. These general trends provide a fundamental framework to the understanding of global health but should be tested and examined for outliers in any specific context.

3.6 The Impact of COVID-19 on the Global Burden of Disease

Because of the challenges of incorporating COVID-19 into their studies, the IHME has not yet published its data for 2020 or 2021 on the Global Burden of Disease and Risk Factors. Nonetheless, preliminary evidence makes it clear that COVID-19 has had a dramatic impact on the global burden of disease [6, 7]. On the one hand, the measures that many countries took to mitigate COVID-19, such as masking and social distancing, dramatically reduced the burden of influenza [8]. However, the large amount of illness, disability, and deaths associated with COVID-19 has led to COVID-19 now being among the top five causes of death in many countries including Brazil, Mexico, France, and Italy [9].

3.7 Risk Factors

A risk factor is "an aspect or personal behavior or lifestyle, an environmental exposure, or an inborn or inherited characteristic, that, on the basis of epidemiologic evidence, is known to be associated with health-related condition(s) considered important to prevent" [10]. Risks factors that relate to health can also be thought of as raising "a probability of an adverse outcome" [11].

Table 3.4 shows the relative importance of different risk factors for deaths by country income groups, and Table 3.5 does the same for DALYs. These risks are generally grouped in three categories: metabolic, behavioral, and environmental and occupational [4].

Table 3.4 Five leading risk factors for deaths, globally, all ages and both sexes, by World Bank country income group, 2019

Risk factor				
Rank	High-income	Upper-middle income	Lower middle-income	Low-income
1	High blood pressure	High blood pressure	High blood pressure	Particulate matter
2	Smoking	Smoking	Particulate matter	High blood pressure
3	High fasting plasma glucose	Particulate matter	High fasting plasma glucose	Low birth weight and short gestation
4	High body-mass index	High fasting plasma glucose	Smoking	Child growth failure
5	High LDL	High body-mass index	High body-mass index	Unsafe water

Acronym: *LDL* low-density lipoprotein. Data from Institute of Health Metrics and Evaluation (IHME). nd GBD. Compare: Viz Hub. Retrieved from https://vizhub.healthdata.org/gbd-compare/

Table 3.5 Five leading risk factors for DALYs, globally, all ages and both sexes, by World Bank country income group, 2019

Risk factor				
Rank	High-income	Upper-middle income	Lower middle-income	Low-income
1	Smoking	High blood pressure	Particulate matter	Low birth weight and short gestation
2	High body-mass index	Smoking	Low birth weight and short gestation	Child growth failure
3	High fasting plasma glucose	High body-mass index	High blood pressure	Particulate matter
4	High blood pressure	High fasting plasma glucose	High fasting plasma glucose	Unsafe water
5	Alcohol use	Particulate matter	Smoking	Unsafe sanitation

Data from Institute of Health Metrics and Evaluation (IHME). nd GBD. Compare: Viz Hub. Retrieved from https://vizhub.healthdata.org/gbd-compare/

3.8 The Demographic Transition

Over time, as a country shifts from lower income to higher income, a phenomenon called the "demographic transition" has historically been observed. The demographic transition can be defined as the shift from a pattern of high fertility and high mortality to low fertility and low mortality, with population growth occurring in between [12].

When we look back historically at the countries that are now high-income, we can see that they had periods of many centuries when fertility was high, mortality was high, and population growth was, therefore, relatively slow, or sometimes even declined during catastrophic events such as epidemics. Beginning around the year 1800, however, mortality in those countries began to decline as hygiene and nutrition improved and the burden of communicable diseases decreased. In most cases, this decline in mortality started before a steep decline in fertility occurred. As mortality declined, but the fertility or birth rate stayed relatively stable, the population increased, and the share of the population of younger ages also increased. Later, after mortality declined, fertility also began to decline. As births and deaths evened out, population growth therefore slowed, and the share of the population that was of older ages increased. There are now some countries, such as Italy and Japan, in which death rates exceed birth rates, and the population is declining. In these populations, an elevated proportion of the population is over age 65.

3.9 The Epidemiologic Transition

The epidemiologic transition [13] is closely related to the demographic transition. The epidemiologic transition can be described as a journey through the following stages, as income increases over time:

1. High and fluctuating mortality, related to famine, poor hygiene, epidemics, and poor access to healthcare.
2. Progressive declines in mortality as epidemics of communicable diseases become less frequent.
3. Declines in mortality, increases in life expectancy, and the predominance of noncommunicable diseases as communicable diseases decline.

This trend can clearly be seen in Table 3.2 above: communicable diseases such as HIV/AIDS and tuberculosis are leading causes of DALYs in low-income countries but are replaced by noncommunicable conditions such as depressive disorders in high-income countries.

Numerous factors related to the determinants of health also affect the pace of the epidemiologic transition in each country. Structural changes such as improvements in hygiene, education, and nutrition, as well as biomedical advancements such as new vaccines and antibiotics, can contribute to the epidemiologic transition [14]. Natural disasters, instability, and war can lead to temporary backtracking, as can be observed through the re-emergence of diseases like cholera in populations displaced by violence [15].

References

1. Lopez AD, et al. The burden of disease and mortality by condition: data, methods, and results for 2001. In: Lopez AD, et al., editors. Global burden of disease and risk factors. New York: Oxford University Press; 2006. p. 45–240.
2. GBD Collaborators 2016. The global burden of disease study 2016. Lancet. 2017;390(10100):1083–464.
3. Institute of Health Metrics and Evaluation (IHME). IHME|GHDx|GBD Compare. *Global Burden of Disease Study 2019 (GBD 2019) Disability Weights*. nd, B. http://ghdx.healthdata.org/record/ihme-data/gbd-2019-disability-weights.
4. Global Burden of Disease. The Lancet. 2020. https://www.thelancet.com/gbd#2019GBDIssue. https://www.thelancet.com/journals/lancet/issue/vol396no10258/PIIS0140-6736(20)X0042-0
5. Institute of Health Metrics and Evaluation (IHME). GBD Compare: Viz Hub. nd, A. https://vizhub.healthdata.org/gbd-compare/.
6. World Health Organization. COVID-19 pandemic triggers 25% increase in prevalence of anxiety and depression worldwide. News release. https://www.who.int/news/item/02-03-2022-covid-19-pandemic-triggers-25-increase-in-prevalence-of-anxiety-and-depression-worldwide. Accessed 2 Mar 2022.
7. Nature. The pandemic's true health cost. News feature. https://www.nature.com/articles/d41586-022-01341-7. Accessed 18 May 2022.
8. Lampejo T. The impact of the COVID-19 pandemic on the global burden of influenza. J Med Virol. 2022;94(6):2357–9. https://doi.org/10.1002/jmv.27653.
9. Troeger C. Just how do deaths due to COVID-19 stack up? https://www.thinkglobalhealth.org/article/just-how-do-deaths-due-covid-19-stack. Accessed 12 May 2022.
10. Kindig DA. Understanding population health terminology. Milbank Q. 2007;85(1):139-61. https://doi.org/10.1111/j.1468-0009.2007.00479.x. PMID: 17319809; PMCID: PMC2690307.
11. Last JM. A dictionary of epidemiology. 4th ed. New York: Oxford University Press; 2001.
12. Lee R. The demographic transition: three centuries of fundamental change. J Econ Perspect. 2003;17(4):167–90.
13. Omran AR. The epidemiologic transition: a theory of the epidemiology of population change. Milbank Q. 2005;83(4):731–57.
14. Jamison DT. Investing in health. In: Jamison DT, Breman JG, Meashem AR, et al., editors. Disease control priorities in developing countries. New York: Oxford University Press; 2006. p. 3–34.
15. Relief International. Four facts about the Cholera Outbreak in Syria and Lebanon. https://www.ri.org/four-facts-about-the-cholera-outbreak-in-syria-and-lebanon/.

The Health Status of the World

4

Emily Briskin

Abstract

Several key indicators are commonly used to compare health status across and within countries, including life expectancy, infant, neonatal, and child mortality rates, and the maternal mortality ratio. From 1990 until the spread of COVID-19 in 2020, life expectancy and health status had improved substantially in many countries worldwide. Despite these improvements on a global level, there remain substantial differences in health status by country, best correlated with the income per capita of a country. The COVID-19 pandemic has had direct and indirect effects on morbidity and mortality and appears to have led to a decrease in life expectancy globally of about 2 years.

Keywords

Child mortality · COVID-19 · Global health status · Infant mortality · Life expectancy · Maternal mortality

E. Briskin (✉)
Epicentre, Paris, France

4.1 The Importance of Data and Key Health Indicators

Data and evidence are essential tools to understand and address key global health issues. They show us what health conditions cause people to be sick, disabled, or die, and how that varies within countries, as well as across countries, regions, and country income groups. We also need data to understand for different settings how long people live, as well as who is at greatest risk of death and at what moments during the life course.

It is important to use a consistent set of indicators to measure health status to make objective comparisons across groups and over time. Therefore, here we will briefly review the "health status of the world" as reflected in several of the most used health indicators: life expectancy; rates of infant, neonatal, and under-five child mortality; and the maternal mortality ratio.

Global health data are often presented by geographic region or by country income group, as classified by the World Bank. Some geographic regions include countries with a wide range of national incomes per capita, but country income group has an even stronger correlation with health status than region does. Therefore, for this chapter, we focus on comparing data across World Bank country income groups [1].

M. C. B. Raviglione et al. (eds.), *Global Health Essentials*, Sustainable Development Goals Series,
https://doi.org/10.1007/978-3-031-33851-9_4

One of the most used indicators of health status is *life expectancy at birth*, a metric used commonly even in the popular media. It is defined by the World Health Organization (WHO) as: "The average number of years that a newborn could expect to live, if he or she were to pass through life exposed to the sex- and age-specific death rates prevailing at the time of his or her birth, for a specific year, in a given country, territory, or geographic area" [2]. Figure 4.1 shows how life expectancy at birth varies by country income group worldwide in the year 2020. A baby born today in a low-income country can expect to live 64 years, while one born in a high-income country can expect to live 25% longer, or 80 years.

Another important indicator is the *infant mortality rate*, shown in Fig. 4.2 and defined as: "the probability of a child born in a specific year or period dying before reaching the age of one, if subject to age-specific mortality rates of that period" [3]. It is expressed as deaths per 1000 live births. In 2020, the average rate ranged from 47 in low-income countries to 4 in high-income countries. In Finland, there were only 2 infant deaths per 1000 live births, while in Central African Republic there were 78 or 39 times as many [4].

While the infant mortality rate is a powerful indicator, most children younger than 1 year of age who die do so during the narrower period of

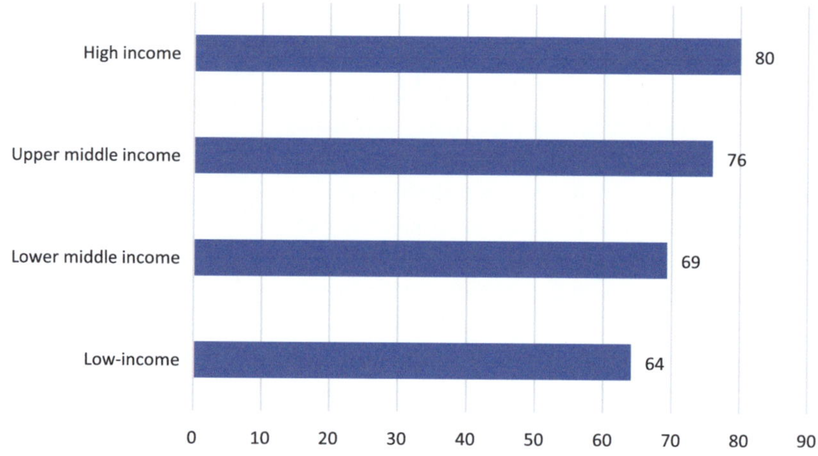

Fig. 4.1 Life expectancy at birth, 2020. (Source: The World Bank Data, Life expectancy at birth, 2020, by World Bank Country Income Group. https://data.worldbank.org/indicator/SP.DYN.LE00.IN)

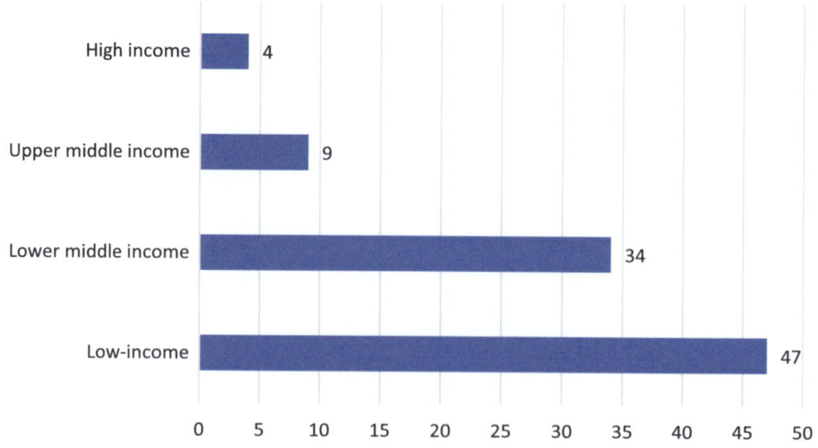

Fig. 4.2 Mortality rate, infant (per 1000 live births), 2020. [Source: The World Bank Data, Mortality rate, infant (per 1000 live births), 2020, by World Bank Country Income Group. https://data.worldbank.org/indicator/SP.DYN.IMRT.IN]

the first month of life, called the neonatal period. Thus, the *neonatal mortality rate* is also important to track and is defined as: "the number of deaths during the first 28 completed days of life per 1000 live births in a given year or other period" [5].

Just as observed with life expectancy and the infant mortality rate, where a person is born has a substantial impact on the neonatal mortality rate, varying from 3 in high-income countries to 26 in low-income countries [6], a difference of almost 9 times.

The *under-5 child mortality rate*, also called the child mortality rate, is defined as: "the probability of a child born in a specific year or period dying before reaching the age of five, if subject to age-specific mortality rates of that period" [7]. As shown in Fig. 4.3 for the year 2020, in the highest-income countries, the rate is generally about 5 per 1000 live births but increases to more than ten times that in some of the lowest-income countries [8].

We have examined health indicators across the life course through infancy and childhood, but one moment in the life course, the period during and immediately after pregnancy, is so risky that it is assigned its own key indicator: the *maternal mortality ratio*, shown in Fig. 4.4. The maternal mortality ratio is defined as: "the number of women who die from pregnancy-related causes while pregnant or within 42 days of pregnancy termination per 100,000 live births" [9]. Where a woman gives birth can have an enormous impact on her likelihood of maternal mortality: in 2017, women in low-income countries had a maternal mortality ratio that was more than 40 times higher than that of women in high-income countries. In Sierra Leone and Chad, the maternal mortality ratios surpassed 1000 maternal deaths per 100,000 live births, meaning that for every 100 live births, we can expect one maternal death [10].

Data for countries and for country income groups are averages, which allow us to compare across countries and groups, but sometimes hide important disparities within countries or groups. For example, while the maternal mortality ratio for the entire United States for the period of 2018–2020 was 20 deaths per 100,000 live births, the maternal mortality ratio for a resident of Alabama was 36, more than triple the maternal

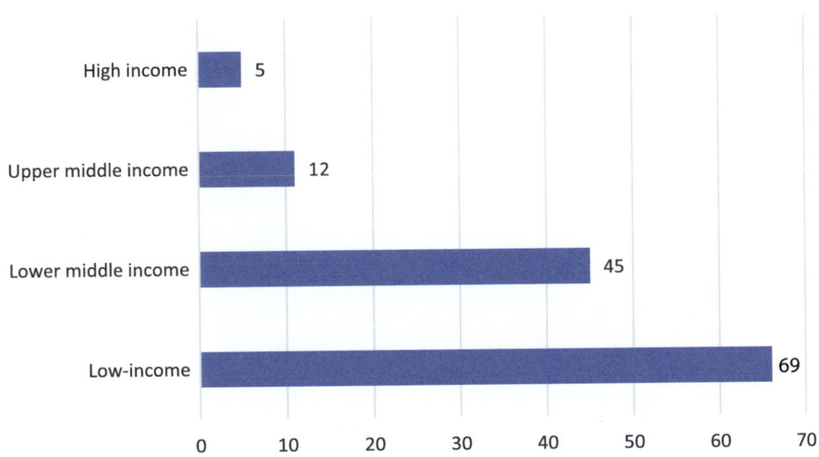

Fig. 4.3 Mortality rate, under-5 (per 1000 live births), 2020. [Source: The World Bank Data, Mortality rate, under-5 (per 1000 live births), 2020, by World Bank Country Income Group. https://data.worldbank.org/indicator/SH.DYN.NMRT]

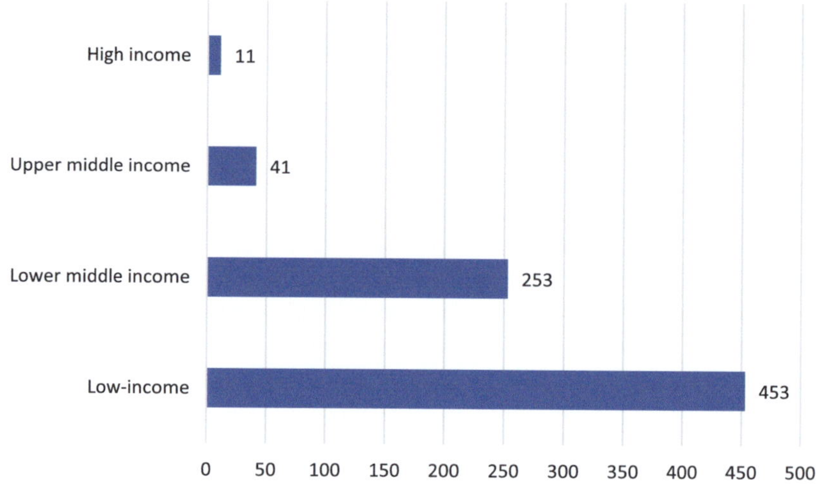

Fig. 4.4 Maternal mortality ratio (modeled estimate, per 100,000 live births), 2017. [Source: The World Bank Data, Maternal mortality ratio (modeled estimate, per 100,000 live births), 2017, by World Bank Country Income Group. https://data.worldbank.org/indicator/SH.STA.MMRT]

mortality ratio of 10 for a resident California [11].

Looking at the key indicators described here can be considered a first step. They help us to understand *what* is going on, hopefully spurring further curiosity and research into *why* such trends might be observed, by digging down into indicators at finer levels and learning more about the political and socioeconomic context of a setting of interest.

4.2 Trends in Key Indicators

From 1990 until the worldwide spread of COVID-19 in 2020, there was dramatic positive change in the key health indicators noted above. Life expectancy worldwide increased from 53 to 73 between 1990 and 2002, an increase of almost 40% and the highest levels recorded to date [2]. During this period, child health indicators also improved substantially: [10] the infant mortality rate fell from 65 to 27 [3]; the neonatal mortality rate fell from 37 to 17 [5]; and the under-five child mortality rate fell from 93 to 37 [7]. From 1990 to 2017, the maternal mortality ratio fell by about half, from 342 to 211 [12].

4.3 Impact of COVID-19 on Population Health

Global data on the indicators above for 2020 and 2021 taking account of the first 2 years of COVID-19 is limited. However, we can expect COVID-19 to influence excess key global health indicators both directly due to deaths from COVID-19 itself and indirectly through effects on the health system and daily life. COVID-19 had an indirect effect on mortality and overall health status, by constraining people's willingness to seek health services and disrupting routine preventive programs. COVID-19 also stressed the health systems in most countries, thus impacting the quality of the care provided. For example, some people with underlying health conditions such as cardiovascular disease or cancer who would have otherwise survived that period may have died due to increased stress or delayed access to routine care.

Unsurprisingly, therefore, one study of the United States and 21 peer countries showed that between 2019 and 2020, life expectancy declined by almost 1.9 years in the US and almost 0.6 years in the peer countries [13]. Another study of 29 countries showed that "life expectancy at birth declined from 2019 to 2020 in 27 out of the 29 countries. Reductions were mostly attributable to increased mortality above age 60 years and to official COVID-19 deaths" [14]. Other estimates have suggested that life expectancy declined by about 2 years globally in the first 2 years of the pandemic [15]. The United Nations Group on Child Mortality Estimation reviewed data to the end of 2020 for ages 0–24. They concluded that about 0.5% of total deaths from COVID-19 in that time were in this age-group. They also concluded that the direct impact of COVID-19 mortality on deaths among those 0–24 years of age was limited. However, experts expect that the indirect effects of COVID-19 on child health might ultimately be substantial, due to delays and disruptions to routine preventive programs such as vaccination and the distribution of anti-malarial bed nets [16]. Reported data showed that from 2020 through mid-2022, COVID-19 contributed to 15% of deaths in the WHO Americas region and 10% of deaths in the Europe region, but only 1% of deaths in the Africa region [17]. Some models suggest that COVID-19 deaths in the Africa region may have been underreported, though factors such as an overall younger population and lower prevalence of underlying chronic conditions can help explain the relatively lower rate of COVID-19 deaths in Africa compared to other regions [17, 18].

References

1. The World Bank. New country classifications by income level:2019–2020.https://blogs.worldbank.org/opendata/new-country-classifications-income-level-2019-2020.
2. World Health Organization. The Global Health Observatory. Life expectancy at birth (years). https://www.who.int/data/gho/indicator-metadata-registry/imr-details/65.
3. World Health Organization. The Global Health Observatory. Infant mortality rate (between birth and 11 months per 1000 live births). https://www.who.int/data/gho/indicator-metadata-registry/imr-details/1.
4. The World Bank. Mortality rate, infant (per 1000 live births). https://data.worldbank.org/indicator/SP.DYN.IMRT.IN.
5. World Health Organization. The Global Health Observatory. Neonatal mortality rate (0–27 days) per 1000 live births (SDG 3.2.2). https://www.who.int/data/gho/indicator-metadata-registry/imr-details/67.
6. The World Bank. Mortality rate, neonatal (per 1000 live births). https://data.worldbank.org/indicator/SH.DYN.NMRT.
7. World Health Organization. The Global Health Observatory. Under-five mortality rate (per 1000 live births) (SDG 3.2.1). https://www.who.int/data/gho/indicator-metadata-registry/imr-details/7.
8. The World Bank. Mortality rate, under-5 (per 1,000 live births). https://data.worldbank.org/indicator/SH.DYN.MORT.
9. World Health Organization. DataBank. Metadata Glossary. https://databank.worldbank.org/metadata-glossary/gender-statistics/series/SH.STA.MMRTci.
10. The World Bank. Maternal mortality ratio (modeled estimate, per 100,000 live births). https://data.world-bank.org/indicator/SH.STA.MMRT.
11. Centers for Disease Control and Prevention. Maternal deaths and mortality rates by state for 2018–2020. https://www.cdc.gov/nchs/maternal-mortality/mmr-2018-2020-state-data.pdf.
12. The World Bank. DataBank. Metadata Glossary. https://databank.worldbank.org/metadataglossary/gender-statistics/series/SH.STA.MMRTci.
13. Woolf SH, et al. Changes in life expectancy between 2019 and 2020 in the US and 21 peer countries. JAMA Netw Open. 2022;5(4):e227–67.
14. Aburto JM, et al. Quantifying impacts of the COVID-19 pandemic through life-expectancy losses: a population-level study of 29 countries. Int J Epidemiol. 2022;51(1):63–74.
15. Marabito M. COVID-19 led to unprecedented decline in global life expectancy. Healio. https://www.healio.com/news/primary-care/20220404/covid19-led-to-unprecedented-decline-in-global-life-expectancy. Accessed 4 Apr 2022.
16. UNICEF for every child. Child mortality and COVID-19. https://data.unicef.org/topic/child-survival/covid-19/.
17. Troeger C. Just how do deaths due to COVID-19 stack up? https://www.thinkglobalhealth.org/article/just-how-do-deaths-due-covid-19-stack. Accessed 12 May 2022.
18. Wamai RG, et al. What could explain the lower COVID-19 burden in Africa despite considerable circulation of the SARS-CoV-2 virus? Int J Environ Res Public Health. 2021;18(16):8638.

5 Demographic Perspectives on Global Health

Raya Muttarak and Simone Ghislandi

Abstract

This chapter focuses on the implications of population dynamics on global health. The chapter describes current and future population trends in terms of population size, composition and distribution. It starts by describing demographic changes and their processes as explained by the demographic transition model. Population pyramids by age, sex and education are employed to illustrate various stages of demographic transition in different world regions. The chapter also presents how accounting for education as another source of demographic heterogeneity helps explain future population trends. Finally, the chapter discusses how changing demographic structure, composition and distribution is linked with future global health.

R. Muttarak (✉)
Department of Statistical Sciences, University of Bologna, Bologna, Italy

Wittgenstein Centre for Demography and Global Human Capital (IIASA, OeAW, University of Vienna), International Institute for Applied Systems Analysis, Vienna, Austria
e-mail: raya.muttarak@unibo.it

S. Ghislandi
Department of Political and Social Sciences, University of Bocconi, Bocconi, Italy

DONDENA, Bocconi University, Bocconi, Italy

Keywords

Demographic transition · Fertility · Mortality · Population dynamics · Urbanisation

5.1 Demographic Transition and Global Demographic Trends

Understanding current and future population size, distribution and composition is fundamental to global health and policy design. Whilst population size indicates the total number of people potentially exposed to health risks and consequently health demand, it is clear that this varies by age structure and population composition. The COVID-19 pandemic, for instance, helps illustrate how underlying demographic heterogeneity may influence a country's health vulnerability. Given a clear evidence that older people, particularly those aged 70 years and over, are highly vulnerable to COVID-19 mortality [1], a country's age structure thus plays a key role in explaining geographical variations in the health impact of the pandemic [2]. Likewise, population distribution also has substantial health implications. While urbanisation often corresponds with better health services and infrastructure, living in an urban area increases exposure to noise, air pollution and

M. C. B. Raviglione et al. (eds.), *Global Health Essentials*, Sustainable Development Goals Series,
https://doi.org/10.1007/978-3-031-33851-9_5

excessive heat. This couples with sedentary behaviour and reduction in physical activity and can cause serious mental and physical health consequences. Therefore, the knowledge of where people live and will live in the future is also vital.

Figure 5.1 presents regional variations in population size, age structure and composition of the current world population (2015) [3]. This represents both the consequences of public health development on human population as well as the global health implications of population dynamics. The varying shapes of the population pyramids illustrate different stages of demographic transition in each continent (see the Box 5.1 for a definition of "demographic transition"). Most African countries, for example, are in stage 2 of the transition, characterised by a decline in mortality (mainly infant and child mortality) due to advancements in agriculture, sanitation and medical technology. Birth rates, however, remain high. As a result, the continent has a young age structure and high dependency ratios.

According to the demographic transition model, at some point, fertility will start falling and the share of the working age population will increase (stage 3), creating a window of economic opportunity—the so-called "demographic dividend". This opportunity, however, can translate in actual economic growth and productivity increases only conditional on appropriate investments in human capital, including health and education [4]. Many countries in Asia and Latin America and the Caribbean are in stage 3 of the demographic transition whereby death rates continue to drop. Increases in female education, access to contraception and urbanisation contribute to fertility decline. As female labour force participation increases, more children survive and the need for a large number of children in agricultural workforce declines. At this stage, the pace of population growth slows down while the number of dependent members, i.e. children, falls, leading to the demographic dividend. East Asian countries were able to harness this opportunity as has been shown that as much as one-third of its economic miracle is attributable to the demographic dividend [5].

Stage 4 of the demographic transition is characterised by low birth rates and death rates, thus population growth is stabilised. As life expectancy increases and fertility starts to fall below the replacement level, population ages. As evident in the population pyramids for Northern America and Europe, in particular, the proportion of those aged 0–19 years is smaller than the proportion of the 20–64 years. As the latter age and enter retirement, their larger size shifts the burden of the economically dependent population from children and adolescents (as in stage 2) to the older persons.

The sources of demographic drivers of population aging have implications on health and socioeconomic development [6]. Population aging driven by mortality decline and increased life expectancy implies health improvements at a societal level [7]. It is possible to draw upon the contribution of the older workforce to sustain economic productivity. Japan is an example of country that actively harnesses its older workers, by extending the retirement age and pension eligibility, coupling them with policies to protect and promote health, which in turn reduces the burden on health care systems and allows people to remain active [8]. Meanwhile, when declining fertility is a major driver of population aging rather than the improvement in life expectancy, population health is not improved [6]. If this is the case, the reduction in the working age population can pose a burden on social welfare and healthcare systems, due to a rising demand for old-age support without the benefit of active participation of the older workforce.

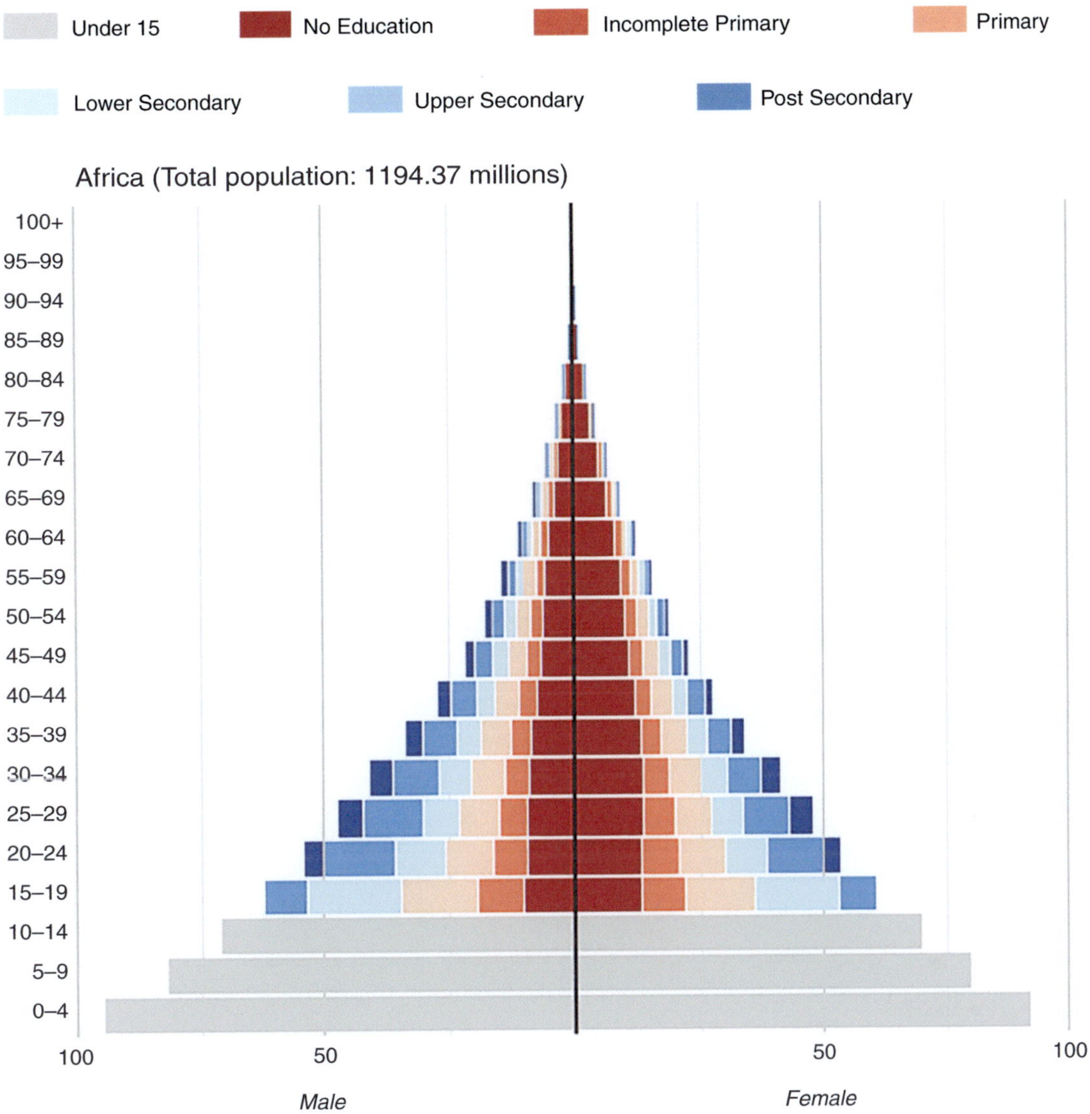

Fig. 5.1 Population of different world regions by age, sex and educational attainment, 2015. (Source: Wittgenstein Centre Human Capital Data Explorer [3])

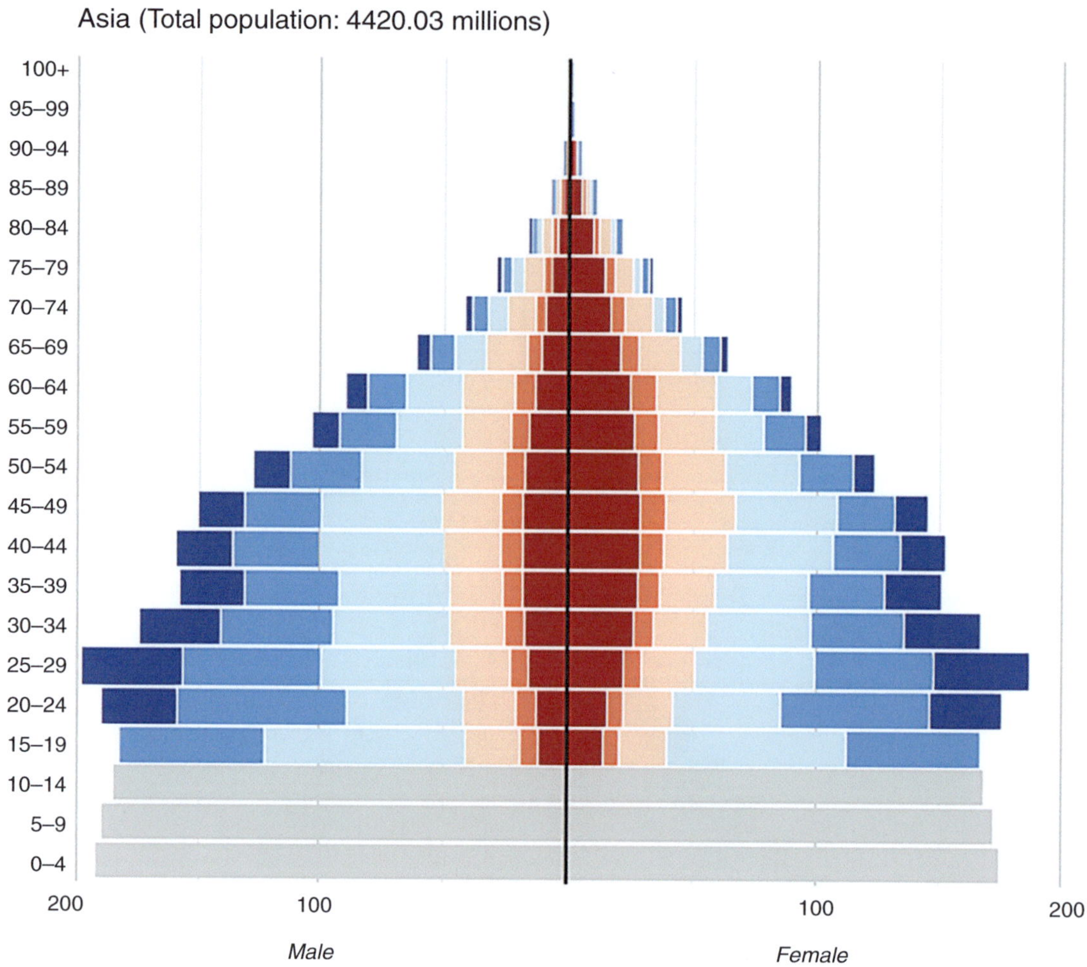

Fig. 5.1 (continued)

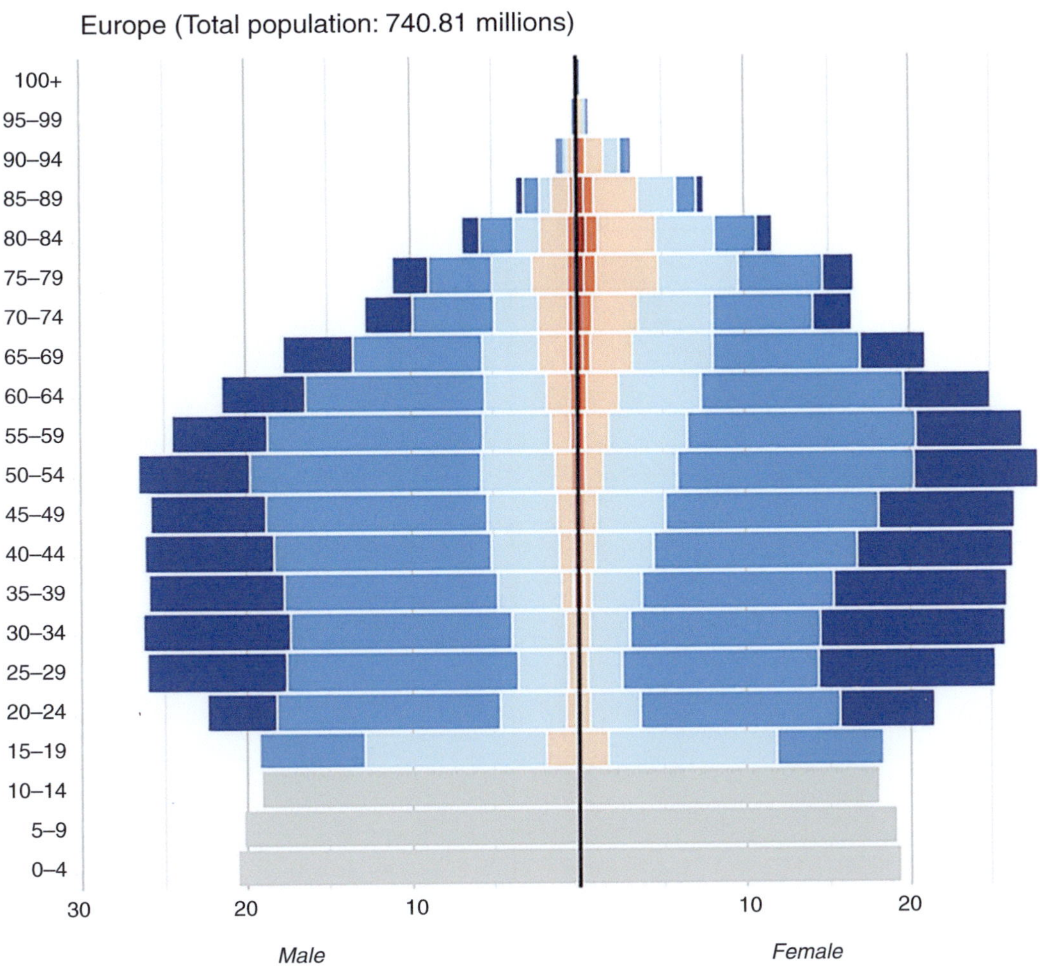

Fig. 5.1 (continued)

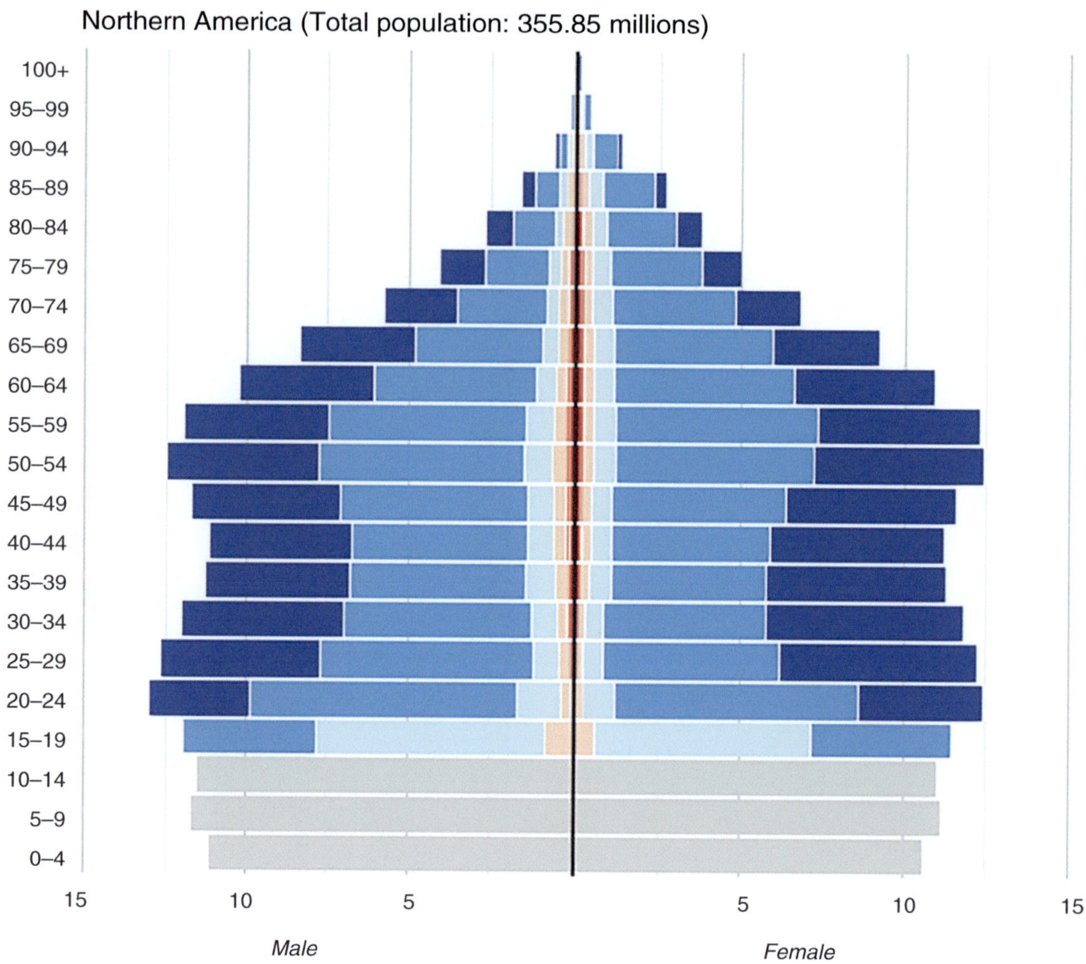

Fig. 5.1 (continued)

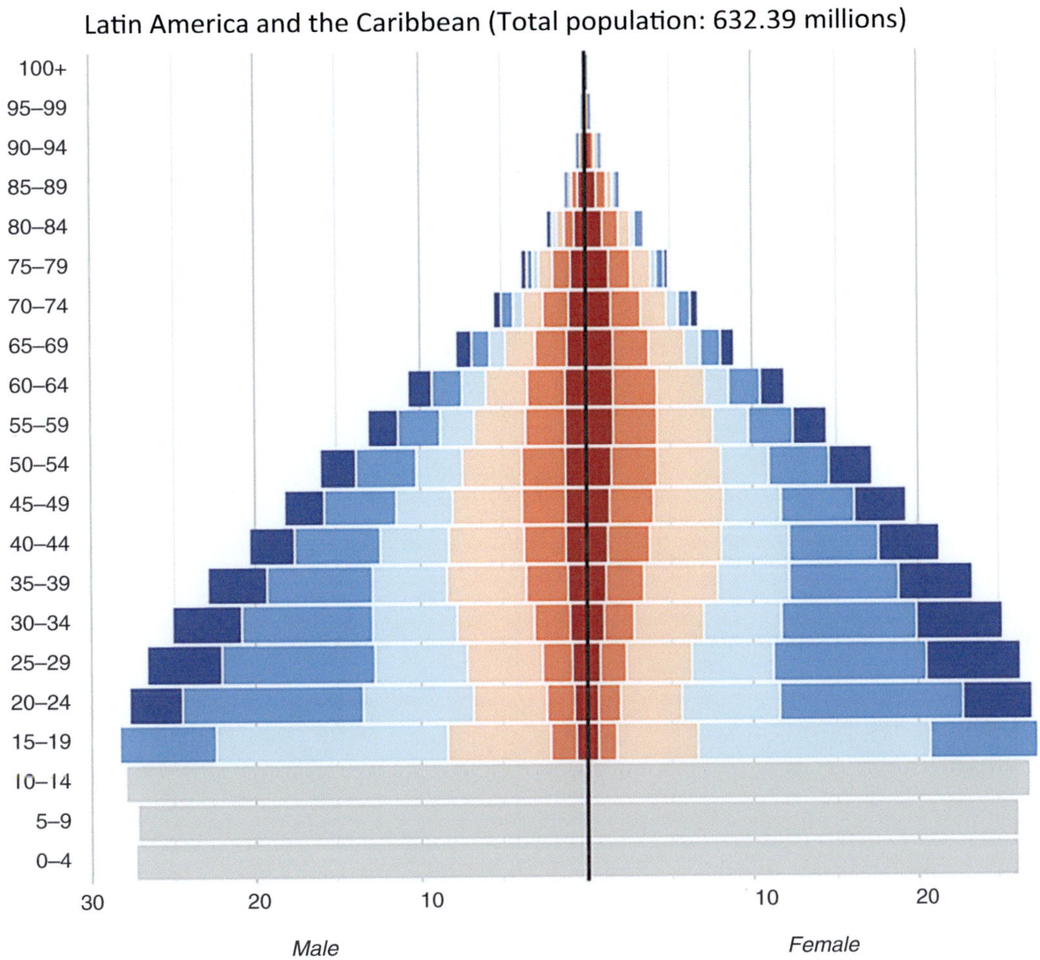

Fig. 5.1 (continued)

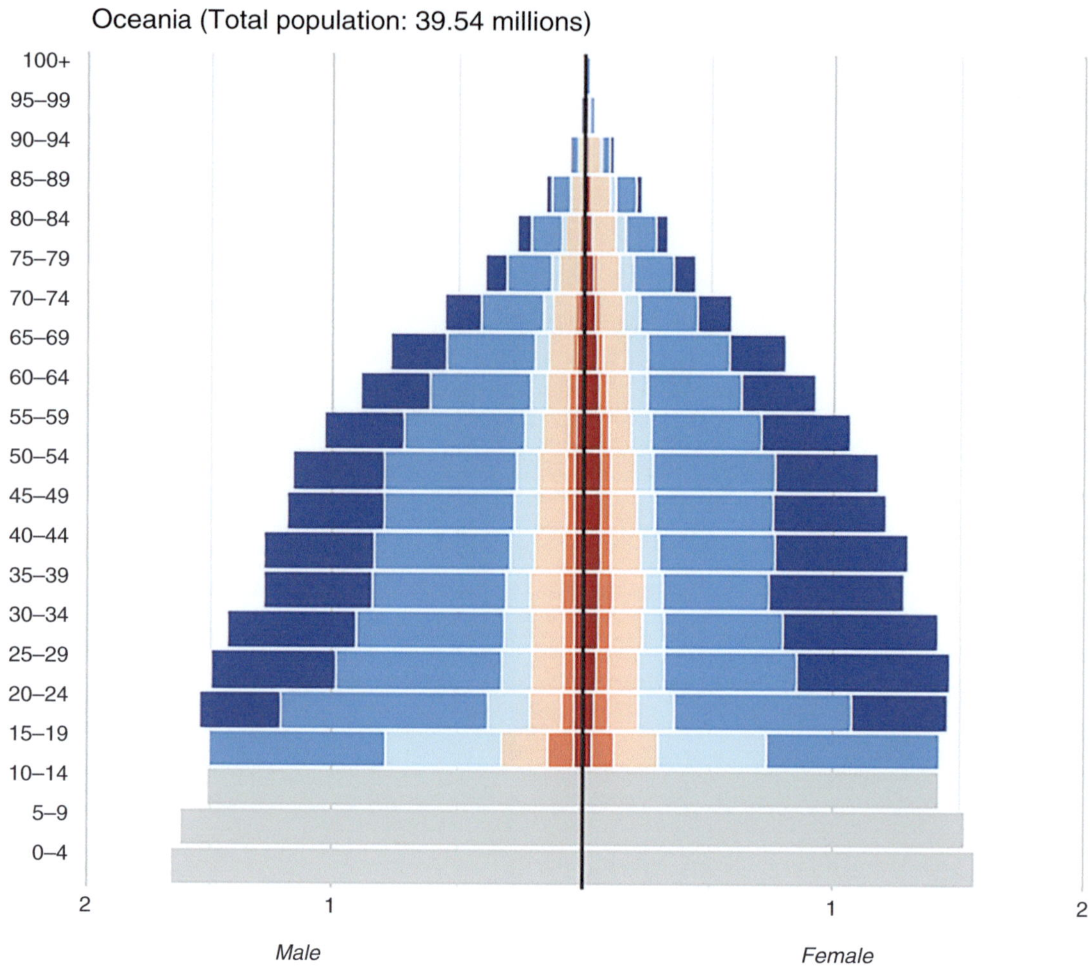

Fig. 5.1 (continued)

5.2 Education as Another Key Source of Demographic Heterogeneity

Unlike most population pyramids, those presented in Fig. 5.1 have a unique feature in presenting the population not only by age and sex but also by the level of educational attainment. Education plays an important role in shaping fertility, mortality and migration patterns. Education directly empowers people with cognitive skills, better risk perception and abstract thinking ability, while indirectly enhances access to socioeconomic resources, social capital and information as well as increasing autonomy in decision making [9, 10]. As a consequence, higher levels of education, especially for women, are associated with lower fertility for a number of reasons, including better access to contraception, ability to exercise reproductive choice and changing desired family size. See Basu [11] and Lutz [12] for an extensive review of the relationship between education and fertility and the mechanisms through which education operates.

Population projections which explicitly account for education disparities in childbearing thus would yield different results to those that do not consider female education. Furthermore, if the global trend of educational expansion will continue (with the exception of the COVID-19 pandemic and conflicts which disrupted the secular trend in many countries [13]), fertility would be on the course of declining further. Depending on the projection methods and assumptions, the world population is projected by the Institute for Health Metrics and Evaluation (IHME), the Wittgenstein Centre/IIASA and the UN Population Division to reach its peak at 9.7 billion in 2064 [14], at 9.8 billion around 2080 [3] and at 10.4 billion around 2080s [15], respectively and then will level off until the end of the century.

5.3 Health Implications of Changing Demographic Structure, Distribution and Composition

Whilst future global population size has direct and indirect implications on health, such as greenhouse gas emissions, land use and food security, where the people will live and who will be part of the population also have health impacts. With 68% of the global population (~6.7 billion) projected to live in the urban areas by the year 2050 [16], differences in infrastructure and services, mobility, housing, lifestyle and consumption between the urban and rural areas will imply changes in population health. On the one hand, urbanization brings about better access to healthcare and services resulting in better health (as measured by e.g. all-cause mortality [17], infant mortality [18] and undernutrition [19]). On the other hand, in poorly planned urban centres, higher exposure to pollutions such as air pollution also leads to higher lung cancer rates among men living in the urban areas as compared to their counterparts in the rural areas [20, 21]. Likewise, a switch to sedentary behaviour associated with urban lifestyles is also responsible for generally higher rates of overweight and obesity in the urban areas, especially in middle-income countries [19]. More generally, disadvantaged segments of the population such as low-income households, people with low level of education and migrants are more likely to develop poorer health due to lack of access to health services and generally lower quality of life e.g. poorer housing conditions and living environments. With the future trend of increasing urbanisation in low- and middle-income countries, health policy needs to ensure that vulnerable subgroups of population are not left behind.

Under the "middle of the road" scenario which assumes a business as usual trajectory where historical patterns of social, economic and technological trends continue based on the Wittgenstein Centre/IIASA projection (see Samir et al. [22] and Samir and Lutz [23, 24] and for further details on assumptions and methods), by the end of the century, the number of world population with at least secondary level of education would increase from about 3.5 billion in 2015 to about 7.5 billion in 2100 (from 48% of the total population 2015 to 81% of total population in 2100). Given the well-established causal relationship between education and health [25–27], if this causal linkage holds over time, then the increasing level of education worldwide would imply better global health in the future. However, at the same time, most countries in the world are on the course of population aging. Increasing longevity coupled with low fertility contribute to a shifting age structure to higher proportion of older people, with the share of population aged 65 years or over projected to rise from 10.0% in 2022 to 16% in 2050 [15]. Age-specific healthcare demand thus needs to be accounted for in policy planning.

Population dynamics and demographic trends are one fundamental determinant of global health. Given that the future health will not match the population of today, it is thus crucial to consider demographic changes in health projections and policy planning. This is feasible because many relevant demographic characteristics have already been quantified and projected and are readily available to be incorporated into health modelling.

Box 5.1 Demographic transition

Demographic transition is a process of demographic changes driven by a shift in birth and death rates as a country goes through the socioeconomic development. The classic demographic transition model describes historical declines in death rates and birth rates in many European societies and the United States since the transformation from an agricultural society into an industrial one in the eighteenth century. In the first stage, before the industrial revolution, because of poor sanitation, limited food supplies and extreme events such as wars, pandemics and famine, death rates were high and so were birth rates. As a consequence, population growth was slow. In the second stage around the period of the industrial revolution, improvement in food production, sanitation and medical technology contributed to lower death rates. However, birth rates remained high and this characterises the period of rapid population growth. In the third stage of the demographic transition, the population was still growing but at a much slower pace since fertility started to decline while mortality remained at a low level. Advancement in several domains such as increasing female education, availability of contraception and declining demand for child labour contributed to lower fertility. In the fourth stage (still ongoing), death rates and birth rates are both low, thus the population is stabilized. Most highly advanced industrial countries are in this stage while some countries have reached stage five, where population decline due to population aging and fertility rate below replacement level.

References

1. Goldstein JR, Lee RD. Demographic perspectives on the mortality of COVID-19 and other epidemics. Proc Natl Acad Sci. 2020;117(36):22035–41.
2. Dowd JB, Andriano L, Brazel DM, Rotondi V, Block P, Ding X, et al. Demographic science aids in understanding the spread and fatality rates of COVID-19. Proc Natl Acad Sci. 2020;117(18):9696–8.
3. Lutz W, Goujon A, Samir KC, Stonawski M, Stilianakis N. Demographic and human capital scenarios for the 21st century: 2018 assessment for 201 countries. New York: EU Science Hub-European Commission; 2018. https://publications.jrc.ec.europa.eu/repository/handle/JRC111148
4. Lutz W, Cuaresma JC, Kebede E, Prskawetz A, Sanderson WC, Striessnig E. Education rather than age structure brings demographic dividend. Proc Natl Acad Sci. 2019;116(26):12798–803.
5. Bloom DE, Canning D, Malaney PN. Population dynamics and economic growth in Asia. Popul Dev Rev. 2000;26:257–90.
6. Lee RD. The demographic transition: three centuries of fundamental change. J Econ Perspect. 2003;17(4):167–90.
7. Ghislandi S, Sanderson WC, Scherbov S. A simple measure of human development: the human life indicator. Popul Dev Rev. 2019;45(1):219–33.
8. Bloom DE, Canning D, Fink G. Implications of population ageing for economic growth. Oxf Rev Econ Policy. 2010;26(4):583–612.
9. Lutz W, Muttarak R, Striessnig E. Universal education is key to enhanced climate adaptation. Science. 2014;346(6213):1061–2.
10. Muttarak R, Lutz W. Is education a key to reducing vulnerability to natural disasters and hence unavoidable climate change? Ecol Soc. 2014;19(1):42.
11. Basu AM. Why does education lead to lower fertility? A critical review of some of the possibilities. World Dev. 2002;30(10):1779–90.
12. Lutz W. Education empowers women to reach their personal fertility target, regardless of what the target is. Vienna Yearb Popul Res. 2017;15:27–31.
13. Meinck S, Fraillon J, Strietholt R, editors. The impact of the COVID-19 pandemic on education international evidence from the responses to educational disruption survey (REDS). Paris: UNESCO Publishing; 2022.
14. Vollset SE, Goren E, Yuan CW, Cao J, Smith AE, Hsiao T, et al. Fertility, mortality, migration, and population scenarios for 195 countries and territories from 2017

to 2100: a forecasting analysis for the global burden of disease study. Lancet. 2020;396(10258):1285–306.
15. United Nations. World population prospects 2022: summary of results. New York: Department of Economic and Social Affairs; 2022. https://www.un.org/development/desa/pd/sites/www.un.org.development.desa.pd/files/wpp2022_summary_of_results.pdf
16. UN DESA. World urbanization prospects: the 2018 revision (ST/ESA/SER.A/420). New York: United Nations; 2019.
17. Cross SH, Califf RM, Warraich HJ. Rural–urban disparity in mortality in the US from 1999 to 2019. JAMA. 2021;325(22):2312–4.
18. Van de Poel E, O'Donnell O, Van Doorslaer E. What explains the rural–urban gap in infant mortality: household or community characteristics? Demography. 2009;46(4):827–50.
19. Arthur SS, Nyide B, Soura AB, Kahn K, Weston M, Sankoh O. Tackling malnutrition: a systematic review of 15-year research evidence from INDEPTH health and demographic surveillance systems. Glob Health Action. 2015;8(1):28298.
20. Guo H, Li W, Wu J, Ho HC. Does air pollution contribute to urban–rural disparity in male lung cancer diseases in China? Environ Sci Pollut Res Int. 2022;29(16):23905–18.
21. Nafstad P, Håheim LL, Oftedal B, Gram F, Holme I, Hjermann I, et al. Lung cancer and air pollution: a 27 year follow up of 16,209 Norwegian men. Thorax. 2003;58(12):1071–6.
22. Samir KC, Potančoková M, Bauer R, Goujon A, Striessnig E. Data and methods. In: Lutz W, Butz WP, Samir KC, editors. World population and human capital in the 21st century. Oxford: Oxford University Press; 2014. p. 434–518. http://ukcatalogue.oup.com/product/9780198703167.do.
23. Samir KC, Lutz W. Demographic scenarios by age, sex and education corresponding to the SSP narratives. Popul Environ. 2014;35(3):243–60.
24. Samir KC, Lutz W. The human core of the shared socioeconomic pathways: population scenarios by age, sex and level of education for all countries to 2100. Glob Environ Change. 2017;42:181–92.
25. Brunello G, Fort M, Schneeweis N, Winter-Ebmer R. The causal effect of education on health: what is the role of health behaviors? Health Econ. 2016;25(3):314–36.
26. Heckman JJ, Humphries JE, Veramendi G. Returns to education: the causal effects of education on earnings, health, and smoking. J Polit Econ. 2018;126(S1):S197–246.
27. Smith WC, Anderson E, Salinas D, Horvatek R, Baker DP. A meta-analysis of education effects on chronic disease: the causal dynamics of the population education transition curve. Soc Sci Med. 2015;127:29–40.

Part III

The Global Burden of Disease: Health Throughout the Life Course

6 Newborn Health

Lulu M. Muhe

Abstract

Newborn health is health of the infant during the period from birth until 28 days of postnatal life. The newborn age group suffers more than infants and older children from under-developed immune system (infections with normal flora), conditions associated with maternal and obstetric risk factors and conditions related to immaturity of vital organs such as the lungs. The newborn period of life is the most vulnerable time of a child's survival. Neonatal mortality accounts for nearly half of the under-5-year mortality and occurs for 98% in low-income countries. Despite the efforts of the past 20 years promoted within the Millennium Development Goals and Sustainable Development Goals, the neonatal period remains the most likely period for a child to die. Most of neonatal deaths (75%) occurs during the first week of life, and about one million newborns die within the first 24 hours every year. Prematurity, birth asphyxia, infections, and birth defects are the main causes.

Keywords

Newborn health · Neonatal mortality · Post-neonatal mortality · Stillbirth · Apgar score

L. M. Muhe (✉)
Addis Ababa University, Addis Ababa, Ethiopia

6.1 Introduction

The newborn period is defined as the period from birth until 28 days of postnatal life. The newborn age group suffers more than infants and older children from under-developed immune system (infections with normal flora), conditions associated with maternal and obstetric risk factors, and conditions related to immaturity of vital organs such as the lungs.

As a result, newborn health is characterized by health problems related to

- Maternal health such as hypertension, diabetes, malnutrition
- Complications of pregnancy, childbirth, and delivery, for example, pre-eclampsia and eclampsia, asphyxia, etc.
- Complications of prematurity (prematurity is defined as those born before 37 completed weeks of gestation) such as immature lungs presenting as respiratory distress syndrome
- Other health problems such as infections, for example, sepsis and pneumonia, and congenital anomalies, for example, congenital heart diseases, chromosomal abnormalities such as Down's syndrome.

The newborn period of life is the most vulnerable time of a child's survival. Neonatal mortality accounts for nearly half of the under-5-year

M. C. B. Raviglione et al. (eds.), *Global Health Essentials*, Sustainable Development Goals Series,
https://doi.org/10.1007/978-3-031-33851-9_6

mortality and occurs for 98% in low-income countries [1].

Important definitions to remember

- Neonatal mortality is defined as the probability of dying within the first month of life per 1000 live births; calculated by dividing the number of infant deaths under 28 days of age in a year per 1000 live births.
- Post-neonatal mortality is defined as the probability of dying after the first month of life but before the first birthday (the difference between infant and neonatal mortality).
- Perinatal mortality rate is defined as the number of born dead + number died at the first 168 h of life (7 days) × 1000 divided by number of born alive and dead.

6.2 Descriptive Epidemiology and International Targets

SDG 3 is specific to health and SDG 3.2 targets child health

- By 2030, end preventable deaths of newborns and children under 5 years of age, with all countries aiming to reduce neonatal mortality to at least as low as 12 per 1000 livebirths and under-5 mortality to at least as low as 25 per 1000 livebirths [2].

Despite the efforts of the past 20 years promoted within the Millennium Development Goals (MDG) and Sustainable Development Goals (SDG), the neonatal period remains the most likely period for a child to die.

While the global Average Annual Rate of Reduction (AARR) of under-5 mortality is going down, the global AARR of neonatal mortality is not declining to meet the SDG 3.2 target by 2030. Every year, from the 130 million live births globally, an estimated 2.4 million neonates die. Over the past decade, substantial progress has been made in newborn health and in preventing stillbirths, including in countries with the highest burdens of mortality. More mothers and their babies can now access effective health care during and after pregnancy. Yet we are far from our goal of ending preventable newborn deaths and stillbirths by 2030.

Stillbirths are deaths of infants in utero, i.e. before delivery. There were nearly two million stillbirths in 2019 globally. Most of the underlying causes of stillbirths and neonatal deaths are the same problems related to maternal health, complications of pregnancy, labour, and delivery.

6.3 Determinants and Risk Factors for Illness and Death

Most of neonatal deaths (75%) occurs during the first week of life, and about one million newborns die within the first 24 h every year. Prematurity, birth asphyxia, infections, and birth defects cause most neonatal deaths in 2017 [3].

Important risk factors to increased neonatal mortality include low and very low birth weight, Apgar* <7 at the 5th min, gestational age ≤37 weeks, caesarean delivery mortality, inadequate and absent prenatal care, presence of complications during pregnancy, congenital malformation, absence of partner, maternal age ≥35 years, male gender, and multiple gestation, [4].

*The APGAR score consists of 5 components scored as 2 (if good), 1 (if not so good) and 0 (if poor): colour, heart rate, reflexes, muscle tone, and respiration.

6.4 Approaches and Strategies for Prevention and Control

Preventive interventions need to bridge the continuum of care from pregnancy, through childbirth and the neonatal period, and beyond. Lack of positive health-related behaviour, education, and poverty is an underlying cause of many neonatal deaths, either through increasing the prevalence of risk factors such as maternal infection, or through reducing access to effective care. Interventions include:

- Pregnant women need to attend antenatal check-up regularly to identify any complications and take immediate measures. Pregnant women need to take immunizations such as for rubella, hepatitis B, and tetanus. In settings where HIV is prevalent, they need to be supported with prevention programs against HIV as well as other sexually transmitted diseases, prevention and treatment of substance use, and smoking cessation. During childbirth, monitoring of progress of labour, maternal and foetal well-being with partograph, immediate newborn care, and antibiotics for preterm premature rupture of membranes (pPROM) should be done.
- In the newborn period, promotion of exclusive breastfeeding, immunizations (BCG, hepatitis B, rotavirus, pentavalent vaccines), thermal care, hygienic cord care and in high HIV settings PMTCT are essential interventions. In countries where the Integrated Management of Childhood Illness (IMCI) strategy is adopted and is being implemented, the component on care of sick newborns provides detailed guidance on how to manage the sick newborn for severe signs, infections, respiratory distress syndrome in addition to the essential newborn care package.

6.5 Responsibilities of Different National and International Institutions

The Partnership for Maternal, Newborn and Child health (PMNCH) hosted by the World Health Organization supports constituencies across the international community including other United Nations (UN) organizations (e.g., UNICEF, UNFPA, WHO, and World Bank) and a multitude of international non-governmental organizations (NGOs) that address the continuum of care for the health of women, newborns (including stillbirths), children, and adolescents. The national-level offices of UN organizations and NGOs, professional associations, and national health bureaus generally support the work of the Ministry of Health of a country.

References

1. United Nations Inter-Agency Group for Child Mortality Estimation (UN IGME). Levels and trends in child mortality. Report 2021. https://data.unicef.org/resources/levels-and-trends-in-child-mortality/#.
2. United Nations. Transforming our world, the Agenda for sustainable development. New York: United Nations; 2030. https://sustainabledevelopment.un.org/content/documents/21252030%20Agenda%20for%20Sustainable%20Development%20web.pdf
3. World Health Organization. https://www.who.int/news-room/fact-sheets/detail/newborns-reducing-mortality.
4. Veloso FCS, Kassar LDML, Oliveira MJC, et al. Analysis of neonatal mortality risk factors in Brazil: a systematic review and meta-analysis of observational studies. J Pediatr (Rio J). 95(5):14. https://doi.org/10.1016/j.jped.2018.12.014.

7 Child and Adolescent Health

Lulu M. Muhe

Abstract

Standard definitions of age groups among children are important because they indicate variations in illness patterns and mortality outcomes. In the first few years of a child, common infections such as pneumonia and diarrhoea are the main causes of illness and death. This trend slowly falls until the age of 5 years. During adolescence (age 10–19 years), mental health and accidents become the main health problems. More than five million children died before reaching their fifth birthday in 2020. Almost half of those deaths, 2.4 million, occurred in the first month of life. Infant and child mortality rates are basic indicators of a country's socioeconomic situation and quality of life. Adolescence is a unique stage of human development and an important time for laying the foundations of good health. Establishing healthy behaviours to prevent chronic diseases in adults is easier and more effective during childhood and adolescence than trying to change unhealthy behaviours during adulthood.

Keywords

Infant mortality rate · Under-5 mortality · Integrated Management of Childhood Illness (IMCI) · Child health · Adolescent health

7.1 Introduction

Standard definitions of the various age groups among children are shown in Fig. 7.1. In the first few years of a child, common infections such as pneumonia and diarrhoea are the main causes of illness and death. This trend slowly falls until the age of 5 years. During adolescence (age 10–19 years) mental health and accidents become the main health problems.

L. M. Muhe (✉)
Addis Ababa University, Addis Ababa, Ethiopia

M. C. B. Raviglione et al. (eds.), *Global Health Essentials*, Sustainable Development Goals Series,
https://doi.org/10.1007/978-3-031-33851-9_7

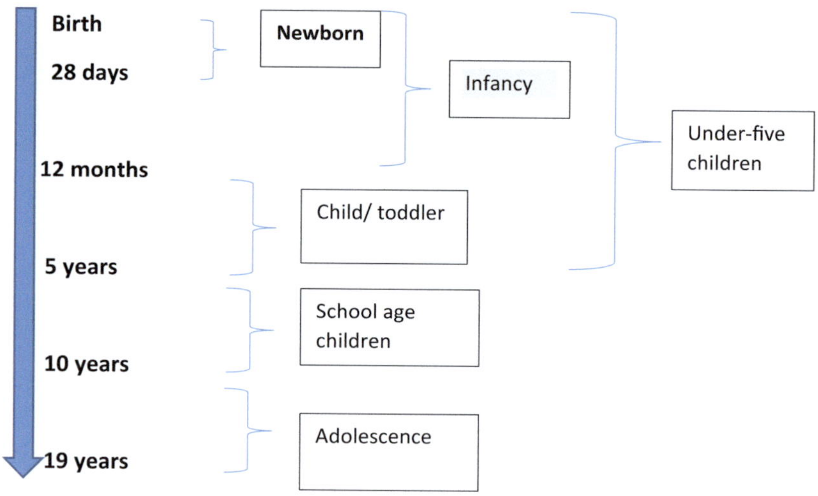

Fig. 7.1 Standard definitions of the various age groups among children

7.2 Global Situation on Child Mortality

More than five million children died before reaching their fifth birthday in 2020. Almost half of those deaths, 2.4 million, occurred among newborns [1]. More than half of these early child deaths are due to conditions that could be prevented or treated with access to simple, affordable interventions. Major causes of child mortality include preterm birth complications, birth asphyxia/trauma, pneumonia, congenital anomalies, diarrhoea, and malaria. Interventions against these conditions include immunization, adequate nutrition, safe water and food and quality care by a trained health provider.

7.3 Indicators on Child Mortality

Infant and child mortality rates are basic indicators of a country's socioeconomic situation and quality of life. The common indicators are defined as below:

- Infant Mortality Rate (IMR): the probability of dying within the first 12 months of life per 1000 live births; calculated by dividing the number of infant deaths under 12 months in a year per 1000 live births.
- Under-5 mortality: the probability of dying between birth and the fifth birthday per 1000 live births.

7.4 Sustainable Development Goals (SDGs)

The Sustainable Development Goal 3 (SDG 3) adopted by the United Nations in 2015 aims to ensure healthy lives and promote well-being for all children [2]. Each SDG has its own targets globally agreed upon. Countries need to set targets and develop specific strategies to address the goal and monitor progress in their own setting. SDG 3 targets include:

> By 2030, end preventable deaths of newborns and children under 5 years of age, with all countries aiming to reduce neonatal mortality to at least as low as 12 per 1000 live births and under-5 mortality to at least as low as 25 per 1000 live births.

Although the world has been accelerating progress in reducing the under-5 mortality rate, differences exist in under-5 mortality across regions and countries. Sub-Saharan Africa remains the region with the highest under-5 mortality rate in the world, with 1 child in 13 dying before his or her fifth birthday, 20 years behind the world average which achieved a 1 in 13 rate already in 1999. In 2019, 122 countries have met the SDG target for under-5 mortality and a further 20 countries are expected to meet the target by 2030 if current trends continue.

7.5 Major Causes and Risk Factors of Child Mortality

Major causes of death child mortality are well-known. These include preterm birth complications including respiratory distress syndrome, sepsis, asphyxia, and congenital anomalies. In older infants and children below 5 years of age, the leading causes of death include acute respiratory infections, acute diarrhoeal illnesses, malaria, measles, meningitis, HIV/AIDS, and non-communicable diseases. Leading causes of under-5 mortality vary from regions to regions of the world. In the African Region, malaria causes up to 10% and congenital anomalies cause only 6% of all under-5 deaths. In Europe, on the other hand, congenital anomalies cause up to 23% of under-5 mortality while malaria is almost negligible.

Low birth weight, malnutrition, non-breastfed children, overcrowded living conditions, lack of antenatal care, lack of immunization are known risk factors for poor outcome from childhood illnesses. Unsafe drinking water and food, poor hygiene practices and malnutrition are significant risk factors for poor outcome from diarrhoea. Ensuring availability and sustainable management of water and sanitation for all is the aim of SDG 6 as these are the determinants of diarrhoeas and its consequences [2].

7.6 Approaches and Strategies for Prevention and Control of Childhood Diseases

To meet the SDG 3.2 target of reducing under-5 mortality, interventions recommended for scale up in a country include

- Integrated Management of Childhood Illness (IMCI) is a strategy promoted by WHO and UNICEF since 1997 on management and prevention of the common causes of under-5 deaths at primary level with guidance on triaging of sick children. It consists of holistic assessment of sick children including for nutrition and immunization status, rapid referral of severely ill children, rational use of diagnostic tools and drugs, and effective communication with caretakers and families.
- Prevention of malaria using insecticide-treated nets (ITNs) and intermittent preventive treatment of malaria (IPT); sleeping under insecticide-treated nets (ITN) and indoor residual spray (IRS), and prevention and management of severe and moderate acute malnutrition are other essential strategies for prevention and control of child mortality.
- Other promotive and preventive interventions are available for infant and young child feeding, including micronutrient supplementation and deworming; immunization, prevention of mother-to-child transmission (PMTCT) of HIV.

7.7 Adolescent Health

Adolescence is the phase of life between childhood and adulthood, from ages 10 to 19. It is a unique stage of human development and an important time for laying the foundations of good health.

Nearly one million adolescents died in 2020. About 43% of the deaths among those aged 5–24 years occurred among adolescents. Over 70% of all deaths among 5–24-year-olds occurred in sub-Saharan Africa (45%) and Central and Southern Asia (27%). Adolescents suffer from injuries, and non-communicable diseases such as chronic respiratory diseases, acquired heart diseases, childhood cancers, diabetes, and obesity, and violence. Injuries (road traffic injuries, drowning, burns, and falls) rank among the top 3 causes of death and lifelong disability among adolescents. Half of all mental health disorders in adulthood start by age 14 [3]. Early onset of substance use and adolescent pregnancy are some of the challenges that need to be addressed in this age group [3].

7.8 Healthy Lifestyle as Prevention of Adult Illness

Establishing healthy behaviours to prevent chronic diseases in adults is easier and more effective during childhood and adolescence than trying to change unhealthy behaviours during adulthood. Examples include reducing obesity, improving healthy food options in school, improving physical education and activity, preventing tobacco use, etc. Adolescents need information, including age-appropriate comprehensive sexuality education; opportunities to develop life skills; and appropriate health services. Detailed guidance is available in the global accelerated action for the health of adolescents (AA-HA!) [4].

References

1. United Nations Inter-Agency Group for Child Mortality Estimation (UN IGME). Levels and trends in child mortality. Report 2021. https://data.unicef.org/resources/levels-and-trends-in-child-mortality/#.
2. United Nations. Transforming our world, the 2030 agenda for sustainable development. New York: United Nations; 2022. https://sustainabledevelopment.un.org/content/documents/21252030%20Agenda%20for%20Sustainable%20Development%20web.pdf
3. World Health Organization. https://www.who.int/news-room/fact-sheets/detail/adolescents-health-risks-and-solutions.
4. World Health Organization. Global accelerated action for the health of adolescents (AA-HA!): guidance to support country implementation. https://www.who.int/publications/i/item/WHO-FWC-MCA-17.05.

Child Health and Nutrition

8

Cristiana Berti, Mattia Baglioni, and Carlo Agostoni

Abstract

Stunting, wasting, hidden hunger, and overweight/obesity are the main nutrition problems affecting, respectively, 149, 45, 340, and 39 million of children. Epidemiological evidence reveals that worldwide the Sustainable Development Goals to eliminate malnutrition by 2030 are far to be reached. Inadequate infant and young child feeding practices, food insecurity, poverty, and limited access to health services contribute to malnutrition, which is also affected by socioeconomic, commercial, and political factors, and occurs in an intergeneration cycle. Furthermore, child malnutrition has been challenged by the economic crisis and food- and health-system disruptions related to the COVID-19 pandemic. The existing key interventions have the potential to be further scaled up to address undernutrition and overnutrition concurrently, notably by cross-cutting education, agriculture, food systems, social safety nets, and "water, hygiene, and sanitation". Despite their positive nutrition outcomes, data on programmes coverage and costs are still lacking. Several stakeholders are called to sustain global nutrition.

Keywords

Children · Stunting · Wasting · Severe acute malnutrition · Hidden hunger · Obesity · Overweight · Non-communicable diseases · Sustainable development goals · COVID-19

C. Berti
Pediatria Immunoreumatologia, Fondazione IRCCS Ca' Granda Ospedale Maggiore Policlinico, Milan, Italy

M. Baglioni
Action Contre la Faim (ACF-France), Paris, France

C. Agostoni (✉)
Pediatria Immunoreumatologia, Fondazione IRCCS Ca' Granda Ospedale Maggiore Policlinico, Milan, Italy

Department of Clinical Sciences and Community Health, University of Milan, Milan, Italy
e-mail: carlo.agostoni@unimi.it

8.1 Definitions, Features, and Epidemiology

Children malnutrition encompasses undernutrition, hidden hunger, and overnutrition. Definitions, main characteristics, and determinants are reported in Table 8.1 [1–4]:

- Undernutrition:
  - Wasting indicates recent and severe weight loss as a result of acute food shortage and/or infections. The conditions causing wasting are related to each other and create a "vicious cycle" with wasting itself. In

M. C. B. Raviglione et al. (eds.), *Global Health Essentials*, Sustainable Development Goals Series,
https://doi.org/10.1007/978-3-031-33851-9_8

Table 8.1 Definition, main features, and determinants of the forms of malnutrition affecting children under 5 years

Form		Definition and main features	Determinants and risk factors
Undernutrition	*Wasting* [1]	• Defined as Z scores of weight-for-height below −2SD • Characterized by a loss of muscle and fat mass • Associated with weakened immunity, increased risk of infectious diseases (diarrhoea, pneumonia), increased risk of disease death • 45.4 million (6.7%) children affected in 2020. Asia, mostly South Asia, is the most affected region in the world	• Poor access to appropriate, timely, affordable health care • Inappropriate caring and feeding practices (e.g. non-exclusive BF; low quantity/quality/variety of complementary food) • Poor food security (e.g. shortage of food quantity/diversity, i.e. monotonous diet); inadequate food knowledge • Lack of a sanitary environment (e.g. no access to safe water, sanitation, hygiene services)
	SAM = Marasmus and Kwashiorkor [2]	• *Marasmus* = Defined as either MUAC <115 mm or Z scores of weight-for-height below −3SD. Due to a significant weight loss in a brief period. Characterized by emaciated and weak appearance • *Kwashiorkor* = Characterized by symmetric bilateral pitting oedema, and "flaky paint" skin depigmentation. Aetiology fairly unknown. Associated with severe complications • SAM accounts for at least 10% of deaths among children, all in LMICs	• Seasonal food insecurity • Environmental enteropathy; chronic and acute infections • Poor complementary feeding practices
	Stunting	• Defined as Z scores of length/height-for-age below −2SD • Characterized by linear growth failure • Associated with poor growth, neuro-cognitive development and educational performance, with lifelong consequences on human capital [3] • 149.2 million children affected in 2020 (decline from 33.1 to 22.0% since 2000–2020). Asia and Africa display the highest prevalence. Africa is the only region where the number of stunted children is not declining [1]	• Poor maternal health and nutrition before/during/after pregnancy; short birth spacing; adolescent pregnancy → Intrauterine growth restriction, LBW, preterm birth, SGA • Wasting • Suboptimal infant and young child feeding practices (e.g. non-exclusive BF; complementary feeding limited in quantity/quality/variety) • Infections, depending on severity, duration, recurrence • Household poverty, food insecurity

Form		Definition and main features	Determinants and risk factors
Hidden hunger		• Defined as deficiencies in essential vitamins and minerals • Associated with poor growth and development; poor immunity and tissue development; poor health and risk of death [3] • At least 340 million children affected [3]. The highest prevalence in LMICs, mostly in Sub-Saharan Africa and Asia [4] • Vitamin A deficiency (29% in 2013): associated with blindness, increased risk of death from infectious disease – Iron deficiency: major cause of anaemia (41.7% in 2016), impaired motor and cognitive development; malaria, helminths, and inflammation as important determinants – Zinc deficiency: associated with reduced linear growth, increased infectious morbidity – Iodine: associated with goitre, neurobehavioural disorders [4]	• Inadequate complementary feeding, nutrition transition, poor food security (e.g. traditional diets relying on a few starch-based staples; global modern diets rich in nutrient-poor ultra-processed foods and drinks) • Infectious morbidity
Overnutrition	*Overweight and obesity* [3]	• Defined as excessive weight-for-height using growth reference standards for children • Associated with early onset of type-2 diabetes, high blood pressure, respiratory problems; psychological and psychosocial disorders; increased risk of NCDs and disability in adulthood; financial burden on health-care systems; lost in economic productivity later in life • Overweight prevalence rose from 33 million (5.4%) in 2000 to 39 million (5.7%) in 2020, with estimates for LMICs showing heterogeneous trends	• Inadequate caring and feeding practices (e.g. non-exclusive BF; early-introduction of complementary food) • Nutrition transition, poor food security (e.g. shortage of nutritious foods; availability of cheap energy-dense foods and beverages); caregivers' inadequate food knowledge • Physical inactivity, sedentary behaviours

SAM severe acute malnutrition, *MUAC* mid-upper arm circumference, *LMICs* low- and middle-income countries, *NCDs* non-communicable diseases, *BF* breastfeeding, *LBW* low birthweight, *SGA* small-for-gestational age

2020, wasting persists at high rates (6.7%) among children under 5 years [1]
- Severe acute malnutrition, including marasmus, kwashiorkor and marasmic kwashiorkor, can be treated with ready-to-use therapeutic food [2]
- Stunting is the result of chronic or recurrent undernutrition. Undernutrition from conception to the second birthday, including maternal nutritional status, is the major contributor. Despite the decline in percentage along the 2000–2020 period, yet 149 million children under 5 suffer of stunting [1]

Child undernutrition exerts both short-term effects on morbidity and mortality, and lifelong effects on non-communicable diseases (NCDs). Paradoxically, early-life undernutrition and the rapid catch-up (weight gain) in childhood likely increase the susceptibility to accumulate fat, predisposing to overweight/obesity and/or NCDs in adulthood, possibly leading to epigenetic, transmissible somatic changes [4, 5]. Further research into mechanisms linking undernutrition in childhood with NCDs is needed to inform policy, programming, and patient management strategies that support long-term health [5].

- Hidden hunger consists of micronutrients' deficiency. It also occurs in absence of an energy-deficit diet, thus an obese child can suffer from hidden hunger, as modern diets are energy-dense but nutrient-poor. At least 340 million children under 5 suffer from micronutrient deficiencies [3]
- Overnutrition, including overweight and obesity, occurs when caloric intake exceeds energy requirements. In recent decades, whilst being plateaued at high levels in high-income countries (HICs), overweight in children under 5 has dramatically risen in low- and middle-income countries (LMICs), reflecting the greater availability of "cheap calories" from fatty- and sugary-foods [3]. Childhood excessive weight has serious short- and long-term consequences.

8.1.1 International Targets and Progress

Current figures reveal that the world is not on course to achieve the Sustainable Development Goals to eliminate malnutrition by 2030. Only one quarter of countries are on track to reach the targets on stunting (i.e. achieve a 40% reduction in the number of children <5 who are stunted), wasting (i.e. reduce and maintain childhood wasting to less than 5%), and overweight (i.e. ensure that there is no increase in childhood overweight) [1]. The greatest progress is being made towards the stunting target, with nearly two thirds of countries getting at least some improvement, and Asia contributing most. In contrast, for overweight, about half of countries have experienced no progress or are worsening, with Latin America and the Caribbean experiencing no progress at all.

8.1.2 Determinants and Risk Factors

The strongest drivers of all the malnutrition forms are poverty, limited access to health services, food insecurity, and inadequate nurturing care (worldwide, only 42% of children under the age of 6 months are breastfed and 29% of children aged 6–23 months eat foods from the minimum number of food groups [3, 4]). Drivers are affected by socioeconomic (e.g. parents' low-income and educational level), commercial (e.g. growing marketing of formula milk and low-cost junk food, mostly unrefined and ultra-processed), and political factors and may occur in an inter-generation cycle [4]. Owing to the nutrition transition, many LMICs are coping with a "triple burden" of malnutrition, i.e. the continuing burden of stunting and wasting, various forms of hidden hunger, and rising rates of overweight, while hidden hunger coexists with overweight/obesity in HICs [3].

8.1.2.1 Challenges

The situation is expected to be exacerbated by the global social and economic crisis triggered by COVID-19 pandemic, due to declines in household incomes; constraints in the availability and affordability of nutritious foods; disruptions of health, nutrition, and protection services; and limited opportunities for physical activities, due to either a dramatic increase of crowded urban settings and pandemic crises (Box 8.1) [6–8].

Box 8.1 The COVID-19 Pandemic Undermining Nutrition Across the World

- **Environmental Background.** The economic crisis and food- and health-system disruptions related to the COVID-19 pandemic, i.e. interruptions in nutrition services and increase in household poverty are amplifying malnutrition, particularly in low- and middle-income countries (LMICs).
- School closures, movement restrictions, and nationwide lockdowns impact food systems by disrupting the production, transportation, and sale of fresh nutrient-rich and affordable foods, leading to price volatility and forcing millions of families to rely on cheap nutrient-poor alternatives [6]. Notably the school closure with its burden of detrimental social and health consequences for children living in poverty has likely aggravating existing inequalities.
- **Undernutrition**. Estimates of the potential impacts of the pandemic-triggered economic, the food and health-system crisis on the early-life undernutrition in 118 LMICs, and the cost of related interventions as well were performed for the 2020–2022 period [7]. In a moderate scenario, among children under 5 years, an estimated 2.6 million additional will be stunted in 2022, the number with wasting will increase by an added 9.3 million, and there will be about 168,000 additional deaths. The majority will be in South Asia and sub-Saharan Africa. These estimated additional burdens would result in future productivity losses of US$29.7 billion.
- An additional US$1.2 billion per annum is expected to mitigate the impacts of COVID-19 on early-life undernutrition. Realigning financing towards a more targeted and balanced mix of interventions will lead to decrease stunting and deaths by 4.9% and 2.2%, respectively.
- **Obesity**. An increase in childhood obesity rates as an indirect effect of COVID-19 can be assumed. The exposure to COVID 19-related measures leading to increased food insecurity and decreased physical activities along with less access to nutrition education may be hypothesized to strongly impact on childhood obesity—risk factors and psychosocial stressors [8].

8.2 Approaches and Strategies for Prevention and Control

Ten key interventions may help addressing undernutrition (Box 8.2) [9]. Throughout the years, research revealed common and modifiable drivers to overnutrition [10, 11]. Early-life nutrition, diet diversity, food environments, and socioeconomic factors are considered as the basis to redesign an overarching strategy that may further scale-up the ten main interventions to tackle both undernutrition and overnutrition [10, 11]. These actions are delivered through platforms both within and outside health facilities (e.g. community-health workers, schools, and mass media) and cross-cutting sectors to nutrition, notably education, agriculture, food systems, social safety nets, and WASH (water, hygiene, and sanitation).

Box 8.2 The Main Ten Nutrition Interventions [9]

- The **Management of severe acute malnutrition (SAM)**, preventive zinc supplementation, and promotion of breastfeeding were deemed the top three interventions able to reduce child mortality.
- Children affected by either SAM or **moderate acute malnutrition** have better chance to recover when treatment is delivered through community-based interventions.
- The latest evidence about **preventive zinc supplementation** to children under 5 years is robust for the incidence of diarrhoea reduction but weak as to the effect on the risk of anaemia, stunting, wasting, and child mortality.
- The **promotion of breastfeeding** and of **appropriate complementary feeding** are considered double-duty key actions. Both interventions contribute to preventing undernutrition, while reducing the risk of overweight and obesity in childhood, and obesity and non-communicable diseases later in life.
- **Folic acid supplementation, or fortification,** and **balanced energy protein supplementation** (defined as nutritional supplementation during pregnancy in which proteins provide less than 25% of the total energy content) remain paramount actions targeting women of reproductive age and during pregnancy because reduce the risk of anaemia, and newborn infants small-for-gestational age (SGA) (including stunting at birth), respectively.
- Several benefits stem from **maternal calcium supplementation**: high doses of calcium (≥1 g per day) limit the risk of pre-eclampsia, high blood pressure, maternal death, preterm birth, and low birthweight.
- **Vitamin A supplementation** proved effective in decreasing the incidence of maternal anaemia, infections, and night blindness, as well as the neonatal mortality in newborn babies of very low weight (>1.5 kg) and in children aged 6–59 months.
- **Multiple micronutrient supplementation** (composed of Vitamin A, B1, B2, Niacin, B6, B12, C, D, E, Folic acid, Iron, Zinc, Copper, Selenium, Iodine) is recommended both for women during the antenatal period and children under 5 years. These prevent the risk of anaemia, stillbirth, low birthweight, preterm birth, and babies born SGA.

8.2.1 Cost-Effectiveness and Financial Considerations

Despite the positive nutrition outcomes of cross-sectoral interventions, a huge data gap concerning programmes coverage and costs exists due to the scarce coordination among sectors and the flaw of the existing information system aimed at tracking the achievements at the national and subnational level against the nutrition global targets (especially for nutritional status and micronutrient intake) [11]. These issues, coupled with the need to improve geographical and individual targeting of nutrition programmes, drew the attention towards the cost-effectiveness of such interventions [4].

However, the analysis commissioned by the World Bank [12] found that to achieve the global nutrition targets regarding stunting, severe wasting, anaemia in women of reproductive age, and exclusive breastfeeding, an additional investment of $70 billion should be needed between 2015 and 2025. This may prevent approximately 65 million cases of stunting, 91 million of severe wasting among under-5 children, 265 million of female anaemia. Moreover, 105 million 0–6 months aged children will be breastfed. Overall, this would translate into at least 3.7 million child deaths averted.

8.3 Responsibilities of Institutions

Prevention and appropriate management of children malnutrition, mostly undernutrition (the ratio of undernourished to overweight children is 5 to 1), must be prioritized to ensure children survival and development, and to avoid the escalation of the NCD burden in the future [5, 13]. Multilateral organizations, governments, United Nations agencies, academic institutions, non-governmental organizations, and private donors are committed to improve global sustainable nutrition by supporting and financing the scale-up of the key interventions [14]. Nevertheless, to date, there is still an open debate as to the legitimacy of the existing governance structure including the private sector with its ability to influence the policy-making aimed at improving global health [15].

References

1. United Nations Children's Fund (UNICEF), World Health Organization, International Bank for Reconstruction and Development/The World Bank. Levels and trends in child malnutrition: key findings of the 2021 edition of the joint child malnutrition estimates. Geneva: World Health Organization; 2021. https://apps.who.int/iris/handle/10665/341135. Assessed 17 Jan 2022.
2. Trehan I, Manary MJ. Management of severe acute malnutrition in low-income and middle-income countries. Arch Dis Child. 2015;100:283–7. https://doi.org/10.1136/archdischild-2014-306026.
3. UNICEF. The State of the World's Children 2019. Children, food and nutrition: growing well in a changing world. New York: UNICEF; 2019. https://www.unicef.org/media/60806/file/SOWC-2019.pdf. Assessed 17 Jan 2022.
4. Victora CG, Christian P, Vidaletti LP, Gatica-Domínguez G, Menon P, Black RE. Revisiting maternal and child undernutrition in low-income and middle-income countries: variable progress towards an unfinished agenda. Lancet. 2021;397:1388–99. https://doi.org/10.1016/S0140-6736(21)00394-9.
5. Grey K, Gonzales GB, Abera M, Lelijveld N, Thompson D, Berhane M, Abdissa A, Girma T, Kerac M. Severe malnutrition or famine exposure in childhood and cardiometabolic non-communicable disease later in life: a systematic review. BMJ Glob Health. 2021;6:e003161. https://doi.org/10.1136/bmjgh-2020-003161.
6. Carducci B, Keats EC, Ruel M, Haddad L, Osendarp SJM, Bhutta ZA. Food systems, diets and nutrition in the wake of COVID-19. Nat Food. 2021;2:68–70. https://doi.org/10.1038/s43016-021-00233-9.
7. Osendarp S, Akuoku JK, Black RE, Headey D, Ruel M, Scott N, Shekar M, Walker N, Flory A, Haddad L, Laborde D, Stegmuller A, Thomas M, Heidkamp R. The COVID-19 crisis will exacerbate maternal and child undernutrition and child mortality in low- and middle-income countries. Nat Food. 2021;2:476–84. https://doi.org/10.1038/s43016-021-00319-4.
8. Knebusch V, Williams J, Yordi Aguirre I, Weber MW, Rakovac I, Breda J. Effects of the coronavirus disease 2019 pandemic and the policy response on childhood obesity risk factors: gender and sex differences and recommendations for research. Obes Rev. 2021;22(Suppl 6):e13222. https://doi.org/10.1111/obr.13222.
9. Keats EC, Das JK, Salam RA, Lassi ZS, Imdad A, Black RE, Bhutta ZA. Effective interventions to address maternal and child malnutrition: an update of the evidence. Lancet Child Adolesc Health. 2021;5:367–84. https://doi.org/10.1016/S2352-4642(20)30274-1.
10. Hawkes C, Ruel MT, Salm L, Sinclair B, Branca F. Double-duty actions: seizing programme and policy opportunities to address malnutrition in all its forms. Lancet. 2020;395:142–55. https://doi.org/10.1016/S0140-6736(19)32506-1.
11. Heidkamp RA, Piwoz E, Gillespie S, Keats EC, D'Alimonte MR, Menon P, Das JK, Flory A, Clift JW, Ruel MT, Vosti S, Akuoku JK, Bhutta ZA. Mobilising evidence, data, and resources to achieve global maternal and child undernutrition targets and the sustainable development goals: an agenda for action. Lancet. 2021;397:1400–18. https://doi.org/10.1016/S0140-6736(21)00568-7.
12. Shekar M, Kakietek J, Dayton Eberwein J, Walters D. Executive summary. An investment framework for nutrition: reaching the global targets for stunting, anemia, breastfeeding, and wasting. Washington, DC: World Bank; 2017. https://openknowledge.worldbank.org/handle/10986/26069. Assessed 10 Feb 2022.
13. Kerac M. Diet and development beyond 1000 days: ensuring children thrive as well as survive. Arch Dis Child. 2022;107(8):701–2. https://doi.org/10.1136/archdischild-2022-323780.
14. The global nutrition report, 2022. https://globalnutritionreport.org. Accessed 8 Apr 2022.
15. Lie AL. 'We are not a partnership'—constructing and contesting legitimacy of global public–private partnerships: the Scaling Up Nutrition (SUN) movement. Globalizations. 2021;18:237–55. https://doi.org/10.1080/14747731.2020.1770038.

Maternal Health

9

Viviana Mangiaterra, Maurice Bucagu, and Flaminia Sabbatucci

Abstract

Maternal health, which encompasses health care for women before, during, and after pregnancy, is a major global health issue. Pregnancy and childbirth complications cause 211 deaths per 100,000 live births worldwide (UNICEF. Maternal mortality. Maternal mortality declined by 38% between 2000 and 2017. 2021. https://data.unicef.org/topic/maternal-health/maternal-mortality/), with strong differences linked to socioeconomic levels. Indeed, women, and girls, living in high-income countries have a lower lifetime risk of maternal death of 1 to 54,000 than those living in low-income countries (1–45). In the context of universal health coverage, Goal 3 of the SDGs increases the focus on ensuring safe motherhood by setting key maternal health targets, such as maternal mortality ratio and access to skilled birth attendant, to be achieved by 2030. In this chapter, we present the multiple factors which impact maternal health outcomes, both within and outside the health field, the current policies, and initiatives which promote access to quality maternal health care services and the available financial resources.

Keywords

Maternal health · Maternal mortality · Antenatal · Intrapartum · Postpartum · Pregnancy

In LMICs, women are often at risk of having poor health outcomes during pregnancy, childbirth, and postnatally. These include severe bleeding, infections, high blood pressure, delivery complications, unsafe abortions, and the aggravation of pre-existing health conditions. These complications account for 70% of maternal deaths globally [1, 2]. More importantly, most of these health conditions are preventable and curable by timely and appropriate access to maternal health care (MHC). The focus on maternal health in recent years has resulted in a significant progress in health outcomes, particularly concerning maternal mortality ratios (MMR). With the set-up of the MDGs (Goal 5), MMR decreased by 38% between 2000 and 2017 globally [3]. Despite the worldwide progress, the burden of maternal morbidity and mortality remains the highest in LMICs. In 2017, the lifetime risk of maternal death ranged from 1 in 5400 in high-income countries (HICs) to 1 in 45 in low-income countries (LICs) [3]. For this

V. Mangiaterra (✉) · F. Sabbatucci
SDA Bocconi, Bocconi University, Milan, Italy
e-mail: viviana.mangiaterra@sdabocconi.it; Flaminia.Sabbatucci@sdabocconi.it

M. Bucagu
World Health Organization, Geneva, Switzerland
e-mail: bucagum@who.int

M. C. B. Raviglione et al. (eds.), *Global Health Essentials*, Sustainable Development Goals Series, https://doi.org/10.1007/978-3-031-33851-9_9

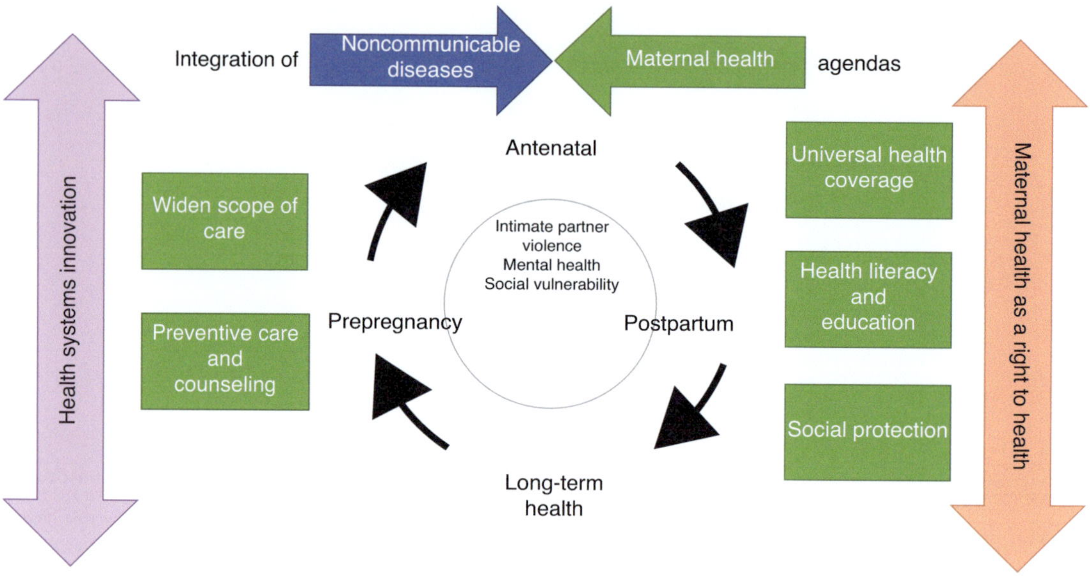

Fig. 9.1 A framework for healthcare interventions to address maternal morbidity [5]. (Intl J Gynecology & Obstet, 141(S1):61–68, First published: 23 May 2018. https://doi.org/10.1002/ijgo.12469)

reason, maternal mortality remains a major public health concern worldwide and a priority under SDG Goal 3—*Ensure healthy lives and promote well-being for all at all ages*—committing to a global reduction in maternal mortality of 70 per 100,000 live births [4]. MHC services cover all interventions addressing women's health during pregnancy, at childbirth and throughout the postnatal period, including antenatal care (ANC), intrapartum care, and postnatal care (PNC). Figure 9.1 illustrates the spectrum of interventions, for maternal health, that influence morbidity and mortality.

9.1 Determinants and Risk Factors for Maternal Deaths

Multiple factors drive maternal mortality and morbidity features. Within the health system sector, timely and appropriate health care during pregnancy and childbirth are the pillars to decrease the risk of adverse maternal health outcomes. The most common medical causes for maternal deaths are hemorrhage (27%), specifically postpartum, hypertension (14%), infection (11%), and abortive outcomes (8%), such as spontaneous or inductive abortions and ectopic pregnancies [6]. Evidence has shown that provision of high-quality antenatal, delivery and postnatal care is an effective strategy to prevent and manage complications and avert maternal deaths. It is assumed that higher MMR in health facilities is due to delays in women's decision of seeking MHC services, leading to patients arriving with advanced pregnancy complications, and in getting the required quality of care. Limited availability of skilled professionals at community and health facility levels and of medical products (e.g., medicines, surgical tools) is important barriers to providing quality care (Box 9.1). Due to the COVID-19 pandemic, delays in the availability and accessibility to MHC services have lately been further exacerbated, hindering the progress in reducing maternal deaths. Outside of the medical sphere, other independent drivers of maternal health outcomes hinder the use and availability of quality MHC services (Box 9.2). These include women's health literacy and education levels, socioeconomic contexts at both household and national levels, and cultural beliefs [7]. A study in sub-Saharan Africa found that access to skilled

ANC in DRC, Ghana, and Zimbabwe showed significant gaps between income levels, with low/high-income ratios of 15, 4.0, and 6.0, respectively [8]. Political and social insecurity, scarce health care resources and infrastructures, linked to low economic development, are critical issues to maternal healthcare accessibility for women in poor living conditions. Access to health insurance, education, and higher community-level SES were associated with a higher likelihood of seeking MHC services among Kenyan women [9]. Furthermore, the perspectives of women, their families, and their communities on the quality of MHC services influence their decision to seek care and are essential components in creating demand and access to high-quality maternal services, even more so in contexts where religion and ethnicity are very important [10]. For instance, in some countries, national policies may prove disadvantageous to unmarried pregnant women by imposing mandatory proof of marital status to access ANC, intrapartum care, and PNC. Given the multiple independent drivers of MH outcomes, a multisectoral approach is required to account for the fundamental interconnectedness of health and improve the quality and availability of MHC services, thus reducing MMRs.

Box 9.1 Socioeconomic Determinants of Maternal Health

Maternal mortality ratios (MMR) are higher among women living in rural areas and in poorer communities. Women living in LMICs have approximately 33 times more odds of dying from a maternal-related cause during their lifetime compared to their counterparts in HICs. Women's utilization of maternal health services (MHS) is affected by several social and economic factors at the individual-, household-, and community levels. Reducing socioeconomic inequalities in pregnancy care and improving public health infrastructure within communities would greatly contribute to reduce the global burden of maternal mortality.

Individual level

Female autonomy increases the probability of receiving MHC through the control of individual and social factors. Women achieve autonomy through financial independence and education. Improving women's literacy levels significantly increases the uptake of MHC, regardless of the socioeconomic status (SES) [8]. Moreover, in Uganda and Kenya, women from wealthier families, living in cities, with high literacy levels, were more likely to utilize MHC services. For this reason, female literacy levels and social protection policies positively contribute to seeking and uptake of MHS by pregnant women. Women can recognize illness symptoms and seek skilled birth attendance and essential obstetric care that is effective and of good quality reducing their chances of maternal mortality and morbidity [2]. However, the extent of the effect of this behavioral change, regarding use of MHC, is limited by social and cultural factors, availability, accessibility, and affordability of health services.

Household level

Family size has been found to be negatively associated with MHC utilization by women, especially in low socioeconomic contexts. Poverty, sociocultural beliefs, and long distances to a health facility emerged as key factors leading to their suboptimal utilization [9]. Furthermore, the marital status of pregnant women can also lead to underutilization of MHS. For instance, in Burundi, a predominantly Christian population, access to ANC services is conditional to the provision of a legal marriage certificate. Maternal health practices encourage pregnant women to be accompanied by their husbands during ANC visits. This can become a barrier for unmarried women to use MHS and deliver in a health facility.

Community level

Public health infrastructure, availability of physical services, and economic development have a strong effect on maternal health. Living in a rural setting reduces the likelihood that a woman delivers in a health facility and receives childbirth assistance by a skilled birth attendant due to long travel distances to the health facility and poor road conditions. For instance, in India, the probability of institutional delivery is double among women in urban settings. Similarly, improved public sector facilities augment utilization of MHS, especially among marginalized women in rural areas. Satisfactory economic development at village level through investment in infrastructure, especially drainage facilities, community electrification, availability of clean water, roads, and transport facilities, increases the use of MHS.

Box 9.2 Quality of Care for Maternal Health

The time of birth is critical to the survival of women and their babies, as the risk of morbidity and mortality could increase considerably if complications arise. It is recognized that high coverage of MHC services is not sufficient to reduce MMRs. Increased coverage should be accompanied by improved quality of MHS throughout the continuum of maternal care (i.e., antenatal, intrapartum, and postnatal), with the purpose of providing a positive childbirth experience to the patient, the newborns, and their families. A positive childbirth experience is defined as one that fulfills the patient's prior personal and sociocultural beliefs and expectations, including giving birth to a healthy baby in a clinically and psychologically safe environment with continuity of practical and emotional support from birth companion(s) and kind, technically competent clinical staff. The quality-of-care framework for pregnant women, set-up by WHO and partners, includes eight factors which increase the likelihood of obtaining the desired outcome from both the patient and the health facility's perspectives. The health system provides the foundation for quality improvement in both the provision and experience of care. Provision of care includes use of (1) evidence-based practices for routine care and management of complications, (2) information systems for record keeping of patient's clinical data, (3) referral systems between different levels of care. Experience of care consists of (4) effective communication with patients and their families about the care provided, (5) their expectations, needs, and rights as well as (6) access to the social and emotional support of their choice. The cross-cutting areas of the framework include the (7) availability of competent, motivated human resources and of the (8) physical resources that are prerequisites for good quality of care in health facilities. Providing high-quality antenatal, intrapartum, and postnatal care should be integral to any quality improvement strategy.

9.2 Approaches and Strategies for Preventing Maternal Mortality and Morbidity

Most maternal deaths are preventable, since the solutions to prevent, diagnose, and manage complications exist. Gaps in the coverage of essential MHC are a barrier that impede progress toward global maternal mortality ratio (MMR) targets. Reducing maternal mortality is one of the international community's top priorities, and both the MDGs and the SDGs have specific targets for ending preventable maternal deaths. The first interventions to address this burden resulted from the MDGs era and included Every *Woman Every*

Child initiative (2010) and *Strategies for Ending Preventable Maternal Mortality* [11] in 2014 [12]. Both initiatives aimed to improve the quality of care for maternal health by ensuring accessibility to MHC services in a safe, effective, timely, efficient, and equitable manner, through education, health system strengthening (infrastructure, governance, referral systems) and establishing national health system information systems. At present, the causes of maternal mortality and morbidity are gradually shifting from predominantly direct obstetric causes to indirect causes largely consisting of noncommunicable disease (e.g., obesity, diabetes). Indeed, findings from a cross-sectional study in Jamaica, Kenya, and Malawi, on women attending ANC and PPC, showed that underlying medical conditions contributed to a large percentage of clinical diagnoses in both ANC (18.0%) and PNC (8.6%) women [13]. In line with the targets of SDG 3, the *Global Strategy for Women's, Children's, and Adolescents' Health,* developed in 2016 by WHO, addresses these changes in global maternal health trends, expanding its focus to ensure that women survive labor complications, thrive, and reach their full potential for health over their lifetime. The strategy sets out three objectives: to survive, to thrive, and to transform [14, 15]. This initiative emphasizes the current need to focus on a life-course approach to women's health, including sexual and reproductive health, as well as NCDs exploiting the pregnancy period as an opportunity for detecting mothers at risk and providing targeted early preventive interventions. In LMICs, most women experience health care for the first-time during pregnancy. Postnatal care services are a fundamental component of the continuum of maternal, newborn, and childcare, and key to achieving the SDGs on reproductive, maternal, and child health, including targets to reduce MMRs and end preventable deaths of newborns. Consequently, future actions should focus on approaches which broaden the scope of MHS. Policy makers should adopt multisectoral measures in dealing with women's health issues, recognizing that women's health is the foundation for social and economic development in all settings.

9.3 Sexual and Reproductive Health Rights and Policies

Maternal health is recognized as a human rights issue that requires the effective promotion and protection of women's and girls' human rights by governmental entities. The SDGs strengthen countries' commitment by ensuring universal access to sexual and reproductive health by 2030. Men are key decision makers, particularly in low-resource contexts, in determining the level of priority of a woman's need for health and access to these services. In a study in Sierra Leone, 68% of mothers explained that decisions on birth delivery were usually made by the husband, despite the launch of the Free Health Care Initiative for ANC and PPC [16]. In some contexts, religious beliefs, misconceptions, and personal convictions can also impede access [17, 18]. For instance, in Burkina Faso, where having many children is also a sign of wealth and social prestige, family planning is associated with infidelity, infertility, and morbidity of women [19]. Access to family planning has a direct impact on women's health and direct socioeconomic benefits. WHO estimates that investing 1 USD in family planning can save up to 4 USD that would otherwise have been spent to subsequently address the complications resulting from unplanned pregnancies. Similarly, abortion bans threaten women's health by targeting health care providers, putting them in legal jeopardy. Comprehensive abortion care (i.e., provision of information, abortion management, and post-abortion care) is comprised in the list of essential health care services published by WHO in 2022. Ban on abortion is considered a form of discrimination against women and violates a range of human rights, including the right to life [17, 18]. Despite these human rights violations, globally approximately 25 million unsafe abortions take place annually, of which 97% take place in LMICs. These 25 million unsafe abortions account for 7.9% of maternal deaths, most of which occur in countries where abortion is severely restricted by law and/or in practice [14, 15].

9.4 Cost-Effectiveness and Financial Considerations

MHS required to meet the SDG 3 target include ANC, skilled birth attendance for normal vaginal delivery and emergency obstetric care, postpartum care, family planning, and post-abortion care. Direct and indirect costs of MHS compromise their accessibility and quality, worsening health disparities, and increasing MMRs [20]. In 2019, the reported total cost of using ANC ranged from 0.01 USD in a public clinic in Rwanda to 78.28 USD in a private hospital in India [21]. Cost implications of MHS lead to neglect of women's health in low-resource settings, such as Nigeria, where the average cost of ANC and delivery at a public facility represented 2% of the average annual income of household leaders in the community [21]. Even in countries where policies guarantee free, universal, access to MHC, many women still pay out-of-pocket for services, such that even when available, they become inaccessible due to high indirect costs. For example, in Tanzania, despite the free delivery services policy, 62.5% of women still pay for delivery services in public facilities [21]. These large out-of-pocket expenses contribute to the overall financial burden of paying for MHS, increasing the vulnerability of poorest populations against catastrophic household expenditures. The health of mothers is vital to the health of their unborn children. Investing in maternal health is therefore an investment in the health of future generations.

References

1. UNICEF. Maternal mortality. Maternal mortality declined by 38% between 2000 and 2017. 2021. https://data.unicef.org/topic/maternal-health/maternal-mortality/.
2. World Health Organization. Standard for improving quality of maternal and newborn care in health facilities. Geneva: World Health Organization; 2016.
3. UNICEF. Maternal mortality. 2019. UNICEF Data: https://data.unicef.org/topic/maternal-health/maternal-mortality/.
4. World Health Organization EUROPE. Fact sheet on sustainable development goals: health targets. 2017.
5. Firoz T, McCaw-Binns A, Filippi V, Magee L, Costa M, Cecatti J, et al. A framework for healthcare interventions to address maternal morbidity. Int J Gynecol Obstet. 2018;141:61.
6. Filippi V, Chou D, Ronsmans C, Graham W, Say L. Chapter 3. Levels and causes of maternal mortality and morbidity. In: Reproductive, maternal, newborn, and child health: disease control priorities, vol. 2, 3rd ed. The World Bank; 2016.
7. Crear-Perry J, Correa-de-Araujo R, Lewis Johnson T, McLemore MR, Neilson E, Wallace M. Social and structural determinants of health inequities in maternal health. J Womens Health (Larchmt). 2021;30:230.
8. Gebeyehu Worku A, Worku Yalew A, Fantahun Afework M. Factors affecting utilization of skilled maternal care in Northwest Ethiopia: a multilevel analysis. BMC Int Health Hum Rights. 2013;13:20.
9. Habonimana D, Batura N. Empirical analysis of socio-economic determinants of maternal health services utilisation in Burundi. BMC Pregnancy Childbirth. 2021;21:684.
10. Tsala Dimbuene Z, Amo-Adjei J, Amugsi D, Mumah J, Izugbara CO, Beguy D. Women's education and utilization of maternal health services in Africa: a multi-country and socioeconomic status analysis. J Biosoc Sci. 2018;50(6):725–48.
11. World Health Organization. Strategies toward ending preventable maternal mortality (EPMM). Geneva: World Health Organization; 2015.
12. Brizuela V, Tunçalp Ö. Global initiatives in maternal and newborn health. Obstet Med. 2017;10(1):21–5.
13. Barreix M, Barbour K, McCaw-Binns A, Chou D, Petzold M, Gichuhi G, et al. Standardizing measurement of maternal morbidity: pilot study results. Int J Gynecol Obstet. 2018;141:10.
14. World Health Organization. Global strategy for women's, children's and adolescents' health data portal. Geneva: World Health Organization; 2021.
15. World Health Organization. (2021). Abortion: fact sheet. Abortion: https://www.who.int/news-room/fact-sheets/detail/abortion.
16. Vallières F, Cassidy E, McAuliffe E, Gilmore B, Bangura A, Musa J. Can Sierra Leone maintain the equitable delivery of their Free Health Care Initiative? The case for more contextualised interventions: results of a cross-sectional survey. BMC Health Serv Res. 2016;16:258.
17. United Nations Human Rights. Contraception and family planning. United Nations Human Rights Office of the High Commissioner; 2020.
18. United Nations Human Rights. Abortion. United Nations Human Rights Office of the High Commissioner; 2020.
19. Romaric Bado A, Badolo H, Robert Zoma L. Use of modern contraceptive methods in Burkina Faso: what

are obstacles to male involvement in improving indicators in the Centre-East and Centre-North regions? Open Access J Contracept. 2020;11:147.
20. Dahab R, Sakellariou D. Barriers to accessing maternal care in low income countries in Africa: a systematic review. Int J Environ Res Public Health. 2020;17(12):4292.
21. Banke-Thomas A, Ifeanyi Ayomoh F, Omolade Abejirinde I-O, Banke-Thomas O, Amaize Eboreime E, Anawo Ameh C. Cost of utilising maternal health services in low- and middle-income countries: a systematic review. Int J Health Policy Manag. 2021;10(9):564–77.

10 Aging and Health: Aiming at Healthy Longevity

Hiroki Nakatani

Abstract

The world is rapidly aging. The demographic changes impact every corner of the society, starting from the population health status and including mortality and morbidity. Such changes necessitate redefining the concept of health versus ill-health, and paying more attention to enhance the intrinsic capacity of individuals through personal and social support. In this context, the public health sector needs to play important roles in realizing healthy longevity. However, not enough attention has been given to this subject and the desirable changes of public health services. This chapter first introduces the current situation and trends of aging and health followed by a brief review of the challenges, international work, and targets. Finally, on-going endeavors to realize better health, well-being, and engagement of older population through multisectoral approaches are described.

Keywords

Aging · Life expectancy · Healthy life expectancy (HALE) · Non-communicable diseases (NCD) · Functional ability

H. Nakatani (✉)
Keio University, Tokyo, Japan
e-mail: nakatanih@keio.jp

10.1 Introduction

People in most countries are living longer, healthier, and wealthier. Life expectancy has improved impressively and accelerated at the beginning of the twenty-first century under the Millennium Development Goals, which set out a new international health development framework. A snapshot of key numbers is shown in Box 10.1. According to WHO, life expectancy has increased by 6.6 years from 2000 to 2019; healthy life expectancy (HALE) has also increased, but only by 5.4 years. The increase in HALE has not kept pace with the rise in life expectancy [1]. This means that more people are living longer but with certain health issues. To narrow the gap between life expectancy and HALE, promotion of the concept of healthy aging (healthy longevity), defined as "the process of developing and maintaining the functional ability that enables well-being in older age" [2] is of paramount importance.

The definition of older people has changed: traditionally UN statistics defined an older person as over 60 years of age, but 65 years is often used. A recent UN publication [3] mentions that globally the 65-and-over population is growing faster than all other age groups and already outnumbered children under 5 years of age. By 2050, 16% of people in the world will be over 65, up from 9% in 2019. The world is rapidly graying. However, the percentage of older people is some-

M. C. B. Raviglione et al. (eds.), *Global Health Essentials*, Sustainable Development Goals Series,
https://doi.org/10.1007/978-3-031-33851-9_10

Box 10.1 Key Data

- Between 2015 and 2050, the proportion of the world's population over 60 years will nearly double from 12 to 22%, and the absolute number will more than double and reach 2.1 billion. In 2050, the number of people aged 80 years and older will triple and reach 426 million.
- By 2020, the number of people aged 60 years and older will outnumber children younger than 5 years.
- In 2050, 80% of older people will be living in low- and middle-income countries.
- The pace of population aging is much faster than in the past.
- Life expectancy has increased by more than 6 years in the past decade, from 66.8 years in 2000 to 73.4 years in 2019.
- Healthy life expectancy has increased by 8%, from 58.3 in 2000 to 63.7 in 2019.

Excerpted from: WHO: Ageing and health, 4 October 2021 (https://www.who.int/news-room/fact-sheets/detail/ageing-and-health) and WHO: The global health observatory (https://www.who.int/data/gho/data/themes/mortality-and-global-health-estimates/ghe-life-expectancy-and-healthy-life-expectancy#:~:text=Globally%2C%20life%20expectancy%20has%20increased,reduced%20years%20lived%20with%20disability.)

times misleading. Japan is already a super-aged society with 28% of the population over 65 years of age. However, in terms of absolute numbers, Japan ranks fourth after China, India, and United States. These three countries have much larger populations, although their percentage of older population is still modest. In addition, the aging speed is very rapid in many mid-income countries in Asia [4]. Therefore, aging and health are a concern of not only selected high-income nations but also many other countries.

10.2 Health Burden: Epidemiology and Assessment

The demographic changes also bring changes in mortality and morbidity. Non-communicable diseases including heart diseases, cerebrovascular diseases, cancers, and diabetes have become the leading causes of death worldwide. However, many health problems in the elderly are not immediately fatal. For example, frailty can cause fractures, leading to long-term disability [5]. Other health problems that significantly impact the daily lives of older persons, such as back and joint pain, cataracts, hearing impairment, depression, and dementia, can impede the quality of life and burden the health care system. Hence, the problem of the older population is often viewed by policymakers as one of increased health care cost and demand for health care service. They are immediate and visible challenges, but as the number of older people increases, there is growing awareness that nurturing a healthy elderly population is critical for maintaining the vitality of the society. Also, an ideal approach should not be limited to medical care in the narrow sense, but should include the prevention of health issues requiring long-term care and, more broadly, active promotion of health and well-being throughout the life course.

10.3 Approaches to Unique Challenges: Determinants and Risk Factors

Two basic concepts help design the public health approach to aging. One is the intrinsic capacity, which is the composite of all the physical and mental capacities of an individual. The other is functional ability, which comprises the individual's intrinsic capacity, environmental characteristics, and their interactions. WHO advocates these concepts as the principal framework of aging strategies [6]. As shown in Fig. 10.1, the two abilities are close together at young ages, but the gap grows as age progresses. Nonetheless, both declines can be delayed by individual health interventions or enrichment of social environ-

Fig. 10.1 Trajectories of functional ability and intrinsic capacity with biological ageing. (Reproduced with permission from World Report on Ageing and Health, World Health Organization, 2015, Fig. 2.3 on page 32. Copyright (World Health Organization 2015) https://apps.who.int/iris/handle/10665/186463)

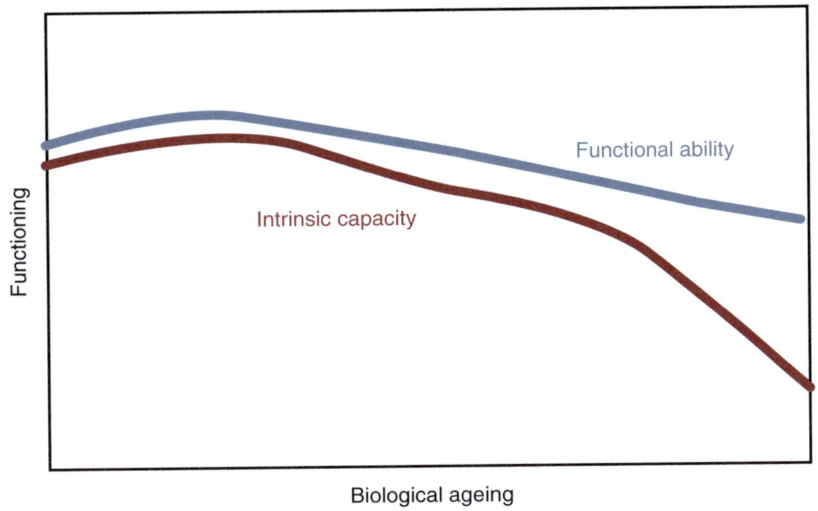

Fig. 10.2 Transformation of Concept of Health. (Translated from Japanese and Reproduced with permission from Hiroki Nakatani: Koshueisei no Kokusaika:Gurobaruka eno Kadai to Tenbo (Globalization in Public Health: Perspectives and Challenges), Koshu Eisei (Public Health) Vol.81 (6), Fig. 2 on p 360, Copyright (Igakushoin 2020))

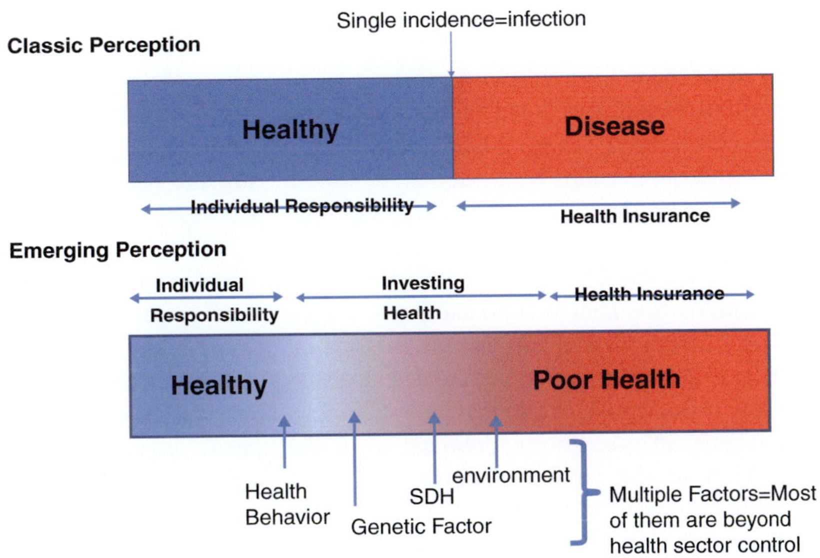

ments. For example, decreased intrinsic capability due to cataracts is reversed by gaining functional ability through eye surgery. Assistive devices and other social services enable physically challenged persons to live and work. However, it should be noted that the characteristics of older people show great individual variations, making it essential to adopt an individualized approach and a group approach.

Moreover, we may need a change in the concept of health itself, as shown in Fig. 10.2. In the past, "health" or "ill-health" was determined by whether or not a person is exposed to pathogens. A typical example is communicable diseases: exposure to a virus is a critical and determining factor. As the disease structure shifts to center on chronic diseases, the incidence that separates health and ill-health becomes less apparent. Instead, health/ill-health is now considered a continuum. Once a person has moved in the direction of ill-health, intervention(s) can pull a person back to the healthy side, thanks to medical and other modalities. The factors involved here are closely related to the social environments in which the individual is placed. Therefore social determinates of health and multisectoral approaches deserve greater attention.

10.4 International Targets

Although many global strategies for diseases such as the Global Strategy for Tuberculosis (WHO) were developed, they were not sufficient to address the more complex challenges that older people face. We need a multisectoral approach to address many factors illustrated in Fig. 10.2. However, such approach often lacked the awareness needed to formulate policies and actions beyond the traditional boundaries of health. These issues were addressed comprehensively in World Health Assembly Resolution 69.3 in 2016: "The global strategy and action plan on aging and health 2016–2020: towards a world where everyone can live a long and healthy life." [7] The strategy (2016–2020) had two goals and five strategic objectives [8]. The goals were as follows: (a) 5 years of evidence-based action to maximize functional ability that reaches every person; and (b) by 2020, establish evidence and partnerships necessary to support a Decade of Healthy Ageing from 2020 to 2030. Based on the 4 years' experience, the World Health Assembly 73 (12) in 2020 decided to extend the action plan to 2030 and proposed the United Nations to start the Decade of Healthy Ageing [9]. The background of the new decision is well documented in the Director-General's report [10]. These efforts culminated in the launching of the United Nations Decade of Healthy Ageing (2021–2030) [11], which addresses four action areas: age-friendly environments, combatting ageism, integrated care, and long-term care.

10.5 Responsibilities in a Multi-sector Approach

To comprehensively promote policies that place the elderly at the center, it is necessary for the public and private sectors, especially local communities and private organizations, to work together to break down the barriers between health care and welfare. To this end, the government must create a platform for cooperation or a new system that supports people needing medical care so that they receive welfare services for living such as long-term care insurance. Furthermore, governments may establish a comprehensive policy to expand public welfare services. As illustrated in the case of Japan [12], the process needs long-term engagement of the whole society, and government stewardship is critical.

10.6 Way Forward

Some countries view the older population as a significant burden that increases the cost of medical care, but they are missing the opportunity to utilize the potential of the older people to maintain a vibrant society, including securing the nation's labor force in a society with declining birthrate. In addition, the recent COVID-19 pandemic has shown that health problems of the older population have a significant impact on the magnitude of the damage caused by infectious diseases. It is expected that older people will increasingly be considered an asset with potential for proactive investment, rather than a heavy burden for the society, as covered comprehensively in the recently published report of the American Academy of Medicine, the Global Roadmap for Healthy Longevity [13]. In this sense, public health activities at national and individual levels must be strengthened to prevent diseases and functional deterioration, and promote well-being. This will require sharing best practices, innovations in problem-solving, and new industries. This is why the importance of promoting a healthy and active aging society has been discussed as a global agenda at G7 and G20 meetings, not only concerning the health-related issue but all issues of the whole society.

References

1. WHO. Life expectancy and healthy life expectancy. https://www.who.int/data/gho/data/themes/mortality-and-global-health-estimates/ghe-life-expectancy-and-healthy-life-expectancy#:~:text=Globally%2C%20life%20expectancy%20has%20increased,reduced%20years%20lived%20with%20disability
2. WHO. World report on aging and health. 2015. https://www.who.int/publications/i/item/9789241565042.
3. United Nations. World population prospects. 2019. https://population.un.org/wpp/.
4. WHO Regional Office for the Western Pacific. Regional action plan for healthy aging in the Western Pacific. 2021. https://www.who.int/publications/i/item/9789290619352.
5. Iwagami M, Taniguchi Y, Jin X, Adomi M, Mori T, Hamada S, et al. Association between recorded medical diagnoses and incidence of long-term care needs certification: a case-control study using linked medical and long-term care data in two Japanese cities. Ann Clin Epidemiol. 2019;1(2):56–68. https://doi.org/10.37737/ace.1.2_56.
6. WHO. World report on ageing and health. 2015. https://apps.who.int/iris/handle/10665/186463.
7. WHO. World Health Assembly 69 (2016). The global strategy and action plan on aging and health 2016–2020: towards a world in which everyone can live a long and healthy life. 2016. https://apps.who.int/iris/handle/10665/252783.
8. WHO. Global strategy and action plan on aging and health. 2017. https://www.who.int/publications/i/item/9789241513500.
9. WHO. WHA73(12) Decade of Healthy Ageing 2020–2030, WHA73/2020/REC/1. https://apps.who.int/gb/or/e/e_wha73r1.html.
10. WHO. Report of the Director-General, Decade of Healthy Ageing Development of a proposal for a Decade of Healthy Ageing 2020–2030, EB146/23. 2019. https://apps.who.int/gb/e/e_eb146.html.
11. United Nations. General Assembly resolution 75/131 United Nations Decade of Healthy Ageing (2021–2030). 2020. https://digitallibrary.un.org/record/3895802?ln=en.
12. Nakatani H. Population aging in Japan: policy transformation, sustainable development goals, universal health coverage, and social determinates of health. Global Health Med. 2019;1(1):3–10. https://doi.org/10.35772/ghm.2019.01011.
13. National Academy of Medicine. The global roadmap for healthy longevity. 2022. https://nam.edu/initiatives/grand-challenge-healthy-longevity/global-roadmap-for-healthy-longevity/.

Part IV

The Global Burden of Disease: Communicable Diseases

11 HIV

Catherine Hankins, Nittaya Phanuphak, Morenike Folayan, and Linda-Gail Bekker

Abstract

The HIV pandemic continues to challenge human health and well-being. Of 84 million people living with HIV (PLHIV), 40 million have died. HIV transmission has slowed in many parts of the world, while scale-up of antiretroviral therapy (ART) access has accelerated, enabling PLHIV to lead longer, healthier lives. The 95-95-95 goals for 2025 refer to 95% of all PLHIV knowing their status, 95% of those diagnosed receiving ART, and 95% of those on treatment achieving viral suppression. This translates to 86% of all PLHIV being virally supressed, but in 2021 this was only 68%. Closing this gap to achieve an AIDS-free world by 2030 requires concerted efforts to address biological, behavioural, and upstream structural determinants of HIV risk, while improving access to effective prevention and treatment tools. HIV testing is the entry point to both prevention and treatment, but pervasive stigma and discrimination against PLHIV and priority populations continue to impede uptake.

Keywords

HIV · AIDS · Condom · Antiretroviral therapy (ART) · Male circumcision · Pre-exposure prophylaxis (PrEP) · Post-exposure prophylaxis (PEP) · T-helper cells · Prevention of mother-to-child trasmission (PMTCT) · UNAIDS

11.1 Introduction

More than four decades after the disease that became known as acquired immune deficiency syndrome (AIDS) was recognised [1] and more than 120 years after its causative infectious agent, human immunodeficiency virus (HIV) [2], crossed species from chimpanzees to humans in the Congo River Basin [3], HIV remains a daunting challenge to human health and well-being. HIV transmission has slowed in many parts of the world, notably in many heavily affected countries in sub-Saharan Africa, while scale-up of access to antiretroviral therapy (ART) has accelerated, enabling people living with HIV (PLHIV) to lead longer, healthier lives.

C. Hankins (✉)
School of Population and Global Health, Faculty of Medicine and Health Sciences, McGill University, Montréal, QC, Canada
e-mail: Catherine.hankins@mcgill.ca

N. Phanuphak
Institute of HIV Research and Innovation (IHRI), Bangkok, Thailand
e-mail: nittaya.p@ihri.org

M. Folayan
Faculty of Dentistry, Obafemi Awolowo University, Ile-Ife, Nigeria
e-mail: toyinukpong@yahoo.co.uk

L.-G. Bekker
The Desmond Tutu HIV Centre, University of Cape Town, Cape Town, Republic of South Africa
e-mail: Linda-Gail.Bekker@hiv-research.org.za

M. C. B. Raviglione et al. (eds.), *Global Health Essentials*, Sustainable Development Goals Series,
https://doi.org/10.1007/978-3-031-33851-9_11

11.2 Epidemiology

UNAIDS estimates that overall 84.2 [64.0–113.0] million people have acquired HIV infection, with 40.1 [33.6–48.6] million having died. Of 38.4 [33.9–43.8] million PLHIV in 2021, 54% were women and girls, while 1.7 [1.3–2.1] million were children under 15 [4]. Among 1.5 [1.0–2.0] million new HIV infections during 2021, 94% of those outside and 51% within sub-Saharan Africa were men who have sex with men, people who inject drugs, transgender people, and sex workers and their clients/sexual partners. With transmission dynamics varying by region, by country, and within countries, the most heavily burdened populations that are key to the epidemic and key to the response differ widely, underpinning principles of co-creation and partnership to tailor accessible, effective prevention, treatment, and mitigation programmes.

11.3 Pathogenesis

The retrovirus HIV is transmitted via bodily fluids through unprotected sexual activity, use of contaminated injecting equipment, or exposure during pregnancy, delivery, or breastfeeding. T-helper cells, found throughout the body but in high concentrations in gastrointestinal tract lymph nodes [5], are its prime target. These immune response 'conductors' activate B-cells to turn into antibody-making plasma cells, stimulate other T-cells to mature into memory cells, and signal macrophages and cytotoxic T-cells to act [6]. T-helper cells express a signature cell-surface marker on their outer membranes, the CD4+ receptor, that is the landing site for HIV to dock using its glycoprotein (GP) 120 envelope spike [7]. Docking causes GP120 configuration changes that give HIV access to CCR5 or CXCR4 chemokine receptors. The ensuing structural change in HIV's gp41 envelope protein permits viral envelope-cell membrane fusion, allowing cell entry. Once inside, HIV uses the cell's genetic machinery to undergo reverse transcription from RNA to DNA. HIV replicates itself and breaks open the T-cell, disseminating to infect T-cells and other cellular targets and setting up chronic immune system activation correlated with disease progression [8]. As blood CD4+ counts fall, capacity to maintain regeneration declines, with HIV steadily weakening immune system defences, increasing susceptibility to opportunistic pathogens that take advantage of immune suppression.

11.4 Determinants of Risk

The biological determinants of HIV acquisition risk include the presence of sexually transmitted infections (STI), cervical ectopy, lack of male circumcision, and genetic factors, with the rare CCR5-delta32 mutation protecting against HIV infection when both gene alleles are affected [9]. Among the behavioural determinants are lack of consistent and correct condom use, early sexual debut, multi-partner and concomitant partnered sex, and lack of access to prevention modalities, including male and female condoms, sterile injecting equipment, and pre- and post-exposure prophylaxis products. Among the upstream structural determinants of HIV exposure are economic dependency among young girls and women, anchored in restricted educational opportunities and constraints to meaningful employment; criminalisation of sexual minority identity, sex work, and drug use; poverty which undermines agency; and stigma and discrimination.

11.5 HIV Prevention and Treatment

Although an HIV vaccine remains elusive, the HIV prevention and treatment toolbox contains many effective tools (Fig. 11.1; Box 11.1), with promising alternative delivery modalities in the pipeline. Translating efficacy seen in randomised controlled trials, for example of medical male circumcision [10], antiretroviral treatment [11], or pre-exposure prophylaxis [12], requires attention to critical implementation considerations, including access, cost, and acceptability. Community- and key population-

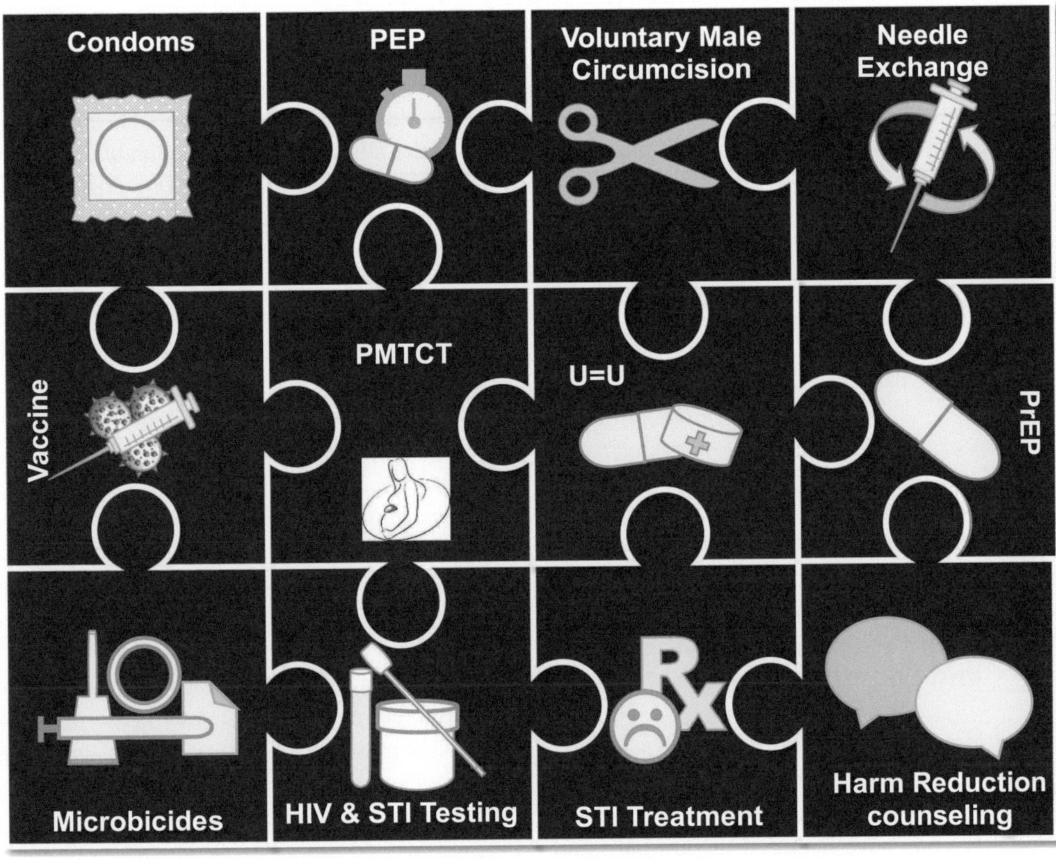

Fig. 11.1 Prevention toolbox. (Source: Landowitz R)

led health services focusing on practical client-centred service delivery can facilitate integration of HIV prevention and treatment services with those tailored to address specific health needs. These include screening for STI and hepatitis; addressing sexual and reproductive health needs, including contraceptive access for women; offering gender affirmation for trans individuals; and providing opioid agonist therapies and sterile injecting equipment for people who use drugs. Access to ART at first diagnosis, regardless of CD4 count, has proven clinically beneficial and reduces HIV transmission when viral suppression is achieved. The latter is reflected in the U=U message: Undetectable equals untransmittable, a message pertinent not only for sexual partners but also for pregnant women. U=U is helping reduce stigma and discrimination while improving mental, physical, and sexual health outcomes [13]. Effective ART has increased longevity for individuals, reflected in progressive restoration of life expectancy in low- and middle-income countries [14]. The challenges of co-morbidities such as hypertension, diabetes, and other chronic conditions as people live longer with HIV underscore the need for differentiated care to better plan needs-based services. HIV testing, including self-testing, is the entry point to both prevention and treatment, but pervasive stigma and discrimination against PLHIV and priority populations continue to impede uptake.

Box 11.1 Antiretroviral Drug Classes (2022)

- Non-nucleoside reverse transcriptase inhibitors (NNRTIs)
- Nucleoside reverse transcriptase inhibitors (NRTIs)
- Protease inhibitors (PIs)
- Fusion inhibitors.
- CCR5 antagonists.
- Integrase strand transfer inhibitors (INSTIs)
- Post-attachment inhibitors.

Source: https://hivinfo.nih.gov/understanding-hiv/fact-sheets/what-start-choosing-hiv-treatment-regimen

11.6 International, Regional, and Country Responses

In 1987, the World Health Programme's Special Programme on AIDS was established, followed by UNAIDS co-sponsored in 1995. Major international funders have included the Global Fund to fight AIDS, TB, and Malaria; the U.S. President's Emergency Plan for AIDS Relief (PEPFAR); the Bill & Melinda Gates Foundation; and others. Countries aiming to achieve the United Nations sustainable development goals [15] have national AIDS programmes with HIV targets. They track their progress towards the 90-90-90 (by 2020) and 95-95-95 (by 2025) goals. The first numbers refer to 90% of all PLHIV knowing their status, 90% of those diagnosed receiving ART, and 90% of those on treatment achieving viral suppression. This translates to 73% of all PLHIV being virally suppressed. In 2021, of all PLHIV, 85% [75–97%] knew their status, 75% [66–85%] were accessing treatment and 68% [60–78%] were virally suppressed. This 5% shortfall in the 2020 target (18% for the 2025 target, see Fig. 11.2) is unevenly distributed geographically, by population at higher risk of exposure, and by age, with many children not being reached, resulting in low viral suppression. Despite great progress worldwide in reducing vertical transmission during pregnancy, childbirth, and breastfeeding, efforts to eradicate paediatric HIV have stalled. Programmes to improve child and adolescent

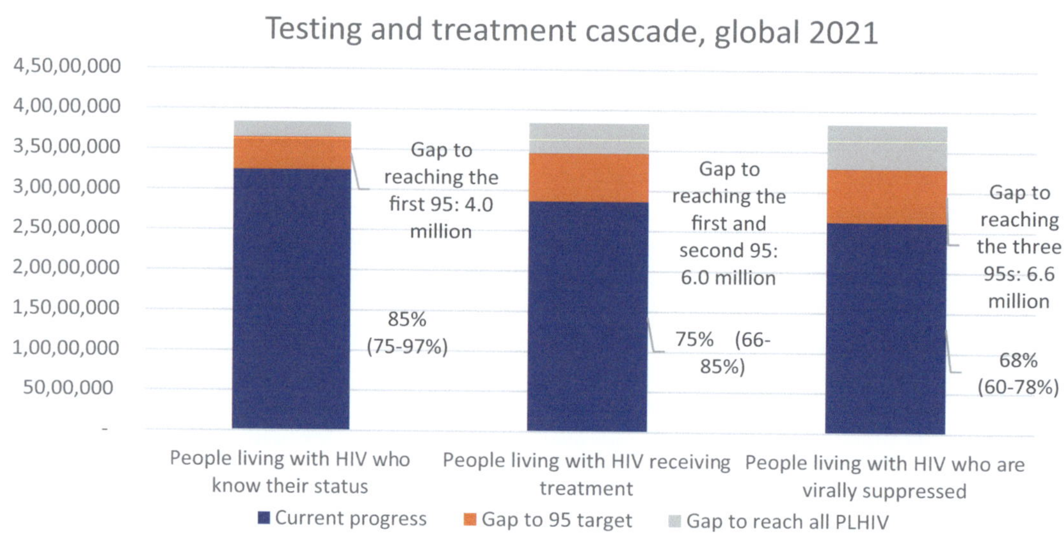

Fig. 11.2 HIV testing and treatment cascade—Global 2021 (permission granted by UNAIDS). (Source: UNAIDS 2022)

health outcomes for those living with HIV, affected by HIV (exposed and uninfected or not exposed but living with family members/care givers with HIV), or at elevated risk for HIV, include adherence support, nutrition, retention, viral load suppression for those with HIV, and support and prevention for all.

11.7 Conclusion

Emerging pandemics such as COVID-19 have taken tolls on health care delivery for all chronic conditions including HIV. The resilient nature of many HIV service delivery services, previously designed and implemented by and with community, fostered immediate adaption and adoption of creative solutions to COVID-19 challenges. Innovations in telehealth and service delivery have helped minimise supply chain disruptions and maintain progress. Given the climate crisis' potential to contribute to future zoonotic pandemics and the looming disaster of antimicrobial resistance, lessons learned during COVID-19 are key to staying on course to achieve the goal of an AIDS-free world by 2030.

References

1. Centers for Disease Control (CDC). Kaposi's sarcoma and Pneumocystis pneumonia among homosexual men—New York City and California. MMWR Morb Mortal Wkly Rep. 1981;30(25):305–8.
2. Barré-Sinoussi F, Chermann JC, Rey F, Nugeyre MT, Chamaret S, Gruest J, Dauguet C, Axler-Blin C, Vézinet-Brun F, Rouzioux C, Rozenbaum W, Montagnier L. Isolation of a T-lymphotropic retrovirus from a patient at risk for acquired immune deficiency syndrome (AIDS). Science. 1983;220(4599):868–71.
3. Worobey M, Gemmel M, Teuwen DE, Haselkorn T, Kunstman K, Bunce M, Muyembe JJ, Kabongo JM, Kalengayi RM, Van Marck E, Gilbert MT, Wolinsky SM. Direct evidence of extensive diversity of HIV-1 in Kinshasa by 1960. Nature. 2008;455(7213):661–4.
4. Joint United Nations Programme on AIDS (UNAIDS). In danger: UNAIDS global AIDS update 2022. 2022. https://www.unaids.org/en/resources/documents/2022/in-danger-global-aids-update.
5. Xu H, Wang X, Veazey RS. Mucosal immunology of HIV infection. Immunol Rev. 2013;254(1):10–33.
6. Douek D, Brenchley J, Betts M, et al. HIV preferentially infects HIV-specific CD4$^+$ T cells. Nature. 2002;417:95–8. https://doi.org/10.1038/417095a.
7. Burton DR, Ahmed R, Barouch DH, Butera ST, Crotty S, Godzik A, et al. A blueprint for HIV vaccine discovery. Cell Host Microbe. 2012;12(4):396–407.
8. Moir S, Chun TW, Fauci AS. Pathogenic mechanisms of HIV disease. Annu Rev Pathol. 2011;6:223–48.
9. Martinson JJ, Chapman NH, Rees DC, Liu YT, Clegg JB. Global distribution of the CCR5 gene 32-basepair deletion. Nat Genet. 1997;16(1):100–3.
10. Weiss HA, Halperin D, Bailey RC, Hayes R, Schmid G, Hankins CA. Male circumcision for HIV prevention: from evidence to action? AIDS. 2008;22(5):567–74. PMID: 18316997. https://doi.org/10.1097/QAD.0b013e3282f3f406.
11. Cohen MS, Chen YQ, McCauley M, Gamble T, Hosseinipour MC, et al. Prevention of HIV-1 infection with early antiretroviral therapy. N Engl J Med. 2011;365(6):493–505.
12. Hankins CA, Dybul MR. The promise of pre-exposure prophylaxis with antiretroviral drugs to prevent HIV transmission: a review. Curr Opin HIV AIDS. 2013;8(1):50–8. PMID: 23201856.
13. Okoli C, Van de Velde N, Richman B, Allan B, Castellanos E, Young B, et al. Undetectable equals untransmittable (U = U): awareness and associations with health outcomes among people living with HIV in 25 countries. Sex Transm Infect. 2021;97(1):18–26.
14. Trickey A, May MT, Vehreschild J-J, Obel N, Gill MJ, Crane HM, et al. Survival of HIV-positive patients starting antiretroviral therapy between 1996 and 2013: a collaborative analysis of cohort studies. Lancet HIV. 2017;4(8):e349–56. PMID: 28501495.
15. Bekker LG, Alleyne G, Baral S, Cepeda J, Daskalakis D, et al. Advancing global health and strengthening the HIV response in the era of the sustainable development goals: the International AIDS Society—Lancet Commission. Lancet. 2018;392(10144):312–58. https://doi.org/10.1016/S0140-6736(18)31070-5. PMCID: PMC6323648.

Tuberculosis 12

Simone Villa, Giovanni Battista Migliori,
Lia D'Ambrosio, and Mario C. B. Raviglione

Abstract

Tuberculosis is an infectious disease caused by bacteria of the *Mycobacterium tuberculosis* complex that are transmitted through air droplets from persons with pulmonary tuberculosis. Once exposed, a person might become infected but only 5–10% of them will, eventually, develop the disease during lifetime. A quarter of the global population is estimated to be infected and, annually, more than ten million develop the disease. Of those only two-thirds are diagnosed and reported. With 1.6 million annual deaths, tuberculosis ranks currently as the second leading cause of death from infectious diseases after COVID-19, the first among those living with HIV. If timely diagnosed and effectively treated, the disease is curable, especially when caused by drug-susceptible strains. In the past three decades, numerous efforts have been made to control and, eventually, eliminate tuberculosis worldwide through global WHO strategies. The current end TB strategy promotes a broad "health and beyond health" approach aligned with the UN Sustainable Development Goals (SDGs) as the root causes of tuberculosis fall beyond the health sector, thus requiring coordinated multi-sectoral interventions.

Keywords

Tuberculosis · Epidemiology · Sustainable Development Goals · Global health · Social determinants

12.1 Introduction and Definitions

Tuberculosis (TB) is an airborne disease caused by bacteria of the *Mycobacterium tuberculosis* complex usually transmitted via droplet nuclei from persons with pulmonary disease. Tuberculosis most often affects the lungs, although other organs are involved in up to 30% of cases. It can be diagnosed within hours using rapid molecular tests; confirmation is obtained through culture that may take up to 4 weeks to yield a positive result. If properly treated, TB caused by drug-susceptible strains is curable in most cases, but if left untreated, it may be fatal in over 2/3 of affected people

S. Villa (✉) · M. C. B. Raviglione
Centre for Multidisciplinary Research in Health Science (MACH), University of Milan, Milan, Italy
e-mail: simone.villa@unimi.it; mario.raviglione@unimi.it

G. B. Migliori
Servizio di Epidemiologia Clinica delle Malattie Respiratorie, Istituti Clinici Scientifici Maugeri IRCCS, Tradate, Italy
e-mail: giovannibattista.migliori@icsmaugeri.it

L. D'Ambrosio
Public Health Consulting Group, Lugano, Switzerland

M. C. B. Raviglione et al. (eds.), *Global Health Essentials*, Sustainable Development Goals Series,
https://doi.org/10.1007/978-3-031-33851-9_12

within 5 years. Through pharmacological prophylaxis, the development of the disease can be prevented in those who have contracted TB infection [1].

12.2 Descriptive Epidemiology and Global Burden of Tuberculosis

Following exposure to an active pulmonary TB case, some individuals will become infected depending on the duration and proximity of contact, degree of infectiousness, and virulence of the strain. The term "TB infection" (formerly "latent infection," an asymptomatic stage) indicates "a continuum" in the process that from inhalation of bacilli may lead to clinically manifested TB disease. Pulmonary TB is usually characterized by chronic cough, fever, night sweats, weight loss, and asthenia. Other symptoms will depend on the organs affected. Among those infected, 5–10% may develop active TB during their lifetime, but generally within the first 12–18 months after exposure. In the remaining >90%, the immune system will contain and eventually block replication of *M. tuberculosis* [2].

It is estimated that about a quarter of the living world's population is infected with *M. tuberculosis* (i.e. about 1.7 billion people) [3]. In 2021, among the 10.6 million people estimated to have had TB, ~2/3 were males, 1.2 million were children, and 6.7% were people living with HIV [4]. Most of the cases occurred in the South-East Asian (45%), African (23%), and Western Pacific (18%) regions of the World Health Organization (WHO), whereas the Eastern Mediterranean (8%), American (3%), and European (2%) regions had a lower burden. Two-thirds of the cases were in eight countries: India (28%), China (7%), Indonesia (9%), the Philippines (7%), Pakistan (6%), Nigeria (4%), Bangladesh (4%), and Democratic Republic of the Congo (3%). Annually, only 2/3 of all cases are diagnosed and reported. An estimated 450,000 cases of multidrug-resistant or rifampicin-resistant TB emerge annually, of which only a third are diagnosed and treated.

In 2019, with 1.5 million estimated deaths annually, TB ranked as the 13th leading cause of death worldwide and the first among people living with HIV [5] and was responsible for around a quarter of all deaths caused by antimicrobial-resistant bacteria [6]. By dramatically reducing access to care and notifications, the COVID-19 pandemic has reversed years of regular decline in TB mortality [7].

12.3 International Targets

International targets (Table 12.1) for TB control were established by the World Health Assembly in 2014 and by the United Nations' General Assembly high-level meeting in 2018 and they were included in the 2030 Sustainable Development Goals (SDG) framework. Most of these targets are currently not on track and COVID-19 further reduced the possibility to reach them [7].

Table 12.1 Global TB targets set in the SDGs framework, the end TB strategy, and the political declaration of the UN high-level meeting on TB, for the period up to the SDG deadline of 2030 [7]

SDG Target 3.3	By 2030, end the epidemics of AIDS, TB, malaria and neglected tropical diseases, and combat hepatitis, water-borne diseases and other communicable diseases
WHO End TB Strategy	80% reduction in the TB incidence rate (new and relapse cases per 100 000 population per year) by 2030, compared with 2015 *2020 milestone:* 20% reduction; *2025 milestone:* 50% reduction
	90% reduction in the annual number of TB deaths by 2030, compared with 2015 *2020 milestone:* 35% reduction; *2025 milestone:* 75% reduction
	No households affected by TB face catastrophic costs by 2020
UN high-level meeting on TB 2018	40 million people treated for TB from 2018 to 2022, including: • 3.5 million children • 1.5 million people with drug-resistant TB, including 115 000 children
	At least 30 million people provided with TB preventive treatment from 2018 to 2022, including: • 6 million people living with HIV • 4 million children under 5 years of age and 20 million people in other age groups, who are household contacts of people affected by TB
	Funding of at least US$ 13 billion per year for universal access to TB prevention, diagnosis, treatment and care by 2022
	Funding of at least US$ 2 billion per year for TB research from 2018 to 2022

AIDS acquired immunodeficiency syndrome, *HIV* human immunodeficiency virus, *SDG* Sustainable Development Goal, *TB* tuberculosis, *UN* United Nations

12.4 Determinants and Risk Factors

The most potent risk factor for developing active TB is HIV infection (relative risk [RR] $\geq$ 18). Other factors and comorbidities include undernutrition (RR = 1.6), diabetes (RR = 1.5), alcohol abuse (RR = 3.3), tobacco smoking (RR = 1.6), and, probably, (indoor) air pollution [7]. Besides direct risk factors, higher-level determinants associated with increased risk to develop TB include poverty and lower socioeconomic status, poor housing conditions, food insecurity, and environmental conditions such as incarceration or working in mines. Poor perception of health problems, care-associated costs, and physical distance to healthcare facilities also hinder access to health services [8].

12.5 Challenges to TB Control and Elimination

TB-specific challenges that national programmes must address in most countries are multiple and include late and missed diagnosis, poor quality of care and treatment outcomes, especially for drug-resistant forms, TB/HIV dual infection, management of drug-resistant TB, and preventive treatment hesitance. However, full TB control and elimination will require a multi-sectorial approach as determinants of TB originate from different development sectors that are well-described within the context of the SDGs [9–12]. Within the health sector itself, lack of universal health coverage is a major issue in most low/middle-income countries precluding access to care. Collaboration with other programmes, hospital services, and non-state providers is also a significant challenge [5]. Lack of sufficient community engagement and strategies for education and stigma removal are impediments in many settings. Under-resourced research efforts and slow uptake of innovations remain hurdles worldwide.

Given the strong links between TB and societal development, one can identify several SDGs where achievements are crucial to achieve TB control and elimination. Poverty reduction (SDG1) is probably the most important goal and availability of social protection in countries is crucial to allow the poor to access care and survive throughout the long treatment period. Other examples of necessary achievements to contain TB include better nutrition (SDG2); education (SDG4); reduction of indoor and outdoor air pollution (SDG7); reduction of urban populations living in slums (SDG11); gender equalities (SDG5) and reduction of income inequalities

(SDG10); finally, mitigation of climate changes (SDG13) and the end of conflicts (SDG16) will alleviate other determinants such as forced migration and increased poverty.

12.6 Strategies for Control and Elimination

During the past three decades, WHO developed global TB control strategies: *DOTS* in 1995, *Stop TB Strategy* in 2006, and the current *End TB Strategy* in 2014 [8]. The *End TB Strategy* 2016–2030/2035 is based on three pillars: (1) integrated, patient-centred TB care, and prevention; (2) bold policies and supportive systems; (3) intensified research and innovation (Box 12.1) [13].

Box 12.1 The Three Pillars and Ten Components of the End Tb Strategy 2016–2030/2035 [7]

1. **Integrated, Patient-Centred Care and Prevention**
   (a) Early diagnosis of tuberculosis including universal drug-susceptibility testing, and systematic screening of contacts and high-risk groups
   (b) Treatment of all people with tuberculosis including drug-resistant tuberculosis, and patient support
   (c) Collaborative tuberculosis /HIV activities, and management of comorbidities
   (d) Preventive treatment of persons at high risk, and vaccination against tuberculosis
2. **Bold Policies and Supportive Systems**
   (a) Political commitment with adequate resources for tuberculosis care and prevention
   (b) Engagement of communities, civil society organizations, and public and private care providers
   (c) Universal health coverage policy, and regulatory frameworks for case notification, vital registration, quality and rational use of medicines, and infection control
   (d) Social protection, poverty alleviation, and actions on other determinants of tuberculosis
3. **Intensified Research and Innovation**
   (a) Discovery, development, and rapid uptake of new tools, interventions, and strategies
   (b) Research to optimize implementation and impact, and promote innovations

The ultimate aim of any strategy for TB control is that of cutting transmission and achieving elimination. Clearly, diagnosing infectious cases rapidly and treating them effectively is a fundamental means. In addition, prevention through pharmacological means or vaccination – should a new more effective vaccine become available – is an essential measure for elimination. To be effective, these interventions require proper health services and systems facilitating access to all in need. A specific TB elimination strategy for low-incidence settings has also been developed by WHO [14].

12.7 Economic Considerations

Progress in reducing the burden of TB disease requires adequate funding for TB diagnostic, treatment, and prevention services sustained over many years. However, funding (especially in low- and middle-income countries accounting for 98% of TB cases) is today insufficient with major gaps in both implementation and research financing.

12.8 Conclusions

Actions solely within the health sector will not allow achievement of the End TB targets if the social and economic determinants of the disease are not effectively addressed. Establishing, developing, and implementing multi-sectoral interventions, backed by bold political commitment, are the way forward to end TB as a global health problem.

References

1. Raviglione MC, Gori A. Tuberculosis. In: Loscalzo J, Jameson JL, Fauci A, Kasper D, Hauser S, Longo D, editors. Harrison's principles of internal medicine. New York: McGraw-Hill Education; 2022.
2. Rieder HL. Epidemiologic basis of tuberculosis control. 1st ed. Paris: International Union Against Tuberculosis and Lung Disease; 1999.

3. Houben RM, Dodd PJ. The global burden of latent tuberculosis infection: a re-estimation using mathematical modelling PLoS Med. 2016;13:p. e1002152.
4. World Health Organization. Global tuberculosis report 2022. Geneva: World Health Organization; 2022.
5. Reid MJA, Arinaminpathy N, Bloom A, et al. Building a tuberculosis-free world: the Lancet Commission on tuberculosis. Lancet. 2019;393(10178):1331–84. https://doi.org/10.1016/S0140-6736(19)30024-8.
6. Knight GM, Raviglione MC, White RG. No antimicrobial resistance research agenda without tuberculosis. Lancet Glob Health. 2020;8(8):e987–8. https://doi.org/10.1016/S2214-109X(20)30309-0.
7. World Health Organization. Global tuberculosis report 2021. Geneva: World Health Organization; 2021.
8. Lönnroth K, Castro KG, Chakaya MJ, Chauhan SL, Floyd K, et al. Tuberculosis control and elimination 2010–50: cure, care, and social development. Lancet. 2010;375(9728):1814–29.
9. WHO Western Pacific. Western Pacific regional framework to end TB: 2021–2030. Manila: WHO Western Pacific Regional Office; 2022. Licence: CC BY-NC-SA 3.0 IGO.
10. Villa S, Kasaeva T, Raviglione MC. A multisectoral approach to tuberculosis control and elimination in the era of the United Nations sustainable development goals. In: Migliori GB, Raviglione MC, editors. Essential tuberculosis. Cham: Springer; 2021.
11. Raviglione M, Uplekar M, Weil D, Kasaeva T. Tuberculosis makes it onto the international political agenda for health…finally. Lancet Glob Health. 2018;6(1):e20–1.
12. World Health Organization. Multisectoral accountability framework to accelerate progress to end tuberculosis by 2030. Geneva: World Health Organization; 2019.
13. Uplekar M, Weil D, Lönnroth K, Jaramillo E, Lienhardt C, et al. WHO's new end TB strategy. Lancet. 2015;385(9979):1799–801.
14. Lönnroth K, Migliori GB, Abubakar I, D'Ambrosio L, de Vries G, et al. Towards tuberculosis elimination: an action framework for low-incidence countries. Eur Respir J. 2015;45(4):928–52.

Malaria

13

Francisco da Conceição Mário Saúte

Abstract

Malaria is caused by a protozoan parasite of the *Plasmodium* genus. Five *Plasmodium* species affect humans: *Plasmodium falciparum, Plasmodium malariae, Plasmodium vivax, Plasmodium ovale and Plasmodium knowlesi.* Malaria symptoms are non-specific and include fever and chills among others. It is transmitted by female anopheline mosquitoes. There is malaria transmission in Africa, South America, the Middle-East, India and South-East Asia. Climate and local ecology are the main determinants of malaria transmission. Children under 5 years of age and pregnant women are at the highest risk.

Preventive methods include vector control and preventive chemotherapies. Recently, WHO endorsed the use of the RTS,S malaria vaccine. Malaria diagnosis is based on symptoms and positive blood smear or rapid malaria diagnostic test (RDTs). Treatment is based on artemisinin-based combination therapies (ACTs). Challenges facing malaria control include vector's resistance to insecticides; parasite's deletion of genes encoding for the histidine-rich protein-2 and the emergence of parasite resistance to the ACTs.

Keywords

Malaria · Epidemiology · Risk factors · Prevention and control · Vector control · Artemisinin-based combination therapy (ACT) · Rapid diagnostic test (RDT) · Plasmodium · Anopheline mosquitoes

13.1 Definitions and Main Features of Malaria

Malaria is one of the oldest diseases of humans [1]. It is caused by a protozoan parasite of the *Plasmodium* genus [2]. Five *Plasmodium* species affect humans: *Plasmodium falciparum (P. falciparum), Plasmodium malariae, Plasmodium vivax (P. vivax), Plasmodium ovale (P. ovale)* and *Plasmodium knowlesi (P. knowlesi). P. falciparum,* the dominant species in Africa, causes most of the severe cases of, and death from, malaria. *P. vivax* and *P. ovale* can remain dormant in the liver and cause relapses months or years later. *P. knowlesi*

F. da Conceição Mário Saúte (✉)
Manhica Health Research Center,
Manhica, Mozambique
e-mail: francisco.saute@manhica.net

M. C. B. Raviglione et al. (eds.), *Global Health Essentials*, Sustainable Development Goals Series,
https://doi.org/10.1007/978-3-031-33851-9_13

affects primarily monkeys but can cause zoonotic malaria in humans. Symptoms of malaria are largely non-specific, including fever and chills, among others. Malaria is transmitted through bites of female anopheline mosquitoes [3].

13.2 Descriptive Epidemiology and Assessment of the Global Burden

Currently, there is regular malaria transmission in Africa, South America, the Middle-East, the Indian sub-continent and South-East Asia [4]. Over 240 million malaria cases and 627 thousand malaria deaths occurred in 2020, of which 95% and 96% of cases and death, respectively, were in Africa.

13.3 International Targets and Progress Towards Their Achievements

In 2015, the World Health Assembly adopted the Global Technical Strategy (GTS) aimed at reducing malaria incidence and mortality, globally, by at least 90% by 2030. A 2020 strategy review found that most countries showed a slow or no progress towards such goal (Fig. 13.1), leading therefore to its update [5].

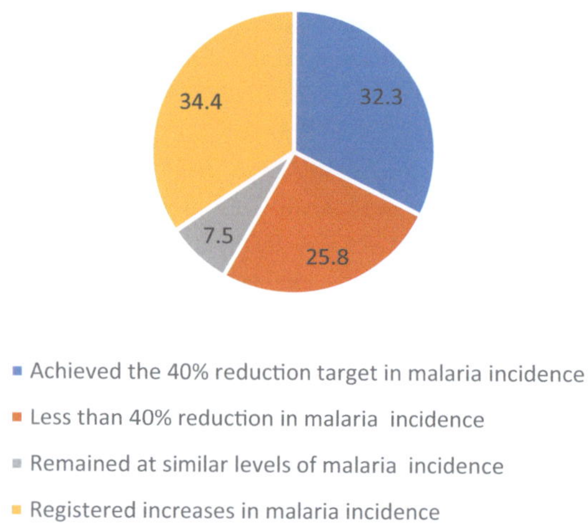

Fig. 13.1 Progress towards the 2020 GTS case incidence milestone, from 2015 baseline (% of countries). (Source of data: 2021 World Malaria Report, WHO)

13.4 Determinants and Risk Factors

Climate and local ecology are by far the main determinants of malaria transmission [6]. In endemic areas, children under 5 years of age and pregnant women are at the highest risk of severe malaria and death. However, other factors can also modify disease distribution [7].

13.5 Approaches and Strategies for Prevention and Control

Preventive methods include vector control (VC) and preventive chemotherapies (PCTs) [8]. The main VC tools include (1) indoor residual spray; which, consists of applying a long-lasting insecticide to internal surfaces of walls, eaves and ceiling of all houses or domestic animal shelters, within a given geographic area, in order to kill mosquitoes when they come into contact with such surfaces); and (2) long-lasting insecticidal nets, which are bed nets treated with safe and long-lasting insecticides, to kill or repel mosquitoes as they try to bite the host sleeping under the net. PCTs include chemoprevention (full course of antimalarial drugs to treat and prevent infections in endemic countries) and chemoprophylaxis (sub-therapeutic dosage of antimalarial drugs to prevent malaria, usually, in non-immune travellers). Recently, WHO endorsed the use of the RTS,S malaria vaccine [9].

Malaria diagnosis is based on clinical history plus a positive blood smear (BS) or rapid malaria diagnostic test (RDTs). Currently, the mainstay of malaria treatment are the artemisinin-based combination therapies (ACTs) [10].

13.6 Challenges to Be Faced for Containment/Control/Elimination

Challenges facing malaria control include vector's resistance to insecticides; parasite's deletion of genes encoding for the histidine-rich protein-2 (HRP2) [11] and the emergence of parasite resistance to the ACTs.

13.7 Cost-Effectiveness and Financial Considerations

Malaria is a *"cause and consequence of poverty"* [12]. It is estimated that malaria is responsible for an annual 1.3% impairment on Africa's economic growth [13]. At the same time, malaria disproportionally affects the poorest of the poor [14].

13.8 Responsibilities of Different National and International Institutions

The cost of malaria control is borne by governments of endemic countries with support from international donors [15]. Among those, particularly important are the Global Fund to Fight AIDS, tuberculosis and malaria as well as the US President's Malaria Initiative.

References

1. Miller RL, Ikram S, Armelagos GJ, Walker R, Harer WB, Shiff CJ, Baggett D, Carrigan M, Maret SM. Diagnosis of *Plasmodium falciparum* infections in mummies using the rapid manual *Para*Sight™-F test. Trans R Soc Trop Med Hyg. 88(11994):31–2. https://doi.org/10.1016/0035-9203(94)90484-7.
2. Sato S. *Plasmodium*—a brief introduction to the parasites causing human malaria and their basic biology. J Physiol Anthropol. 2021;40:1. https://doi.org/10.1186/s40101-020-00251-9.
3. Sinka ME. Global distribution of the dominant vector species of malaria. In: Manguin S, editor. Anopheles mosquitoes—new insights into malaria vectors [Internet]. London: IntechOpen; 2013 [cited 2022 Jun 23]. https://www.intechopen.com/chapters/43624. https://doi.org/10.5772/54163.
4. World Health Organization. World Malaria report 2021.
5. Global technical strategy for malaria 2016–2030, 2021 update. Geneva: World Health Organization; 2021. Licence: CC BY-NC-SA 3.0 IGO.
6. Caminade C, Kovats S, Rocklov J, Tompkins AM, Morse AP, Colón-González FJ, Stenlund H, Martens P, Lloyd SJ. Impact of climate change on global malaria distribution. Proc Natl Acad Sci U S A. 2014;111(9):3286–91. https://doi.org/10.1073/pnas.1302089111. Epub 2014 Feb 3. PMID: 24596427; PMCID: PMC3948226.
7. Snow RW, Sartorius B, Kyalo D, Maina J, Amratia P, Mundia CW, Bejon P, Noor AM. The prevalence of Plasmodium falciparum in sub-Saharan Africa since 1900. Nature. 2017;550(7677):515–8. https://doi.org/10.1038/nature24059. Epub 2017 Oct 11. PMID: 29019978; PMCID: PMC5660624.
8. https://www.who.int/news/item/03-06-2022-Updated-WHO-recommendations-for-malaria-chemoprevention-among-children-and-pregnant-women.
9. World Health Organization 2021. https://www.who.int/news/item/06-10-2021-who-recommends-groundbreaking-malaria-vaccine-for-children-at-risk.
10. World Health Organization. Guidelines for the treatment of malaria. 3rd ed. Geneva: World Health Organization; 2015. https://apps.who.int/iris/handle/10665/162441.
11. Agaba BB, Yeka A, Nsobya S, et al. Systematic review of the status of *pfhrp2* and *pfhrp3* gene deletion, approaches and methods used for its estimation and reporting in *Plasmodium falciparum* populations in Africa: review of published studies 2010–2019. Malar J. 2019;18:355. https://doi.org/10.1186/s12936-019-2987-4.
12. Ettling MB, Shepard DS. Economic cost of malaria in Rwanda. Trop Med Parasitol. 1991;42(3):214–8. PMID: 1801149.
13. Roll Back Malaria. https://www.malariaconsortium.org/userfiles/file/Malaria%20resources/RBM%20Economic%20costs%20of%20malaria.pdf.
14. Affiah N, Fadoju S, James I, James N, Uzoma C, Opada E, Jasini J. Economic impact of malaria treatment on resource-constrained households in Akwa Ibom: a case study on selected local government areas. World J Public Health. 2022;7(2):39–45. https://doi.org/10.11648/j.wjph.20220702.11.
15. Rannan-Eliya RP. Financing malaria. PLOS Glob Public Health. 2022;2(6):e0000609. https://doi.org/10.1371/journal.pgph.0000609.

Hepatitis

14

Daniel Low-Beer and Fuqiang Cui

Abstract

A decade ago, viral hepatitis was a largely neglected disease burden. Since then, three factors have led to a global effort for eliminating viral hepatitis as a public health threat by 2030.

First, the approach and burden have been consolidated with a comprehensive strategy to tackle the 1.1 million deaths and three million new infections per year. Second, five strategic interventions were integrated covering hepatitis B vaccination, blood and injection safety, harm reduction, and testing and treatment for hepatitis B and cure for hepatitis C, which when scaled to universal coverage result in elimination as a public health threat. Thirdly, viral hepatitis was included in the Sustainable Development Goals from 2015, and ambitious targets set for 2030 endorsed by 194 countries.

This section assesses this transformation in the global response for what is now recognised as a major global disease burden for which elimination as a public health threat is feasible.

The views are those of the authors and not necessarily of the institutions of which they are part.

D. Low-Beer (✉)
World Health Organization, Geneva, Switzerland

F. Cui
Peking University, Peking, China

Keywords

Viral hepatitis · SDGs · Universal access · Liver cancer · Public health · Elimination · Immunisation · Harm reduction · Costing · Injection safety · Investment case

14.1 Introduction

A decade ago, viral hepatitis was a largely neglected disease burden, dispersed under cancer, immunisation and communicable disease [1]. Since then, three factors have led to a global effort for eliminating viral hepatitis as a public health threat by 2030.

First, the approach and burden have been consolidated with a comprehensive strategy to tackle the 1.1 million deaths and three million new infections per year [2, 3].

Second, the foundation in prevention and immunisation has been supplemented with a cure for Hepatitis C and commitment to universal access for effective treatment for Hepatitis B to address the 354 million people infected by these two viruses [4].

Thirdly, viral hepatitis has been included in the United Nations Sustainable Development

M. C. B. Raviglione et al. (eds.), *Global Health Essentials*, Sustainable Development Goals Series,
https://doi.org/10.1007/978-3-031-33851-9_14

Goals since 2015, and ambitious targets set for 2030 [5]. This section assesses this transformation in the global response for what is now recognised as a major global disease burden for which elimination as a public health problem is feasible.

Yet there is no room for complacency. With a huge cohort of 354 million people infected and low baseline coverage of testing and treatment (10% of people with hepatitis B and 22% with hepatitis C diagnosed in 2019), hepatitis remains one of the major challenges in global public health [2].

14.2 Epidemiological Background

Hepatitis is the inflammation of the liver. Heavy alcohol use, toxins, some medications, and autoimmune diseases can cause hepatitis. However, five hepatitis viruses A, B, C, D, and E are responsible for most cases of hepatitis [6].

All hepatitis viruses can cause acute hepatitis. Hepatitis B (HBV) and C (HCV) most commonly lead to progressive liver fibrosis (the first stage of scarring of the liver which does not heal), cirrhosis (severe scarring) and increased risk of liver cancer (hepatocellular carcinoma). Hepatitis B and C account for over 95% of all deaths from hepatitis.

Hepatitis A and E are mostly transmitted through consumption of contaminated water and food. They can be prevented through improved sanitation and vaccination, although Hepatitis E is increasingly recognised as an important cause of disease and outbreaks in developed countries [7]. Hepatitis D is an incomplete virus and can only replicate and cause infection in those who are already infected with HBV. Co-infection can cause worse outcomes, but Hepatitis B vaccine provides protection against Hepatitis D.

WHO estimates there are 296 million people living with chronic HBV infection, 1.5 million new infections and 820,000 deaths per year, or 75% of all hepatitis deaths in 2019 [2, 8]. HBV is transmitted through exposure to infected blood, semen and other body fluids and can be transmitted from infected mothers to infants, contaminated blood and blood products, unsafe injections, injecting drug use and sexually. The increasing coverage of HBV vaccination has been one of the major successes in recent decades on which the elimination agenda is built [9].

There are 58 million people living with chronic HCV infection, 1.5 million new infections and 288,000 deaths per year or approximately 25% of total hepatitis deaths [2]. HCV is mostly transmitted through exposure to infected blood, through contaminated blood and blood products, unsafe injections and through injecting drug use. Sexual transmission is also possible but is less common. There is no vaccine but there is a cure for HCV with a twelve-week course of direct acting antiviral agents (DAA) curing over 90% of cases.

14.3 Towards Global Elimination

The global response to hepatitis was fragmented at the beginning of the twenty-first century. Estimates of the mortality from viral hepatitis due to cirrhosis and cancer were consolidated from 2000 [1] and improved with each iteration of the Global Burden of Disease [8]. Coverage of immunisation against HBV increased from 2000 with the support from the Global Alliance for Vaccines and Immunisation (GAVI).

In 2010 the World Health Assembly adopted its first resolution on viral hepatitis. Despite a vaccine, effective treatment for HBV and the breakthrough of a cure for HCV from 2013 [6], there was hesitation to commit to universal access and hepatitis elimination. In a series of meetings, civil society alongside countries like Egypt and China were crucial in declaring "Don't ask whether but how to eliminate viral hepatitis" [2].

The first integrated Global Health Sector Strategy on viral hepatitis was adopted by the World Assembly in 2016, with 194 countries committing to ambitious targets to eliminate viral hepatitis as a public health threat by 2030 [5]. When WHO and UNAIDS were asked to present on HIV in preparation for the SDGs framework, WHO promoted the notion of the huge burden of viral hepatitis. As a result, it was included as part of the SDGs.

Table 14.1 Targets for 5 core interventions which when scaled to universal access result in major declines in incidence and mortality by 2030

Impact/Intervention	Indicator	2015 baseline	2020 target	2030 target
Impact	Reduction in HBV/HCV incidence	5 million new infections p.a.	30%	90%
Impact	Reduction in HBV/HCV mortality	1.4 million deaths	10%	65%
1. Hepatitis B vaccination	Three dose vaccination coverage of Hepatitis B vaccine	84%	90%	90%
HBV PMTCT	Hepatitis B vaccine birth dose coverage	39%	50%	90%
2. Blood safety	Donations screened with quality assurance	97%	97%	100%
Injection safety	Proportion of unsafe injections	5%	0%	0%
3. Harm reduction	Syringes and needles distributed/PWID/year	27	200	300
4. Testing services	% HBV infected diagnosed	9%	30%	90%
	% HCV diagnosed	20%	30%	90%
5. Treatment	% HBV treatment	8%	8 million people	80%
	% HCV cure	7%		80%

The integrated set of interventions across hepatitis B vaccination (1), blood and injection safety (2), harm reduction (3) and testing and treatment (4 and 5) which when scaled to universal access achieve the impact targets (shaded in orange) are shown in Table 14.1 [5, 10, 11]. Rather than stand-alone components, they are also strongly integrated with HIV, immunisation, and primary health care strategies:

14.4 How to Make Public Health Elimination Feasible

The question of how to make public health elimination feasible is probably more difficult than whether it is feasible. Public health elimination of viral hepatitis is not business as usual and remains one of the great public health challenges of the 2020s.

The first stage of implementation 2015–2020 had modest coverage targets recognising the need for upfront work on market dynamics to radically reduce treatment costs, simplify delivery, and innovation before rapid scale up of 10% p.a. coverage in testing and treatment from 2020 to 2030 [2]. The main innovations and challenges identified are shown in Box 14.1:

Box 14.1 Innovations and Challenges to Meet the Public Health Elimination Agenda

1. **Scale up of prevention now**
   (a) **Innovation in approaches to eliminate mother to child transmission**, given the gap in delivery of birth dose (critical to reduce HBV incidence)
   (b) **Scale up of blood and injection safety in and beyond health settings** (critical to reduce HCV incidence)
   (c) **Harm reduction** in coordination with HIV programs (critical to HCV and HIV incidence)
2. **Treatment access and preparation now for universal access** by 2030 (critical to reduce HBV and HCV mortality and over time incidence and prevalence)
   (a) **Innovations in diagnostics**, including point of care testing and new case finding
   (b) **Radical reductions in treatment costs** now, and innovations in curative HBV treatment over time

(c) **Preparation of a simplified, standard package** of delivery and access, leveraging health and community workers, simplifying access, eligibility and delivery

3. **Strong linkages of hepatitis interventions** to HIV, maternal and child health, NCDs, harm reduction and primary health and community systems to make it affordable. Financing gap, particularly in poorer settings where domestic finance is limited. Significant investment in country surveillance to reduce the uncertainty in estimates and targets.

The health sector costing of the next steps of the strategy, 2022–2030, show costs will double to eight billion p.a. by 2028 from 2020. Costs will then decline associated with major returns in terms of reduced incidence and mortality [3], and as shown with country investment cases, for example, in China in terms of returns on investment of over two dollars for every dollar invested [12]. Yet the costing depends on significant shared costs with HIV for testing and harm reduction, leveraging health and community systems, domestic financing, and radical simplification of diagnosis, eligibility, delivery of services, and innovations in HBV cure [3]. For the costing to be affordable, implementation needs to leverage existing testing platforms, outreach to populations at risk, HBV treatment synergies with HIV, and integrated approaches like triple elimination of mother to child transmission of HBV, HIV and syphilis.

Where are we now? The latest data shows 10% of the estimated 296 million people with chronic HBV are diagnosed (and 2% on treatment) and 21% of people with chronic HCV are diagnosed (and 13% initiated curative treatment). Even the progress in the SDG indicator for hepatitis B, which achieved its 2020 target, hides the huge cohort of over 290 million people already chronically infected, who are not yet receiving care.

There is no room for complacency and public health elimination will be at the end of a difficult decade of scaling up access, simplification, linkage and innovation, the groundwork of universal access. The trajectory and targets to 2030 are shown in Fig. 14.1 for HBV (above) and HCV (below).

Yet viral hepatitis remains one of the most compelling and exciting global health challenges this decade, based in strong prevention and immunisation, effective and increasingly affordable treatments, and a cure for HCV. It is a question not of whether but how we can make universal access and public health elimination feasible in the coming years to 2030.

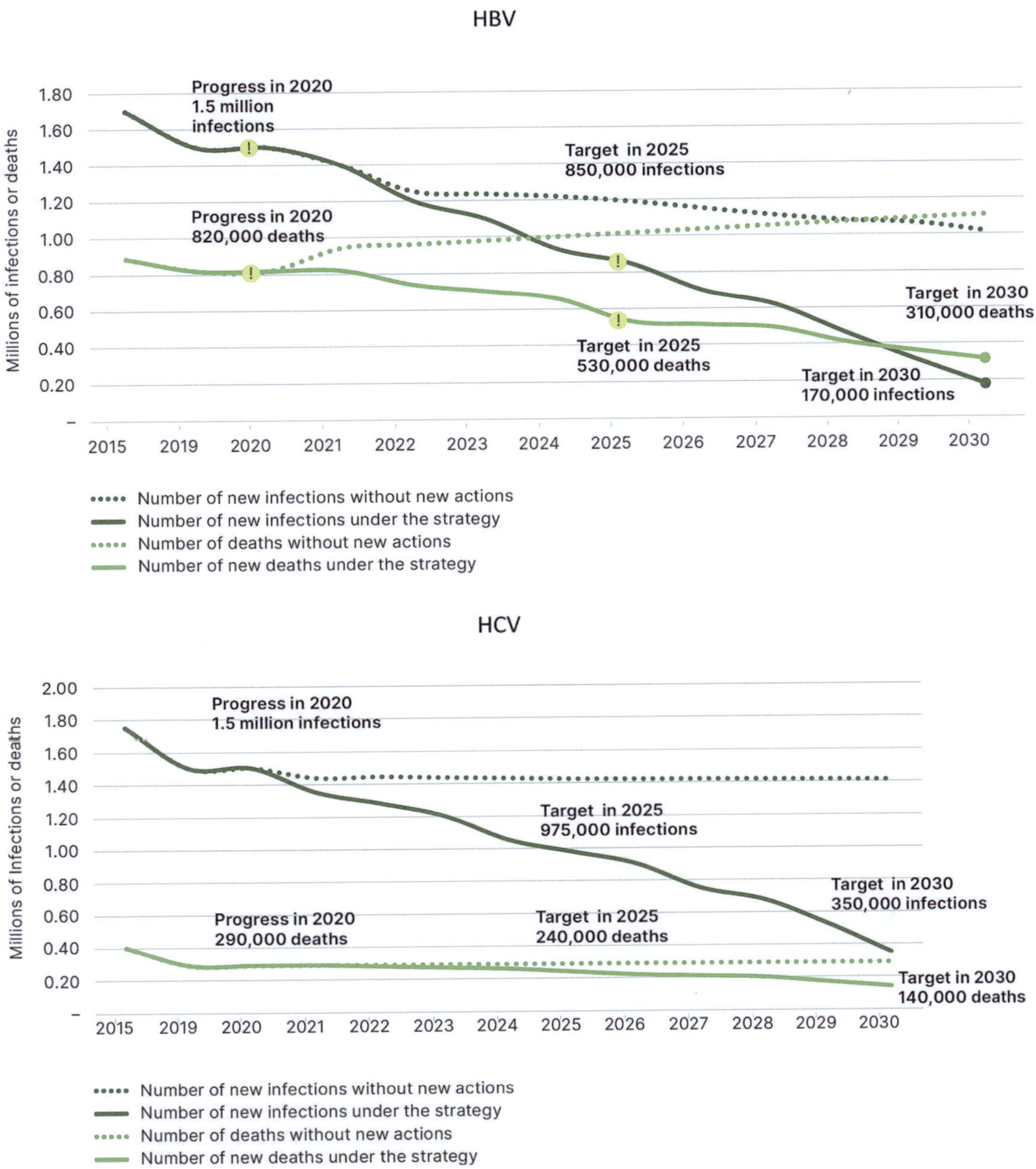

Fig. 14.1 Hepatitis incidence (green) and mortality (blue) trends and targets 2015–2030 (HBV above, HCV below), comparing implementation of strategy (fixed line) compared to no new actions (dotted line)

References

1. Perz JF, Armstrong GL, Farrington LA, Hutin YJ, Bell BP. The contribution of hepatitis B virus and hepatitis C virus infections to cirrhosis and primary liver cancer worldwide. J Hepatol. 2006;45:529–38.
2. World Health Organization. Global progress report on HIV, viral hepatitis and sexually transmitted infections. Geneva: WHO; 2021.
3. World Health Organization. Global health sector strategies on HIV, viral hepatitis and sexually transmitted infections, 2022–2030. Geneva: WHO; 2022.
4. Cox AL, El-Sayed MH, Jia-Horng K, Lazarus JV, Lemoine M, Lok AS. Progress towards elimina-

tion goals for viral hepatitis. Nat Rev Gastroenterol Hepatol. 2020;17(9):533–42.
5. World Health Organization. WHO global health sector strategy on viral hepatitis. Geneva: WHO; 2016.
6. Wiktor S. In: Homes K, Bertozzi S, Bloom B, Jha P, editors. Viral hepatitis in major infectious diseases. Washington, DC: World Bank; 2017.
7. Raji YE, Toung OP, Taib NM, Sekawi ZB. Hepatitis E virus: an emerging enigmatic and underestimated pathogen. Saudi J Biol Sci. 2022;29(1):499–512.
8. Sheena BS, Hiebert L, Han H, Ippolito H. Global, regional, and national burden of hepatitis B, 1990-2019: a systematic analysis for the global burden of disease study 2019. Lancet Gastroenterol Hepatol. 2022;7(9):796–829.
9. Cui F. Strategies to increase timely uptake of hepatitis B vaccine birth dose. Lancet. 2020;8:e869–70.
10. Heffernan A, Cooke GS, Nayagam S, Thursz M, Hallett T. Scaling up prevention and treatment towards the elimination of hepatitis C: a global mathematical model. Lancet. 2019;393(10178):1319.
11. Nayagam S, Thursz M, Sicuri E, Conteh L, Wiktor S, Low-Beer D, Hallett T. Requirements for global elimination of hepatitis B: a modelling study. Lancet Infect Dis. 2016;16(12):1399–408.
12. Nayagam S, Chan P, Zhao K, et al. Investment case for a comprehensive package of interventions against hepatitis B in China. Clin Infect Dis. 2021;72(5):743–52.

Poliomyelitis

15

Michel Zaffran

Abstract

Poliomyelitis is the second human disease after smallpox which could be eradicated. This chapter briefly describes the disease, the status of the 37 years eradication effort, and remaining challenges.

Keywords

Poliomyelitis · Polio · Poliovirus · Eradication · GPEI · OPV · IPV · cVDPV · Vaccines · Immunization

15.1 Introduction

Poliomyelitis (polio) is a viral infection of cranial nerve nuclei in the brain stem that can cause paralysis. The poliovirus is transmitted through the fecal-oral route and generally affects children under 5. Humans are the only reservoir for the virus. Most people infected become asymptomatic carriers of the virus (1 in 300 develops irreversible acute flaccid paralysis). This makes surveillance more complex than for other infectious diseases with mostly symptomatic cases such as smallpox or measles.

15.2 Global Polio Eradication

In 1988, building on the smallpox achievement (declared eradicated by WHO in 1980), as well as on progress with the Expanded Programme on Immunization, the World Health Assembly adopted a resolution to eradicate poliomyelitis. The poliovirus was then endemic in 125 countries causing approximately 350,000 cases yearly. Much progress has been made since by the Global Polio Eradication Initiative (GPEI). Five of six regions of the world have been certified as polio-free: the region of the Americas in 1994, followed by the Western Pacific (2000), European (2002), Southeast Asia (2014), and African (2020) regions. Polioviruses type 2 and type 3 were also declared eradicated in 2015 and 2019, respectively. Only type 1 survives and remains endemic in two countries: Pakistan and Afghanistan where, as of 24 June, 11 cases had been reported for 2022, with one additional case in Mozambique caused by a virus exported from Pakistan (Table 15.1).

M. Zaffran (✉)
Divonne les Bains, France

M. C. B. Raviglione et al. (eds.), *Global Health Essentials*, Sustainable Development Goals Series,
https://doi.org/10.1007/978-3-031-33851-9_15

Table 15.1 Wild poliovirus cases since 2016

Country	Wild virus type 1 confirmed cases								
	Full year total						1 Jan–21 June[a]		
	2016	2017	2018	2019	2020	2021	2021	2022	Date of most recent case
Pakistan	20	8	12	147	84	1	1	10	27-May-22
Afghanistan	13	14	21	29	56	4	1	1	14-Jan-22
Mozambique	0	0	0	0	0	0	0	1	25-Mar-22
Malawi	0	0	0	0	0	1	0	0	19-Nov-21
Nigeria[b]	4	0	0	0	0	0	0	0	21-Aug-16
Total (Type 1)	**37**	**22**	**33**	**176**	**140**	**6**	2	12	
Tot. in endemic countries	37	22	33	176	140	5	2	11	
Tot. in non-end countries	0	0	0	0	0	1	0	1	
No. of countries (infected)	3	2	2	2	2	3	2	3	
No. of countries (endemic)	2	2	3	3	3	2	2	2	
Total female	13	7	18	72	59	2	0	5	
Total male	24	15	15	104	81	4	2	7	

[a] Data reported to WHO HQ on 22 June 2021 for 2021 data and 21 June for 2022 data

15.3 Risks to the Eradication Goal

Since 2016, the programme is facing outbreaks caused by *circulating vaccine derived polioviruses* (cVDPV). The programme relies on the Sabin live attenuated oral polio vaccine which is effective at stopping person-to-person transmission. However, when allowed to circulate in areas with insufficient vaccination coverage and poor sanitation, the live attenuated virus can mutate, revert to virulence, and cause paralytic cases. Type 2 cVDPVs cause the largest number of such outbreaks. In April 2016, the GPEI coordinated the global withdrawal[1] of the trivalent oral vaccine (tOPV) to replace it with the bivalent oral polio vaccine(bOPV) containing only types 1 and 3 attenuated viruses thus removing all type 2 viruses. The objective was to eliminate the risk of type 2 cVDPV outbreaks. This approach was deemed necessary for programmatic and ethical reasons. Type 2 wild poliovirus had not been detected since 1999 and had been officially declared eradicated in 2015. This made the continued use of the vaccine in mass immunization campaigns unnecessary. In some countries however, the inadequate implementation of the withdrawal resulted in outbreaks. Since 20 16, waning population immunity against type-2 combined with low levels of immunization coverage with the injectable inactivated poliovirus vaccine (IPV) have made these outbreaks increasingly difficult to interrupt. GPEI therefore started to roll out a novel type 2 oral polio vaccine (nOPV2) with a genetically modified, more stable, live attenuated virus. The use of this vaccine under the WHO Emergency Use Listing mechanism started in March 2021. In addition, countries that still use bOPV are encouraged to introduce at least two doses of IPV in their immunization schedule.

Furthermore, as final eradication gets closer, complacency can result in increased risks of international circulation to previously polio-free areas as illustrated by recent cases in Malawi and Mozambique.

15.4 Challenges

Since 1988, many difficulties have arisen, including complex terrain and logistics, vaccine refusal, anti-vaccination narratives (now spreading

[1] This globally synchronized withdrawal of tOPV was conducted over a two-week period in April 2016 and is known as "the Switch".

through social media), access issues exacerbated by unrest and war, antigovernment groups banning immunization, violence targeting vaccinators, as well as the lack of political commitment by some countries and occasional managerial problems within GPEI. Independent monitoring, regular questioning, and sustained innovation have helped address them.

Two challenges remain:

Effective poliovirus containment must be in place globally to avoid post eradication release into the population. The poliovirus remains present in a large number of laboratories, manufacturing sites and in potentially infected materials (specimen collected for research purposes other than polio in countries where the wild virus was still in circulation). The GPEI has developed a thorough containment strategy backed by a World Health Assembly resolution. Its implementation requires strong engagement of all parties.

Additionally, the use of the bivalent oral vaccine will have to cease soon after the certification of wild virus eradication. Lessons from the relative failure of the 2016 "switch" will inform this critical step. A refined strategy, suitable tools (including possibly novel types 1 and 3 vaccines), together with stronger routine immunization coverage in at-risk areas will be required.

15.4.1 Approaches and Strategies

Eradication efforts have relied on high levels of coverage with three doses of OPV through routine immunization complemented with under-5 campaigns (National Immunization Days) in order to reach all children. Most countries have eradicated polio with this approach. In others, NIDs intensification has not been sufficient, and more efforts were required to strengthen routine immunization programs. Following eradication and withdrawal of OPV, the world will need to continue vaccinating with IPV for at least 10 years (Box 15.1).

Box 15.1 IPV Vs OPV

Two types of vaccines exist to protect against poliomyelitis: The Sabin live attenuated virus oral polio vaccine (OPV) and the Salk Inactivated poliovirus vaccine (IPV).

Sabin OPV contains live attenuated Sabin poliovirus strains and is administered orally. OPV vaccine induces mucosal immunity which makes it a good tool to stop person-to-person transmission. OPV vaccinated individuals shed Sabin poliovirus which can be transmitted passively and immunize persons not directly reached through immunization programmes. Because it is oral, it is easy to administer by non-medical volunteers. It is also relatively cheap (US $ 0.15 per dose). For many years, it has been the vaccine of choice for the immunization and eradication programmes.

Two rare but serious adverse events are, however, associated with OPV: Vaccine associated Polio Paralysis (VAPP) (which occurs among OPV recipients and their contacts) and vaccine derived polioviruses (VDPVs) when the attenuated Sabin polioviruses replicate over a prolonged period, mutate and re-acquire the characteristics of WPV. With the progress of polio eradication, the risk-benefit analysis has been shifting toward a discontinuation of the use of OPV.

IPV contains wild poliovirus strains which are inactivated with formaldehyde. It is given by injection. IPV is safe and effective at protecting against polio infection. IPV, however, induces limited intestinal mucosal immunity. Infected individuals can therefore become asymptomatic carriers of the virus. Silent transmission of WPV in Israel in 2013 demonstrated that polio transmission can be sustained for months in spite of very high IPV coverage. IPV is substantially more costly than OPV (over US $ 2 per dose) and requires medically trained personnel for its administration.

Since 2014, the GPEI has supported the introduction of at least one dose of IPV in the immunization programme of all countries where OPV continues to be used. As of 2021 two doses of IPV are recommended and financially supported by Gavi, The Vaccine Alliance.

It is anticipated that, after the certification of the eradication of the wild poliovirus, OPV will be withdrawn. Vaccination with IPV will however likely continue.

The decision to interrupt the eradication effort and move to a control strategy has often been debated, particularly when financing was seen to be in danger. An investment case recently released by the GPEI posits that investing in polio eradication may cumulatively save US$ 33.1 billion by 2100 whereas the combined costs involved in controlling polio, and treating survivors, would amount to over US$ 1 billion per year for decades (Fig. 15.1).

15.4.2 Responsibilities

GPEI partners have provided crucial technical and financial support to countries' eradication effort: Rotary International provided the vision of World free of polio and plays a strong fund raising and advocacy role; WHO represents member-states and provides technical leadership; UNICEF procures vaccines, secures logistics, and supports social mobilization; The US Centers for Disease Control provides technical expertise, particularly in surveillance and genetic sequencing; The Bill and Melinda Gates Foundation supports political advocacy, provides funding and helps introduce innovative strategies and tools; Gavi, the Vaccine Alliance finances the IPV and its introduction while supporting the strengthening of routine immunization services.

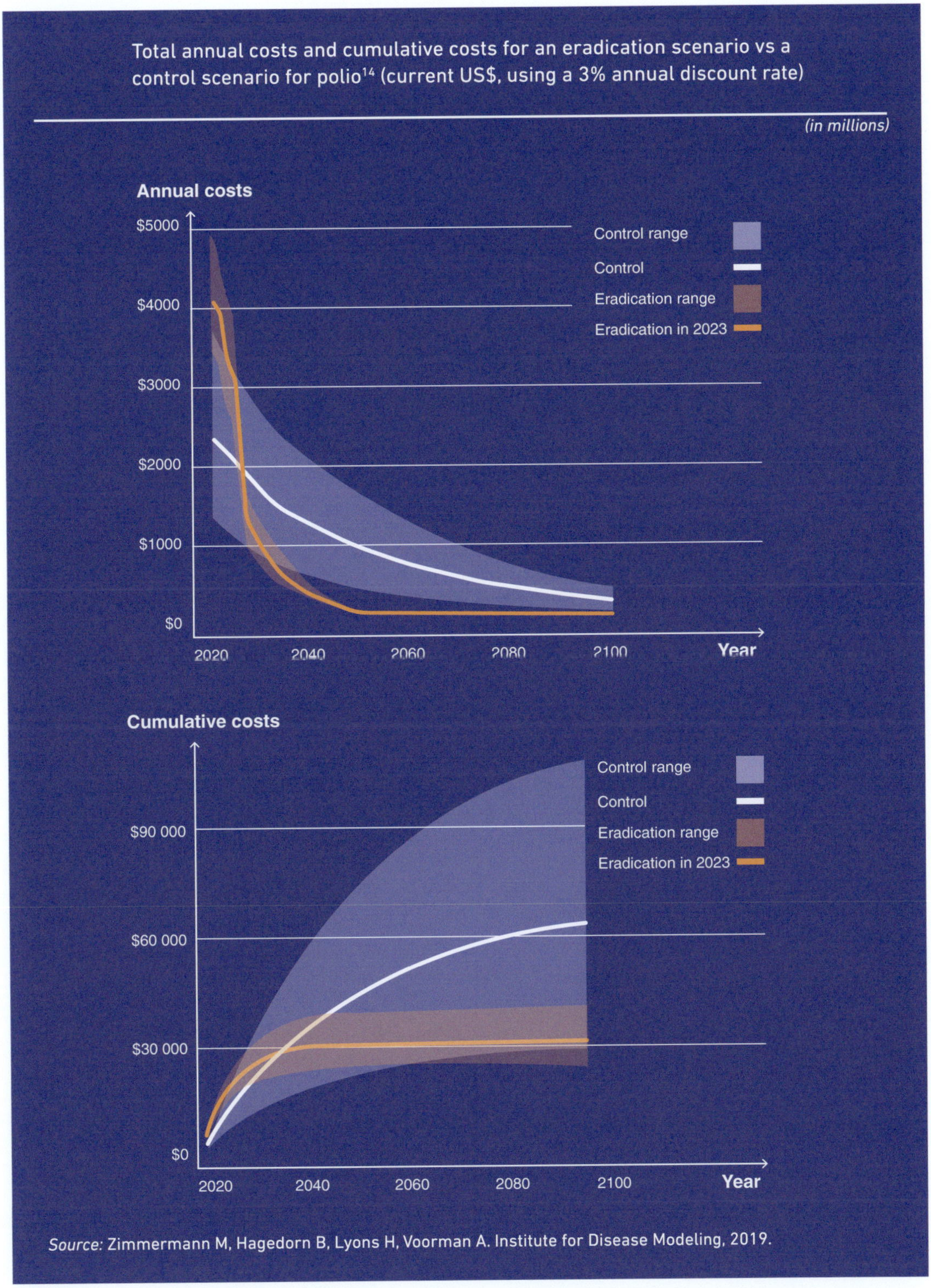

Fig. 15.1 Cost of control versus eradication (reproduced with permission of the the GPEI—The Global Polio Eradication Initiative)

Further Reading

Donaldson L, Alwan A, Frieden T, Goldstein S, Pate M. Highs and lows in the quest for zero: 21st report of the Independent Monitoring Board. https://polioeradication.org/wp-content/uploads/2022/05/21st-IMB-report-20220430.pdf. Accessed 17 Aug 2022.

Garon J, Seib K, Orenstein WA, Ramirez Gonzalez A, Chang Blanc D, Zaffran M, Patel M. Polio endgame: the global switch from tOPV to bOPV. Expert Rev Vaccines. 2016;15(6):693–708. https://doi.org/10.1586/14760584.2016.1140041. Epub 2016 Feb 2. PMID: 26751187.

Global Polio Eradication Initiative investment case 2022–2026: investing in the promise of a polio-free world. Geneva: World Health Organization; 2022. License: CC BY-NC-SA 3.0 IGO.

Polio Eradication Strategy 2022–2026: delivering on a promise. Geneva: World Health Organization; 2021. License: CC BY-NC-SA 3.0 IGO.

Weekly epidemiological record—24 June 2022, 97th year/24 June 2022, 97e ANNÉE No 25, 2022, 97, 277–300. https://apps.who.int/iris/bitstream/handle/10665/357167/WER9725-eng-fre.pdf. Accessed 17 Aug 2022.

World Health Assembly, 41. Global eradication of poliomyelitis by the year 2000. World Health Organization; 1988. https://apps.who.int/iris/handle/10665/164531. Accessed 17 Aug 2022.

World Health Assembly, 71. Poliomyelitis: containment of polioviruses. World Health Organization; 2018. https://apps.who.int/gb/ebwha/pdf_files/WHA71-REC1/A71_2018_REC1-en.pdf#page=25. Accessed 17 Aug 2022.

World Health Assembly, 75. Poliomyelitis eradication—report by the director general; 2022. World Health Organization. https://apps.who.int/gb/ebwha/pdf_files/WHA75/A75_23-en.pdf. Accessed 17 Aug 2022.

16 Neglected Tropical Diseases

Antonio Montresor

Abstract

Neglected tropical diseases (NTDs) are a diverse set of 20 diseases caused by different groups of pathogens (virus, bacteria, fungi, protozoa, helminths, toxins) that affect populations living in poverty. Approximately 1.8 billion people worldwide live in areas where they are transmitted. NTDs have been chronically overlooked by global policymakers and donor agencies but grouping them as a single entity of high morbidity diseases that are preventable and treatable with relatively simple, low-cost control interventions has facilitated the expansion of control measures which in 2020 reached over 800 million individuals.

Five core interventions are recommended by WHO for the control of NTDs: preventive chemotherapy, innovative and intensified disease management, vector control, veterinary public health measures and provision of safe water and sanitation.

The WHO Department of Control of Neglected Tropical Diseases has been preparing guidelines and recommendations for NTD control and conducting advocacy and technical support activities to promote control and elimination of NTDs in countries where they are endemic.

Keywords

Neglected tropical diseases · Control · Morbidity · DALYs · Vector control · Safe water · Preventive chemotherapy · Veterinary public health

16.1 Introduction

Neglected tropical diseases (NTDs) are a heterogeneous set of 20 diseases and disease groups (Table 16.1) that are transmitted in tropical and subtropical areas where they affect impoverished populations [1]. NTDs thrive in areas where sanitation is poor, and populations have close contact with infectious vectors and infected animals. More than 1 billion people are infected with one or more NTD [1].

A. Montresor (✉)
Department of Control of Neglected Tropical Diseases, World Health Organization (WHO), Geneva, Switzerland
e-mail: montresora@who.int

M. C. B. Raviglione et al. (eds.), *Global Health Essentials*, Sustainable Development Goals Series,
https://doi.org/10.1007/978-3-031-33851-9_16

Table 16.1 The 20 NTDs, their main causative agent and the WHO target for 2030

Disease	Main causative agent	WHO target for 2030
Buruli ulcer	*Mycobacterium ulcerans* (bacteria)	Control
Chagas disease	*Trypanosoma cruzi* (protozoa)	Elimination as a public health problem
Dengue and Chikungunya	*Flaviviridae* and *Alphavirus* (virus)	Control
Dracunculiasis	*Dracunculus medinensis* (helminths)	Eradication
Echinococcosis	*Echinococcus* spp. (helminths)	Control
Foodborne trematodiases	*Clonorchis sinensis*, *Opisthorchis felineus*, *O. viverrini*, *Fasciola hepatica*, *F. gigantica*, *Paragonimus* spp. (helminths)	Control
Human African trypanosomiasis	Gambiense form: *Trypanosoma brucei gambiense* (protozoa)	Elimination (interruption of transmission)
	Rhodesiense form: *Trypanosoma brucei rhodesiense* (protozoa)	Elimination as a public health problem
Leishmaniasis	Cutaneous forms: *Leishmania* spp. (protozoa)	Control
	Visceral forms: *Leishmania* spp. (protozoa)	Elimination as a public health problem
Leprosy	*Mycobacterium leprae* (bacteria)	Elimination (interruption of transmission)
Lymphatic filariasis	*Wuchereria bancrofti*, *Brugia malayi*, *B. timori* (helminths)	Elimination as a public health problem
Mycetoma, chromoblastomycosis and other deep mycoses	Several microorganisms of bacterial and fungal origin (bacteria and fungi)	Control
Onchocerciasis	*Onchocerca volvulus* (helminths)	Elimination (interruption of transmission)
Rabies	Rabies virus (virus)	Elimination as a public health problem
Scabies and other ectoparasitoses	*Sarcoptes scabiei* (mite)	Control
Schistosomiasis	*Schistosoma haematobium*, *S. mansoni*, *S. japonicum* (helminths)	Elimination as a public health problem
Soil-transmitted helminthiases	*Ascaris lumbricoides*, *Trichuris trichiura*, Hookworms, *Strongyloides stercoralis* (helminths)	Elimination as a public health problem
Snakebite envenoming	Toxin following a bite of a venomous snake	Control
Taeniasis and cysticercosis	*Taenia solium* (helminths)	Control
Trachoma	*Chlamydia trachomatis* (bacteria)	Elimination as a public health problem
Yaws	*Treponema pallidum* subspecies *pertenue* (bacteria)	Eradication

16.2 Global Burden and Challenges

NTDs have been chronically overlooked by global policymakers and donor agencies, by the national health agendas of endemic countries and, sometimes, even by affected communities themselves for two main reasons:

1. NTDs cause relatively low numbers of deaths compared with the "three big killers" (malaria, HIV and TB) which, since the 1990s, have attracted the largest share of attention from global policymakers and, consequently, most of the financial investment by donors.
2. Each of the 20 NTDs "individually" causes limited morbidity.

16.3 Strategic Approach

Under the guidance of the WHO Department of Control of Neglected Tropical Diseases, that was created in 2005 with the aim of reverting this situation, intensive advocacy has been organized to promote that:

1. Despite their relatively low mortality, NTDs cause significant morbidity: they debilitate, deform and blind infected individuals. They disable through both overt (skin and eye lesions, internal organ lesions, limb deformation, impairment and retardation of mental functions) and silent morbidity (energy deficits, anaemia, growth retardation, chronic pain, exercise intolerance), with the potential to stunt the social, educational and professional lives of affected individuals.
2. Collectively, NTDs cause a loss of DALYs that is in the same order of magnitude as the three big killers (Fig. 16.1) [2].
3. Interventions to control NTDs are simpler and of lower cost than those to control the three big killers; in addition, they can be easily integrated among themselves or with existing platforms to further reduce control costs.

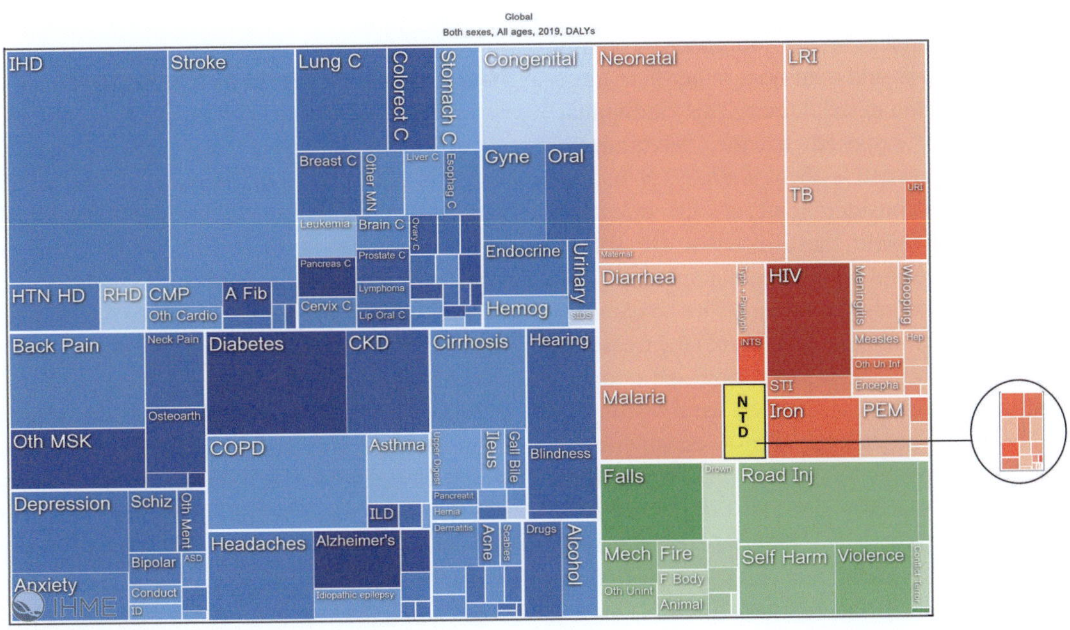

Fig. 16.1 Relevance of NTDs in the global burden of diseases; the total weight of NTDs is presented in yellow; the circles present the individual weights of each NTD. (Source: Institute for Health Metrics Evaluation [2]. Used with permission. All rights reserved)

This advocacy effort has resulted in a progressive intensification of the control activities that reach over a billion people every year [3].

16.4 Interventions for Prevention and Control

WHO recommends five core interventions to control NTDs.

Preventive chemotherapy is the regular, large-scale administration of medicines to entire population groups with the aim of reducing transmission or associated morbidity. Individual diagnosis is not necessary: surveys are conducted to assess if the disease is endemic in the area (community diagnosis), and if so, community treatment is organized. This approach is effective and easy to administer using safe, low-cost medicines; the treatment of uninfected individuals is without risk [4]. This approach is recommended for the following NTDs: lymphatic filariasis, onchocerciasis, schistosomiasis, soil-transmitted helminthiases, trachoma and yaws.

Innovative and intensified disease management is applicable to diseases which require a more traditional clinical approach entailing proper diagnosis and treatment rather than large-scale distribution of medicines. This "individual" approach (as opposed to the "community" approach of preventive chemotherapy) is justified by two main considerations: (1) the infectious agents that transmit these diseases are able to produce severe and possibly lethal outcomes, and infected individuals should therefore be carefully cared for and completely cured; (2) the treatment of such diseases necessitates long and complex treatment courses, specialized equipment and highly toxic medicines. These considerations mandate an approach involving close, individual, clinical case-management and follow-up of the patient by an experienced physician or nurse [5]. This approach is recommended for the following NTDs: Buruli ulcer, Chagas disease, human African trypanosomiasis, leishmaniasis, leprosy and snakebite envenoming.

Vector control is the reduction or elimination of the vectors that transmit infectious diseases using multiple strategies that entail environmental, chemical and biological control, and reduction of contacts between vectors and humans. This approach is recommended for the following vector-borne NTDs: Chagas disease, dengue, chikungunya, dracunculiasis, human African trypanosomiasis, lymphatic filariasis, onchocerciasis, schistosomiasis and trachoma.

Veterinary public health measures, such as vaccination or treatment of livestock and domestic animals, safe slaughtering and rodent control, are used to target NTDs for which animals play an active role in transmission. This approach is recommended for diseases such as rabies, echinococcosis, foodborne trematodiases, human African trypanosomiasis, leishmaniasis, taeniasis and cysticercosis.

Provision of safe water and sanitation is the improvement of water and sanitation services to levels that improve general hygiene living conditions and impede environmental contamination with human excreta. This approach is applicable to most of the NTDs because it reduces not only NTD-associated morbidity but also that of several other infections.

16.5 Role of WHO in the Control of NTDs

WHO is the specialized agency of the United Nations responsible for directing and coordinating international public health. Aside from its normative role in developing technical guidance and recommendations, WHO has two additional main tasks: advocacy and technical support to Member States.

NTD advocacy consists in raising the international level of attention and interest for NTDs: documenting the burden of NTDs and the benefits resulting from their control; promoting the inclusion of NTDs into public health agendas at national and international levels; sensitizing potential supporting institutions (bilateral cooperation agencies, public and private foundations and pharmaceutical companies or firms interested in corporate social responsibility); and coordinating all the actors involved in combating NTDs through the establishment of global partnerships and the organization of regular meetings [5].

WHO provides technical support to Member States upon request by national governments. This support concerns the development of national plans of action based on WHO strategies and recommendations but adapted to the country's prevailing conditions and specificities; the implementation of disease-control activities; and the supervision, monitoring, evaluation and validation of such activities. Technical support is a key role of WHO, which has to be considered as a technical support agency rather than a funding agency. This implies that WHO does not cover the expenses related to implementation of national policies but does assure that implementation meets agreed technical standards. Furthermore, by leveraging its network of partners, WHO can facilitate resource mobilization from third parties willing to support the efforts of national governments [5].

References

1. Ending the neglect to attain the sustainable development goals: a road map for neglected tropical diseases 2021–2030. Geneva: World Health Organization; 2020. https://apps.who.int/iris/handle/10665/338565.
2. GBD compare: Viz Hub. Seattle: Institute for Health Metrics and Evaluation; 2022. https://vizhub.healthdata.org/gbd-compare/.
3. Crossing the billion: preventive chemotherapy for neglected tropical diseases. Geneva: World Health Organization; 2017. https://apps.who.int/iris/handle/10665/255498.
4. Gabrielli A, Montresor A, Engels D, Savioli L. Preventive chemotherapy in human helminthiasis: theoretical and operational aspects. Trans R Soc Trop Med Hyg. 2011;105:683–93. https://doi.org/10.1016/j.trstmh.2011.08.013.
5. Gabrielli AF, Mariotti SP, Montresor A, Rio F, Savioli L. Neglected tropical diseases: an introduction for the Italian medical and scientific community. Ital J Trop Med. 2008;13:1–7.

17 HPV Infection and Cervical Cancer

Elisabetta Tanzi and Marta Canuti

Abstract

Cancer cases attributed to Human Papillomavirus (HPV) represent approximately 4.5% of all cancers. High-risk HPV types cause nearly 100% of cervical cancer (CC) cases, the fourth most frequent female cancer and the fourth leading cause of cancer mortality worldwide. The burden of CC is greater in low- and middle-income countries, reflecting global inequities in the access to vaccination and screening programs, health services, and high-quality treatments.

In May 2018, WHO announced a global action to eliminate CC as a public health problem, a goal defined as achieving and maintaining in all countries an incidence rate of <4 per 100,000 women-years, and established intermediate targets (90-70-90) to be achieved by 2030 in all countries, based on the implementation of primary (HPV vaccination), secondary (screening), and tertiary (precancer and cancer treatment and management) prevention strategies. This is the first time the world has committed to eliminate a cancer.

Keywords

Human papillomavirus · HPV prevalence · Cervical cancer incidence · Cervical cancer elimination · HPV vaccination · Cervical cancer screening · Cervical cancer treatment

17.1 HPV and Cervical Cancer

Human papillomavirus (HPV) is a species-specific double-stranded DNA (dsDNA) epitheliotropic virus responsible for the world most common sexually transmitted infection. There are several types of HPV with the potential to induce both benign and malignant lesions [1] (Box 17.1). Both sexes are susceptible to the infection, but the risk of disease outcomes is higher in women.

E. Tanzi (✉)
Department of Health Sciences, University of Milan, Milan, Italy
e-mail: elisabetta.tanzi@unimi.it

M. Canuti
Centre for Multidisciplinary Research in Health Science (MACH), University of Milan, Milan, Italy

M. C. B. Raviglione et al. (eds.), *Global Health Essentials*, Sustainable Development Goals Series,
https://doi.org/10.1007/978-3-031-33851-9_17

Box 17.1 Characteristics of HPV Types

- There are over **200 HPV types**, which have distinct genetic, epidemiological, and clinical features. The International Agency for Research on Cancer (IARC) has classified HPV types from the **HR-clade into**:
  - 12 high-risk (HR-HPV) types (HPV-16, 18, 31, 33, 35, 39, 45, 51, 52, 56, 58, and 59) into Group 1 of human carcinogens
  - 13 types as probable (Group 2A: HPV-68) and possibly (Group 2B: HPV-26, 30, 34, 53, 66, 67, 69, 70, 73, 82, 85, 97) carcinogenic for humans.
- **HR-HPVs** can cause persistent infections and several types of cancer (~4.5% of all cancers worldwide, with ~620,000 and ~70,000 HPV-related cancers each year in women and men, respectively); **LR-HPVs** (low-risk HPVs) are mostly associated with no or mild disease (warts on or around the genitals, anus, mouth, or throat). Among the latter, HPV-6 and HPV-11 are responsible for ~90% of anogenital warts cases.
- **HPV-16** is the most frequently detected type in all stages of infection/disease and in all geographic regions. After HPV16, the most prevalent HPV types are **HPV 18/45/31/33/52/58**, but there are variations among different geographic regions. HPV-16, along with HPV-18, is associated with the highest risk of progression to cancer and together they are responsible for ~70% of all CC. HPV16 is also detected more frequently in squamous cell carcinoma (SCC) cases than in adenocarcinoma (ADC), which is more frequently attributed to HPV18 and HPV45 infections.
- All currently available **vaccines** protect against HPV-16 and HPV-18. While the **bivalent** vaccine is only directed against these two types, the **quadrivalent** vaccine protects also against types 6 and 11 and the **nine-valent** vaccine protects against five additional oncogenic types (31, 33, 45, 52, and 58) that cause an additional ~20% of CC.

About 4.5% of all cancers worldwide are attributed to HPV. It is causally associated with CC and is also involved in anogenital (anus, vulva, vagina, and penis) and oral (particularly the oropharynx) cancers [2].

Most HPV infections are asymptomatic and clear within 6–24 months, while infection persistence is necessary to initiate the oncogenic process. Clinical manifestations in the cervix are classified into ASCUS (Atypical Squamous cells of Undetermined Significance), low-grade lesions (LSILs/CIN1), ASC-H (Atypical Squamous cells-cannot exclude HSIL), high-grade lesions (HSILs/CIN2–3), and cancer.

17.2 Epidemiology and Global Burden

Among women with normal cervical cytology, overall HPV prevalence is estimated around 10% [3]. HPV prevalence peaks (~24.0%) in women younger than 25 years and declines with age [3, 4]. In Africa and Asia, this marked decline is not observed and, in some regions (i.e. West Africa, Central and South America), a second modest peak is observed in older women. HPV prevalence increases with increasing lesion severity (~50% of ASCUS, 75% of L-SIL, 89% of H-SIL, and almost 100% in CC) [3]. Table 17.1 shows the prevalence of the most oncogenic HPV types.

CC is the fourth most common cancer (second in women aged 15–44 years) and the fourth leading cause of cancer death in women globally [3], with an estimated 8.96 million disability-adjusted life years (DALYs) lost in 2019 [6].

More than 600,000 new cases have been estimated for 2020 globally [3, 5], and the disease burden is higher in low- and middle-income countries (LMICs) compared to high-income countries (HICs) (Table 17.1; Fig. 17.1a). More than 85% of affected women are young and live in resource-limited countries. Age-standardized incidence rates vary from 84.5 to <7 per 100,000 women worldwide. Nearly 90% of the estimated yearly 342,000 CC-related deaths occur in LMICs (Fig. 17.1b). The global burden of CC is projected to increase in future years, especially in LMICs.

Table 17.1 Prevalence of HPV-16 and HPV-18 broken down by cytological status and cervical cancer incidence in different geographical regions and high (HIC), middle (MIC) and low (LIC) income countries

	Prevalence of HPV-16 and HPV-18								Estimated number of new cervical cancer cases in 2020			
	Normal cytology		Low-grade lesions		High-grade lesions		Cervical cancer					
	N.	P	N.	P	N.	P	N.	P	Number of cases	Uncertainty interval	ASR[a] (World)	Cumulative risk[b]
World	453,184	3.9	38,191	25.8	50,202	51.9	453,184	69.4	604,127	[582030.8–627062.1]	13.3	1.82
Africa	19,726	3.8	465	24.9	399	38.6	19,726	67.2	117,316	[105998.6–129841.8]	25.6	3.86
Eastern Africa	4115	4.7	150	30	138	45.7	4115	67.9	54,560	[48276.6–61661.3]	40.1	5.67
Middle Africa	–	–	24	12.5	–	–	–	–	15,646	[13437.4–18217.6]	31.6	5.01
Northern Africa	2224	3.0	24	20.8	–	–	2224	78.9	6971	[6061.2–8017.3]	6.3	1.1
Southern Africa	8661	3.2	57	21.1	98	33.7	8661	62.5	12,333	[11952.0–12726.2]	36.4	5.66
Western Africa	4726	4.3	210	24.3	163	35.6	4726	55.6	27,806	[23307.1–33173.3]	22.9	3.83
Americas	105,042	4.5	9893	26.7	13,590	56.9	105,042	68.2	74,410	[56232.0–62828.9]	11.3	1.56
Caribbean	323	15.8	263	7.6	285	32.6	323	60.2	3857	[3427–4341]	13.7	2.29
Central America	16,786	4.1	1424	15	559	40.8	16,786	63.1	13,848	[13283.5–14436.5]	13.8	2.21
Northern America	77,952	4.4	6015	27.1	10,230	58.6	77,952	71.4	14,971	[14703.2–15243.7]	6.1	0.72
South America	10,180	5.8	2191	35.6	2516	56.3	10,180	62.6	41,734	[38925.2–44745.5]	15.4	2.34
Asia	142,676	3.4	7959	21.2	13,444	42.1	142,676	68.9	351,720	[339675.0–364192.1]	12.7	1.82
Central Asia	–	–	–	–	–	–	–	–	4945	[4667.0–5882.9]	12.7	1.32
Eastern Asia	111,548	3.4	6981	20.3	10,551	41	111,548	65.0	129,567	[126381.1–132833.1]	10.8	1.33
South-Eastern Asia	8755	3.0	474	27.4	1044	33.4	8755	70.4	68,623	[64656.6–72832.8]	17.8	2.66
Southern Asia	14,520	4.4	225	30.2	287	63.4	14,520	80.3	143,183	[138883.0–160300.8]	15.4	1,72
Western Asia	7853	2.5	279	24	1562	52.3	7853	72.4	5402	[4559.0–6400,8]	4.14	0.45
Europe	180,090	3.8	19,401	27.1	21,140	54.5	180,090	74	58,169	[56344.7–60052.4]	10.7	1.25
Eastern Europe	7818	9.7	1058	31.8	661	60.5	7818	84.7	32,348	[31583.5–33131.0]	14.5	1.42
Norther Europe	86,821	4.2	4949	30.6	8448	54.9	86,821	77	6666	[6414.5–6927.3]	10.4	1.07
Southern Europe	31,831	3.8	10,519	25.4	5866	53.2	31,831	68	9053	[8181.3–10017.5]	7.7	0.93
Western Europe	56,074	2.6	2875	25.2	3062	59.4	56,074	78.7	10,102	[9650.9–10574.2]	7.0	0.88

(continued)

Table 17.1 (continued)

	Prevalence of HPV-16 and HPV-18								Estimated number of new cervical cancer cases in 2020			
	Normal cytology		Low-grade lesions		High-grade lesions		Cervical cancer					
	N.	P	N.	P	N.	P	N.	P	Number of cases	Uncertainty interval	ASR[a] (World)	Cumulative risk[b]
Oceania	2997	8.3	473	27.1	1629	59.1	2997	76.6	2512	[2299.4–2744.2]	10.1	1.11
Australia & New Zealand	2271	8.5	473	27.1	1517	58.4	2271	76.1	1094	[1021.2–1172.0]	5.6	0,63
Melanesia	726	7.7	–	–	112	68.8	726	82.9	1330	[975.5–1813.4]	28.3	4.23
Micronesia	–	–	–	–	–	–	–	–	53	[33.3–84.4]	18.7	2.76
Polynesia	–	–	–	–	–	–	–	–	35	[20.2–60.7]	9.7	1.16
HIC	–	–	–	–	–	–	–	–	71,624	[69708.5–73592.1]	8.4	1.01
Upper MIC	–	–	–	–	–	–	–	–	247,840	[240358.8–255554.1]	12.8	1.72
Lower MIC	–	–	–	–	–	–	–	–	236,828	[224,446,0-249,893,0]	16.9	2.72
LIC	–	–	–	–	–	–	–	–	47,571	[42451.1–53308.4]	23.8	3.34

N. number of individuals tested, *P* HPV-16 and HPV-18 prevalence

Data source: ICO/IARC HPV Information Centre, Bruni L et al. *2021* [3] *and Global Cancer Observatory: Cancer Today, Ferlay J* et al. *2020* [5]

[a] *ASR* rates per 100,000 women per year

[b] Cumulative risk (Incidence): probability of individuals getting from the disease during ages 0–74 years

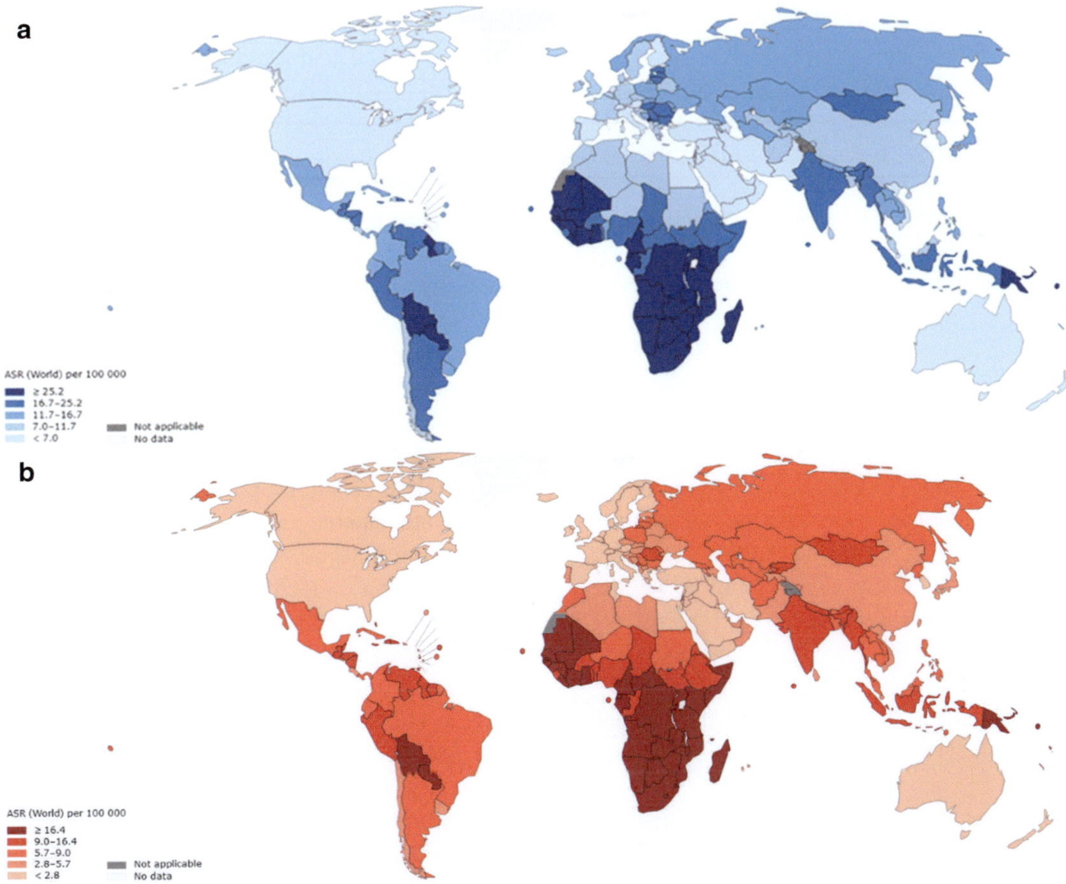

Fig. 17.1 Estimated age-standardized cervical cancer incidence (**a**) and mortality (**b**) rates, 2020. (Reprinted with permission from Global Cancer Observatory: Cancer Today, Ferlay J et al., 2020 [5])

17.3 International Targets

As a result of effective screening and early treatment, HICs experienced a marked decrease in CC incidence and mortality. High HPV vaccination coverage contributed to decreasing HPV and cervical lesion prevalence in countries with well-established immunization programs. However, CC remains a major cause of morbidity and mortality worldwide, especially in LMICs.

In May 2018, WHO announced a global initiative to eliminate CC as a public health problem by achieving an incidence rate <4 per 100,000 women-years [7]. By 2030, the 90-70-90 intermediate targets, which focus on vaccinations, screening, and treatment, are expected to be met (Box 17.2).

Box 17.2 The WHO Global Strategy to Eliminate Cervical Cancer as a Public Health Problem

- **May 2018**: The WHO Director-General announced a **Global call for action** to eliminate CC
- **August 2020**: The World Health Assembly adopted the **Global Strategy for cervical cancer elimination**
- **Goals**
  - A vision of a world where cervical cancer is eliminated
  - Achieving and maintaining an incidence rate of 4 per 100,000 women-years in all countries

- **90-70-90** interim targets to be met by 2030:

  90% of girls fully vaccinated with HPV vaccine by the age of 15 years

  70% of women screened with high-performance tests by 35 years and again by 45 years of age

  90% of women identified with cervical disease receive treatment: 90% of women with precancer treated and 90% of women with invasive cancer managed

- Identified interventions must be implemented simultaneously and on a large scale to achieve acceleration of the expected outcomes:
  - immediate reduction in mortality rates resulting from CC treatment
  - gradual decrease in CC incidence rates from implementation of screening and treatment services
  - protection against CC for girls and future generations from HPV vaccination
- **Expected benefits** from achieving interim targets:
  - in LMICs a 2% reduction in median incidence rate by 2030, 42% by 2045 and 97% by 2120, averting more than 74 million new cases of CC
  - in LMICs 300,000 CC deaths averted by 2030, over 14 million by 2070, over 62 million by 2030
  - for every dollar invested through 2030 to meet the 90-70-90 targets, up to US$ 26.00 (estimated including social benefits) will be returned to the economy

The global commitment to achieving these targets is in line with the 2030 Agenda for Sustainable Development (Goals 1, 3, 5, 10) [8] and the principle of leaving no one behind, and it is a component of the UN Secretary-General's Global Strategy for Women's, Children's and Adolescents' Health (2016–2030) [9].

17.4 Determinants and Risk Factors

Morbidity factors include viral characteristics and environmental/exogenous (geographical area, socioeconomic and cultural status) and individual determinants. Young age, early sexual onset, high number of sexual partners, and related sexual behaviours are all risk factors for infection. Persistence and progression of infection are largely attributable to characteristics of the infecting virus (type, viral load, multiple infections) although co-factors related to the individual (e.g. co-infections with other sexually transmitted agents, multiparity, use of oral contraceptives, smoking) may contribute significantly to increase the risk of progression [3].

In LMICs, factors such as cultural diversity, poverty, early onset of sexual activities, and early marriage are associated with a high risk of infection. Access to screening programs, health services and high-quality treatments remain a critical issue in many LMICs. Moreover, many LMICs are heavily affected by HIV, which gives a higher risk of persistent HPV infection and a six times higher risk of CC, even at a very young age [10].

17.5 Challenges to Control and Elimination

Measures for eliminating CC have not been widely implemented in regions of the world with the highest disease burden. These strategies must be implemented nationwide, using person-centred health service delivery systems that are responsive to the women's needs in their social context, breaking down all barriers (individual, cultural, economic, etc.) that hinder their access to health services.

Access to HPV vaccination has been a prerogative of young women in HICs since 2006 but in 2019 more than 65% of vaccinated girls lived in LMICs. However, only 55% of LMICs have introduced HPV vaccination compared to the 85% of HICs. Similar percentages are observed for CC screening programs (about 55% LMICs have a national program, as of 2020). Additionally, 30% LICs and 90% HICs report having CC management services (pathology, surgery, chemotherapy, radiotherapy) [7].

Countries experiencing difficulties (financial, social, organizational) in implementing vaccination programs must improve access to secondary/tertiary prevention strategies for women with or at risk of CC (HR-HPV infected and/or with precancer).

It is also imperative to implement integrated prevention, screening, and treatment services for HIV and HPV to increase efficiency and maximize impact.

17.6 Strategies for Prevention and Control

Primary prevention aims to protect against HPV infection, mainly by administering the vaccine (see Box 17.1) to girls before sexual life onset (9–14 years) and through sex education. Screening is a secondary prevention intervention aimed at early detection and treatment of precancerous lesions. Treatment and palliative care for CC are tertiary prevention interventions. Monitoring and evaluating key indicators of the prevention programs should be carried out regularly to ensure effectiveness [11].

17.7 Economic and Financial Considerations

In HICs, with well-established screening programs, the highest expense is for prevention; in LMICs the highest costs are incurred for treatment. Treatment expenses vary depending on the lesion type and on the cancer stage at diagnosis, with more advanced CC requiring the highest managing costs. HPV vaccination campaigns would allow to spare many resources that are now invested in management [12].

Financial resources (~US$ 10.5 billion) for scaling up HPV vaccination, CC screening, and managing invasive CC need to be allocated in LMICs to achieve the 90-70-90 targets. WHO is providing support to health ministries in various countries to prepare costing plans and mobilize resources to create cost-effective strategies tailored to countries' needs [7].

17.8 Role of National and International Institutions

WHO global strategy to accelerate CC elimination will be successful only if all Member States, already committed to reaching universal health coverage and the SDGs, mobilize.

Political support, availability of funding and their distribution based on concerted action plans, global solidarity, partnerships, health systems strengthening, and health promotion will permit CC elimination, which is also the result of social inequalities and the lack of women's right to health.

According to the WHO Global Action Plan for the Prevention and Control of Non-Communicable Diseases 2013–2020 [13], HPV vaccination and CC screening and treatment are highly valuable and are among the interventions recommended by WHO for inclusion in Member States' national health plans.

CC screening and treatment are also among the integrated services set in the Political Declaration on HIV and AIDS (UN General Assembly) [14] to address co-infections and comorbidities to guarantee the sustainability of HIV prevention, treatment, care, and support services.

References

1. International Agency for Research on Cancer (IARC). Human papillomaviruses. IARC monographs on the evaluation of carcinogenic risks to humans. 2012;100B:255–313. https://publications.iarc.fr/119. Accessed 30 Aug 2022.
2. de Martel C, Georges D, Bray F, Ferlay J, Clifford GM. Global burden of cancer attributable to infections in 2018: a worldwide incidence analysis. Lancet Glob Health. 2020;8:e180–90. https://doi.org/10.1016/S2214-109X(19)30488-7.
3. Bruni L, Albero G, Serrano B, Mena M, Collado JJ, Gómez D, Muñoz J, Bosch FX, de Sanjosé S. ICO/IARC Information Centre on HPV and Cancer (HPV Information Centre). Human papillomavirus and related diseases in the world. Summary report. 2021. https://www.hpvcentre.net/statistics/reports/XWX.pdf. Accessed 30 Aug 2022.
4. Bruni L, Diaz M, Castellsague X, Ferrer E, Bosch FX, de Sanjosé S. Cervical human papillomavirus prevalence in 5 continents: meta-analysis of 1 million women with normal cytological findings. J Infect Dis. 2010;202(12):1789–99. https://doi.org/10.1086/657321.
5. Ferlay J, Ervik M, Lam F, Colombet M, Mery L, Piñeros M, Znaor A, Soerjomataram I, Bray F. Global cancer observatory: cancer today. Lyon: International Agency for Research on Cancer; 2020. https://gco.iarc.fr/today. Accessed 30 Aug 2022.
6. Zhang X, Zeng Q, Cai W, Ruan W. Trends of cervical cancer at global, regional, and national level: data from the global burden of disease study 2019. BMC Public Health. 2021;21(1):894. https://doi.org/10.1186/s12889-021-10907-5.
7. WHO cervical cancer elimination initiative. Global strategy to accelerate the elimination of cervical cancer as a public health problem. 2020. https://www.who.int/initiatives/cervical-cancer-elimination-initiative#cms. Accessed 30 Aug 2022.
8. Resolution adopted by the General Assembly on 25 September 2015. Resolution 70.1: transforming our world: The 2030 agenda for sustainable development. New York: United nations General Assembly, Seventieth session. 2015. https://sdgs.un.org/publications/transforming-our-world-2030-agenda-sustainable-development-17981. Accessed 30 Aug 2022.
9. Global strategy for women's, children's and adolescents' health (2016–2030): survive, thrive, transform. New York: United Nations. 2015. https://globalalliancematernalmentalhealth.org/wp-content/uploads/2017/12/globalstrategyreport2016-2030-lowres.pdf. Accessed 30 Aug 2022.
10. Stelzle D, Tanaka LF, Ken Lee K, Khalil AI, Baussano I, Shah ASV, et al. Estimates of the global burden of cervical cancer associated with HIV. Lancet Glob Health. 2021;9:e161–9. https://doi.org/10.1016/S2214-109X(20)30459-9.
11. WHO. Comprehensive cervical cancer control: a guide to essential practice, 2nd ed. https://apps.who.int/iris/bitstream/handle/10665/144785/9789241548953_eng.pdf. Accessed 30 Aug 2022.
12. Ngcamphalala C, Östensson E, Ginindza TG. The economic burden of cervical cancer in Eswatini: societal perspective. PLoS One. 2021;16(4):e0250113. https://doi.org/10.1371/journal.pone.0250113.
13. Global action plan for the prevention and control of noncommunicable diseases 2013–2020. Geneva: World Health Organization; 2013. https://apps.who.int/iris/handle/10665/94384. Accessed 30 Aug 2022.
14. Resolution adopted by the General Assembly on 8 June 2016. Resolution 70/266: political declaration on HIV and AIDS: on the fast track to accelerating the fight against HIV and to ending the AIDS epidemic by 2030. New York: United Nations General Assembly, Seventieth session; 2016. https://undocs.org/en/A/RES/70/266. Accessed 2 Oct 2020.

18 Vaccine-Preventable Diseases

Antonella Amendola and Marta Canuti

Abstract

The burden of vaccine-preventable diseases (VPDs), diseases for which vaccination is recommended by national immunization programs, decreased significantly in the last decades but it is still high in low-middle income countries (LMICs), particularly in Africa and Southeast Asia. While vaccine coverage increased in LMICs, also thanks to the support of the Vaccine Alliance (GAVI), it has declined in fully self-funded middle-income countries (MICs).

Immunization is among the greatest advances in global health as, for over two centuries, vaccination programs have succeeded to reduce the burden of diseases like smallpox, polio, and measles. High and equitable vaccination coverage is essential to control/prevent and eliminate VPDs and vaccination is part of 14 of the 17 SDGs. The 2030 Agenda for Immunization was endorsed by all WHO member states in 2020 to achieve "a world in which everyone, everywhere, at every age, can fully benefit from vaccines to improve health and well-being."

Keywords

Vaccine-preventable diseases · Expanded Program on Immunization (EPI) · Vaccine Alliance (GAVI) · Global Vaccine Plan (GVP) · Immunization Agenda 2030 · Vaccine coverage · Measles · Poliomyelitis · Maternal and neonatal tetanus

18.1 Introduction

Vaccines save over five lives every minute, preventing up to five million deaths a year [1]. WHO, with the support of UNICEF and global donors, introduced in 1974 the Expanded Program on Immunization (EPI), which brought substantial increases in routine childhood vaccine coverage. Vaccine-preventable diseases (VPDs) include all diseases for which vaccination is recommended by national immunization programs. The most common and serious VPDs tracked by WHO are listed in Table 18.1. Surveillance for VPDs is critical to identify outbreaks and unreached or under-immunized populations and to monitor regional and global

A. Amendola (✉)
Department of Health Sciences, University of Milan, Milan, Italy
e-mail: antonella.amendola@unimi.it

M. Canuti
Centre for Multidisciplinary Research in Health Science (MACH), University of Milan, Milan, Italy

M. C. B. Raviglione et al. (eds.), *Global Health Essentials*, Sustainable Development Goals Series,
https://doi.org/10.1007/978-3-031-33851-9_18

Table 18.1 Summary of vaccine-preventable disease (VPDs)

Disease	Etiological agent	Symptoms	Transmission	Disease burden
Poliomyelitis	Poliovirus type 1, 2 and 3 (*Picornaviridae*)	Fever, headache, vomiting, pharyngitis, nonparalytic aseptic meningitis, paralytic poliomyelitis	Fecal-oral	Cases caused by wild-type poliovirus (WPV) decreased from 350,000 in 1988 to 19 in August 2022. Poliomyelitis is still endemic in Afghanistan and Pakistan; 2 cases of WPV1 were registered in Mozambique and Malawi. Vaccine-derivated poliovirus type 1 cases (cVDPV1) were registered in Madagascar; cVDPV2 were registered in Africa and Yemen; one cVDPV3 was registered in Israel. In August 2022, a VDPV2-related flaccid paralysis case was observed in New York in an unvaccinated adult and related viral strains were detected in Jerusalem and in the wastewaters of New York and London
Diphtheria	*Corynobacterium diphtheriae* (Corynebacteriaceae)	Sore throat, cough, painful swallowing, swollen glands in the neck, pseudomembranes in respiratory tract	Respiratory droplets, contact with cutaneous lesions or contaminate objects	Global deaths (2019): 4368 Incidence (2019): – High SDI (0.00); – high-middle SDI (0.01); – middle SDI (0.03); – low-middle SDI (0.07); – low SDI (0.84). In 2021, the highest number of cases was reported in Ethiopia (51.5%), India (20.5%) and Yemen (17.5%)
Whooping cough	*Bordetella pertussis* (Alcaligenaceae)	Paroxysms of coughs followed by a high-pitched "whoop" sound, encephalopathy, bronchopneumonia, asphyxia (in babies)	Respiratory droplets	Global deaths (2019): 116510 Incidence (2019): – High SDI (69.18); – high-middle SDI (82.20); – middle SDI (184.18); – low-middle SDI (305.71); – low SDI (692.88) In 2021, the highest number of cases was reported in China (33.3%) and USA (21.2%)

Table 18.1 (continued)

Disease	Etiological agent	Symptoms	Transmission	Disease burden
Tetanus	*Clostridium tetani* (Clostridiaceae)	Jaw cramping or the inability to open the mouth, muscle spasms, trouble swallowing, seizures, headache, fever, and sweating changes in blood pressure or fast heart rate	Contact with soil and contaminated material through deep cuts, wounds, or burns	Global deaths (2019): 34684 Incidence (2019): – High SDI (0.03); – high-middle SDI (0.14); – middle SDI (0.59); – low-middle SDI (1.56); – low SDI (2.63) In 2021, the highest number of cases was reported in Afghanistan (31.7%), Africa (30.2%), and south-east Asia (23%). In Afghanistan, cases increased 40 times more than in 2020
Rotavirus gastroenteritis	Rotavirus (*Sedoreoviridae*)	Diarrhea, vomiting, fever, often followed by abdominal pain and dehydration	Fecal-oral, interpersonal contact, contaminated surface	Global deaths (2019): 235331 WHO estimated that >25 million outpatient visits and >2 million hospitalizations are attributable to rotavirus infections each year. In developing countries, three-quarters of children acquire their first episode of rotavirus diarrhea before the age of 12 months
Hepatitis B	Hepatitis B virus (*Hepadnaviridae*)	Nausea, vomiting, abdominal pain, and jaundice. People with acute hepatitis can develop acute liver failure. A subset of persons develops advanced liver diseases such as cirrhosis and hepatocellular carcinoma	Sexual, perinatal, parenteral	Global deaths (2019): 555487 Incidence (2019): – High SDI (414.09); – high-middle SDI (833.18); – middle SDI (1197.20); – low-middle SDI (1096.03); – low SDI (1459.34) The WHO Western Pacific Region and the WHO African Region were the most affected with, respectively, 116 million and 81 million people chronically infected

(continued)

Table 18.1 (continued)

Disease	Etiological agent	Symptoms	Transmission	Disease burden
Meningitis	*Neisseria meningitidis* (Neisseriaceae), *Streptococcus pneumoniae* (Streptococcaceae), *Hemophilus influenzae* (Pasteurellaceae)	Neck stiffness, fever, severe headache, vomiting, nausea, seizure, sepsis, impaired consciousness, rash, cold hands and feet	Respiratory droplets and direct contact	Global deaths (2019) for *N. meningitidis*: 54427 Global deaths (2019) for *S. pneumoniae*: 82842 Global deaths (2019) for *H. influenzae*: 30440 Meningitis is highly prevalent in the African meningitis belt. In 2021, 24 of the 26 countries in the meningitis belt have conducted mass preventive campaigns, and half of them have introduced vaccinations into their national immunization schedule routines
Measles	Measles virus (*Paramyxoviridae*)	High fever, runny nose, cough, red watery eyes, rash, diarrhea, ear infections, pneumonia	Respiratory droplets and direct contact	Global deaths (2019): 83392 Incidence (2019): – High SDI (6.17); – high-middle SDI (64.62); – middle SDI (119.66); – low-middle SDI (194.43); – low SDI (488.37) In 2021, the highest number of cases was reported in Africa (72.2%) and eastern Mediterranean (21%). The most affected country was the Democratic Republic of the Congo with 44% of the global cases
Mumps	Mumps virus (*Paramyxoviridae*)	Fever, headache, muscle aches, tiredness, parotitis, pancreatitis, encephalitis	Respiratory droplets and direct contact	In 2021, the highest number of cases were reported in China (53.4%) and in Africa (37.7%)
Rubella	Rubella virus (*Matonaviridae*)	Rash, fever, nausea, mild conjunctivitis, swollen lymph glands behind the ears and in the neck, arthritis and painful joints (infected adults)	Respiratory droplets and direct contact	In 2021, the highest number of cases was reported in Africa (43.1%) and in Yemen (22%)

Table 18.1 (continued)

Disease	Etiological agent	Symptoms	Transmission	Disease burden
Chickenpox	Varicella-zoster virus (*Herpesviridae*)	Rash, fever, nausea, papules, pustules, neurological infection	Respiratory droplets and direct contact	Global deaths (2019): 14553 Incidence (2019): – High SDI (908.41); – high-middle SDI (854.29); – middle SDI (1012.61); – low-middle SDI (1143.79); – low SDI (1598.52) In 2019, 24.9% of the global cases were reported in South-East Asia region
Cervical cancer	Human Papillomavirus (*Papillomaviridae*)	Warts in genital areas, skin lesions	Sexual, skin contact	Global deaths (2019): 280479 Incidence (2019): – High SDI (6.30); – high-middle SDI (7.91); – middle SDI (7.65); – low-middle SDI (7.14); – low SDI (6.98) In 2020, the highest incidence was registered in Africa
Influenza	Influenza virus (*Orthomyxoviridae*)	Fever, cough, headache, muscle and joint pain, sore throat, runny nose, bronchitis, pneumonia	Respiratory droplets	Global deaths (2019): 243671. Cases between 2020 and 2021 are very low and may have been affected by the Covid-19 pandemic. In 2022, cases have risen, especially in Europe and America
COVID-19	SARS-CoV-2 (*Coronaviridae*)	Cough, fever, anosmia, ageusia, headaches, runny nose, muscle pain, sore throat, diarrhea, eye irritation, shortness of breath, vomiting, mild pneumonia, dyspnea, hypoxia	Respiratory droplets	Global deaths (2021): 3869997 In 2021–2022, the highest number of cases was reported in Europe and Americas
Tuberculosis	*Mycobacterium tuberculosis* (Mycobacteriaceae)	Prolonged cough, chest pain, weakness or fatigue, weight loss, fever, night sweats	Respiratory droplets	Global deaths (2020): 1.5 million Incidence: – High SDI (12.24); – High-middle SDI (52.97); – Middle SDI (101.38); – Low-middle SDI (179.44); – Low SDI (178.72) In 2020, the highest number of cases was reported in south-east Asia (43.3%). The most affected country was India with 26.2% of global cases

(continued)

Table 18.1 (continued)

Disease	Etiological agent	Symptoms	Transmission	Disease burden
Yellow fever	Yellow fever virus (*Flaviviridae*)	Fever, muscle pain with prominent backache, headache, loss of appetite, nausea, vomiting, jaundice, dark urine and abdominal pain	Bites of infected *Aedes* and *Haemagogus* mosquitoes	Global deaths (2019): 4283 Incidence (2019): – High SDI (0.00); – high-middle SDI (0.14); – middle SDI (0.27); – low-middle SDI (1.48); – low SDI (6.80) In 2021, the infection is endemic in Africa and south America. Worldwide, 281 cases were reported
Cholera	*Vibrio cholera* (Vibrionaceae)	Severe acute watery diarrhea with severe dehydration, leg cramps.	Fecal-oral	Global deaths (2019): 117241 In 2020, the global number of reported cholera cases was 65% lower than in 2019. In the same year, Yemen experienced endemic cholera due to the explosive beginning of the persistent outbreak in 2017; the number of reported cases (275,712) was 68% lower than in 2019
Typhoid fever	*Salmonella* typhi (Enterobacteriaceae)	Prolonged fever, fatigue, nausea, headache, rash, abdominal pain, and constipation or diarrhea	Contaminated food or water	Global deaths (2019): 110029 Incidence (2019): – High SDI (1.33); – high-middle SDI (22.06); – middle SDI (78.64); – low-middle SDI (243.99); – low SDI (240.64) WHO estimated 11–20 million people getting sick from typhoid. Poor communities and vulnerable groups including children are at highest risk

Incidence is expressed per 100,000 population, divided into Socio-Demographic Index (SDI). Data from Global Burden of Disease 2019 (https://www.healthdata.org/gbd/2019)

elimination and eradication targets. Particularly, measles is considered "the canary in the mine" of vaccine-preventable diseases (Box 18.1).

Box 18.1 Measles: The Canary in the Coal Mine

- Before vaccinations were introduced (1963), measles caused >2.5 million deaths each year, especially among children. Immunization program has led to a significant reduction in burden and measles-associated deaths. However, this has caused a reduction in the perceived risk of the disease and a lowering of vaccination coverage due to unjustified fear of adverse reactions (e.g., autism). Because the disease is highly contagious (R0 between 9 and 18), more than 95% immunization is required to interrupt transmission, and this is the most crucial obstacle to measles elimination/eradication. In countries with suboptimal vaccination coverage, measles occurs among young adults, with an increased risk of complications and death. Measles outbreaks can serve as a "canary in the coal mine" of health inequities and can help identify gaps in immunization programs and primary health care systems.
- In 1998, WHO declared the goal to eliminate measles through the Measles Initiative, a collaboration with American Red Cross, United Nations, and UNICEF. In 2012, the Health Assembly endorsed the Global Vaccine Action Plan, which included the objective of eliminating measles in four WHO regions by 2015 and in five by 2020. Despite a total of 82 countries having been certified as having eliminated measles at the end of 2018 and the enormous progress made in implementing surveillance and increasing vaccination coverage with a sizeable reduction in measles disease burden, the regional elimination target provided by the Global Measles and Rubella Strategic Plan 2012–2020 has not been achieved. Globally, the number of measles cases has more than doubled from 2017 to 2018, and several countries experienced large outbreaks in 2019. A new goal of measles elimination has been defined with the 2021–2030 strategic framework [2].

18.2 The Global Burden of Vaccine Preventable Diseases

The epidemiology and burden of VPDs vary across countries and regions, mainly due to differences in immunization coverage. Unvaccinated or partially vaccinated populations are at higher risk of morbidity and mortality. Other factors contributing to disease burden are geography, crowding, nutritional status, travel to and from other countries, genetic differences, and socioeconomic status of populations.

Although immunization coverage increased in recent decades, the global coverage of the three doses of diphtheria-tetanus-pertussis (DTP3) vaccination, an indicator for immunization outcomes, has remained stagnant at 85% since 2010. While vaccine coverage increased in low-income countries (LMICs), also thanks to the support of the Vaccine Alliance (GAVI) [3], it has declined in fully self-funded middle-income countries (MICs). Meanwhile, the burden of VPDs decreased significantly in the last decades but it is still high in LMICs, particularly in the African and South-East Asian WHO regions. Figure 18.1 shows the burden of the principal VPDs and the coverage of DTP3 and measles immunizations in the various WHO regions.

Disruptions due to the COVID-19 pandemic, growing inequalities in access to vaccines, and detour of resources away from routine immunization are leaving children unprotected. In addition, with millions of people displaced by conflicts and crises, disruptions in routine and emergency

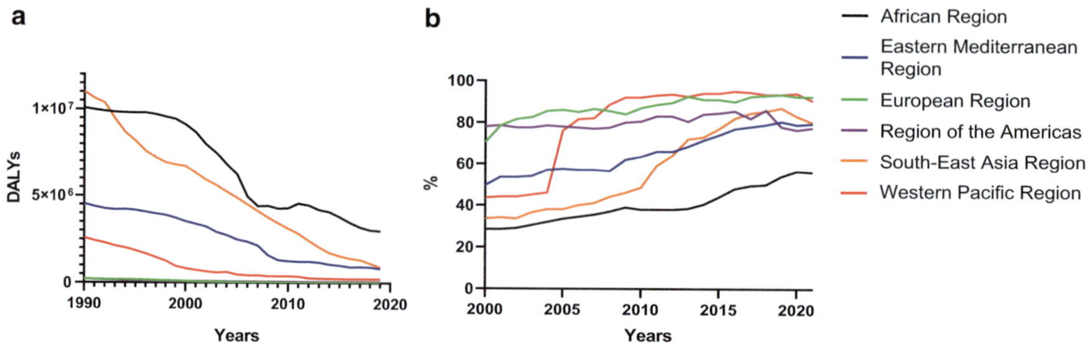

Fig. 18.1 (**a**) Disability-adjusted life years (DALYs) of measles, diphtheria, tetanus, and pertussis; (**b**) three doses of diphtheria-tetanus-pertussis (DTP3) and measles vaccination coverage broken down by WHO regions. (Data from Global Burden of Disease 2019 (https://www.healthdata.org/gbd/2019) and WHO (https://www.who.int/news-room/fact-sheets/detail/immunization-coverage))

immunizations, lack of safe water and sanitation, and overcrowding increase the risk of VPD outbreaks [4].

18.3 Progress Toward Achievement of International Targets

Thanks to EPI, global coverage of DTP3 increased from >20% in 1980 to >75% in 1990. These achievements, along with the eradication of smallpox in 1980, inspired similar goals, including the eradication of poliomyelitis, elimination of maternal and neonatal tetanus, and elimination of measles and rubella in all WHO regions [4]. The Global Vaccine Plan (GVP) was launched in 2012 by WHO with the aim of preventing millions of deaths by 2020 through access to vaccines in all countries. However, only the target for introduction of new vaccines was met (Box 18.2). GVP was further reinforced by target 3.8 of the Sustainable Development Goal (SDGs) for access to vaccines for all by 2030 [5].

In 2020, all WHO member states endorsed the 2030 Agenda for Immunization (IA2030), a global strategy to guarantee that everyone can benefit from vaccines [6].

Box 18.2 Progress Toward Meeting Core Global Vaccine Action Plan Indicators

- **Goal 1. Achieve a world free of poliomyelitis**. Wild-type poliovirus (WTP) types 2 and 3 were officially certified as globally eradicated in 2015 and 2019, respectively. With the certification of Africa as WTP free (August 2020) only Pakistan and Afghanistan continue to have endemic WTP transmission. In 2015, the "Switch" global initiative made 156 countries still using a trivalent oral polio vaccine (OPV) switch to a bivalent vaccine. In 126 countries with an OPV-only program, this was accompanied by the introduction of at least 1 dose of inactivated polio vaccine. Since 2016 a global shortage of IPV contributed to lower immunization coverages and to the emergence of vaccine-derived poliovirus type 2 (cVDPV2) cases. In 2022, cVDPV (93% were cDPV2) have been detected in 15 countries with the disease re-emerging after decades in USA, Europe, and the Middle East [7, 8].
- **Goal 2. Meet global and regional elimination targets** through the elimination of maternal and neonatal tetanus, measles, and rubella/congenital rubella

syndrome (CRS). In 1999, the Maternal and Neonatal Tetanus Initiative was launched to reduce neonatal tetanus incidence to <1/1000 live births in 59 endemic countries [9]. By 2019, 80% of these countries achieved elimination with an estimated reduction of the number of deaths from ~171,000 in 2000 to ~25,000 in 2018 [18]. Neonatal tetanus afflicts the most marginalized populations, signaling that harsh social and economic inequalities have yet to be overcome.

From 2000 to 2019, ~25.5 million measles deaths were prevented by vaccination. First-dose vaccination coverage increased globally from 72 to 84% between 2000 and 2010 but, between 2011 and 2019, it settled at 84–85% [2]. The global number of reported cases more than quadrupled from 2017 (170,000) to 2019 (863,000). The Americas, the only WHO region to verify measles elimination (2016), lost its measles-free status in 2018 due to the reestablishment of endemic transmission for >12 months in some Latin American countries; the other 5 WHO regions did not meet the elimination targets. Rubella is still endemic in many countries, and CRS is still reported.

- **Goal 3. Meet vaccination coverage targets in every region, country, and community**: the first step was to reach DTP3 90% national coverage and 80% in every district or equivalent administrative unit by 2015; the second was to achieve the same with all vaccines in national programmes by 2020, unless otherwise recommended. The DPT3 coverage remained constant at 86% between 2010 and -2018, but only about one-third of countries in 2018 have met the target. The lag in the introduction of new vaccines between rich and poor countries has shortened. Globally, vaccination coverage has increased for many vaccines but there are still many inequities between the countries [4].
- **Goal 4. Develop and introduce new and improved vaccines and technologies**: between 2010 and 2017, 116 LMIC have introduced at least one vaccine. The number of childhood vaccines in immunization programs has increased remarkably since 2000 and now immunization programs include vaccines also for older age-groups. These include measles-containing vaccines after the first year of life, booster DTP doses in preschool and school-age children, HPV vaccines in the preadolescents and adolescents, seasonal influenza vaccines, pneumococcal and shingles vaccines in the elderly, and COVID-19 vaccines. Additionally, several vaccinations are recommended for pregnant women [4].
- **Goal 5. Exceed the MDG 4 target for reducing child mortality and integration indicators**: immunizations have contributed to MDG 4 to reduce childhood mortality. All-cause mortality in children younger than 5 years decreased by 47% between the year 2000 (9.7 million deaths) and 2019 (5.2 million deaths) [4].

18.4 Determinants of Incomplete Vaccination Coverage

Globally, immunization coverage remains variable between and within countries and some populations are disproportionately under-immunized. Low and unequal vaccination coverages are the main drivers of VPDs. In 2019, an estimated 14 million infants, 62% of these residing in just ten countries, did not receive an initial DTP dose [10]. These children are from families and communities most likely also to be left out from other essential health services, to be impoverished, and to live in rural areas, urban slums, or in settings of conflict, fragility, or vulnerability.

Vaccine hesitancy, defined as "delayed acceptance or refusal of vaccination despite the availability of immunization services," has recently emerged causing sometimes large outbreaks of VPDs, leading WHO to include vaccine hesitancy among the top ten threats to global health in 2019 [11].

Finally, as a result of impaired immunization campaigns due to the COVID-19 pandemic, the global community is at risk of resurgence in VPD cases [4].

18.5 Challenges to Achieve Full Vaccination Coverage

Achieving and sustaining high and equitable vaccination coverage is the first challenge to prevent, control, and eliminate VPDs. Access to sufficient and predictable financing is essential to sustain vaccination coverage, service quality, and access to newer vaccines [12, 13]. In addition, policies that deny refugee or migrant populations immunization services as well as gender barriers (e.g., the inability of unaccompanied women to seek immunization services, the male gender of door-to-door vaccinators, prioritization of male health, gender norms, or stigmatization) must be countered. In many countries, there is a need to strengthen the capacity of human resources to manage and implement immunization programs. Limitations in the quality and use of vaccination and surveillance data have been major additional obstacles to filling current immunization gaps [4].

Finally, immunization systems must be able to recover quickly from acute shocks, such as prolonged epidemics, conflicts, and other health and social emergencies that cause their disruption [4].

18.6 Strategies for Prevention and Control

The core elements of any strategy to fight VPDs include: (1) commitment of national governments and sufficient financing; (2) adequate and sustained supply of safe and effective vaccines at free or affordable prices; (3) improved supply chain and logistics systems to ensure uninterrupted availability of vaccines; (4) focus to reach the unimmunized by promoting extraordinary approaches to reach marginalized and partially served communities; (5) improvements in delivery infrastructure, surveillance systems, and regional and global laboratory networks; (6) community engagement and advocacy on the value of vaccines; and (7) vaccine research and coordination of vaccine safety monitoring and regulatory systems.

18.7 Economic Gains

Vaccinations have a positive impact on economic growth and on the sustainability and efficiency of health systems, and economic growth, in turn, is favored by effective public health. Immunization helps end poverty and reduces hunger and inequalities. It plays a central role toward SDG achievement, particularly in LMIC. Vaccination is part of 14 of the 17 SDGs [14].

Since EPI started, novel and more expensive vaccines have been introduced and immunization costs increased. In GAVI-supported countries, public investment increased, but governmental funding represented only 37% of total immunization costs [13]. However, as the role of LMIC manufacturers in vaccine supply increases, prices of key vaccines decline [15]. UNICEF, GAVI, and the Pan American Health Organization Revolving Fund, through predictable financing and innovative procurement mechanisms, further contribute to reduce vaccine pricing.

18.8 Responsibilities of Different National and International Institutions

In 2020, all WHO Member States endorsed the IA2030 and country engagement ensured that goals and strategies are aligned with country needs. One of the most impactful weapons in the fight against VPDs is the national government commitment to prioritizing immunization programs. Many LMICs have increased their national expenditures on immunization and instituted national immunization technical advisory groups (NITAGs) to advice on vaccine and immunization-related policies. NITAGs have been established in all six WHO regions to help adapting global policies at a national level [5].

References

1. UNICEF. Immunization. https://www.unicef.org/immunization. Accessed 30 Aug 2022.
2. Measles and Rubella strategic framework: 2021–2030. https://www.who.int/publications-detail-redirect/measles-and-rubella-strategic-framework-2021-2030. Accessed 30 Aug 2022.
3. GAVI. https://www.gavi.org/. Accessed 30 Aug 2022.
4. Lindstrand A, Cherian T, Chang-Blanc D, Feikin D, O'Brien KL. The world of immunization: achievements, challenges, and strategic vision for the next decade. J Infect Dis. 2021;224(4):S452–67. https://doi.org/10.1093/infdis/jiab284.
5. WHO. Strategic Advisory Group of Experts on Immunization. The global vaccine action plan 2011–2020. Review and lessons learned 2019. https://www.who.int/publications/i/item/the-global-vaccine-action-plan-2011-2020-review-and-lessons-learned-strategic-advisory-group-of-experts-on-immunization. Accessed 30 Aug 2022.
6. WHO. Immunization agenda A 2030. https://www.who.int/teams/immunization-vaccines-and-biologicals/strategies/ia2030. Accessed 30 Aug 2022.
7. WHO. Poliomyelitis (polio). https://www.who.int/health-topics/poliomyelitis#tab=tab_1. Accessed 30 Aug 2022.
8. GPEI. GPEI strategy for the response to cVDPV2 2020–2021. https://polioeradication.org/wp-content/uploads/2020/12/cVDPV2-strategy-nOPV-rollout-fact-sheet-20201211.pdf. Accessed 30 Aug 2022.
9. WHO. Progress toward maternal and neonatal tetanus elimination—worldwide, 2000–2018. https://www.who.int/publications/i/item/WER9518. Accessed 30 Aug 2022.
10. Ozawa S, Clark S, Portnoy A, Grewal S, Brenzel L, Walker DG. Return on investment from childhood immunization in low- and middle-income countries, 2011-20. Health Aff (Millwood). 2016;35(2):199–207. https://doi.org/10.1377/hlthaff.2015.1086.
11. WHO. Ten threats to global health in 2019. https://www.who.int/news-room/spotlight/ten-threats-to-global-health-in-2019. Accessed 30 Aug 2022.
12. WHO. Global vaccine action plan 2011–2020. https://www.who.int/teams/immunization-vaccines-and-biologicals/strategies/global-vaccine-action-plan. Accessed 30 Aug 2022.
13. WHO. Intensification of routine immunization. https://www.who.int/southeastasia/activities/intensification-of-routine-immunization. Accessed 30 Aug 2022.
14. GAVI. Sustainable development goals. https://www.gavi.org/our-alliance/global-health-development/sustainable-development-goals. Accessed 30 Aug 2022.
15. WHO. Global vaccine action plan. Monitoring, evaluation & accountability. Secretariat Annual Report 2018. https://cdn.who.int/media/docs/default-source/immunization/strategy/gvap/gvap2018/gvap2018-secretariatreport_final.pdf?sfvrsn=b5211b_1. Accessed 30 Aug 2022.

19 Influenza

Donato Greco

Abstract

Influenza is an acute upper respiratory illness caused by a virus member of the Orthomyxoviridae family affected by minor annual mutations and more infrequently major genome mutations with dramatic pandemic potential. An infection with very high transmission rate that occurs in seasonal winter epidemics worldwide and affects a significant proportion of the whole population and develops severe pulmonary complications in the elderly and in high-risk groups; this resulting in high levels of work/school absenteeism and productivity losses; clinics and hospitals can be overwhelmed during peak periods of illness. Estimated cost of those seasonal epidemics can significantly affect the national budget. Global influenza surveillance has been conducted through WHO's Global Influenza Surveillance and Response System (GISRS). Prevention of influenza is based on moderately effective influenza vaccines reformulated annually according to virus type circulation and non-medical interventions. Therapy is recommended in high-risk individuals with dedicated antivirals.

Keywords

Influenza (flu) · Orthomyxoviridae · Influenza pandemics · Influenza surveillance · Influenza prevention

Influenza ("flu") is an acute viral infection of the respiratory tract presenting with fever, cough, headache, and myalgias; sometimes gastrointestinal symptoms. Rarely it can start directly with a viral pneumonia. Most cases are mild and resolve within 5–7 days, but pulmonary complications often occur and may be fatal specially among the elderly and patients with chronic conditions.

Causative agents are influenza viruses, a family of negative-sense, single-stranded, segmented RNA viruses, members of the Orthomyxoviridae. Influenza is a zoonotic disease; it is most frequent in mammals and birds. However, mainly tree types named A,B, and C affect humans with a large number of subtype combinations identifiable by the surface glycoproteins neuraminidase (N) and haemagglutinin (H). The genes of these glycoproteins are constantly changing through mutations during viral replication (a process named "drift"). The A type can also undergo dramatic change combinations with infrequent types of glycoproteins, thus leading to a completely unknown virus with high pandemic potential.

D. Greco (✉)
Istituto Superiore di Sanità, Former General Director Prevenzione Sanitaria, Ministerio della Salute, Roma, Italy

M. C. B. Raviglione et al. (eds.), *Global Health Essentials*, Sustainable Development Goals Series,
https://doi.org/10.1007/978-3-031-33851-9_19

Box 19.1 Global Influenza Surveillance

Global influenza surveillance has been conducted through WHO's Global Influenza Surveillance and Response System (GISRS) since 1952. FluNet is the web tool for both virological and epidemiological influenza data globally. Viral surveillance of influenza is performed by a network of 160 WHO-accredited influenza laboratories worldwide. They monitor in the Southern and Northern hemispheres the emergence of new influenza viruses through "drift" leading to an annual revision of effective vaccines recipes based on the constant monitoring of circulating types [1]. Several thousands of viral isolates are identified each year [2, 3]. In many countries, clinical influenza incidence is monitored through sentinel sites based on general practitioners reporting weekly ILI cases (Influenza-Like Illness) as it is done, for example, in Italy (Fig. 19.1) [2]. Mortality and morbidity of influenza are estimated with excess pneumonia mortality studies and through hospital discharge cards studies. The illness ranges from mild to severe and death. Hospitalization and death occur mainly among high-risk groups. Worldwide, these annual epidemics are estimated to result in about three to five million cases of severe illness, and about 250,000–500,000 deaths. Reported ILI incidence can go up to 10% of the whole population within 3 winter months. This results in high levels of work/school absenteeism and productivity losses. Clinics and hospitals can be overwhelmed during peak periods of illness. Estimated cost of those seasonal epidemics can significantly affect the national health budget. The effects of seasonal influenza epidemics in developing countries are not fully known, but estimates indicate that 99% of deaths in children under 5 years of age with influenza-related lower respiratory tract infections are in developing countries [4].

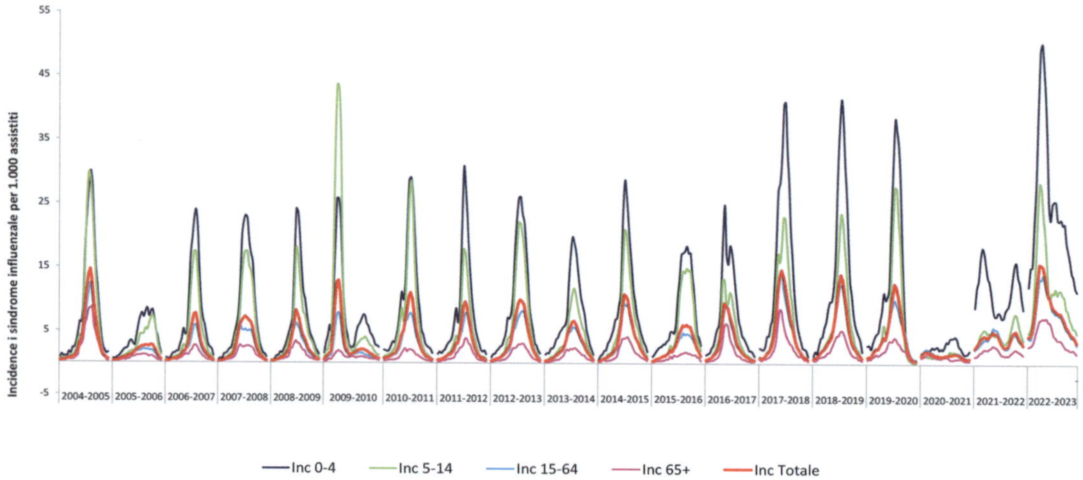

Fig. 19.1 Weekly Incidence of Influenza-Like Illness (ILI) from 1000 general practitioners nationwide in Italy

19.1 Influenza Pandemic

An influenza pandemic is a global epidemic caused by a new influenza virus to which there is little or no pre-existing immunity in the human population. Most influenza pandemics have been caused by an A type virus shifted from the seasonal one and with a genome resulting from a combination of human, avian and mammal genes. Severe disease may occur in certain risk groups, which may correspond to those at risk of severe disease due to seasonal influenza. However, healthy persons may also experience more serious disease than that caused by seasonal influenza. Influenza pandemics are impossible to predict and may be mild, or cause severe disease or death: in the twentieth century, influenza pandemics occurred three times (1918, 1957, 1968) with devastating effects [5]. The most recent pandemic occurred in 2009 and was caused by an influenza A (H1N1) virus, it is estimated to have caused between 100,000 and 400,000 deaths globally in the first year alone [6].

19.2 Prevention and Treatment

Influenza vaccines are yearly prepared according to the predicted circulating vaccine strains. They offer a significant protection (up to 80%) against severe disease and death, but they are much less effective against asymptomatic infection [7]. In the European WHO region, vaccines are recommended for people over 65 years, health workers, pregnant women and individuals with chronic conditions; while in the USA they are recommended for the entire population over 6 months of age. The WHO European Regional Office target of 75% coverage for the elderly population was recently achieved by only one country in the region. Many European Union (EU) countries expanded the recommendations for influenza vaccines to other categories such as teachers, police staff and workers in essential social services. Existing antiviral drugs proved effective in reducing disease length and frequencies of complications when administered in the first few days of disease [8].

19.3 Strategies for Control

Preparedness for pandemic influenza has been strongly promoted by WHO since 1997. Countries have been invited to produce influenza pandemic plans according to WHO guidelines and update them every 4 years [9]. Most high-income countries have produced such plans and many also conduct field exercises regularly. The EU Parliament has issued a preparedness specific deliberation asking Member States to update preparedness plans every 3 years (EU 082/2013) [10]. Unfortunately, many EU countries have been neglecting regular updates and they have been largely unprepared to cope with the recent 2020 COVID-19 pandemic.

Influenza is one of the most transmissible infections known with a basic reproduction number (R0) ranging between 1.2 and 2.7 [11] and a minimal infection dose estimated at <1 TCID50 of influenza virus [12]. These make eradication, elimination or control approaches not applicable to this disease while containment and mitigation can successfully be performed reducing substantially the disease burden. Education, vaccination, appropriate use of face masks, social distancing and school closure during seasonal peaks have been proven to reduce disease burden [13]. The needed step to more effectively cope with the influenza virus is to adopt a One Health approach globally. This implies viral and clinical surveillance of the natural virus reservoirs combined with human surveillance. These measures can lead to a predictive approach for seasonal and pandemic influenza. Finally, strengthening the existing laboratory networks for both human and animal surveillance is a condition to improve control efforts [14].

References

1. Organization mondiale de la Santé & World Health Organization. Recommended composition of influenza virus vaccines for use in the 2021–2022 northern hemisphere influenza season–Composition recommandée des vaccins antigrippaux pour la saison grippale 2021-2022 dans l'hémisphère Nord. Wkly Epidemiol Rec. 2021;96(11):77–88.
2. WHO Global Influenza Surveillance and Response System (GISRS). https://www.who.int/initiatives/global-influenza-surveillance-and-response-system.
3. Trentini F, Pariani E, Bella A, et al. Characterizing the transmission patterns of seasonal influenza in Italy: lessons from the last decade. BMC Public Health. 2022;22(1):19. https://doi.org/10.1186/s12889-021-12426-9.
4. Yazdanbakhsh M, Kremsner PG. Influenza in Africa. PLoS Med. 2009;6(12):e1000182. https://doi.org/10.1371/journal.pmed.1000182.
5. Kilbourne ED. Influenza pandemics of the 20th century. Emerg Infect Dis. 2006;12(1):9–14. https://doi.org/10.3201/eid1201.051254.
6. Wiley SK. The 2009 influenza pandemic: 10 years later. Nursing. 2020;50(1):17–20. https://doi.org/10.1097/01.NURSE.0000615128.93339.22.
7. Kissling E, Rondy M, I-MOVE/I-MOVE+ Study Team. Early 2016/17 vaccine effectiveness estimates against influenza a(H3N2): I-MOVE multicentre case control studies at primary care and hospital levels in Europe. Euro Surveill. 2017;22(7):30464. https://doi.org/10.2807/1560-7917.ES.2017.22.7.30464.
8. Ruf BR, Szucs T. Reducing the burden of influenza-associated complications with antiviral therapy. Infection. 2009;37(3):186–96. https://doi.org/10.1007/s15010-009-8241-1.
9. World Health Organization. WHO global influenza preparedness plan: the role of WHO and recommendations for national measures before and during pandemics (No. WHO/CDS/CSR/GIP/2005.5); 2005.
10. Guglielmetti P. Decision no 1082/2013/EU of the European Parliament and of the Council of 22 October 2013 on serious cross-border threats to health. 2016.
11. Biggerstaff M, Cauchemez S, Reed C, et al. Estimates of the reproduction number for seasonal, pandemic, and zoonotic influenza: a systematic review of the literature. BMC Infect Dis. 2014;14:480. https://doi.org/10.1186/1471-2334-14-480.
12. Yezli S, Otter JA. Minimum infective dose of the major human respiratory and enteric viruses transmitted through food and the environment. Food Environ Virol. 2011;3(1):1–30. https://doi.org/10.1007/s12560-011-9056-7.
13. Lafond KE, Porter RM, Whaley MJ, et al. Global burden of influenza-associated lower respiratory tract infections and hospitalizations among adults: a systematic review and meta-analysis. PLoS Med. 2021;18(3):e1003550. Published 2021 Mar 1. https://doi.org/10.1371/journal.pmed.1003550.
14. Sullivan S. Challenges in reducing influenza-associated mortality. Lancet. 2018;391(10127):1242–4. https://doi.org/10.1016/S0140-6736(17)33292-0.

20 Recent Pandemics: SARS, MERS, Ebola, and Zika

Donato Greco and Emmanuel Ochola

Abstract

The third millennium started with the Severe Acute Respiratory Syndrome outbreak in Hong Kong: an event with very peculiar characteristics fully profiting of globalization of rapid information's exchange, newly molecular diagnostic techniques and international travel, thus quickly leading to a global concern as promptly declared by World Health Organization (WHO) Public Health Emergency of International Concern (PHEIC 2002). The Middle East respiratory syndrome coronavirus (MERS) outbreak, despite its limited expansion, confirmed the international threat, but it was the large Zika outbreak with another WHO PHEIC 2015 to mark the urgent need of international cooperation and national plans to cope with emerging epidemics. In the middle of the decade (2014-16), Ebola virus broke the gates of the Ebola river traditional endemic triangle to assault large towns in west Africa counting to many thousands cases, more than half fatal. It was clear to the world the risk of newly recognized epidemics with a social and economic impact much greater than the health impact on human beings.

Keywords

Pandemics · SARS · MERS · Ebola · Zika

20.1 Epidemics Caused by Coronaviruses: SARS and MERS

In November 2002, an outbreak of severe respiratory infection (i.e., Severe Acute Respiratory Syndrome or SARS) occurred in Hong Kong and in a few weeks expanded to involve eventually 29 countries. In the end, it resulted in 8096 confirmed cases with 774 deaths. The virus responsible for the severe pneumonia was identified as the coronavirus named SARS-CoV [1]. The transmission was airborne but environmental transmission was also observed. Super-spreader individuals were associated with up to 30 secondary cases [2]. In a year time, the disease spread in many Asian countries and severely affected Canada. Among the over 8000 cases, the case fatality was 9% [3, 4]. Since then, SARS has practically disappeared despite intensive worldwide surveillance. The reasons for the disappearance are not fully understood. However, SARS-CoV-1 was mostly transmissible when patients were seriously ill. Therefore, by isolating those with symptoms, one could effectively prevent onward spread. The strong response to SARS-CoV-1 led to the extinction of that lineage of viruses in humans (Table 20.1).

D. Greco (✉)
Istituto Superiore di Sanità, Former General Director Prevenzione Sanitaria, Ministerio della Salute, Rome, Italy

E. Ochola
Lacor Hospital, Gulu, Uganda

M. C. B. Raviglione et al. (eds.), *Global Health Essentials*, Sustainable Development Goals Series,
https://doi.org/10.1007/978-3-031-33851-9_20

Table 20.1 Characteristics of recent epidemic infections

Name	Agent	Clinical features	Incubation	Reservoir	Transmission	Occurrence	Lethality	Burden	Treatment	Prevention
SARS	SARS CoV	URTI	2–10 days	Civets , bats, and other mammals	Respiratory	From Middle East to 29 coutries up to 10.000 cases from 2002 to 2020	5–10%	Severe social and economic impacts	No specific	Non-medical measures
MERS	MERS-CoV	URTI	2–14 days	Bats, camels	Respiratory	Outbreaks in Middle East but sporadic cases worldwide	6–20%	Moderate social impact	No specific	Non-medical measures
Ebola	Ebola virus	Severe haemorragic fever	5–15 days	Bats, primates	Direct contact and respiratory	More than 20 outbreaks from 1976 to 2020 all in Central Africa	30–80%	Severe social and economic impacts	No specific	Non medical measures
Zika	ZIKAV	URTI, in pregnancy preterm birth, stillbirth, microenchephaly	3–14 days	Bats and many domestic animals	Infected Aedes aeqypti and Aedes albopictus	At 2022, 89 Latin America and Southern Pacific countries reported hundreds of thousands cases	Very rare	Great impact on pregnancy in endemic countries	No specific	Mosquito control and personal protection against mosquito bites

In 2012, a new severe pneumonia associated with dromedary camels spread in southern Arabia. It was found to be caused by a new coronavirus named Middle East respiratory syndrome coronavirus (MERS)CoV virus. Small clusters and sporadic cases were identified in many countries in the following years. Overall, 27 countries have reported cases since 2012, of which 858 are known to have died due to the infection and related complications, mainly in the Middle East [5].

Both these coronavirus infections have no specific treatment. However, SARS vaccines are under development. Therefore, infection control measures constitute the main response. They rely on prompt identification and isolation of cases, respiratory droplet control with face masks, social distancing, and hand hygiene. These are the principles of the currently well-known TTT acronym (Trace, Test, Treat). Despite the limited number of cases globally, those two Coronavirus diseases had a great impact on the economy and social life of the affected countries [6].

20.2 Zika Virus Disease

Already known to be endemic in Africa and Southeast Asia as cause of acute febrile illness, Zika virus (ZIKV) arose from obscurity when an Asian genotype caused an outbreak of mild febrile illness in 2007 in Micronesia. It then became internationally well-known following a very large outbreak in Brazil in 2017 from where several hundred thousand cases were reported [7]. As of 2022, 89 countries have reported confirmed Zika virus disease cases mainly in Central and South America and in the Pacific region [8].

Zika virus, a Flaviviridae virus, spreads to people primarily through the bite of an infected mosquito (*Aedes aegypti*, *Aedes albopictus*, and other *Aedes* species). The mosquitoes that spread Zika virus can bite during day- and night-time but transmission can also occur through sexual contact, blood transfusion and from mother to foetus. While most Zika infections occur without or with very mild respiratory symptoms, Zika virus disease acquired during pregnancy can lead to severe complications including preterm birth, foetal death, and stillbirth, as well as congenital malformations such as microcephaly and other abnormal cranial morphologies [9].

Infection control measures are similar to those for malaria. They include mainly mosquito control and personal protection against mosquito bites. In endemic areas, travel recommendations for pregnant women have been adopted, and safe sex has been recommended. There is no specific treatment for Zika virus infection but several Zika vaccines are in advanced phase of development.

20.3 Ebola Virus Disease (EVD)

In October 2000, a devastating disease rapidly swept through the Gulu district, Uganda. On 28th February 2001, the outbreak was declared as 'controlled'. By then, Ebola virus disease had infected at least 425 people and killed at least 224 including 13 health workers [10]. This outbreak at the turn of the century was regarded by many as the first major Ebola outbreak contained through implementation of rapid and effective control measures thanks also to an early multisectoral government approach and the prompt engagement of WHO. Forty Ebola virus disease outbreaks, mostly in Africa, have been recorded from the first reported outbreaks in 1976 and a major epidemic in Kikwit, D.R. Congo, in 1995, through the largest epidemic in west Africa in 2014–2016. The latter resulted in 11,308 reported deaths out of the 28,610 notified cases, although real numbers may have been much higher; lately, recurrent small outbreaks in D.R. Congo kept occurring [11, 12]. Following an incubation period of 2–21 days, Ebola virus disease presents with sudden onset of fever, asthenia, myalgias, headache, and sore throat. The disease can then progress rapidly towards vomiting, diarrhoea, rash, and in the most severe cases, internal and external bleeding and features of liver and kidney failure. Ebola virus crosses species barriers to be transmitted from its suspected reservoirs—the fruit-eating bats of the Pteropodidae family—to humans through hunters or bushmeat consumers who enter in contact with body fluids of infected bats, primates, or even porcupine and antelopes. Thereafter, human-to-human transmission occurs, mainly via unprotected contact with blood, faeces, vomitus, and mucosal secretions from infected, symptomatic persons, or through infected objects and fomites. Health workers therefore are at very high risk of transmission, as are family and other contacts of infected persons. Handlers of the corpse and burial ceremonies are at specially increased risk, given religious and cultural ritual cleaning of the dead body [13]. Risk of international spread increases in the absence of prompt screening. Case fatality has ranged from 20 to 90%. The control of Ebola depends on prompt local, national, and international surveillance, preparedness, and multisectoral response. Following an outbreak, infection prevention practices in health care settings are crucial and include basic hygiene measures, personal protective equipment, availability of safe disposal of waste, precaution of handling and disposal of dead bodies, and isolation of suspected and confirmed cases [14].

Box 20.1 Epidemics of the New Millennium

The new millennium started with the emergence of SARS-CoV, a newly identified member of the well-known Coronavirus family. This was the first new disease of the twenty-first century that posed a threat to global health with its pandemic potential. It opened the Pandora's box of global pandemic risk. The initially observed very high case fatality led to an international alarm and to the prompt revision of the WHO's International Health Regulations 2005 with the new definition of Public Health Emergency of International Concern (PHEIC). The emergence of a similar Coronavirus disease, MERS, in 2012 inevitably rang the bell of a PHEIC despite the geographically limited spread. Much greater concern followed the emergence of Ebola, known to be sporadic in Africa, that evolved from its traditional pattern of village spread to assaulting large towns of west Africa. Similarly, great concern was raised by the Zika virus epidemic in 2015, an infection already known but that started spreading at high speed in several countries with the horrible complication of microcephaly in neonates from infected mothers: this prompted another PHEIC declaration.

Finally, we entered the COVID-19 era with the largest pandemic since the Spanish flu of a century before and all its multisectoral implications.

References

1. Chan-Yeung M, Rui-Heng X. SARS: epidemiology. Respirology (Carlton, Vic.). 2003;8(Suppl 1):S9–14. https://doi.org/10.1046/j.1440-1843.2003.00518.x.
2. Small M, Tse CK, Walker DM. Super-spreaders and the rate of transmission of the SARS virus. Phys D Nonlinear Phenom. 2006;215(2):146–58. https://doi.org/10.1016/j.physd.2006.01.021.
3. Chan-Yeung M, Xu RH. SARS: epidemiology. Respirology. 2003;8:S9–S14.
4. Al-Omari A, Rabaan AA, Salih S, Al-Tawfiq JA, Memish ZA. MERS coronavirus outbreak: implications for emerging viral infections. Diagn Microbiol Infect Dis. 2019;93(3):265–85. https://doi.org/10.1016/j.diagmicrobio.2018.10.011. Epub 2018 Oct 18
5. WHO MERS situation update. 2022. http://www.emro.who.int/health-topics/mers-cov/mers-outbreaks.html.
6. Keogh-Brown MR, Smith RD. The economic impact of SARS: how does the reality match the predictions? Health Policy. 2008;88(1):110–20.
7. Hills SL, Fischer M, Petersen LR. Epidemiology of Zika virus infection. J Infect Dis. 2017;216(suppl_10):S868–74. https://doi.org/10.1093/infdis/jix434.
8. WHO Zika epidemiology update. 2022. https://www.who.int/publications/m/item/zika-epidemiology-update%2D%2D-february-2022.
9. Halani S, Tombindo PE, O'Reilly R, et al. Clinical manifestations and health outcomes associated with Zika virus infections in adults: a systematic review. PLoS Negl Trop Dis. 2021;15(7):e0009516. https://doi.org/10.1371/journal.pntd.0009516.
10. Francesconi P, Yoti Z, Declich S, Onek PA, Fabiani M, Olango J, et al. Ebola hemorrhagic fever transmission and risk factors of contacts, Uganda. Emerg Infect Dis. 2003;9(11):1430.
11. Qureshi AI. Ebola virus disease epidemic in light of other epidemics. Ebola Virus Disease. 2016:39–65.
12. González PA, Camporro ÁF, Eriksson A, Llada CA. The epidemiological presentation pattern of Ebola virus disease outbreaks: changes from 1976 to 2019. Prehosp Disaster Med. 2020;35(3):247–53.
13. Manguvo A, Mafuvadze B. The impact of traditional and religious practices on the spread of Ebola in West Africa: time for a strategic shift. Pan Afr Med J. 2015;22(Suppl 1):9.
14. World Health Organization. Ebola and Marburg virus disease epidemics: preparedness, alert, control, and evaluation. World Health Organization; 2014.

Coronavirus Disease 19 (COVID-19) 21

Andrea Gori, Federico Fama, and Camilla Genovese

Abstract

The COVID-19 pandemic represents one of the greatest threats to economies and health systems worldwide.

As of August 2022, more than 600 million people had been infected with SARS-CoV-2, causing an unprecedented health emergency that shattered health systems on a global level.

This catastrophic phenomenon can be explained not only by the biological features of the virus, but most importantly by the social, economic, and cultural changes that society has been experiencing in the last decades.

The international response was coordinated by the WHO, even if national governments applied diverse public health measures, with very different outcomes. Vaccine coverage, evidence-based public health measures and policy designed to protect the most vulnerable populations are the three main tools that international and national organizations must implement in order to end this emergency.

A. Gori (✉) · F. Fama · C. Genovese
Centre for Multidisciplinary Research in Health Science (MACH), University of Milan, Milan, Italy
e-mail: andrea.gori@unimi.it; camilla.genovese@unimi.it

Keywords

COVID-19 pandemic · Public Health Emergency of International Concern (PHEIC) · Global governance · Zoonotic diseases

21.1 The COVID-19 Pandemic

The Severe Acute Respiratory Syndrome Coronavirus 2 (SARS-CoV-2) virus is the etiologic agent of Coronavirus disease 2019 (COVID-19), resulted from a spillover supposedly from bats and via other animals [1]. COVID-19 is a respiratory disease that may evolve into an interstitial pneumonia and, in 5% of the cases, might result in respiratory failure and death. It was firstly reported in China in December 2019; on 30 January 2020, the SARS-CoV-2 outbreak was declared Public Health Emergency of International Concern (PHEIC) by the WHO, and on March 11th the Director General officially declared the COVID-19, a pandemic [2].

The unexpectedly rapid explosion of COVID-19, with ≈630 million cases and more than 6.5 million deaths (by end of October 2022), represents one of the greatest threats to economies and health systems of our century [3] (Fig. 21.1).

SARS-CoV-2 has some biological features that promoted its unprecedented spread throughout the globe:

M. C. B. Raviglione et al. (eds.), *Global Health Essentials*, Sustainable Development Goals Series,
https://doi.org/10.1007/978-3-031-33851-9_21

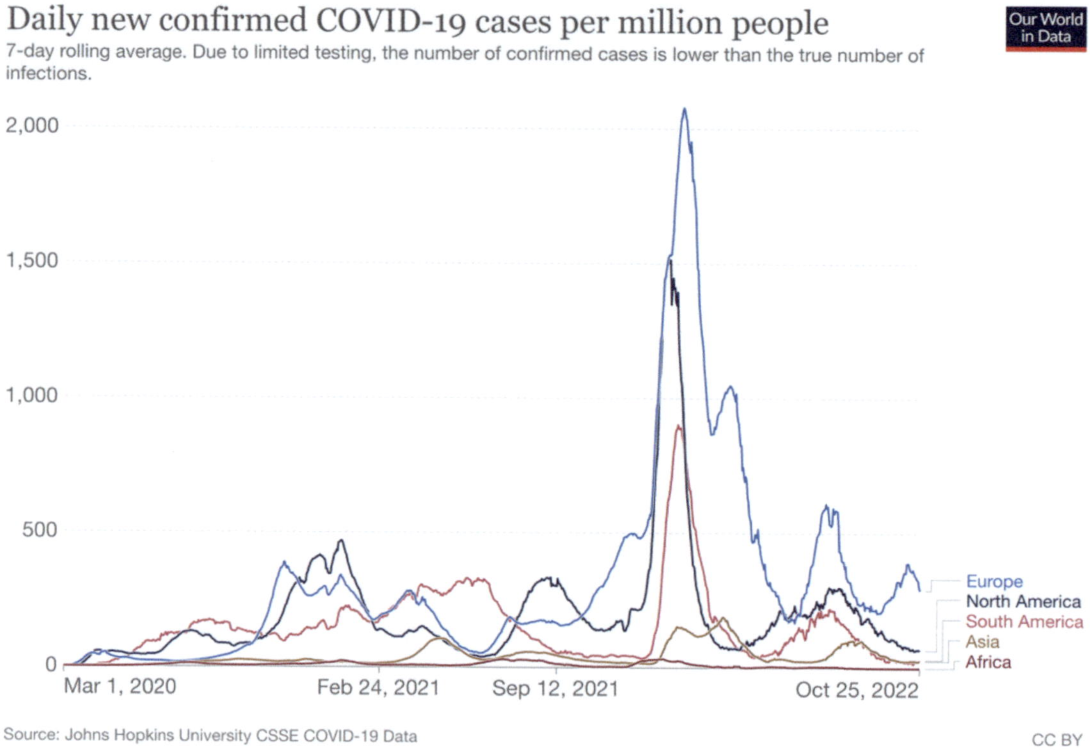

Fig. 21.1 Incidence of confirmed COVID-19 cases per continent (as of end-October 2022). Source: Edouard Mathieu, Hannah Ritchie, Lucas Rodés-Guirao, Cameron Appel, Charlie Giattino, Joe Hasell, Bobbie Macdonald, Saloni Dattani, Diana Beltekian, Esteban Ortiz-Ospina and Max Roser (2020) – 'Coronavirus Pandemic (COVID-19)'. Published online at OurWorldInData.org. Retrieved from: 'https://ourworldindata.org/coronavirus' [Online Resource]

- Airborne transmission with a high R0 index
- Long prodromal period
- Age-dependent severity/mortality
- 1/3 of the cases remain asymptomatic but are still infectious [4]

21.2 Socioeconomical Impact

However, the socioeconomical changes that society underwent in the last decades and the relative weaknesses of national health systems and supranational health organizations were crucial to boost the magnitude of this phenomenon. Globalization led the world to unprecedented levels of human interconnectivity, mobility, and sociodemographic transformations: it is reasonable to think that the rise of world population, the increased density in urban population, especially in low- and low-middle income countries facilitated the spread of the infection.

Moreover, COVID-19 had a greater impact on vulnerable populations: groups that have experienced increased rates of COVID-19 morbidity and mortality include poorer people, marginalized and discriminated minorities, low-paid essential workers, migrants, and homeless [5].

Furthermore, over the last decade, it was demonstrated how climate change has been having an impact on the emergence and spread of infectious diseases, especially zoonoses. By altering the human–environment–animal interface, climate change contributes to pathogen mutations and transmission, as well as new dis-

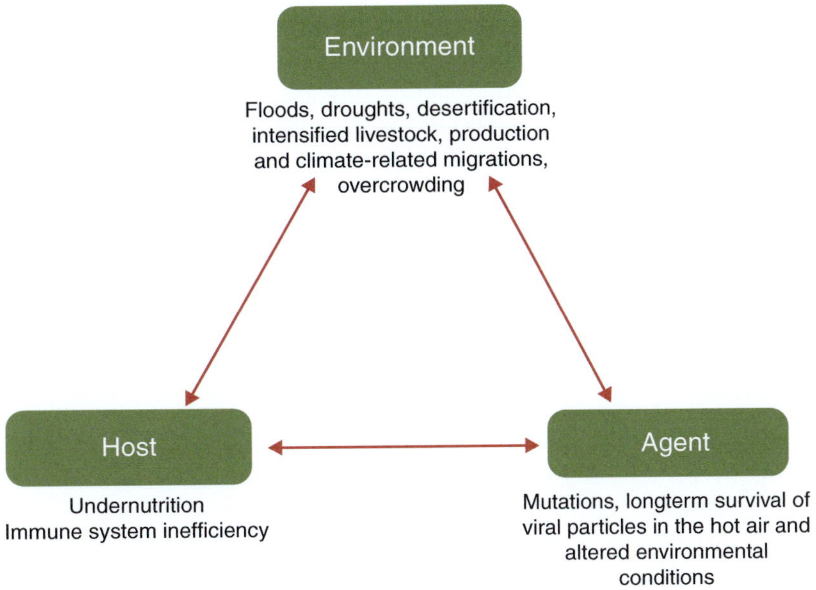

Fig. 21.2 Environmental, host, and agent dependent factors that have contributed to spread of COVID-19

tribution of reservoirs, carriers, and exposure to new and wider ranges of host population [6, 7]. These principles are the cornerstone of the so-called *One Health* approach, an integrated and holistic perspective that recognizes the intrinsic link between the health of humans, animals, and ecosystems [8] (Fig. 21.2).

21.3 Containment and Elimination

In general, considering the response overall, it is noteworthy that almost all countries were unprepared with respect to the spread of the pandemic. In particular, the national governments' response to this phenomenon all around the globe established different Public Health (PH) strategies that varied in terms of stringency such as social distancing, contact tracing, stay-at-home, use of sanitizing solutions and disposable masks, lockdowns; national governments adopted more restrictive strategies (i.e. lockdowns), during the first waves of the pandemic in 2020, later shifting towards less severe restrictions as vaccines, monoclonal and antiviral therapies started to be massively administrated to the public (more in high-income than in low- and middle-income countries (LMICs)) and the emergence of less pathogenic but more infectious variants.

Some measures showed a significant effectiveness only during the first waves of the pandemic and during periods with reduced incidence of infection, such as lockdowns and contact tracing, while later on they showed to be less effective due to the emergence of new highly contagious variants; other measures such as social distancing and the promotion of masks are still strongly recommended by supranational health authorities, such as the WHO, the CDC and ECDC [9].

21.4 An International Issue: The Role of Supranational Organizations

On a larger scale, the WHO is the main institution that led the COVID-19 response: its contribution not only was limited to share medical expertise, data, and fight misinformation, but also pushed forward the development of vaccines and therapeutics against coronaviruses [3]. An important milestone was reached with the resolution adopted at the 77th WHA in

December 2021 that authorizes the formulation of an international agreement on pandemic prevention, preparedness, and response (the so-called Pandemic Treaty); the project is ongoing and should be completed by 2024 [10].

However, the WHO was heavily criticized for its relatively slow response and scarce preparation, and its mild initial countermeasures regarding China's approach to control the epidemic, causing exacerbations of geopolitical tensions [11].

Also, in order not only to counteract to the COVID-19 pandemic but also to improve preparedness for future health threats, national and regional initiatives and organizations were instituted; some significant examples are listed in Box 21.1.

Box 21.1 Distinctive Features and Functions of the Main National and Regional Initiatives Against COVID-19

Institution	Country	Functions	Main features
BARDA (US Biomedical Advanced Research and Development Authority)	United States of America	Prepare and maintain system of medical countermeasures for PH emergencies, providing a systematic approach to the R&D of vaccines, diagnostics, and therapeutic tools	Founded in 2006, during the COVID-19 pandemic became part of public–private partnerships to sponsor and develop medical countermeasures
HERA (EU Health Emergency Preparedness and Response Authority)	European Union	Ensuring the rapid development of medicines, vaccines and other medical countermeasures for EU citizens, aiming to fill the gaps in the EU preparedness towards health emergencies	Launched in 2021 with a prospected budget of six billion euros for its first 6 years
ARIA (UK Advanced Research and Invention Agency)	United Kingdom	Focus on projects with potential to produce transformative technological change	Created in 2021, with an initial budget of 2.4% of GDP on R&D by 2027
SCARDA (Strategic Center of Biomedical Advanced Vaccine Research and Development for Preparedness and Response)	Japan	Data collection and analysis focused on vaccine R&D to deliver safe and effective vaccines for a priority list of infectious diseases	Set up in March 2022 within the Japan Agency for Medical Research, it will have a budget of 420 million USD for infrastructure and 1.22 billion USD for R&D
BRICS Vaccine Research and Development (R&D) Center	Brazil, Russia, India, China, South Africa	Strengthen vaccine cooperation to ensure the accessibility and affordability of vaccines in developing countries through their equitable distribution as global public goods	Launched in March 2022, creates a network between the agencies of the BRICS countries
AFTCOR (Africa Task Force for Novel Coronavirus)	African Union	Ensure better coordination with existing regional structures (Africa CDC). It is supposed to provide an incident management system to its Member States and to support technical assistance	Founded in February 2020 by African Health Ministers and Africa CDC to respond to manage the COVID-19 response

What became clear is the importance of the cooperation between the public and the private health sectors. The Bill and Melinda Gates Foundation played a decisive role in the pandemic management, providing more than two billion dollars in the fight against COVID-19 [12] and sponsoring WHO, several NGOs, and pharmaceutical companies [13].

This new perception led to the creation of two new institutions: ACT-A (Access to COVID-19 tools Accelerator) [14], a global collaboration to accelerate the development, production, and equitable access to COVID-19 tests, treatments, and vaccines and its subordinate COVAX [15], led by WHO, GAVI, UNICEF, and CEVI in order to provide equitable access to COVID-19 vaccines.

21.5 An Open Issue: Challenges and Future Prospects

Despite the important global community effort, the pandemic has still revealed alarming structural and social inequalities within and between countries worldwide.

Vaccine coverage is very heterogeneous across the globe: as of end October 2022, ≈68% of world population had received at least one dose of COVID-19 vaccine, but the coverage ranged from less than 1% in some low-income countries, to over 85% in wealthier countries [16]. Possible reasons include restricted funding and financial constraints, reduced supply because of violent political backgrounds, reduced capacity for vaccine production and distribution, inconsistent access because of vaccine misinformation [17].

Beyond its direct effect on health, COVID-19 has had dramatic and unequal socio-economic consequences: economic disruptions and growing rates of unemployment have reduced the income of billions of people and drove almost 100 million people into extreme poverty, particularly in LMICs [18].

This vicious circle exacerbates health inequities, not only in the current pandemic but also many years into the future.

Furthermore, the scarcity of health resources and redirection of healthcare professionals towards COVID-19 departments strongly impacted the access to health services, thereby influencing the overall mortality for all causes (i.e., failed cancer screenings, lost to follow-up patients with chronic diseases, decreased access to emergency rooms), especially in low-resource settings [19].

In conclusion, the impact of the SARS-CoV-2 pandemic has been mitigated through mass vaccinations, new treatments, free mass testing, and PH control measures. However, this is a virus that is destined to become endemic, and the COVID-19 pandemic as of today is far to be over.

The main steps needed to be taken in order to end this global phenomenon are:

1. **Extending vaccine, monoclonal and antiviral treatments coverage**: it is imperative to promote an equitable production, supply and distribution of COVID-19 vaccines in LMICs, therefore building capacity for locally produced vaccines.
2. National governments need to **design evidence-based PH plans**, designed to easily adapt to the circumstances and new events. WHO and global health agencies should coordinate the implementation of these plans.
3. **Safeguard vulnerable populations**: COVID-19 is a severe disease but proved to impact more certain populations, that need to be taken into consideration and to have specifically designed PH strategies to protect them [20].

References

1. Gupta S, Rouse BT, Sarangi PP. Did Climate Change Influence the Emergence, Transmission, and Expression of the COVID-19 Pandemic? Front Med. 2021;8:2549.
2. World Health Organization. COVID-19 Public Health Emergency of International Concern (PHEIC) Global research and innovation forum 2020. https://www.who.int/publications/m/item/covid-19-public-health-emergency-of-international-concern-(pheic)-global-research-and-innovation-forum.

3. World Health Organization & R&D Blueprint. COVID-19 Research and innovation achievements. 2021. https://cdn.who.int/media/docs/default-source/documents/r-d-blueprint-meetings/r-d-achievements-report_v42.pdf?sfvrsn=c4728b39_10&download=true.
4. Gates B. Responding to Covid-19—a once-in-a-century pandemic? N Engl J Med. 2020;382:1677–9.
5. World Health Organization. COVID-19 and the social determinants of health and health equity: evidence brief. World Health Organization; 2021.
6. Volkov V. System analysis of the fast global coronavirus disease 2019 (COVID-19) spread. Can we avoid future pandemics under global climate change? Commun. Integr Biol. 2022;15:150–7.
7. Mirsaeidi M, et al. PERSPECTIVES Climate Change and Respiratory Infections. Ann Am Thorac Soc. 2016;13:1223–30.
8. One health. https://www.who.int/health-topics/one-health#tab=tab_1.
9. Girum T, et al. Optimal strategies for COVID-19 prevention from global evidence achieved through social distancing, stay at home, travel restriction and lockdown: a systematic review. Arch Public Heal. 2021;79:1–18.
10. Parliamentary question | WHO pandemic treaty | P-000921/2022 | European Parliament. https://www.europarl.europa.eu/doceo/document/P-9-2022-000921_EN.html.
11. The World Health Organization and Pandemic Politics | Think Global Health. https://www.thinkglobalhealth.org/article/world-health-organization-and-pandemic-politics.
12. Funding commitments to fight COVID-19 | Bill & Melinda Gates Foundation. https://www.gatesfoundation.org/ideas/articles/covid19-contributions.
13. Tchiombiano S. L'influence à double tranchant de Bill Gates sur la santé mondiale. AOC; 2022.
14. The Access to COVID-19 Tools (ACT) Accelerator. https://www.who.int/initiatives/act-accelerator.
15. World Health Organization. COVAX—working for global equitable access to COVID-19 vaccines. https://www.who.int/initiatives/act-accelerator/covax.
16. Coronavirus (COVID-19) vaccinations—our world in data. https://ourworldindata.org/covid-vaccinations.
17. Wells CR, Galvani AP. The global impact of disproportionate vaccination coverage on COVID-19 mortality. Lancet Infect Dis. 2022;22(9):1254–5. https://doi.org/10.1016/S1473-3099(22)00417-0.
18. International Monetary Fund. Global prospects and policies. World Econ Outlook. 2020;2020:1–60.
19. COVID-19 continues to disrupt essential health services in 90% of countries. https://www.who.int/news/item/23-04-2021-covid-19-continues-to-disrupt-essential-health-services-in-90-of-countries.
20. Perkins J, et al. The distinct impacts of race and genetic ancestry on health. Nat Med. 2022;28:890–3. https://doi.org/10.1038/s41591-022-01796-1.

22 Antimicrobial Resistance

Haileyesus Getahun

Abstract

Antimicrobial Resistance (AMR) occurs when bacteria, viruses, fungi and parasites no longer respond to antimicrobial agents. Antimicrobials are used in humans, animals and plants for both treatment and prevention purposes, and they are continuously released into the environment. Although the true global burden of AMR across humans, animals and plants is not known, there is growing evidence of increasing trend due to the overuse and misuse of antimicrobials. Antibacterial drug resistance alone is estimated to cause 1.27 million human deaths annually. AMR is a complex challenge that require a comprehensive response through a "One Health" approach so that antimicrobials are preserved.

Keywords

Antimicrobial resistance (AMR) · Antimicrobial agents · Antimicrobials · Drug resistance · One Health

22.1 Definitions and Main Features

Antimicrobials—including antibiotics, antivirals, antifungals and antiparasitic drugs—are drugs used to prevent, control and treat infectious diseases in humans, animals and plants. Antimicrobial Resistance (AMR) occurs when bacteria, viruses, fungi and parasites no longer respond to antimicrobial agents [1]. As a result of drug resistance, antibiotics and other antimicrobial agents become ineffective and infections become difficult or impossible to treat, increasing the risk of disease spread, severe illness and death. The capability to select for resistance to at least some antimicrobial agents is a natural phenomenon that is shared among pathogens. Generally, the drug resistance mechanisms of bacteria are well studied compared with those for viruses, fungi and parasites. Several mechanisms exist that facilitate the selection for drug resistance by bacteria: limiting the uptake of the drug; facilitating the active efflux of the drug; modifying the target of the drug; and inactivation of a drug [2]. Mechanisms for antifungal resistance include interference with the antifungal mechanism of the respective drug often through action on the fungal cell wall and cell membrane [3]. These mechanisms for bacteria and fungi may be native to the microorganisms or acquired from other microorganisms when environmental factors lead to colonization or replacement of a susceptible species with a resistant one [2, 3].

H. Getahun (✉)
World Health Organization, Geneva, Switzerland
e-mail: getahunh@who.int

M. C. B. Raviglione et al. (eds.), *Global Health Essentials*, Sustainable Development Goals Series,
https://doi.org/10.1007/978-3-031-33851-9_22

22.2 Global Burden of Antimicrobial Resistance

The true global burden of AMR across all pathogens and classes of drugs as well as across humans, animals and plants is not known. However, there is evidence of increasing trend of development and transmission of drug-resistant infections among humans, animals and plants largely due to the overuse and misuse of antimicrobials.

It was estimated that in 2019, 1.27 million deaths occurred due to drug resistant bacterial infections and that AMR indirectly contributed to 4.9 million deaths [4]. A study from point prevalence surveys reporting AMR rates in animals focusing on *Escherichia coli, Campylobacter* spp., *non-typhoidal Salmonella* spp., *and Staphylococcus aureus* showed that between 2000 and 2018 the proportion of antimicrobial compounds with resistance higher than 50% increased from 0.15 to 0.41 in chickens and from 0.13 to 0.34 in pigs and plateaued between 0.12 and 0.23 in cattle [5].

There is no comprehensive global burden data about drug resistant viral, fungal or parasitic infections. However, there is evidence that non-invasive fungal diseases are rising overall and particularly among immunocompromised populations. The diagnosis and treatment of invasive fungal diseases are challenged by limited access to quality diagnostics and treatment as well as emergence of antifungal resistance in many settings. These further limit the ability to understand the true burden. The case of multidrug-resistant *Candida auris* highlights the challenge of drug-resistant fungal infections: in fact, it not only causes increased morbidity and mortality for hospitalized patients, but this pathogen is also difficult to eradicate from hospitals, even with intensive infection-prevention strategies [6].

The COVID-19 pandemic has exacerbated the misuse of antibiotics and other antimicrobials including antifungals and it is expected to further worsen the global burden of antimicrobial resistance [7]. A review of studies published on hospitalized COVID-19 patients identified that while 72% (1450/2010) of patients received antibiotics, only 8% (62/806) demonstrated superimposed bacterial or fungal co-infections [8]. The US Centre for Diseases Control reported that nearly 30,000 people died from antimicrobial-resistant infections during the first year of the COVID-19 pandemic, and nearly 40% of the infections were acquired in hospital [9]. Similarly, there was a widespread use of azithromycin among COVID-19 patients, although there was no evidence of any benefit and an association with adverse events [10].

22.3 Determinants and Challenges of Antimicrobial Resistance

Although antimicrobial resistance can develop naturally, misuse and overuse of antimicrobial agents in humans, terrestrial and aquatic animals, plants and crops are greatly accelerating its development and spread. Concomitantly inadequate access to quality and affordable antibiotics alone kills nearly six million people annually, including a million children who die of preventable sepsis and pneumonia [11]. Poor medical prescribing practices and patient adherence to therapies, weak regulations and oversight including over-the-counter sales, and the proliferation of substandard and falsified antimicrobials are all contributing to the problem both in humans and animals [12].

Many low- and middle-income countries face a higher burden of disease and increased risk of antimicrobial resistance due to poor access to basic water, sanitation and hygiene in health care facilities, farms, schools, households and community settings and weak infection prevention and control in health facilities, farms and food and feed production. Similarly weak waste management and environmental protection facilities further accelerate the transmission and spread of drug-resistant infections. (see panel).

The use of antimicrobials to promote growth and routinely prevent disease in healthy animals and plants, without appropriate veterinary or phytosanitary indication and in the absence of good agricultural practices, to prevent infectious diseases in farms are further contributing to the development and spread of antimicrobial resistance including risk of transmission of drug resistant infections to humans [13]. Similarly, studies suggest that as global and local temperatures rise due to the climate changes, antimicrobial resistance and rates of infection are increasing in humans, animals, plants and the environment [14].

Key challenges in the AMR response include the exit of major pharmaceutical companies from new antibiotic research and development due to market failure, the absence of effective regulations and antimicrobial stewardship programmes in humans, animals and plants and limited access to quality and affordable antimicrobials and their alternatives.

22.4 International Goals and Targets on Antimicrobial Resistance

At the moment, there are no international targets to guide the global response on AMR agreed by all countries. Although antimicrobial resistance has no specific targets in the Sustainable Development Goals (SDGs), it is recognized as a barrier to the achievement of several SDGs including on human health and other SDGs related to food security, clean water and sanitation, and responsible consumption and production. Due to cascading impacts on economic development and inequality, antimicrobial resistance also indirectly threatens progress against the SDGs that aim to reduce poverty and inequality. More recently, the 2020 comprehensive review of the SDGs indicator framework resulted in the inclusion of a new indicator on bloodstream infections due to selected antimicrobial-resistant organisms among patients seeking care and blood sampled [15]. The first set of microorganisms included for the measurement are methicillin-resistant *Staphylococcus aureus* (MRSA) and *Escherichia coli* resistant to third-generation cephalosporins. Despite these pathogens being already captured by the WHO GLASS (Global Antimicrobial Resistance and Use Surveillance System), the inability to get representative data to inform policy and programmatic action is a major challenge. The WHO 13th General Programme of Work 2019–2023 includes a country-level target of having at least 60% of total antibiotic consumption being in the access group antibiotics (a category of antibiotics that are affordable, safe and have a low AMR risk) [16] employing the WHO AWaRe (Access, Watch, Reserve) categorization of antibiotics. The other categories of the AWaRe categorization include Watch (a category of antibiotics with higher resistance potential) and Reserve (a category of antibiotics which should be treated as the last resort of treatment options) [17].

However, there are several commitments and political declarations on AMR. AMR has been a constant agenda item in political discussions like those at G7 and G20 meetings as well as Ministerial Conferences. The First and Second Ministerial Conferences on AMR organized by the Government of the Netherlands in 2014 and 2019 have been instrumental in catalysing the global response to address AMR. The key outcome of the first ministerial conference was accelerated political commitment and action that facilitated the development of the WHO Global Action Plan on AMR in 2015 as well as the UN General Assembly High Level Meeting on AMR in September 2016. The Second Ministerial Conference led to the establishment of the AMR Multipartner Trust Fund with a five million US dollars initial financial commitment from the Government of the Netherlands. The Third Ministerial Conference was hosted by the government of Oman in November 2022 with the outcome of the Muscat Ministerial Manifesto. This also includes three global targets on AMR for the first time: (1) reduce the total amount of antimicrobials used in the agri-food system at least by 30–50% by 2030 from the current level; (2) zero use of medically important antimicrobials for human medicine in animals for non-veterinary medical use and in crop production for non-phytosanitary use in the agri-food systems; and (3) ensure that access group antibiotics are at least ≥60% of overall antibiotic consumption in humans by 2030. These targets are intended to inform the next UN General Assembly High Level Meeting on AMR scheduled for 2024.

22.5 The Quadripartite Collaboration for AMR

The UN Food and Agriculture Organisation (FAO), the United Nations Environment Programme (UNEP); the World Health Organisation (WHO); and the World Organisation of Animal Health (WOAH, founded as OIE) represent the four intergovernmental agencies with mandate and competencies to address the multisectoral aspects of AMR using the "One Health" Approach.

The 2016 political declaration of the United Nations High Level Meeting on Antimicrobial Resistance emphasized the need for a coordinated approach that engages the human, animal, plant and environmental health sectors and requested that the Secretary-General of the United Nations establish an *ad hoc* Interagency Coordination Group (IACG) on AMR. In its 2019 report, the IACG made several recommendations around global governance including strengthened collaboration and leadership by the Quadripartite Organizations to respond to the complex challenges of AMR.

Although the four organisations have a long history of working together on AMR and other issues, their commitment on AMR was formalized with the signature of a Memorandum of Understanding in 2018 between FAO, WOAH and WHO, which was later updated with the inclusion of UNEP in 2022. Furthermore, in 2019 the four organisations established the Quadripartite Joint Secretariat on AMR led by a director and hosted at WHO with full time Liaison Officers from FAO, UNEP and WOAH. The activities of the Quadripartite Organisations are guided by a Strategic Framework that defines their shared vision and purpose of collaboration: to preserve antimicrobial efficacy and ensure sustainable and equitable access to antimicrobials for responsible and prudent use in human, animal and plant health, thus contributing to achieving the Sustainable Development Goals [18].

References

1. WHO. Antimicrobial Resistance. 2020. https://www.who.int/news-room/fact-sheets/detail/antimicrobial-resistance.
2. Reygaert WC. An overview of the antimicrobial resistance mechanisms of bacteria. AIMS Microbiol. 2018;4(3):482–501.
3. Denning DW. Antifungal drug resistance: an update. Eur J Hosp Pharm. 2022;29(2):109–12.
4. Antimicrobial Resistance Collaborators. Global burden of bacterial antimicrobial resistance in 2019: a systematic analysis. Lancet. 2022;12(399):629–55.
5. Van Boeckel TP, et al. Global trends in antimicrobial resistance in animals in low- and middle-income countries. Science. 2019;365(6459):eaaw1944.
6. Lockhart SR, Etienne KA, Vallabhaneni S, Farooqi J, Chowdhary A, Govender NP, et al. Simultaneous emergence of multidrug-resistant Candida auris on 3 continents confirmed by whole-genome sequencing and epidemiological analyses. Clin Infect Dis. 2017;64(2):134–40.
7. Getahun H, Smith I, Trivedi K, Paulin S, Balkhy HH. Tackling antimicrobial resistance in the COVID-19 pandemic. Bull World Health Organ. 2020;98(7):442–442A.
8. Rawson TM, Moore LSP, Zhu N, Ranganathan N, Skolimowska K, Gilchrist M, et al. Bacterial and fungal co-infection in individuals with coronavirus: a rapid review to support COVID-19 antimicrobial prescribing. Clin Infect Dis. 2020;71(9):2459–68. https://doi.org/10.1093/cid/ciaa530.
9. US Centers for Disease Control and Prevention. Covid-19 & antibiotic resistance: impact report. 2022. https://www.cdc.gov/drugresistance/covid19.html.
10. Antonazzo IC, et al. Azithromycin use and outcomes in patients with COVID-19: an observational real-world study. Int J Infect Dis. 2022;124:27–34.
11. Laxminarayan R, et al. Access to effective antimicrobials: a worldwide challenge. Lancet. 2016;387:168–75.
12. WHO. Interagency Coordination Group on Antimicrobial Resistance Report. No time to wait. 2019.
13. Vieira AR, et al. Association between antimicrobial resistance in Escherichia coli isolates from food animals and blood stream isolates from humans in Europe: an ecological study. Foodborne Pathog Dis. 2011;8(12):1295–301.
14. McGough S, et al. Rates of increase of antibiotic resistance and ambient temperature in Europe: a cross-national analysis of 28 countries between 2000 and 2016. Euro Surveill. 2020;25(45):1900414.
15. UN. Global indicator framework for the Sustainable Development Goals and targets of the 2030 Agenda for Sustainable Development. https://unstats.un.org/sdgs/indicators/indicators-list/.

16. WHO. Thirteenth General Programme of Work 2019–2023. https://www.who.int/about/what-we-do/thirteenth-general-programme-of-work-2019-2023.
17. Sharland, et al. The WHO essential medicines list AWaRe book: from a list to a quality improvement system. Clin Microbiol Infect. 2022;28(12):1533–5.
18. FAO, OIE, WHO and UNEP. Strategic framework for collaboration on antimicrobial resistance https://www.who.int/publications/i/item/9789240045408.

23 Foodborne Diseases

Mirella Pontello and Maria Gori

Abstract

The category of foodborne diseases (FBDs) includes all diseases whose causative agent, often of zoonotic origin, may be carried—although not exclusively—by food. This chapter will focus only on biological agents, responsible for approximately 600 million FBDs cases yearly. Globally, a disease burden of >33 million DALYs was calculated based on a selection of 11 agents causing diarrhoea, 8 agents responsible for invasive forms and 10 helminths. Over 80% of the burden is attributable to bacteria. The median DALYs rates are particularly high in three WHO regions, AFR, SEAR and EMR, where the occurrence of FBDs is strongly influenced by poverty and lack of essential sanitation facilities (drinking water supply and adequate sewage disposal). Several targets included in the SDGs 2015–2030 call for interventions to reduce the enormous global health impact of FBDs, for which the set goal is control and not elimination.

Keywords

Foodborne diseases (FBDs) · Biological agents · Diarrheal disease or diarrhoea · Invasive diseases · Helminths

M. Pontello (✉) · M. Gori
Department of Health Sciences, University of Milan, Milan, Italy
e-mail: mirella.pontello@unimi.it; maria.gori@unimi.it

23.1 Definition

According to the WHO, a foodborne disease (FBD) is simply defined as 'a disease commonly transmitted through ingested food'. However, this is a very complex topic that also closely intersects with waterborne diseases and is of great interest for global health. The over 200 FBDs of various aetiologies have a significant impact on the morbidity and mortality worldwide and on the health systems and socio-economic development of different countries [1]. This chapter will only focus on biological agents, excluding other causative agents (e.g., chemical or physical agents).

23.2 Descriptive Epidemiology and Global Burden Assessment

The epidemiology of FBDs is influenced by the broad spectrum of agents involved, the great variety of clinical manifestations (from asymptomatic to life-threatening), their burden in the general population and in at-risk groups, and transmission pathways. For many foodborne pathogens, also transmission through water, soil, air, direct contacts between people, and between people and animals may be involved.

Data obtained from passive surveillance systems generally only represent the tip of the iceberg. For a FBD case to be diagnosed and reported to health authorities, after the consumption of

M. C. B. Raviglione et al. (eds.), *Global Health Essentials*, Sustainable Development Goals Series, https://doi.org/10.1007/978-3-031-33851-9_23

contaminated food, a series of conditions must be met, and this causes an underestimation (underdiagnosis and/or underreporting) of the number of cases. Underestimations vary considerably in relation to the type of disease and the sensitivity of the surveillance systems of the various countries. The need for more reliable estimates of global FBDs burden was highlighted in 2007 by the WHO, which established the Foodborne Disease Burden Epidemiology Reference Group (FERG) [1]. The FERG has estimated the global, regional and sub-regional burden for 11 diarrhoeal disease agents (1 virus, 7 bacteria, 3 protozoa), 8 invasive infectious disease agents (1 virus, 6 bacteria and 1 protozoon), 10 helminths (3 cestodes, 2 nematodes and 5 trematodes) and 3 chemicals (Table 23.1 and Box 23.1). Of all biological agents, only 10 are exclusively transmitted via food vehicles. The proportion of cases attributable to transmission via food is approximately 29% for the group of diarrhoeal diseases, 34% for invasive diseases, and 45%, 72% and 100% for the helminthic FBDs caused by nematodes, cestodes and trematodes, respectively [2–4].

Box 23.1 Global Burden of Foodborne Illnesses Estimates: Key Points from Table 23.1

Above all, what emerges is the burden of bacterial agents, which account for 64% of cases and over 80% for both mortality and Disability Adjusted Life Years (especially EPEC among diarrhoeal forms and *S. Typhi* among invasive diseases).

Although invasive forms and helminthiasis account for only 6% and 2% of total FBD cases, respectively, their burden in terms of mortality (30% and 12%) and DALYs (26% and 18%) is considerably higher than that of viral diseases.

Among viral agents, while Noroviruses are relevant as the number of cases in the group of diarrhoeal diseases (almost 125,000 cases corresponding to more than 20% of illnesses), the hepatitis viruses are relevant among invasive diseases (about 13,700 cases, almost 40%).

It was estimated that 600 million FBD cases occurred globally in 2010, with a high proportion (92%) being diarrhoeal diseases. The total global burden of FBD is estimated to 33 million DALYs (Disability Adjusted Life Years), but—given the high frequency of cases among children under 5 years of age—almost 83% of this number is given by the YLLs (*Years of Life Lost*), while DALYs (*Disability Adjusted Life Years*) represent only 17% of the total burden [2]. FBDs distribution is non-homogeneous among the six WHO regions, with a higher burden in AFR, SEAR and EMR (Fig. 23.1).

Table 23.1 Global burden of foodborne illnesses, deaths and disability adjusted life: % of the total of the group (diarrheal illness, invasive diseases, helminthiasis) with the exception of the % of the subtotals indicated with[a]. The highest percentage values are indicated in bold. (Adapted from references [2–4])

	foodborne hazard	proportion foodborne %	foodborne illnesses	foodborne deaths	foodborne DALYs
diarrheal diseases	**Viruses**		22,8%	15,2%	14,1%
	Norovirus	18	**22,7%**	15,2%	14,1%
	Bacteria		63,7%	81,4%	82,1%
	Campylobacter spp	58	17,4%	9,3%	12,1%
	Enteropathogenic E. coli– EPEC	30	4,3%	**16,1%**	**16,6%**
	Enterotoxigenic E. coli-ETEC	36	15,8%	11,4%	11,8%
	Shiga toxin-producing E. coli-STEC	48	0,2%	0,1%	0,1%
	Non-typhoidal S. enterica (NtS)^	52	14,3%	12,5%	12,4%
	Shigella spp	27	9,3%	6,6%	7,0%
	Vibrio cholera	24	0,1%	10,7%	9,8%
	Protozoa		12,2%	2,4%	2,8%
	Cryptosporidium spp	13	1,6%	1,6%	1,7%
	Entamoeba histolytica	28	5,1%	0,6%	0,8%
	Giardia spp	15	5,1%	0,0%	0,1%
invasive diseases	**Viruses**		38,3%	23,7%	16,8%
	Virus hepatitis A	30	**38,3%**	23,7%	16, 8%
	Bacteria		28,9%	72,7%	70,6%
	Brucella spp.	47	1,1%	1,7%	1,5%
	Listeria monocytogenes	100	0,0%	2,7%	1,5%
	Mycobacterium bovis	100	0,3%	9,0%	7,5%
	Salmonella Typhi	37	21,2%	**44,8%**	**46,1%**
	Salmonella Paratyphi A	37	4,9%	10,3%	10,6%
	Salmonella enterica iNtS^	48	0,8%	25,1%	22,2%
	Protozoa		28,7%	0,6%	10,3%
	Toxoplasma gondii	49	28,7%	0,6%	10,3%
Helminths	**Cestodes**		3,3%	80,7%	54,4%
	Echinicoccus granulosus	21	0,3%	1,1%	0,7%
	Echinicoccus multilocularis	48	0,1%	17,2%	5,4%
	Taenia solium	100	2,9%	**62,2%**	**48,0%**
	Nematodes		95,0%	2,2%	10,4%
	Ascaris lumbricoides	46	**95,0%**	2,2%	10,4%
	Trichinella spp.	100	<0,1%	<0,1%	<0,1%
	Trematodes		1,7%	16,7%	34,8%
	Clonorchis sinensis	100	0,2%	12,8%	9,0%
	Fasciola spp.	100	0,1%	0,0%	1,5%
	Intestinal flukes°	100	0,1%	0,0%	2,7%
	Opistorchis spp,	100	0,1%	3,3%	3,2%
	Paragonimus spp.	100	1,1%	0,6%	18,1%
Subtotal	**Diarrheal disease agents***		**91,8%**	**58,6%**	**56,0%**
	Invasive diseases or Invasive infections*		**6,0%**	**29,9%**	**25,6%**
	Helminths*		**2,2%**	**11,5%**	**18,4%**

^ non typhoidal Salmonella serotypes are agents of both diarrheal (NtS) and invasive diseases (iNtS)

°*intestinal flukes* included diseases caused by several species of Trematodes

*For the subtotal of the three diseases groups the % are calculated on the total of the 31 hazards (597.294.786 foodborne illnesses, 392.560 foodborne deaths, 31.535.396 foodborne DALYS)

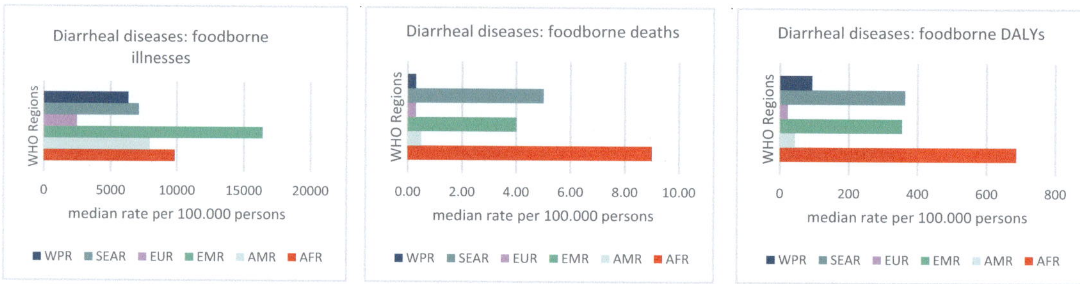

Fig. 23.1 Foodborne diarrheal illnesses: median rates Disability Adjusted Life Years (DALYs) per 100,000 population, by region. (Adapted from reference [3])

23.3 International Targets

The importance of the prevention and control of FBDs for global health was recognised by the WHO as early as 2000 (WHA53.15) [5]. Nowadays, among the 169 targets included in the 17 Sustainable Development Goals (SDGs, 2016–2030, available at https://www.globalgoals.org/goals/), many are interconnected with food- and waterborne diseases. In fact, FBDs are considered 'multifactorial', being widely influenced by (1) poverty and malnutrition, especially in children from low- and middle-income countries; (2) levels of food security and food safety; (3) accessibility to primary care and availability of health service resources; and (4) presence of sanitation infrastructure (drinking water supply, sewage disposal). Reducing FBDs burden involves different targets included in the SDGs and requires the commitment of different international players (WHO, United Nations, FAO).

Since globalisation has made food safety a concern also for middle- and high-income countries, an International Food Safety Authority (INFOSAN) was established on the initiative of the WHO and the FAO, to deal with food-related epidemic emergencies.

23.4 Determinants and Risk Factors

The occurrence of FBDs is influenced by host and external factors. Host factors consist of (1) age (people aged <5 and >65 years are the most at-risk); (2) nutritional deficiencies and eating habits, (3) underlying diseases, (4) immunodepression (primary or secondary), and (5) concomitant therapies [6]. Environmental risk factors vary in relation to the natural habitat/reservoir of the agents involved (environmental, animal, or human source), transmission routes, and food chain characteristics. The spread of FBDs in lower income countries is mainly influenced by food and water quality, given the high risk of faecal contamination of food due to the difficulties to access potable water and the lack of hygiene services. In higher income countries, global trade (long food chain and large-scale distribution) and the frequency of travel are more important. Additionally, climatic (e.g., temperature, humidity, natural events such as floods) and sociodemographic (e.g., migration, inequalities, vulnerable population groups, precariousness of health services) factors play a key role in FBDs occurrence [5, 7, 8].

23.5 FBD Control Challenges

Elimination and/or eradication can be hypothesised only for diseases with an exclusive human reservoir or strictly referable to a faecal-oral circuit (e.g., typhoid fever, hepatitis A). Otherwise, zoonotic diseases (e.g., salmonellosis) are controllable, but not eliminable, by multiple approaches along the food chain (from farm to fork) and public health interventions. The former includes control activities on primary production (e.g., hygiene on farms, slaughtering, and plant supply chain) and on the subsequent stages of food processing, to reduce the risk of contamination as well as the survival and multiplication of pathogens in food (e.g., self-control, Hazard Analysis Critical Control Point—HACCP). Today, the food safety approach is based on risk assessment, risk management and risk communication, which involve producers, stakeholders and consumers, and must consider the presence of vulnerable groups in the populations [6, 9]. Surveillance based on national and international networks is one of the fundamental public health activities and was already the focus of WHO's attention in the early 2000s (Resolution WHO Assembly, May 2000). The purposes of surveillance are to: (1) identify causative agents (also through metagenomics); (2) describe characteristics of cases ('who-where-when'); (3) recognise clusters of cases and conduct epidemiological investigation on outbreaks and epidemics; and (4) implement measures necessary to interrupt transmission chains (e.g., alerts, withdrawal of contaminated foods recognised) [9–11].

Given the characteristics of FBDs, it is preferable to base their control on a combination of 'non-specific' measures rather than on immunoprophylaxis, which can help to control only a small number of FBDs (e.g., typhoid fever, hepatitis A, cholera, rotavirus). Vaccines for other etiological agents (including parasites) are under development [12]. The sometimes-secondary role that immunoprophylaxis can have for FBDs control is exemplified by the case of cholera, whose elimination in many countries is primarily attributable to the interruption of the faecal-oral transmission chain thanks to environmental sanitation measures. Overall, the control (but not the elimination) of FBDs is based on a 'One Health' approach and involves multiple activities concerning animal reservoir, environment, food chains and employing public health measures.

23.5.1 Cost-Effectiveness

FBDs are also complex to assess in terms of associated costs. Besides direct costs (diagnosis, treatment and care of the individual case) and indirect costs (absence from work, loss of productivity), there are also costs for the society and businesses. Costs for surveillance activities, outbreak investigations, control over supply chains and for food withdrawals must be considered. Unfortunately, available data (mostly from high-income countries) are not easily comparable. In the United States, a recent analysis estimated yearly costs of USD10-83 billion [13, 14].

23.6 Responsibilities

In the 'One Health' perspective, many national and international institutions are involved. All processes that from primary production, through processing and distribution phases, reach the final consumer must be managed. Nowadays, the consumer may have access to food produced elsewhere, which may have been contaminated during any phase 'from farm to fork'. To improve safety, quality and equality of international food trade, the FAO and the WHO established in 1963 a Commission to draft a *Codex Alimentarius* that collects and updates internationally standardised good practice guidelines [15]. Of particular importance are the Codex Principles and Guidelines for National Food Control Systems (CAC/GL 82-2013). A Food Control System—defined as 'the integration of regulatory activities across all responsible competent authorities to achieve the key objectives of food control, including preventive and educational strategies that protect the whole food chain'—should be evaluated with respect to the objectives of the system, control programme effectiveness, and legislative and regulatory requirements, to allow further improvements and favour the interest of all players along the whole food production chain, including the final consumer [15].

References

1. Kuchenmüller T, Abela-Ridder B, Corrigan T, Tritscher A. World Health Organization initiative to estimate the global burden of foodborne diseases. Rev Sci Tech. 2013;32(2):459–67. https://doi.org/10.20506/rst.32.2.2249.

2. Havelaar AH, Kirk MD, Torgerson PR, Gibb HJ, Hald T, Lake RJ, et al. World Health Organization global estimates and regional comparisons of the burden of foodborne disease in 2010. PLoS Med. 2015;12(12):e1001923. https://doi.org/10.1371/journal.pmed.1001923.
3. Kirk MD, Pires SM, Black RE, Caipo M, Crump JA, Devleesschauwer B, et al. World Health Organization estimates of the global and regional disease burden of 22 foodborne bacterial, protozoal, and viral diseases, 2010: a data synthesis. PLoS Med. 2015;12(12):e1001921. https://doi.org/10.1371/journal.pmed.1001921.
4. Torgerson PR, Devleesschauwer B, Praet N, Speybroeck N, Willingham AL, Kasuga F, et al. World Health Organization estimates of the global and regional disease burden of 11 foodborne parasitic diseases, 2010: a data synthesis. PLoS Med. 2015;12(12):e1001920. https://doi.org/10.1371/journal.pmed.1001920.
5. Lake IR, Barker GC. Climate change, foodborne pathogens and illness in higher-income countries. Curr Environ Health Rep. 2018;5(1):187–96. https://doi.org/10.1007/s40572-018-0189-9.
6. Lund BM. Microbiological food safety for vulnerable people. Int J Environ Res Public Health. 2015;12(8):10117–32. https://doi.org/10.3390/ijerph120810117.
7. Antunes P, Novais C, Peixe L. Food-to-humans bacterial transmission. Microbiol Spectrum. 2020;8:1. https://doi.org/10.1128/microbiolspec.MTBP-0019-2016.
8. Semenza JC, Lindgren E, Balkanyi L, Espinosa L, Almqvist MS, Penttinen P, Rocklöv J. Determinants and drivers of infectious disease threat events in Europe. Emerg Infect Dis. 2016;22(4):581–9. https://doi.org/10.3201/eid2204.
9. Schlundt J. New directions in foodborne disease prevention. Int J Food Microbiol. 2002;78(1–2):3–17. https://doi.org/10.1016/s0168-1605(02)00234-9.
10. Carleton HA, Besser J, Williams-Newkirk AJ, Huang A, Trees E, Gerner-Smidt P. Metagenomic approaches for public health surveillance of foodborne infections: opportunities and challenges. Foodborne Pathog Dis. 2019;16(7):474–9. https://doi.org/10.1089/fpd.2019.2636. Epub 2019 Jun 6
11. Hoelzer K, Moreno Switt AI, Wiedmann M, Boor KJ. Emerging needs and opportunities in foodborne disease detection and prevention: from tools to people. Food Microbiol. 2018;75:65–71. https://doi.org/10.1016/j.fm.2017.07.006. Epub 2017 Jul 11
12. Hasso-Agopsowicz M, Lopman BA, Lanata CF, Rogawski McQuade ET, Kang G, Prudden HJ, Khalil I, Platts-Mills JA, Kotloff K, Jit M, Riddle MS, Pavlinac PB, Luz PM, Pitzer VE, Breiman RF, Giersing BK. World Health Organization expert working group: recommendations for assessing morbidity associated with enteric pathogens. Vaccine. 2021;39(52):7521–5. https://doi.org/10.1016/j.vaccine.2021.11.033. Epub 2021 Nov 24.
13. McLinden T, Sargeant JM, Thomas MK, Papadopoulos A, Fazil A. Component costs of foodborne illness: a scoping review. BMC Public Health. 2014;14:509. https://doi.org/10.1186/1471-2458-14-509.
14. Scharff RL. Economic burden from health losses due to foodborne illness in the United States. J Food Prot. 2012;75(1):123–31. https://doi.org/10.4315/0362-028X.JFP-11-058.
15. FAO and WHO. Food control system assessment tool: Introduction and glossary. Food safety and quality series No. 7/1. Rome; 2019.

Part V

The Global Burden of Disease: Non-communicable Diseases

24 Cardiovascular Diseases

Astrid Berner-Rodoreda, Cecilia Kanyama, Alexander Supady, and Till Bärnighausen

Abstract

Cardiovascular diseases (CVDs) are the leading cause of death globally. They reduce the function of vital organs and can lead to major conditions like heart attack or stroke, yet they often remain undetected until a life-threatening event occurs. Major risk factors for CVDs are hypertension, lipid disorders, diabetes mellitus, smoking, physical inactivity and alcohol consumption. CVDs also have a gender, age and income dimension. Further social determinants include pollution, low-level education, poor working conditions, stress and restricted access to health care. Challenges range from insufficient CVD prevalence data to reaching people with correct and culture- and gender-sensitive information and ensuring community access to the treatment of CVDs. Gender and age-targeted screening, counselling and treatment for patients at risk are cost-effective. Quitting smoking, a healthier diet, increased physical activity and alcohol reduction may reduce the risk of CVDs. Adoption of WHO recommendations and their implementation should be increased globally.

Keywords

Hypertension · Heart attack · Stroke · Social determinants · WHO recommendations · Reduction strategies

A. Berner-Rodoreda (✉)
Heidelberg Institute of Global Health, University of Heidelberg, Heidelberg, Germany
e-mail: astrid.berner-rodoreda@uni-heidelberg.de

C. Kanyama
University of North Carolina – Malawi, Lilongwe, Malawi
e-mail: ckanyama@med.unc.edu

A. Supady
Medical Center, Interdisciplinary Medical Intensive Care, University of Freiburg, Freiburg, Germany
e-mail: alexander.supady@uniklinik-freiburg.de

T. Bärnighausen
Africa Health Research Institute (AHRI), Durban, South Africa
e-mail: till.baernighausen@uni-heidelberg.de

24.1 Definitions and Main Disease Features

Cardiovascular diseases (CVDs) comprise a broad array of pathologies of the heart and the blood vessels, including coronary and valvular heart disease, cardiomyopathies, peripheral artery disease, cerebrovascular disease, congenital heart disease, venous and pulmonary thromboembolism [1]. Thus, CVDs represent one of the largest groups of noncommunicable diseases (NCDs). Whether

M. C. B. Raviglione et al. (eds.), *Global Health Essentials*, Sustainable Development Goals Series,
https://doi.org/10.1007/978-3-031-33851-9_24

caused by a congenital defect or developed over time through fat deposits in the arteries, CVDs reduce and may eventually block the blood supply to the heart (heart attack) or brain (stroke) or reduce the function of vital organs, yet often remain undetected until the person experiences life-threatening signs and symptoms (ibid).

24.2 Descriptive Epidemiology and Assessment of the Global Burden

CVDs are the leading cause of death globally for both men and women [2], accounting for one-third of all deaths with the majority (~80%) of CVD-related deaths occurring in low- and middle-income countries (LMICs) [1]. In most high-income countries (HICs), the incidence of CVDs has declined since 1990, whereas in many LMICs, the burden of CVDs has increased in recent years [3]. CVDs are associated with premature death or a lower quality of life as expressed in daily adjusted life-years (DALYs). A higher occurrence of CVD-related DALYs is recorded for African and Asian countries with some East, Central and Southern African countries exceeding 1000 DALYs per 100,000 population [4]. In particular, infection with viral hepatitis [5] or HIV [6] showed a heightened risk for developing CVDs leading to a double-disease burden for many countries.

24.3 International Targets and Progress Towards Their Achievements

Acknowledging the impact of NCDs, including CVDs, on global morbidity and mortality, the WHO recommended nine targets to control and reduce NCDs by 2025, see Fig. 24.1 [7]. In 2015, United Nations members agreed to reduce by the year 2030 premature deaths due to NCDs by one-third [8]. These targets were affirmed by the Political Declaration on NCDs [9] with a view to control CVDs.

A global analysis of WHO NCD country progress reports showed that, on average, only less than half of WHO's recommended policies were adopted by countries. Most frequently implemented policies related to clinical guidelines, warning signs on tobacco packages and conducting surveys, whereas the least implemented related to providing medical treatment for CVDs and banning of alcohol advertising [10]. A systematic review on salt reduction showed policy improvements, but no country attaining the recommended 30% reduction [11].

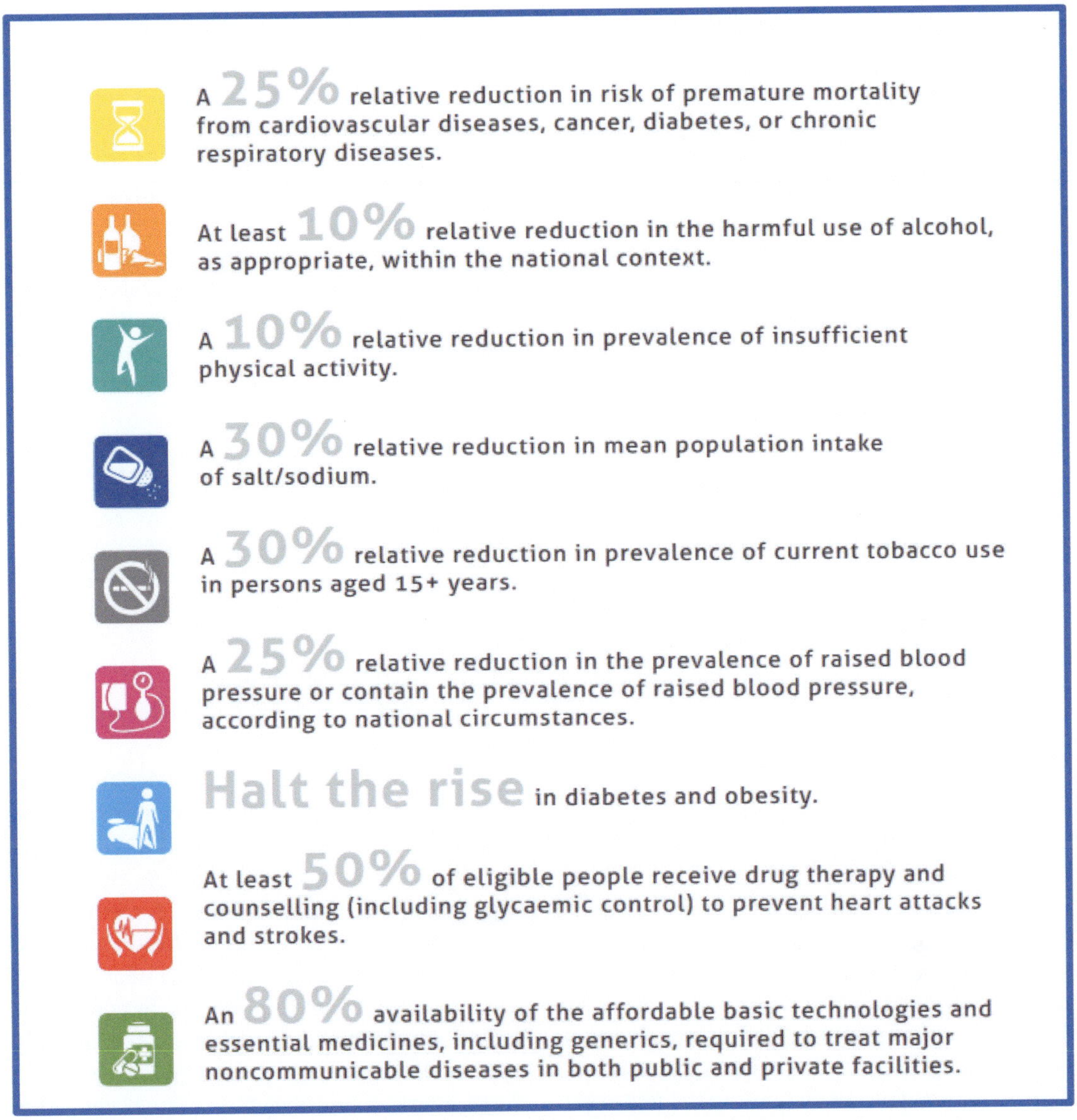

Fig. 24.1 Voluntary Global Targets reproduced from Global Action Plan for the Prevention and Control of Noncommunicable Diseases 2013–2020, WHO, Voluntary Global Targets, page 5, Copyright (2013). Reproduced with permissions from Global Action Plan for the Prevention and Control of Noncommunicable Diseases 2013–2020, WHO, Voluntary Global Targets, page 5, Copyright (2013)

24.4 Determinants and Risk Factors

The most relevant risk factors for CVDs are hypertension, tobacco use, lipid disorders, diabetes mellitus and a sedentary lifestyle [12]; with food and physical inactivity-related factors showing varying levels of association with CVDs in different national contexts [13]. Social determinants for CVDs include lower level education, low income, unfavourable working conditions and stress and limited access to health care [14]. CVDs also have a gender, age and income dimension: ischemic heart disease (with the danger of a heart attack) affects more men than women globally up to the age of 80, with a reversal of the gender-pattern above 80 years [4]; strokes are predominantly a disease burden in LMICs (ibid). A study comparing six LMICs found angina (ischemic chest pain) more common in women and stroke more common in men and urban areas [13].

24.5 Challenges to Be Faced for Containment, Control and Elimination

Major challenges impeding progress in reducing global cardiovascular morbidity and mortality range from insufficient data on the scale of the problem in a particular setting (necessitating more population-based surveys) to reaching people with correct information about prevention and treatment of CVDs, ensuring access to and utilization of health facilities for all (irrespective of income and gender) and identifying and treating CVDs in the realm of primary health care. A recent cross-sectional study of 45 countries identified under-usage of hypertension medicines in clients with a heightened CVD risk (particularly in men) and over-usage in clients with a lower CVD risk [3], calling for more targeted interventions.

24.6 Approaches and Strategies for Prevention and Control

Quitting smoking, a healthier diet (reducing salt intake, increasing fruit and vegetable intake), more physical activity and alcohol reduction may reduce the risk of CVDs [1]. A recent Lancet Commission report [2] suggested additional measures for women, such as, access to education and culturally-tailored communication about health and well-being, culture-sensitive prevention programs, support through community health workers, strengthening women's health self-care and self-management.

24.7 Cost-Effectiveness and Financial Considerations

Gender- and age-targeted CVD screening is more cost-effective than general population screening programs [15]. Community-based interventions, such as community health workers monitoring hypertension in clients and linking them to care at the nearest facility, training of health personnel at local facilities on diagnosis and treatment and regular patient education sessions at community and health centre level would be further cost-effective interventions. As the most cost-effective CVD interventions listed as part of the "Best Buys", WHO recommends counselling and drug treatment for patients at high risk ($\geq$30%) of a stroke or heart attack in the next 10 years and for those who have already experienced such an event [16]. Figure 24.2 summarizes major risk factors, social determinants and approaches to improve the CVD disease burden globally.

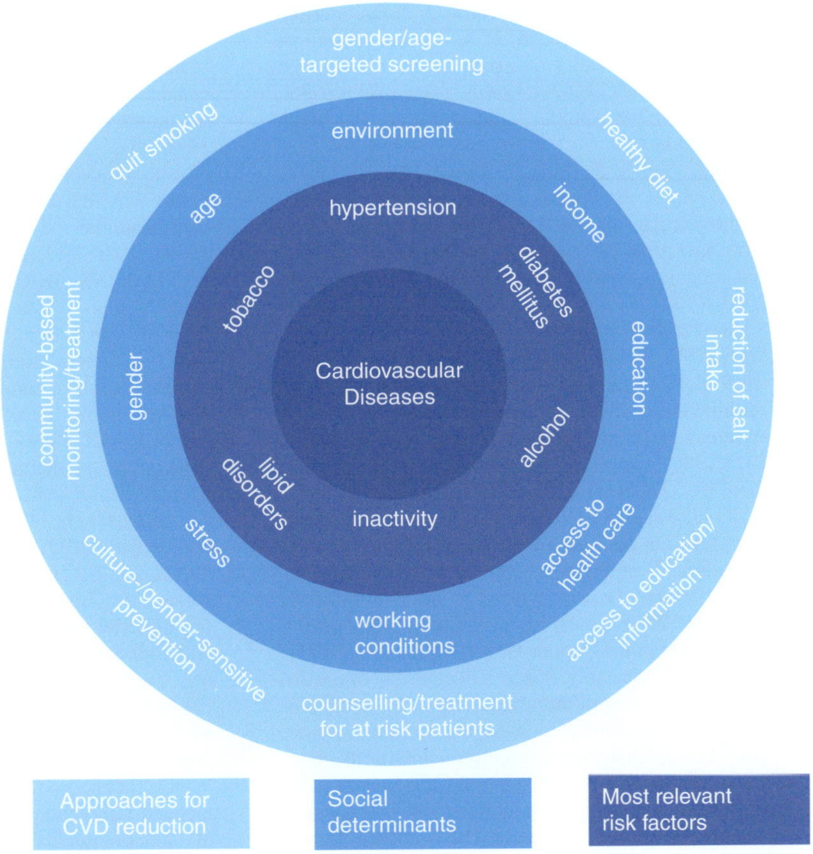

Fig. 24.2 Major CVD risks and approaches for risk reduction

24.8 Responsibilities of Different National and International Institutions

WHO develops guidelines and recommendations for evidence-based CVD policies and interventions, and the UN General Assembly garners global political commitment for actions, policies and targets and provides visibility in the form of political declarations. However, national governments are responsible for developing and implementing national and context-specific guidelines based on global guidance.

References

1. WHO. Fact sheet Cardiovascular Diseases (CVDs). 2021. https://www.who.int/en/news-room/fact-sheets/detail/cardiovascular-diseases-(cvds). Accessed 29 Apr 2022.
2. Vogel B, Acevedo M, Appelman Y, Merz CNB, Chieffo A, Figtree GA, et al. The lancet women and cardiovascular disease commission: reducing the global burden by 2030. Lancet. 2021;397(10292):2385–438. https://doi.org/10.1016/S0140-6736(21)00684-X.
3. Peiris D, Ghosh A, Manne-Goehler J, Jaacks LM, Theilmann M, Marcus ME, et al. Cardiovascular disease risk profile and management practices in 45 low-income and middle-income countries: a cross-sectional study of nationally representative individual-level survey data. PLoS Med. 2021;18(3):e1003485.

4. Roth GA, Mensah GA, Johnson CO, Addolorato G, Ammirati E, Baddour LM, et al. Global burden of cardiovascular diseases and risk factors, 1990-2019: update from the GBD 2019 study. J Am Coll Cardiol. 2020;76(25):2982–3021. https://doi.org/10.1016/j.jacc.2020.11.010.
5. Lee KK, Stelzle D, Bing R, Anwar M, Strachan F, Bashir S, et al. Global burden of atherosclerotic cardiovascular disease in people with hepatitis C virus infection: a systematic review, meta-analysis, and modelling study. Lancet Gastroenterol Hepatol. 2019;4(10):794–804. https://doi.org/10.1016/S2468-1253(19)30227-4.
6. Shah ASV, Stelzle D, Lee KK, Beck EJ, Alam S, Clifford S, et al. Global burden of atherosclerotic cardiovascular disease in people living with HIV: systematic review and meta-analysis. Circulation. 2018;138(11):1100–12. https://doi.org/10.1161/CIRCULATIONAHA.117.033369.
7. WHO Global action plan for the prevention and control of NCDs 2013-2020. WHO; 2013. https://www.who.int/publications-detail-redirect/9789241506236.
8. United Nations General Assembly. Transforming our world: the 2030 agenda for sustainable development. New York: United Nations General Assembly; 2015.
9. UN General Assembly. Political declaration of the 3rd high-level meeting of the general assembly on the prevention and control of non-communicable diseases. 2018. https://digitallibrary.un.org/record/1648984.
10. Allen LN, Nicholson BD, Yeung BY, Goiana-da-Silva F. Implementation of non-communicable disease policies: a geopolitical analysis of 151 countries. Lancet Glob Health. 2020;8(1):e50–8.
11. Santos JA, Tekle D, Rosewarne E, Flexner N, Cobb L, Al-Jawaldeh A, et al. A systematic review of salt reduction initiatives around the world: a midterm evaluation of Progress towards the 2025 global non-communicable diseases salt reduction target. Adv Nutr. 2021;12(5):1768–80. https://doi.org/10.1093/advances/nmab008.
12. Fuchs FD, Whelton PK. High blood pressure and cardiovascular disease. Hypertens Dallas Tex 1979. 2020;75(2):285–92. https://doi.org/10.1161/HYPERTENSIONAHA.119.14240.
13. Ruan Y, Guo Y, Zheng Y, Huang Z, Sun S, Kowal P, et al. Cardiovascular disease (CVD) and associated risk factors among older adults in six low-and middle-income countries: results from SAGE wave 1. BMC Public Health. 2018;18(1):778. https://doi.org/10.1186/s12889-018-5653-9.
14. Roger VL. Medicine and society: social determinants of health and cardiovascular disease. Eur Heart J. 2020;41(11):1179–81. https://doi.org/10.1093/eurheartj/ehaa134.
15. Selvarajah S, Haniff J, Kaur G, Guat Hiong T, Bujang A, Chee Cheong K, et al. Identification of effective screening strategies for cardiovascular disease prevention in a developing country: using cardiovascular risk-estimation and risk-reduction tools for policy recommendations. BMC Cardiovasc Disord. 2013;13(1):10. https://doi.org/10.1186/1471-2261-13-10.
16. WHO. Tackling NCDs: 'best buys' and other recommended interventions for the prevention and control of noncommunicable diseases (No. WHO/NMH/NVI/17.9).

25 Chronic Obstructive Lung Diseases

Surendra K. Sharma, Jai P. Narain, and Alladi Mohan

Abstract

Chronic obstructive lung diseases (COLD), also referred to as chronic obstructive pulmonary disease (COPD), are a group of diseases characterised by persistent and progressive cough and airflow limitation. As the third leading cause of mortality globally causing 3.2 million deaths annually, these constitute a substantial socio-economic burden. The prevalence is significantly higher among men aged ≥40 years and in tobacco smokers. Exposure to ambient and indoor air pollution, and occupational exposures are other important risk factors. The key strategies to prevent COLD include smoking cessation and avoiding exposure to air pollutants, adopting gas for cooking, and switching to motor vehicles run on compressed natural gas or to electric cars. In addition, early diagnosis, access to high quality healthcare, life-saving medications including oxygen, and influenza and pneumococcal vaccinations are an integral part of national programmes. High priority must be accorded to strengthening capacity in low-income and middle-income countries to enable collectively achieve the related Sustainable Development Goal 3.4 by 2030.

Keywords

Chronic obstructive lung diseases (COLD) · Chronic obstructive pulmonary disease (COPD) · Tobacco smoking · Air pollution exposure · Occupational exposure

25.1 Introduction

Chronic obstructive lung diseases (COLD), also referred to as chronic obstructive pulmonary disease (COPD), are a group of pulmonary diseases including chronic bronchitis and emphysema that are characterised by persistent and progressive cough leading to airflow limitation. The Global Initiative for Chronic Obstructive Lung Disease (GOLD) [1] defines COLD as "a common, pre-

S. K. Sharma (✉)
Department of Molecular Medicine, Jamia Hamdard (Deemed to be University), New Delhi, India

Department of Pulmonary Medicine, Jawaharlal Nehru Medical College, Datta Meghe Institute of Medical Sciences, Sawangi (Meghe), Wardha, Maharashtra, India

Department of General Medicine, Jawaharlal Nehru Medical College, Datta Meghe Institute of Medical Sciences, Sawangi (Meghe), Wardha, Maharashtra, India

Formerly at Department of Internal Medicine (WHO Collaborating Centre for Research & Training in Tuberculosis, Centre of Excellence for EPTB, MoH & FW, GoI), All India Institute of Medical Sciences, New Delhi, India

J. P. Narain
University of New South Wales, Sydney, Australia

A. Mohan
Department of Medicine, Sri Venkateswara Institute of Medical Sciences, Tirupati, India

M. C. B. Raviglione et al. (eds.), *Global Health Essentials*, Sustainable Development Goals Series,
https://doi.org/10.1007/978-3-031-33851-9_25

ventable, and treatable disease that is characterized by persistent respiratory symptoms and airflow limitation that is due to airway and/or alveolar abnormalities usually caused by significant exposure to noxious particles or gases and influenced by host factors including abnormal lung development". Cough with mucus production, shortness of breath, wheezing and airflow limitations are cardinal features of COLD [2].

25.2 Epidemiology and Disease Burden

According to the World Health Organization (WHO), COLD is the third leading cause of death worldwide, causing 3.2 million deaths annually; most of these deaths occur in those <70 years living in low-and middle-income countries (LMICs) where prevention and control measures are either not implemented or are not accessible [1, 3–6].

The global prevalence is ~12% with a considerable regional variation; Americas (14.5%) have the highest prevalence, South-East/Western Pacific regions have the lowest prevalence (Fig. 25.1) [4, 5]. Prevalence is substantially higher among men than women (15.7% vs. 9.1%) [7], among persons aged ≥40 years, among smokers and ex-smokers than non-smokers [1], and in rural areas [8]. As one of the prominent non-communicable diseases (NCDs), COLD form part of the agenda for United Nations (UN) Sustainable Development Goals (SDGs), in particular target 3.4 which aims to reduce by one-third premature mortality from NCDs through prevention and treatment by 2030 [9].

25.3 Determinants and Risk Factors

Tobacco smoking remains the most important risk factor for development of COLD globally. While an overall "dose-response curve" for tobacco smoking and lung function has been observed, severe disease may develop in some patients with fewer pack-years and others may not develop disease despite smoking. Other factors include ambient (outdoor) air pollution [especially, fine particulate matter <2.5 mm in

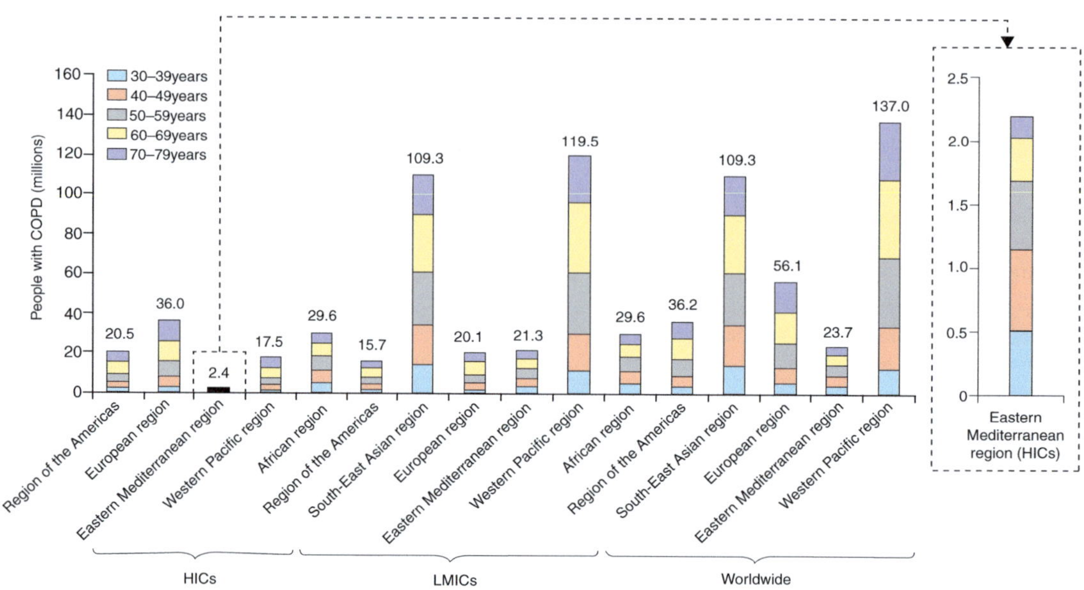

Fig. 25.1 Number of people with GOLD-COPD by region and age groups in 2019. COPD = chronic obstructive pulmonary disease; GOLD = Global Initiative on Chronic Obstructive Lung Disease; HICs = high income countries; LMICs = low- and middle-income countries. GOLD-COPD is defined as forced expiratory volume in the first second (FEV_1)/forced vital capacity (FVC) < 0.7. Reproduced with kind permission from "Adeloye D, Song P, Zhu Y, Campbell H, Sheikh A, Rudan I; NIHR RESPIRE Global Respiratory Health Unit. Global, regional, and national prevalence of, and risk factors for, chronic obstructive pulmonary disease (COPD) in 2019: a systematic review and modelling analysis. Lancet Respir Med 2022;10:447–58" [4]

Table 25.1 Determinants and risk factors for COLD development and progression

- Exposure to tobacco smoke from smoking or exposure to second-hand tobacco smoke
- Exposure to atmospheric particulate matter
  - Indoor and outdoor air pollution (e.g., from biomass fuel used for cooking and heating for, e.g. burning coal, wood, dried leaves, twigs, firewood, animal dung cakes, crop residues)
  - Occupational exposures (organic and inorganic dusts, chemicals, fumes, etc.)
- Genetic factors
  - Alpha-1 antitrypsin deficiency, suboptimal lung development during gestation or childhood, asthma, and airway hyperreactivity
- Demographic factors
  - Older age, male gender, low socio-economic status
- Infections
  - Severe childhood respiratory infections
  - Repeated viral, bacterial upper and lower respiratory tract infections
  - Tuberculosis
  - Human immunodeficiency virus infection

COLD = chronic obstructive lung diseases

aerodynamic diameter ($PM_{2.5}$)], household (indoor) air pollution (domestic and biomass fuel) and occupational exposures, which are important determinants especially in LMICs (Table 25.1). Given the higher exposure of these risk factors, the most disadvantaged groups of society such as the poor are more vulnerable to develop COLD. They, in addition, have limited access to information and healthcare services.

25.4 Approaches and Strategies for Prevention and Control

Various strategies include early diagnosis, effective management of stable disease and acute exacerbations, prevention of exposures and future exacerbations, as well as investigations to monitor complications (Box 25.1). At individual level, smokers must quit tobacco smoking and avoid exposure to other air pollutants, by refraining from burning firewood or trash in the vicinity, and by individuals planning various outdoor activities based on local air quality index. Households should resort to cooking gas and must refrain from using firewood or biomass for cooking. Cooking gas should be made available at subsidised rates to the disadvantaged groups of the society by the national governments, as has been done in India [10]. Use of compressed natural gas (CNG) for motor vehicles, switching to electric cars and/or shifting industries away from urban areas can help reduce outdoor air pollution. Pulmonary rehabilitation should also be encouraged.

Box 25.1 Key Strategies for Prevention and Control

- Tobacco smoking cessation counselling
- Avoiding exposure to various air pollutants
- Implementing various measures for ensuring good quality of air
- Ensuring availability of various medications, drug delivery devices (e.g., metered dose inhalers, dry powder inhalers, nebulisers. positive airway pressure devices, mechanical ventilation, heart-lung/lung transplantation)
- Facilitating access to quality health care (including, but not limited to oxygen therapy, emergency and intensive care for rational management and prevention of acute exacerbations of COLD) and health insurance coverage for COLD and its complications in national health schemes/ programmes
- Carrying out investigations[a] periodically for early detection of complications (type I and type II respiratory failure, pulmonary artery hypertension and congestive cardiac failure, detection of co-existing coronary artery disease)
- Management of other comorbid conditions and correction of nutritional deficiencies
- Vaccination for SARS-CoV-2, seasonal influenza, pneumococcal infection, pertussis (for American adults who were not vaccinated during adolescence) and herpes zoster
- Education and training in various techniques of pulmonary rehabilitation

[a]Arterial blood gas analysis, HRCT of the chest, 2-dimensional echocardiography and NT-Pro BNP, among others
COLD = chronic obstructive lung diseases; HRCT = high resolution computed tomography; NT-Pro BNP = N-terminal Pro B-type natriuretic peptide; SARS-CoV-2 = severe acute respiratory syndrome coronavirus 2

Disease awareness programmes on prevention and control should be held. There is a need for creating community awareness through information and communication campaigns, focussing on: (1) various risk factors associated with chronic respiratory diseases and avoiding exposure to these risk factors and (2) early detection of the disease. These strategies can help in prevention and management of various chronic respiratory diseases including COLD. Access to emergency and out-patient medical care for sick and disabled patients, oral, inhalational drugs, various devices (inhalers, nebulisers), supplemental oxygen and delivery devices should be facilitated by programmes and governments at district levels [11, 12]. Concurrent presence of comorbidities, multimorbidity (≥2 chronic conditions) should be identified for better management of COLD. The potential of artificial intelligence and machine learning should be explored in management and predicting exacerbations of COLD.

Vaccinations against severe acute respiratory syndrome coronavirus 2 (SARS-CoV-2) virus, seasonal influenza and pneumococcal infections for all COLD patients aged 65 years and in younger patients with significant comorbidities are recommended [1]. The US Centers for Disease Control (CDC) also recommends vaccination to protect against pertussis for American adults who were not vaccinated during adolescence and zoster vaccine for COLD patients >50 years [1].

25.5 Cost-Effectiveness and Financial Considerations

Cost-effective strategies for disease prevention, e.g., tobacco smoking cessation, vaccination, and for early case detection and management are already available. These need to be implemented urgently and widely in order to reduce the disease burden and try to achieve the UN SDG target relating to NCDs. The socio-economic burden of COLD is enormous globally, especially in the developing world, although precise estimates are lacking. More research on the socio-economic burden of COLD in developing countries is required. The disability-adjusted life years (DALYs) lost globally from COLD continues to increase, from being the 11th leading cause of total DALYs lost in 1990, to the fourth rank in 2019. It clearly is a major contributor to disability globally, and LMICs account for 62·6% of the global burden of COLD [6].

25.6 Challenges Faced by National Programmes

Despite being the third most common cause of death and fourth in terms of DALYs lost, COLD is not given due priority by both policy makers and public health managers. The political will to combat this NCD is lacking and is often limited to token attention. Consequently, in most cases, no resources are available in government healthcare facilities in LMICs for COLD. Serious efforts to systematically collect COLD surveillance data required for evidence-based public health policy and program planning are presently lacking. In most countries, no national guidelines on COLD exist [13, 14].

As COLD is not listed among the UN SDG indicators/targets, hence there is no mechanism in place to monitor or measure progress in mortality or morbidity reduction. Population groups too are unaware that COLD is a preventable and treatable disease and what they can do individually and collectively to ameliorate the problem. Healthcare technologies, including spirometry, drugs including antibiotics, corticosteroids, bronchodilators and delivery devices, supplemental oxygen and vaccines are generally not available at district level and below.

25.7 National and International Efforts

There is an urgent need for implementing a national programme for surveillance and control of COLD globally with adequate financial and human resources to manage it. A compelling evidence exists that COLD is a cause of increased global morbidity and mortality, producing a huge socio-economic impact and is a serious impediment to social and national development. To achieve the 2030 agenda for UN SDG 3.4 and reduction of one-third premature mortality from NCDs including COLD by 2030, we must ensure urgently a sustained scaling up of efforts towards prevention and healthcare interventions, universal health coverage for COLD, with technical and financial capacity building support to LMICs. There is also an urgent need to develop partnerships, multisectoral co-ordination, including with tuberculosis elimination and tobacco control programmes, both at national and international levels. To mobilise national and international efforts, a Global Alliance against Chronic Respiratory Diseases has been established as a voluntary alliance of national and international organizations which contributes to WHO's global work to prevent and control chronic respiratory diseases [15].

References

1. Global initiative for chronic obstructive lung disease. Global strategy for the diagnosis, management, and prevention of chronic obstructive pulmonary disease. 2022 Report. https://goldcopd.org/. Accessed 20 Aug 2022.
2. Rabe KF, Watz H. Chronic obstructive pulmonary disease. Lancet. 2017;389:1931–40.
3. Ruvuna L, Sood A. Epidemiology of chronic obstructive pulmonary disease. Clin Chest Med. 2020;41:315–27.
4. Adeloye D, Song P, Zhu Y, Campbell H, Sheikh A, Rudan I, NIHR RESPIRE Global Respiratory Health Unit. Global, regional, and national prevalence of, and risk factors for, chronic obstructive pulmonary disease (COPD) in 2019: a systematic review and modelling analysis. Lancet Respir Med. 2022(10):447–58.
5. World Health Organization. Chronic obstructive pulmonary disease. https://www.who.int/news-room/fact-sheets/detail/chronicobstructive-pulmonary-disease-(copd). Accessed 25 June and 29 August 2022.
6. GBD 2019 Diseases and Injuries Collaborators. Global burden of 369 diseases and injuries in 204 countries and territories, 1990–2019: a systematic analysis for the Global Burden of Disease Study 2019. Lancet. 2020;396:1204–22.
7. Varmaghani M, Dehghani M, Heidari E, Sharifi F, Moghaddam SS, Farzadfar F. Global prevalence of chronic obstructive pulmonary disease: systematic review and meta-analysis. East Mediterr Health J. 2019;25:47–57.
8. Urban-Rural differences in COPD. https://www.cdc.gov/copd/features/copd-urban-rural-differences.html. Accessed 29 Aug 2022.
9. United nations. Department of Economic and Social Affairs. Sustainable development. https://sdgs.un.org/goals. Accessed 29 Aug 2022.
10. Government of India. Ministry of Petroleum and Natural Gas. Pradhan Mantri Ujjwala Yojana 2.0. https://www.pmuy.gov.in/about.html. Accessed 17 Oct 2022.
11. Brakema EA, Vermond D, Pinnock H, Lionis C, Kirenga B, An PL, et al. FRESH AIR collaborators. Implementing lung health interventions in low- and middle-income countries: a FRESH AIR systematic review and meta-synthesis. Eur Respir J. 2020;56:2000127.
12. Tabyshova A, Hurst JR, Soriano JB, Checkley W, Wan-Chun Huang E, Trofor AC, et al. Gaps in COPD guidelines of low- and middle-income countries: a systematic scoping review. Chest. 2021;159:575–84.
13. Yorgancioglu A, Khaltaev N, Bousquet J, Varghese C. The global Alliance against chronic respiratory diseases: journey so far and way ahead. Chin Med J. 2020;133:1513–5.
14. The COPD National Action Plan. https://www.nhlbi.nih.gov/health-topics/education-and-awareness/COPD-national-action-plan. Accessed 20 Aug 2022.
15. Khaltaev N, Akselrod S. Role of global Alliance against chronic respiratory diseases (GARD) in achievement of the UN sustainable development goals (SDG) and targets. J Thorac Dis. 2021;13:5117–22.

Cancer

26

Andreas Ullrich and Jalid Sehouli

Abstract

Cancer is a leading cause of death worldwide. A broad range of known risk factors open effective ways to prevent cancer on population basis such as vaccination against HPV and HBV and tobacco control. Compared to other NCDs, many cancers are curable if detected early and treated adequately. Although knowledge about effective ways to prevent and to treat cancer is constantly increasing, the translation to national health systems is mostly limited to high-income countries. In the context of the emerging efforts to set up NCD plans, countries will need to invest in cancer-specific interventions to achieve the target as defined by the Sustainable Development Goal three relating to NCDs. International cooperation is needed to support low- and middle-income countries in their efforts to strengthen national health systems to provide equal access to cancer prevention, early detection, treatment, and palliative care at all ages. Long-term cooperation is particularly crucial for the training of health care providers in comprehensive cancer care.

A. Ullrich (✉) · J. Sehouli
Department of Gynecology with Center for Oncological Surgery, Charité Universitätsmedizin, Berlin, Germany
e-mail: andreas.ullrich@charite.de; jalid.sehouli@charite.de

Keywords

Cancer · Cancer control · Cancer risks/hazards · Cancer prevention · Healthy behaviour

26.1 Introduction to the Issue, Background, and Aims of the Chapter

Cancer is the leading and second-leading cause of death for people aged 30–69 years in 134 countries [1] (Fig. 26.1) imposing major challenges to health systems and national economies worldwide. The term "cancer" or malignant tumour refers to a group of over 100 distinct diseases which have the common feature of uncontrolled proliferation of abnormal cells due to exposure to cancer risks and genetic factors.

Originating from one single altered cell, cancer is spreading by local proliferation through the lymphatic and vascular system leading to metastasis across the body. The five most common cancers among men include: lung, prostate, colorectal, stomach, and liver cancer. Among women the five most common cancers include: breast, colorectal, lung, cervical, and gastric cancer.

Progress in knowledge about the various causes of cancer and their tumour biology has opened multiple new opportunities for a broad range of cancer prevention measures and thera-

M. C. B. Raviglione et al. (eds.), *Global Health Essentials*, Sustainable Development Goals Series,
https://doi.org/10.1007/978-3-031-33851-9_26

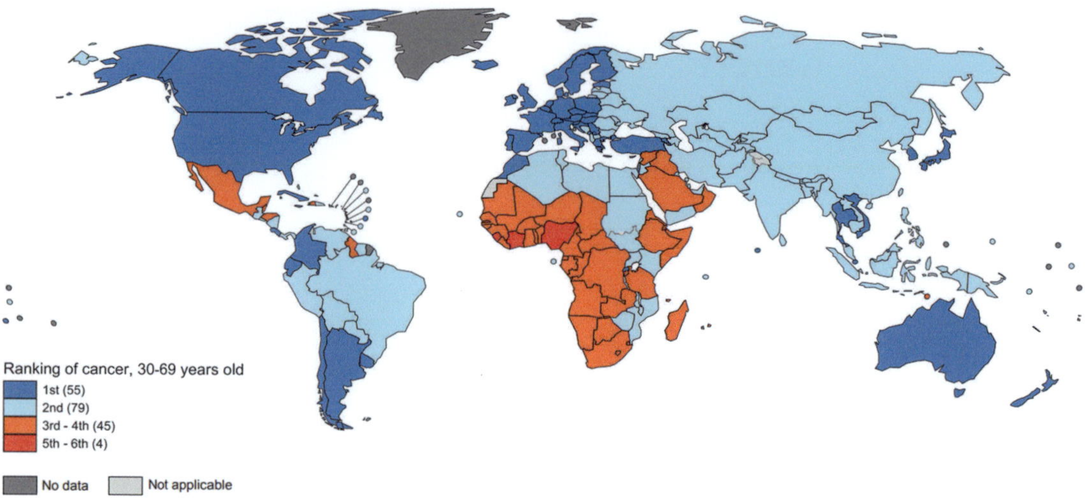

Fig. 26.1 Global map of cancer as a leading cause of premature death (i.e., at ages 30–69 years), indicating the rankings, with the numbers of countries in parentheses [1]

peutical interventions. Cancer treatment modalities are complex and evolving rapidly. Many cancer types are curable if detected early and treated adequately. Despite this, progress in reducing national cancer burdens is still limited to higher-income countries (HICs).

This chapter aims at highlighting the specificities of cancer control in the context of noncommunicable diseases (NCDs). It emphasizes the need for contextualizing cancer prevention and control measures to the needs of low- and middle-income countries, their health care systems, so that all patients benefit from progress in cancer research. It also provides perspectives for progress in cancer control at the crossroad of women's health, communicable diseases, and NCDs.

26.2 Description of the Issue

26.2.1 Descriptive Epidemiology and Assessment of the Cancer Burden

Population-based cancer registries play an eminent role in assessing cancer burden and trends. They are, however, limited in lower-income countries (LICs). According to WHO estimates, there were 18.1 million new cases of cancer and 9.6 million deaths in 2018 [2]. The WHO identifies cancer and other NCDs mortality data as "premature deaths" for those aged 30–69 to highlight the impact on productivity loss and economic development. Of the 15.2 million premature deaths from NCDs worldwide in 2016, 4.5 million (29.8%) were due to cancer [1]. The global cancer burden is projected to double by 2040, with the greatest increase in LICs [2]. Population growth and ageing will be the primary reasons for this.

26.2.2 International Targets and Progress Toward Their Achievements

There are no globally agreed cancer-specific targets except for cervical cancer (see chapter on cervical cancer). In 2017, the World Health Assembly (WHA) resolution on cancer urged governments to implement a set of comprehensive cancer prevention and control measures as part of National Cancer Control Programmes (NCCPs) [3]. Furthermore, cancer control is integral part of WHO's Global Action Plan for the Prevention and Control of NCDs (2013–2030) and its corresponding implementation roadmap (2023–2030) [4] with its globally agreed NCD targets and indicators [5]. The Sustainable Development Goal 3 (SDG3) specifies with its sub-goal 3.4 to reduce by 2030 premature mortality from NCDs by one-third compared to 2015 [6]. The Global NCD Report to the WHA in 2022 found that progress had been achieved in many countries regarding setting up NCDs prevention strategies that target tobacco and unhealthy diets, however, NCDs management remains a major challenge in LICs [7].

26.2.3 Determinants and Risk Factors

The chance to develop cancer depends on a great variety of risk factors. These include individual genetic susceptibility, age, unhealthy behaviour, and exposures to cancer hazards (carcinogens) and determine the transformation from normal to abnormal cells (carcinogenesis). National cancer burden, therefore, largely relates to population ageing, lifestyle, socioeconomic factors, and exposures to environmental and occupational carcinogens. Over 100 well-defined agents can induce cancerogenic cell mutations [8]. Physical agents (e.g., UV radiation), chemical agents (e.g., tobacco smoke components), and biological agents (e.g., hepatitis B virus—HBV, human papilloma virus—HPV, and human immunodeficiency virus—HIV) can cause cancers. The most important behavioural risk factors are tobacco use, unhealthy diet, alcohol use, and a lack of physical activity. Between one-third and half of all cancers are preventable [2]. In HICs, tobacco use and other behavioural cancer risk factors are predominant, whereas in LICs, infections are a major cause of cancer. With increasing urbanization in LICs, behavioural risk factors are increasing. Cancer case fatality rates largely depend on health care system preparedness to detect cancer early and treat patients. Nevertheless, there is a need to define and assess further risk factors, within the clinical, sociocultural, and translational perspectives of the care systems by using large real-world databases.

26.3 Approach to Solutions

26.3.1 Challenges to Be Faced for Containment/Control/Elimination

The planning and implementation of a Nationwide Cancer Control Programme (NCCP) is the WHO gold standard to reduce the burden of cancer [2]. A NCCP is defined as the continuum of interventions from prevention to early detection, treatment, and palliative care [2]. A step wise planning and implementation cycle is essential to achieve progress in cancer control. In 2015, 87% of all countries had developed a NCCP [9]. However, NCCPs often lack key elements to be successfully identified, developed, validated, and implemented.

Gaps in situation analysis, priority setting, budgeting, and health workforce planning are hampering progress in cancer control in many parts of the world. Investments in cancer prevention and palliative care are often scarce. With the adoption of the Global Action Plan for the Prevention and Control of NCDs and its implementation roadmap [4], the promotion of NCCPs as a distinct entity of interventions requires more attention. Although some elements of a NCCP overlap with the Global Action Plan, effective cancer control needs investments in cancer-specific prevention, early detection, treatment, and palliative care which are tailored to country priorities. Governments committed to making progress in reducing the national cancer burden are encouraged to develop both NCDs and NCCP plans that will benefit from cross-over synergies such as tobacco control. Building upon women's health and infections control programs (such as HIV) are important opportunities for scaling up cancer control. Planning a comprehensive NCCP can be one of the pacemaker steps to catalyse broad cross-talks within the care systems between prevention, early detection, treatment, and palliative care and the larger spectrum of NCDs, communicable diseases, and women's health.

26.3.2 Approaches and Strategies for Prevention and Control

Cancer prevention consists of strategies to lower modifiable risks by reducing exposure to cancer hazards and by encouraging healthy behaviour. However, there are major challenges in overcoming unhealthy behaviour because individual choices are strongly linked to social determinants such as socioeconomic status and education.

The WHO Framework Convention on Tobacco Control (FCTC) is the only legally binding strategy to prevent cancer and other NCDs [10]. It consists of a series of the most effective strategies to reduce the supply and demand of tobacco products. By 2022, 182 countries had ratified the treaty and are legally bound to implement it. In the last 20 years, there has been a constant decline in tobacco consumption worldwide [11].

Laws and regulations can play an integral role in preventing environmental exposures to cancer hazards. The control of air pollution and exposure to cancer hazards at the workplace are examples of possible governmental regulations that have a major positive impact on the health of populations. In addition, vaccination programmes against hepatitis B and HPV and the control of HIV through medical advancements have major cancer preventive potential in LICs.

The early detection of cancer increases the chance for cure. Promoting awareness among populations about the early signs and symptoms of cancer increases early diagnosis. Early detection of breast, cervical, and colorectal cancer is best achieved by organized population-based screening programmes. Substantial investment is needed to achieve high coverage of the target population and to guarantee follow-up for all screened individuals who may have cancer. Early detection and treatment of breast and cervical cancer is part of the broader context of women's health and can build upon already established care systems in low-and middle-income countries (LMICs). Adequate cancer diagnosis and treatment require specific health services including radiology, pathology, surgery, medical oncology, and radiotherapy which, however, are scarce in LICs [12]. Primary health care systems can play an important role in cancer prevention, early detection, and palliative care. For example, trained health care providers in primary health centres (PHCs) can detect and treat pre-cancer of the cervix.

It is fundamental that early detection services are integrated into a functional referral system that links to secondary and tertiary care. Curative treatment for breast, colorectal, cervix, and childhood cancers is affordable in LICs [2]. A diagnosis of cancer often is associated with major psychosocial distress among patients, their families and their caregivers which require special attention by the care team.

26.3.3 Cost-Effectiveness and Financial Considerations

Productivity loss due to cancer morbidity and mortality and the cost of cancer-related health services comprise up to 2% of the total global Gross Domestic Product (GDP) [13]. In LICs, cancer and other NCDs are playing an increasing burden on national economic development. There is urgency that international development aid funders and national governments prioritize cancer control and other NCDs. Several cancers are preventable through the implementation of a series of cost-effective interventions [14], such as increasing tobacco taxes and HBV and HPV vaccination programmes. Cervical cancer screening and the early detection of breast cancer that is linked to referral systems for management are cost-effective in low resource settings [15]. In addition, investments in palliative care programmes are feasible and inexpensive and are effective in increasing the quality of life of patients from diagnosis to advanced stages. Despite the limitations to define the direct and indirect cost-effectiveness of cancer control interventions, there is a large consensus in the scientific community that a multimodal prevention and treatment program is also beneficial from the economic perspective.

26.3.4 Responsibilities of Different National and International Institutions

National governments are responsible for developing a NCCP. NCCP planning and implementation requires a multi-stakeholder platform. Governmental representatives should include Ministries of Health, Finance, Labour and Agriculture, and Social Affairs. Civil society such as the Union for International Cancer Control (UICC), professional organizations such as the European Society for Gynaecological Oncology (ESGO), the European Society of Medical Oncology (ESMO), and foundations such as Global Surgery Foundation (GSF) are important stakeholders to support national cancer control planning. Governments can rely on guidance by WHO and other UN agencies in the planning and priority setting for evidence-based interventions. Patient advocacy organizations have a key role in creating political will and advocating on behalf of patients to gain equal access to quality services.

26.4 Main Conclusions and Recommendations

There is an urgent need to set up comprehensive and effective NCCPs to respond to the increasing cancer burden worldwide. Inequalities in access to cancer prevention and care result in millions of cancer deaths every year, many of which could be avoided. Countries will need to invest in cancer-specific interventions to achieve SDG 3.4. Effective cancer control requires national priority setting and budgeting in cost-effective and feasible interventions under the umbrella of a well-organized and financed NCCP. An assessment of the prevailing cancer risks and cancer types along with quality health care system's strengths and weaknesses is the first step to develop a NCCP that is tailored to specific country needs. Prioritizing interventions that are most cost-effective is key. Programs aimed at women's health—one of the key quality indicators of health care systems—are best positioned to be synergized with the prevention and control of women's cancers. International cooperation is needed to support LMICs in their efforts to strengthen health systems to enable them to provide equal access to cancer prevention, early detection, treatment, and palliative care at all ages. Such support is particularly crucial for the training of health care providers in comprehensive cancer care.

References

1. International Agency for Research on Cancer (IARC), Wild C, Weiderpass E, Stewart B. Editors. World cancer report. Cancer research for cancer prevention. IARC Lyon; 2020. p. 16. https://www.iarc.who.int/cards_page/world-cancer-report/. Accessed 30 June 2023.
2. World Health Organization. WHO report on cancer: setting priorities, investing wisely, and providing care for all. Geneva: World Health Organization; 2020. p. 13–4. https://www.who.int/publications/i/item/9789240001299. Accessed 30 June 2023.
3. 70th World Health Assembly. Cancer prevention and control in the context of an integrated approach. WHA70.12 agenda item 15.6 31. Geneva; 2017. https://apps.who.int/gb/ebwha/pdf_files/WHA70/A70_R12-en.pdf. Accessed 30 June 2023.
4. 75th World Health Assembly. Follow-up to the political declaration of the third high-level meeting of the general assembly on the prevention and control of non-communicable diseases A75/10. Geneva; 2022. https://apps.who.int/gb/ebwha/pdf_files/WHA75/A75_10Add8-en.pdf. Accessed 30 June 2023.
5. World Health Organization. Noncommunicable Disease Surveillance, Monitoring and Reporting. NCD global monitoring framework. https://www.who.int/teams/ncds/surveillance/monitoring-capacity/gmf. Accessed 30 June 2023.
6. World Health Organization. The Global Health Observatory. SDG Target 3.4 Noncommunicable diseases and mental health: by 2030, reduce by one third premature mortality from non-communicable diseases through prevention and treatment and pro-

mote mental health and well-being. https://www.who.int/data/gho/data/themes/topics/indicator-groups/indicator-group-details/GHO/sdg-target-3.4-noncommunicable-diseases-and-mental-health. Accessed 30 June 2023.
7. WHO Executive Board. Political declaration of the third high-level meeting of the general assembly on the prevention and control of noncommunicable diseases report by the director-general. EB150/7 150th session. Geneva; 2022. https://apps.who.int/gb/ebwha/pdf_files/EB150/B150_7-en.pdf. Accessed 30 June 2023.
8. International Agency for the Research in Cancer (IARC). IARC Monographs for the identification of carcinogenic hazards to humans. https://monographs.iarc.who.int/. Accessed 30 June 2023.
9. Romero Y, Trapani D, Johnson S, et al. National cancer control plans: a global analysis. Lancet Oncol. 2018;19:e546–55.
10. World Health Organization. WHO Framework Convention on Tobacco Control. https://fctc.who.int/who-fctc/overview. Accessed 30 June 2023.
11. World Health Organization. WHO global report on trends in prevalence of tobacco use 2000–2025, fourth edition. Geneva; 2021. https://www.who.int/publications/i/item/9789240039322. Accessed 30 June 2023.
12. Ullrich A, et al. Gynecologic oncology on the global health agenda: a wake-up call. Gynecol Oncol. 2021;161(2):336–8.
13. International Agency for Research on Cancer (IARC). Stewart B. Wild C. Editors. World cancer report 2014. Geneva: IARC Lyon, disseminated by WHO Press; 2014. p. 67. https://publications.iarc.fr/Non-Series-Publications/World-Cancer-Reports/World-Cancer-Report-2014. Accessed 30 June 2023.
14. World Health Organization. Tackling NCDs: 'best buys' and other recommended interventions for the prevention and control of noncommunicable diseases. Geneva: WHO; 2017. https://apps.who.int/iris/handle/10665/259232. Accessed 30 June 2023.
15. Ralaidovy A, et al. Cost-effective interventions for breast cancer, cervical cancer, and colorectal cancer: new results from WHO-CHOICE. Cost Eff Resour Alloc. 2018;16:38. https://doi.org/10.1186/s12962-018-0157-0. Accessed 30 June 2023.

27 Diabetes

Chittari V. Harinarayan and Akhila Harinarayan

Abstract

Diabetes mellitus (DM) is a metabolic vascular disorder affecting carbohydrate, protein and lipid metabolism. Type 1 DM is due to the inability of the body to produce enough insulin while type 2 DM is due to not being able to utilize the insulin it produces. The term prediabetes is used to describe Impaired Glucose Tolerance (IGT) or Impaired Fasting Glucose (IFG), and gestational diabetes mellitus (GDM) is diabetes detected for the first time in the antenatal period. Diabetes affects all the organs in the body, and complications can be vascular or metabolic. While the microvascular disease is specific to diabetes, macrovascular disease gets accelerated and increases morbidity and mortality. This chapter deals with the prevalence, health expenditure above type of diabetes as of 2021 and its projection in 2045. It also deals with the various ongoing prevention programs and the possible measures to be taken to prevent morbidity and mortality due to diabetes and also emphasizes the role of information technology in addressing the pandemic of diabetes.

Keywords

Diabetes mellitus · Type 1 · Type 2 · Gestational diabetes · Microvascular complications · Macrovascular complications · Diabetes prevention program · Diabetes-related expenditure

27.1 Introduction

Diabetes (DM) is a metabolic cum vascular disorder affecting carbohydrate, protein and lipid metabolism either due to the inability of the body to produce enough insulin (type 1 diabetes—T1DM) or not being able to utilize the insulin it produces (type 2 diabetes—T2DM). T1DM mostly occurs in children and also adults. They require insulin for survival. T2DM is common between 20 and 79 years of age. T2DM can also occur in adolescent children. T2DM can be prevented or delayed, and sometimes remission is possible. The term prediabetes is used to describe Impaired Glucose Tolerance (IGT) or Impaired Fasting Glucose (IFG). It indicates a high risk of developing T2DM and related complications. Gestational diabetes mellitus (GDM) is detected

C. V. Harinarayan (✉)
Institute of Endocrinology, Diabetes, Thyroid and Osteoporosis Disorders, Sakra World Hospitals, Bangalore, Karnataka, India

Department of Medicine & Endocrinology, Saveetha Medical College, Saveetha Institute of Medical and Technical Sciences University, Chennai, Tamil Nadu, India

A. Harinarayan
Information Services Group (ISG), Bangalore, Karnataka, India

M. C. B. Raviglione et al. (eds.), *Global Health Essentials*, Sustainable Development Goals Series,
https://doi.org/10.1007/978-3-031-33851-9_27

for the first time in the antenatal period. It disappears post-partum. Diabetes affects all the organs in the body. While the microvascular disease is specific to diabetes, macrovascular disease gets accelerated. Complications can be vascular or metabolic. It increases morbidity and mortality.

27.2 Descriptive Epidemiology and Assessment of the Global Burden [1, 2]

27.2.1 Prevalence and Global Burden

As described in detail in Table 27.1 and Box 27.1.

Box 27.1 Depicting the Epidemiology and Burden of Diabetes Mellitus: A Fact Sheet

Global:

- Diabetes Mellitus (DM) is a major health issue affecting nearly half a billion people worldwide.
- Type 2 diabetes (T2DM) accounts for 90% of all diabetes worldwide.
- Between 20 and 79 years, 537 million (10.5%) adults are living with diabetes, and this number is estimated to increase to 783 million (12.2%) by 2045.
- Currently, 1 in 2 adults lives with undiagnosed diabetes (~240 million). Among them, 3 in 4 adults (90% of them) live in low- and middle-income countries. More than half of these people are in Africa, Southeast Asia and the Western Pacific regions.
- Between the ages of 0 and 19 years, 1.2 million children and adolescents have type 1 diabetes (T1DM) and 54% of them are under the age of 15. The number of newly diagnosed cases is 186,100 per year.
- 541 million people (10.6%) between the age of 20 and 79 years are living with Impaired Glucose Tolerance (IGT).
- 319 million people (10.6%) are having Impaired Fasting Glucose (IFG)
- 21.1 million live births (16.7%) (1 in 6 live births) between the age of 20 and 49 years are affected by hyperglycaemia in pregnancy (HIP).
- 16% growth in the prevalence of diabetes. Of this 94% will be from low- and middle-income countries where the population growth is likely to be greater.

Africa:

- Lowest prevalence rate (4.5%) of diabetes among the International Diabetes Federation (IDF) regions.
- Undiagnosed diabetes is the highest 53.6% (1 in 5 people). The highest proportion of all IDF regions.
- The predicted increase in Impaired Glucose Tolerance (IGT) by 107% (117 million) by 2045.
- Second lowest diabetes-related expenditure is $13b (1% of global expenditure).

Europe:

- The highest number of people with type 1 diabetes mellitus (T1DM) (295,000) and the highest increase annually per year (31,000 new cases/year).
- In 2021, the expenditure spent on diabetes was 189.3 billion USD which is 19.6% of the total spent worldwide.
- Second highest treatment cost worldwide per person of diabetes aged 20–79 years ($3086).

Middle-East and North Africa:

- The highest prevalence of DM among IDF regions (16.2%).
- 13.6% of people with diabetes worldwide reside here.
- Second highest increase by 18% of all IDF regions is predicted to reach 136 million by 2045.

Table 27.1 Describing the prevalence (age group 20–79 years) of diabetes mellitus, impaired glucose tolerance, hyperglycaemia in pregnancy, number of undiagnosed diabetes, diabetes-related deaths, diabetes between 0 and 19 years of age in 2021 and projected for 2045

	2021 Prevalence (%)				No of adults with DM 20–79 years	No of undiagnosed DM 2021	Diabetes-related deaths 2021	0–19 years	Health expenditure ($) 2021 billions	2045 prevalence (%)			Health expenditure ($) 2045 billions	Predicted increase by 2045 (age 20–79 years)
	20–79 years									20–79 years				
	DM	IGT	IFG	HIP in live births						DM	IGT	IFG		
Global	10.5	10.6	6.2	16.7	536.6 m	240 m	6.7 m	1.2 m	966	12.5	11.4	6.9	1054	12.25% n = 783 m
Africa	4.5(5.3)	9.9(12.6)	7.8(8)	1 in 8	1 in 22 n = 24 m	1 in 5 (54%)	4,16,000	59,500	12.6	5.2(5.6)	11.1(14.1)	8(7.6)	46.7	129% n = 55 m
Europe	9.2(7)	8.2(7.1)	3.8(3.3)	1 in 7	1 in 11 n = 61 m	1 in 3 (36%)	1,11,100	294,000	189.3	10.4(8.7)	8.3(7.8)	4(3.7)	185.3	13% n = 69 m
Middle East and North Africa	16.2(18.1)	10.6(11.2)	6.5(6.1)	1 in 7	1 in 6 n = 73 m	1 in 3 (37.6%)	7,96,000	192,500	32.6	19.3(20.4)	11.5(11.7)	6.8(6.3)	46.3	86% n = 136 m
North America and Caribbean	14(11.9)	13(11.2)	8.8(8.3)	1 in 6	1 in 7 n = 51 m	1 in 4 (24.1%)	9,31,000	192,500	414.5	15.2(14.2)	13.7(11.7)	9.1(8.7)	408.7	24% n = 63 m
South and Central America	9.5(8.2)	11.6(10.9)	13.8(10)	1 in 6	1 in 11 n = 33 m	1 in 3 (32.9%)	4,10,000	121,300	65.3	11.9(9.8)	12.8(11.7)	15.3(10.6)	81.6	48% n = 49 m
Southeast Asia	8.7(10)	4.5(5.4)	9.2(8.8)	1 in 4	1 in 11 n = 90 m	1 in 2 (51.2%)	7,47,000	244,500	10.1	11.3(11.3)	5.7(5.8)	9.4(9.3)	15	69% n = 152 m
Western Pacific	11.9(9.9)	14.6(12.9)	2.9(2.5)	1 in 7	1 in 8 n = 206 m	1 in 2 52.9%	2.3 m	107,900	241.3	14.4(11.5)	16.1(14)	3.1(2.7)	269.5	27% n = 260 m

The prevalence values given are in percentage
Values given in brackets are age-adjusted comparative prevalence. *DM* diabetes mellitus; *IGT* impaired glucose tolerance; *IFG* impaired fasting glucose; *HIP* hyperglycaemia in pregnancy; *m* million; *b* billion; $ US dollars [1]

- 32.6 billion USD spent on diabetes (3% of the total spent worldwide)
- The highest percentage of diabetes-related deaths among the working-age group (25.4%).

North America and the Caribbean:
- Second highest prevalence of DM among IDF regions.
- The highest number of children and adults with T1DM (193,000).
- The highest diabetes-related expenditure is $415b—which is 43% of global expenditure.
- The highest average cost per person with DM 20–79 years ($ 8208).

South and Central America:
- 65.3 billion USD spent representing 6.7% of the total spent worldwide.
- By 2045, the prevalence of DM will increase by 25% reaching 49 million.

South-East Asia:
- 16.8% of diabetes worldwide reside here.
- India accounts for 90% of all diabetes worldwide which is 1 in 7 adults worldwide.
- Total diabetes-related expenditure in the region is 10 billion USD—second lowest in all IDF regions (1% of the total spent worldwide).

Western Pacific
- 38% of adults (one-third) with DM live in this region.
- China accounts for 1 in 4 adults living in DM worldwide.
- Diabetes-related expenditure 241b $—25% of global expenditure.

Based on the World Bank Income Classification:
- In 2021 worldwide, in high-, middle-, and low-income countries, the prevalence and comparative prevalence (given in brackets) of DM (20–79 years) in percentage are 10.5(9.8), 11(8.4), 10.8(10.5), 5.5(6.7) and in 2045 it is expected to be 12.2(11.2), 12.4(10.3), 13.1(12) and 6.1(7), respectively.
- The proportion of undiagnosed DM in 2021 is 44.7, 28.8, 48.4 and 50.5, respectively.
- Among adults 20–79 years of age, the prevalence (comparative prevalence) in % is 10.5(9.8) in 2021 and is predicted to rise to 12.2(11.2) by 2045.
- As a result of globalization, the prevalence of DM in urban areas is expected to increase from 360 million-12.1% (2021) to 596.5 million-13.9% (2045) due to population ageing.
- The top 5 countries with the number of adults with diabetes in 2021 are China, India, Pakistan, the USA and Indonesia, they would maintain the same order in 2045.
- The comparative prevalence in Pakistan at 30.8%, French Polynesia at 25.2%, Kuwait at 24.9%, New Caledonia at 23.4% and Northern Mariana Island at 23.4%. In 2045, it will be Pakistan at 33.6%, Kuwait at 29.8%, French Polynesia at 28.2%, Mauritius at 26.6% and New Caledonia at 26.2%.

27.2.2 Incidence

Incidence is the key element in tracking the progress of the diabetes epidemic. It is an appropriate measure of the population at risk. A systematic review of trends in the incidence of T2DM showed the trends peaked in 1990–1999. Between 1960 and 1989, 36% had increased, 55% had stable and 9% had decreasing trends; from 1990 to 2005, 66% had increased, 32% stable and 2% had decreasing trends; from 2006 to 2014, 33% increased trends, 30% stable and 36% had decreasing trends [3]. The falling and stable incidence hint at the success of prevention strategies implemented in regions. The stable or declining trend may also be because of the reduction in undiagnosed diabetes which is due to changing diagnostic criteria in previous decades and the intensification of diagnostic and screening activities. The incidence data for T1DM shows the highest in northern European regions and Middle-East and North Africa.

Analysis of trends of diabetes—global, regional and national between 1995 and 2005 shows diabetes as a leading cause of reduced life expectancy and mortality. Since 1990, global burden has increased significantly. The magnitude of diabetes-related disease burden and trends varies across different regions and countries. The global prevalence, death, disability-adjusted life years (DALY) and incidence in 2017 (in millions) were 476, 1.37, 67.9, 22.9 are projected to be 570.9, 1.59, 79.3 and 56.6, respectively. For T1DM DALY and global age-standardized mortality declined. The metabolic risk factors contributing to DALY and attributable deaths in diabetes are high body mass index (BMI), inappropriate diet, smoking and low physical activity (Box 27.2) [4, 5].

27.3 Approaches and Strategies for Prevention and Control of the Diabetes

Diabetes is a growing public health challenge globally. Around 70% of the cases occur in low- and middle-income countries (LMICs) because of decreasing physical activity (due to urbanization and mechanization) and consumption of high-calorie food [5]. Prediabetics are a set of populations who have dysglycemia not meeting conventional criteria for diabetes but higher than normal. They are at risk of developing diabetes approximately 5–10% compared to below 1% of normoglycemic individuals. Early recognition of prediabetes in high-risk individuals, crucial lifestyle modifications as well as medications has effectively reduced the progression to diabetes. Hence, early identification of prediabetes helps intensive management to delay progression to diabetes and delay progression of diabetes and its complications.

T2DM develops because of the interaction between genetic and environmental risk factors. T2DM is a long-latency disease which casts it effects of dysglycemia in later life as vascular and metabolic complications. Good glycaemic control in the early course of the disease reduces the risk of complications known as the "Legacy Effect" (metabolic memory).

Primary prevention of DM is defined as controlling the modifiable risk factors like overweight, obesity, sedentary lifestyle, unhealthy diet, previous IFG or IGT, alcohol and tobacco consumption and the adverse intrauterine environment through population prevention programs.

Primary prevention strategies are: (a) downstream strategies targeting individuals with IFG or IGT (population with the highest risk of diabetes); (b) midstream strategies targeting defined populations who are at increased risk, like Pima Indians and Asian Indians; and (c) upstream strategies by public policy and environmental interventions targeting the whole population to maintain a healthy lifestyle [6, 7].

The downstream strategy is simple and cost-effective. Major lifestyle modifications (LSM) addressing diet regulations and increased physical activity have shown beneficial effects in reducing conversion to diabetes. These outcomes are supported by the China Da Qing Study, the Finnish diabetes prevention program, the Diabetes Prevention Program (DPP) (USA), the India DPP (IDPP) and the Japanese Diabetes Prevention Study. Pharmacological studies in the prevention of DM are DPP (metformin), IDPP-1 (Metformin), STOP-NIDDM (Acarbose), TRIPOD (Troglitazone), DREAM (Rosiglitazone), IDPP-2 (LSM + Pioglitazone) and CANOE (Rosiglitazone + Metformin). Except for metformin, all other drugs have had long-term adverse effects limiting their long-term use in prevention programs. The DPPOS study (LSM + Metformin), Finnish DPS (LSM), and China Da Qing Study (CDQDPS) have shown the durability of the programs through their sustained improvement in insulin sensitivity, and beta-cell function has been reported from these studies. Except for metformin other drugs used for DPP did not show an acceptable long-term safety profile. Also, they are costly. Monitoring safety adds to the cost [8, 9].

Box 27.2 describes in detail upstream strategies by community interventions and policies for the prevention of T2DM and the burden of complications of this disease.

Box 27.2 Upstream Strategies by Community Interventions and Policies for the Prevention of Type 2 Diabetes

- The healthcare system focuses on care and not prevention. At the community level—complementary clinical and public health strategies are needed.
- Clinical sector—identifying risk status and referring to community-based lifestyle programs for high-risk individuals. They are provided nutrition counselling and medications to prevent diabetes.
- The public health sector—monitors the risk of diabetes, establishes diabetes prevention services and mobilizes partnerships for these services.
- Diabetes Prevention Program (DPP)—Lifestyle interventions initially weekly sessions—help learn skills to reduce calories and increase physical activity to achieve weight loss.
- Focus on translational research—significantly decreases the incidence of diabetes and health cost associated with T2DM by best utilizing limited resources for delivering lifestyle interventions.
- Meta-analysis of various translational studies based on United States DPP has shown an average of 4% weight loss from baseline after 12 months after the intervention.
- Finnish DPP showed it was possible to prevent T2DM in primary healthcare settings.
- The Life—program in Australia is successful—a good example of translating prevention research to intervention programs in adults.
- In addition to the durability of the program, it is important to assess the cost associated with intervention programs.
- At the population level, intervention programs require collaboration among community-based organizations, healthcare and public health professionals, insurance players, academia and others. DPP brings together the above groups and unifies the delivery of the program.
- Community–civic partnership [8–10] is provided by
  - At the population level: Community—encompassing strong community organizations, informed populations, healthy public policy, insurance players and a supportive environment. This helps the population prevent entering the prediabetes phase.
  - At the clinic level: proactive practice, informed and activated patients, information system and decision support. This helps established diabetics prevent diabetes-related complications.
  - The partnership between the community and clinical levels established the preventive zone—where prediabetics can be prevented to become established diabetes patients. This involves screening for high-risk, diagnosing prediabetes, structured lifestyle prevention programs, regular glucose monitoring and reimbursement facilities made available.
- **Other proposals:**
  - Emphasizing primary prevention of diabetes in medical graduates, post-graduate training and allied health care providers.
  - Enhancing the emphasis on primary prevention in medical and scientific societies and primary care.

- Prevention modules like continuing medical education—webinars, scientific meeting and so on.
- Third-party reimbursement with referrals from health care professionals to conduct community-based prevention programs.
- Incentivising primary prevention programs.
- Screening of high-risk populations for prediabetes and diabetes at the community level.
- Establishing academically based prevention and treatment programs in the hospitals.

Burden of complications:

- DM is a cause of prematurity mortality. Approximately 50% of T2DM die due to cardiovascular disease, and 10% due to renal failure. Global mortality is estimated to be 3.8 million deaths. Under 35 years of age—75% of all deaths were due to DM, decreases to 50% and 29% between the ages of 35 and 64 years and 64 years and older, respectively. The risk is high for women with diabetes. DM is the 8th out of 10 leading causes of death in high- and middle-income countries.
- Coronary heart disease (CHD) is the leading complication of T2DM. Diabetes doubles the risk of CHD in men and quadruples in women. Prevalence ranges from 5 to 36% depending on the setting. Smoking, dyslipidaemia, hypertension and other determinants of vascular risk are further risks for IGF and IGT. Cerebrovascular accidents (CVA) prevalence ranges from 4 to 12% (clinic-based population) and 4 to 5% (population-based studies). The risk of CVA is three times more than the general population.
- Nephropathy, retinopathy, neuropathy and small vessel vasculopathy leading to amputations are the principle microvascular complications of diabetes. DM is the cause of end-stage renal failure (ESRD) in many developed countries and accounts for 50% of renal replacement therapy. The incidence rate of ESRD is approximately 6 per 1000 person-years, with two-thirds becoming dialysis dependant and a third dying. Changes in referral and acceptance rates for renal replacement therapy are caused by a real increase in incidence. Microalbuminuria, a predictor of early renal disease ranges from 3 to 57% (clinic-based) and 19–42% (population-based) in various studies. Overt nephropathy prevalence ranged from 5 to 20% and 9 to 33%, respectively. Nephropathy is higher among men and increases with age.
- Diabetic retinopathy (DR) is the common cause of blindness among diabetics between 30 and 69 years of age. Prevalence ranges from 11 to 65% (clinic-based) and 10 to 55% (population-based) studies. Prevalence ranges from 11 to 65% (clinic-based) and 10 to 55% (population-based) studies. It is projected to triple from 5.5 to 16 million (DR) and 1.2 to 3.4 million (vision-threatening DR) between 2005 and 2050.
- Diabetic neuropathy and lower limb amputations—Diabetics are at 25 times greater risk. Prevalence ranges from 6 to 68% (clinic-based) and 13 to 45% (population-based) studies. It increases with the duration of DM and age.

27.4 Cost-Effectiveness and Financial Considerations

In diabetes prevention program studies (DPP), to prevent one case of DM by lifestyle modification (LSM) the cost was $15,700 and with metformin $31,000. In India DPP (IDPP), the cost for LSM was $1,052. Finnish DPP showed the initial phase of 4 years of LSM had an extended benefit for another 3 years lowering the risk for DM. This shows the durability of the program. Translating this knowledge to action at the community level is the need of the hour. It is not a simple task for LMICs where the disease is anticipated to reach epidemic proportions.

In the past 15 years, there is a 316% increase in the direct cost of diabetes healthcare expenditure for adults 20–79 years of age. It has grown from $232 billion in 2007 to $ 966 billion in 2021. It is estimated to reach $ 1.03 trillion by 2030 (66.4% increase) and $1.05 by 2045 (9.1% increase compared to 2021 estimates). The highest diabetes-related health expenditure ($8,209 per adult diabetic) is from North America and the Caribbean (NAC). About 11.5% of global spending is due to diabetes. The highest is 18.4% from the South and Central America, and the lowest is 8.6% observed in Europe. The cost of treatment of DM with the macrovascular disease is three times higher than patients without the macrovascular disease and it is seven times higher compared to those without DM or macrovascular disease. The cost for microvascular disease is two times higher than those with no complications. Inpatient costs are the maximum drive in those with macrovascular complications and the component of pharmacy costs are the maximum of all [6].

Table 27.2 Describing the role of information technology in addressing the pandemic of diabetes mellitus

	Personal health approach [11–13]	Public health approach [11–13]
Description	Services are provided for the benefit of an individual or for the specific treatment of DM for the individual	Activities are aimed to provide goods and services for a set of population segment
Target audience	Individuals including adults, children, and aged persons	Targets a set of population depending on region or endemic issues
Industry players involved	• Healthcare service provider • Public health service	• Public service departments • Non-profit organizations • Government initiatives
Some approaches using it	• Tailored web-based lifestyle intervention • Telemedicine application to reach to DM patients • Targeted services through smartphone apps • Use of social media for weight-loss related interventions	• DM prevention programs through mass media using social media channels. • Mobile-health interventions targeted to specific set of population • Government initiatives through mobile-based apps

27.5 Information Technology as Means of Addressing the Diabetes Pandemic

With numerous strategies for the control, management and prevention of DM, healthcare information technology has acted as a catalyst to accelerate the strategies and have a positive outcome for technology-based interventions [12]. Some of the technology interventions include telemedicine, automated insulin delivery and smartphone applications [13]. These interventions can be categorized into personal health approaches and public health approaches (see Table 27.2).

Many approaches use technology as a lever to deliver services. Web-based tailored lifestyle intervention delivers lifestyle adjustments required for DM through a web based on the conditions of the patient. This method has a low intervention cost and wider reach. These web-based programs deliver positive behaviour change at low costs. Telemedicine application for the care of DM patients delivers services through a video call or a telephonic call with a medical graduate monitoring at the patient end. Doctors can connect to remote regions to provide services to patients. The telemedicine approach for DM care has had some impact on managing diabetes. Building sustainable business models around telemedicine which can be scaled is yet to see the light. Mobile applications are also sought by many as it enables easy access to self-manage certain aspects of day-to-day care for DM patients. Mobile-health apps support self-management for both Type 1 and 2 DM patients. While the cost of development of these apps is minimal, most of these apps are targeted at providing education and support for individuals. The tangible benefits of these apps are yet to be realized completely and established.

27.6 Responsibilities of Different National and International Institutions

Prevention programs require the integration of community, government, healthcare services, media and education with healthcare services. Financial support from institutional and national organizations is a must. Technology has been solving multiple challenges across the world and is a means to reach to a wider audience to solve challenges faced by DM patients.

References

1. IDF Diabetes Atlas 2021. https://diabetesatlas.org/atlas/tenth-edition/.
2. Sun H, Saeedi P, Karuranga S, Pinkepank M, Ogurtsova K, Duncan BB, et al. IDF Diabetes Atlas: global, regional and country-level diabetes prevalence estimates for 2021 and projections for 2045. Diabetes Res Clin Pract. 2022;183:109119. https://doi.org/10.1016/j.diabres.2021.109119. Epub 2021 Dec 6
3. Magliano DJ, Islam RM, Barr ELM, Gregg EW, Pavkov ME, Harding JL, et al. Trends in incidence of total or type 2 diabetes: systematic review. BMJ. 2019;366:l5003. https://doi.org/10.1136/bmj.l5003.
4. Wild S, Roglic G, Green A, Sicree R, King H. Global prevalence of diabetes: estimates for the year 2000 and projections for 2030. Diabetes Care. 2004;27(5):1047–53. https://doi.org/10.2337/diacare.27.5.1047.
5. Lin X, Xu Y, Pan X, Xu J, Ding Y, Sun X, et al. Global, regional, and national burden and trend of diabetes in 195 countries and territories: an analysis from 1990 to 2025. Sci Rep. 2020;10(1):14790. https://doi.org/10.1038/s41598-020-71908-9.
6. van Dieren S, Beulens JW, van der Schouw YT, Grobbee DE, Neal B. The global burden of diabetes and its complications: an emerging pandemic. Eur J Cardiovasc Prev Rehabil. 2010;17(Suppl 1):S3–8. https://doi.org/10.1097/01.hjr.0000368191.86614.5a.
7. Bergman M, Buysschaert M, Schwarz PE, Albright A, Narayan KV, Yach D. Diabetes prevention: global health policy and perspectives from the ground. Diabetes Manag (Lond). 2012;2(4):309–21. https://doi.org/10.2217/dmt.12.34.
8. Uusitupa M, Khan TA, Viguiliouk E, Kahleova H, Rivellese AA, Hermansen K, et al. Prevention of type 2 diabetes by lifestyle changes: a systematic review and meta-analysis. Nutrients. 2019;11(11):2611 https://doi.org/10.3390/nu11112611.
9. Hussain A, Claussen B, Ramachandran A, Williams R. Prevention of type 2 diabetes: a review. Diabetes Res Clin Pract. 2007;76(3):317–26. https://doi.org/10.1016/j.diabres.2006.09.020. Epub 2006 Oct 27.
10. Diabetes Prevention Program Research Group. 10-year follow-up of diabetes incidence and weight loss in the Diabetes Prevention Program Outcomes Study. Lancet. 2009;374(9702):1677–86. https://doi.org/10.1016/S0140-6736(09)61457-4. Epub 2009 Oct 29. Erratum in: Lancet. 2009 Dec 19;374(9707):2054.
11. Kaufman N, Mel E. Using digital health technology to prevent and treat Diabetes. Diabetes Technol Ther. 2020;22(S1):S63–78. https://doi.org/10.1089/dia.2020.2505.
12. Knox ECL, Quirk H, Glazebrook C, Randell T, Blake H. Impact of technology-based interventions for children and young people with type 1 diabetes on key diabetes self-management behaviours and prerequisites: a systematic review. BMC Endocr Disord. 2019;19(1):7. https://www.ncbi.nlm.nih.gov/pmc/articles/PMC6329145/. Accessed 22 Oct 2022.
13. Abbot. New Diabetes Technology: Improving Care Through Innovation. https://www.abbott.com/corpnewsroom/diabetes-care/new-diabetes-technology-improving-care-through-innovation.html. Accessed 22 Oct 2022.

Endocrinological Disorders of Population-Level Importance

28

Chittari V. Harinarayan and Akhila Harinarayan

Abstract

Iodine is a trace element essential for nervous and skeletal development during pregnancy. Iodine deficiency during pregnancy can cause spontaneous abortions, stillbirths and an irreversible form of mental retardation—cretinism. Calcium and vitamin D are complementary twin nutrients essential for bone health. Worldwide, 88% of households consume iodized salt. Since 1990, the iodine-deficient countries have fallen from 113 to 21. Improved surveillance and mandatory iodization of salt are required to achieve 100% coverage of the population. Global calcium and vitamin D deficiency (twin nutrient deficiency) is described along with various measures to combat the same. Though there are various measures to combat the twin nutrient deficiency, it has a long way to go. Use of information technology to address the problem will be very useful.

C. V. Harinarayan (✉)
Institute of Endocrinology, Diabetes, Thyroid and Osteoporosis Disorders, Sakra World Hospitals, Bangalore, Karnataka, India

Department of Medicine & Endocrinology, Saveetha Medical College, Saveetha Institute of Medical and Technical Sciences University, Chennai, Tamil Nadu, India

A. Harinarayan
Information Services Group (ISG), Bangalore, Karnataka, India

Keywords

Iodine · Salt iodization · Deficiency · Recommended daily/dietary allowances · Calcium · Vitamin D · Rickets · Osteomalacia · Osteoporosis

28.1 Introduction

Iodine is a micronutrient essential for the mental development of the foetus in pregnancy and can cause stillbirths, spontaneous abortions, and cretinism. Iodine deficiency in infants can affect cognitive development and healthy growth of infants. Calcium and vitamin D are essential twin nutrients for bone health to achieve peak bone mass and preserve bone with advancing age. Deficiency of these nutrients causes diseases—rickets/osteomalacia which are short/long latency diseases. This section deals with the global deficiency of these nutrients and the remedial measures undertaken and their impact.

28.2 Iodine

Iodine is an essential trace element found in some food. It is necessary to make thyroid hormones, triiodothyronine and thyroxin, a critical determinant of metabolic activity. It helps regulate biochemical reactions, protein synthesis and

M. C. B. Raviglione et al. (eds.), *Global Health Essentials*, Sustainable Development Goals Series,
https://doi.org/10.1007/978-3-031-33851-9_28

enzymatic activity. Thyroxin is also vital for the proper development of the nervous and skeletal systems in foetuses and infants.

Iodine is found in dairy products, sea foods (fish-cods and tuna), shrimps, seaweeds and iodized salt. People who do not eat dairy products or seafood might not get enough iodine. People living in mountainous areas like the Himalayas, the Alps, the Andes, and river valleys in South-East Asia have iodine-poor soil and may have an iodine deficiency.

The Recommended Daily/Dietary Allowance (RDA) for iodine for different age groups of both genders are—adequate intake (AI) in mcg: Birth to 6 months 110; 7–12 years 130; 1–8 years 90; 9–13 years 120; >14 years above 150; pregnancy 220 and lactation 290.

A median urinary iodine concentration of 100–199 μg/L is defined as an adequate iodine level for the population. In pregnant women, it is 150–249 μg/L and in lactating women ≥100 μg/L. Iodine deficiency is defined based on the mean urinary iodine concentration (μg/L) as severe <20, moderate iodine deficiency 20–49; as mild iodine deficiency 50–99, and insufficient <100.

Iodine deficiency in preterm births jeopardizes the mental health of children and their very survival. Iodine deficiency during pregnancy results in stillbirth, spontaneous abortions and cretinism, an irreversible form of mental retardation. Iodine deficiency during pregnancy can lead to mental impairment with reduced intellectual capacity at school and work. Excess iodine can be harmful and can cause enlargement of the thyroid gland (goitre) and the same symptoms as iodine deficiency. Getting several grams of iodine can cause burning of the throat and mouth, stomach ache, nausea, vomiting, diarrhoea and weak pulse. The daily upper limits of iodine (in mcg) are children 1–3 years 200; 4–8 years 300; 9–13 years 600; 14–18 years 900 and adults 1100.

Currently, about 88% of households worldwide consume iodized salt (Table 28.1) [1–3]. Mandatory and voluntary fortification of various regions and their socioeconomic data is shown in Box 28.1 [1–3]. The iodine-deficient countries have fallen from 113 to 21 since 1990 [4]. To achieve 100% iodization of the population and sustain the achievements, refinements like improved motoring and surveillance in salt iodization programs are required.

Box 28.1 Box Showing Mandatory and Voluntary Fortification—Percentage Covered—Based on Region and Socioeconomic Status [1, 2]

Region	Country
Mandatory fortification	
Low income	
	4–25% Coverage
• Africa	Guinea-Bissau, Somalia, Guinea, Ethiopia, Gambia, Central African Republic
• Americas	Haiti
	25–50% Coverage
• Africa	Guinea-Bissau, Ethiopia, Gambia, Mozambique, Guinea, Niger
• Asia	Tajikistan, Yemen
	50–75% Coverage
• Africa	Benin, Burkina Faso, Chad, Democratic Republic of the Congo, Ethiopia, Gambia, Madagascar, Mali, Mozambique, Niger, Tanzania, Togo, Uganda
• Asia	Afghanistan, Yemen, Tajikistan
	75–100% Coverage
• Africa	Benin, Burkina Faso, Burkina Faso, Central African Republic, Chad, Democratic Republic of the Congo, Ethiopia, Guinea, Guinea-Bissau, Liberia, Madagascar, Malawi, Mali, Niger, Rwanda, Tanzania, Togo, Uganda
• Americas	Haiti
• Asia	Nepal, Tajikistan
Lower middle income	
	4–25% Coverage
• Africa	Mauritania, Djibouti, Sudan, Gabon
• Asia	Cambodia, Philippines
	25–50% Coverage
• Africa	Ghana, Senegal, Sudan, Morocco, Dominican Republic,

Region	Country
• Asia	Mongolia, Uzbekistan
	50–75% Coverage
• Africa	Zambia, Egypt, Angola, Senegal, Cote d'Ivoire, Ghana, Lesotho, Sao Tome and Principe,
• Asia	Bangladesh, Cambodia, India, Myanmar, Philippines, Vietnam
• Europe	Moldova
	75–100% Coverage
• Africa	Angola, Cabo Verde, Cameroon, Congo, Cote d'Ivoire, Egypt, Eswatini, Ghana, Kenya, Lesotho, Mauritania, Nigeria, Sao Tome and Principe, Sudan, Zambia, Zimbabwe
• Americas	Bolivia
• Asia	Bangladesh, Cambodia, India, Indonesia, Kyrgyzstan, Lao PDR, Mongolia, Myanmar, Palestine, Uzbekistan
• Europe	Moldova
• Oceania	Solomon Islands
Upper middle income	
	25–50% Coverage
• Asia	Malaysia, Kazakhstan
•	**50–75% Coverage**
• Africa	Namibia
• Americas	Guatemala
• Asia	Thailand, Turkey
• Asia	Azerbaijan
• Europe	Albania
•	**75–100% Coverage**
• Africa	Algeria, Gabon, South Africa
• Asia	Armenia, Azerbaijan, China, Georgia, Jordan, Kazakhstan, Lebanon, Sri Lanka, Thailand, Turkey, Turkmenistan
• Europe	Albania, Bulgaria
• Oceania	Samoa
High income	
	50–75% Coverage
• Asia	Saudi Arabia
•	**75–100% Coverage**
• Asia	Oman
Voluntary fortification	

Region	Country
Low income	
• Africa	Sierra Leone *(40–92% COVERAGE)*
Lower middle income	
• Asia	Pakistan *(69% COVERAGE)*
• Europe	Ukraine *(33–36% COVERAGE)*
High income	
• Americas	Trinidad and Tobago *(14–63% COVERAGE)*
Low income	
	4–25% Coverage
• Africa	Guinea-Bissau, Somalia, Guinea, Ethiopia, Gambia, Central African Republic
• Americas	Haiti
	25–50% Coverage
• Africa	Guinea-Bissau, Ethiopia, Gambia, Mozambique, Guinea, Niger
• Asia	Tajikistan, Yemen
	50–75% Coverage
• Africa	Benin, Burkina Faso, Chad, Democratic Republic of the Congo, Ethiopia, Gambia, Madagascar, Mali, Mozambique, Niger, Tanzania, Togo, Uganda
• Asia	Afghanistan, Yemen, Tajikistan
	75–100% Coverage
• Africa	Benin, Burkina Faso, Burkina Faso, Central African Republic, Chad, Democratic Republic of the Congo, Ethiopia, Guinea, Guinea-Bissau, Liberia, Madagascar, Malawi, Mali, Niger, Rwanda, Tanzania, Togo, Uganda
• Americas	Haiti
• Asia	Nepal, Tajikistan
Lower middle income	
	4–25% Coverage
• Africa	Mauritania, Djibouti, Sudan, Gabon
• Asia	Cambodia, Philippines
	25–50% Coverage
• Africa	Ghana, Senegal, Sudan, Morocco, Dominican Republic,

Region	Country
• Asia	Mongolia, Uzbekistan
	50–75% Coverage
• Africa	Zambia, Egypt, Angola, Senegal, Cote d'Ivoire, Ghana, Lesotho, Sao Tome and Principe,
• Asia	Bangladesh, Cambodia, India, Myanmar, Philippines, Vietnam,
• Europe	Moldova
	75–100% Coverage
• Africa	Angola, Cabo Verde, Cameroon, Congo, Cote d'Ivoire, Egypt, Eswatini, Ghana, Kenya, Lesotho, Mauritania, Nigeria, Sao Tome and Principe, Sudan, Zambia, Zimbabwe
• Americas	Bolivia
• Asia	Bangladesh, Cambodia, India, Indonesia, Kyrgyzstan, Lao PDR, Mongolia, Myanmar, Palestine, Uzbekistan
• Europe	Moldova
• Oceania	Solomon Islands
Upper middle income	

Region	Country
	25–50% Coverage
• Asia	Malaysia, Kazakhstan
•	**50–75% Coverage**
• Africa	Namibia
• Americas	Guatemala
• Asia	Thailand, Turkey
• Asia	Azerbaijan
• Europe	Albania
•	**75–100% Coverage**
• Africa	Algeria, Gabon, South Africa
• Asia	Armenia, Azerbaijan, China, Georgia, Jordan, Kazakhstan, Lebanon, Sri Lanka, Thailand, Turkey, Turkmenistan
• Europe	Albania, Bulgaria
• Oceania	Samoa
High income	
	50–75% Coverage
• Asia	Saudi Arabia
•	**75–100% Coverage**
• Asia	Oman
• Americas	Trinidad and Tobago *(14–63% COVERAGE)*

Table 28.1 Data showing health status before and after fortification—based on region and socioeconomic status [1–2]

Region	Country	Population group	Post-fortification assessment year	Pre-fortification value µg/L	Post-fortification value µg/L
High-income countries					
		1993–1999			
Europe	Austria	SAC	2012	148.9	111[a]
Asia	Oman	SAC	2012	91	192
Europe	Croatia	SAC	2009	62.4	248
Americas	Chile	SAC	2006	91.7	252
Europe	Poland, Slovenia	SAC	2009, 2017	88.2	119.8
		2007–2009			
Asia	Bahrain, United Arab Emirates	SAC	2014	81–185	162–247
Oceania	Australia, New Zealand	SAC	2011, 2015	38–96	113–175
Upper middle-income group					
		1990–1995			
Africa	Namibia, South Africa	SAC	1999	54.5–162	215–216
Americas	Brazil, Colombia, Paraguay, Belize	SAC	2015–16	48–88	277–407
Asia	China, Iran, Sri Lanka, Thailand, Turkmenistan	SAC	2014	58–82	156–233
Europe	Bulgaria, Macedonia	SAC	2008	68–117	182–216

Table 28.1 (continued)

Region	Country	Population group	Post-fortification assessment year	Pre-fortification value μg/L	Post-fortification value μg/L
Oceania	Fiji	SAC	2016	49.1	207
		2001–2008			
Asia	Azerbaijan, Armenia, Kazakhstan, Georgia	SAC	2007	67.8–88.2	183–298
Europe	Belarus, Romania, Serbia, Albania	SAC	2018	44.5–158	102–195
Lower middle-income group					
		1990–1995			
Africa	Nigeria, Morocco	SAC	2004, 2018	68–88.2	71–130
Asia	Indonesia, Bangladesh, Lao PDR	SAC	2012–13	11 to 60	103–215
Oceania	Papua New Guinea	SAC	2005	58.2	170
		1996–2000			
Africa	Senegal, Eswatini, Ghana, Cote d'Ivoire, Tunisia, Lesotho	SAC	2009	73.5–121	104–220
Africa	Zimbabwe	SAC	2013	245	130[a]
Asia	Philippines, India, Myanmar, Viet Nam	SAC	2018	32–92	84–183
		2001–2005			
Africa	Cabo Verde, Mauritania	SAC	2010–12	52–55	115–179
Asia	Kyrgyzstan, Cambodia, Mongolia	SAC	2007	68–98	114–236
Africa	Egypt	SAC	2015	183.57	170[a]
Africa	Angola	SAC	2019	93.7	107
Americas	Nicaragua	SAC	2018	121.3	90[a]
Asia	Uzbekistan	SAC	2017	141	135[a]
Europe	Moldova	SAC	2012	165	204
Low Income Countries					
		1995–2000			
Africa	Guinea, Togo, Chad, Malawi, Uganda, Mali	SAC	2003	80.5–104	69–139
Africa	Mozambique	SAC	2004	67.8 μg/L	60[a]
		1999–2016			
Asia	Nepal	WRA, PLW	2016	114–134	241–286
Asia	Nepal	SAC	2016	143.8	314.1
		2000–2015			
Africa	Burkina Faso, Somalia	SAC	2014	73.5–101	99–147
Asia	Tajikistan	SAC	2007	67.8	139
Asia	Yemen	SAC	2015	173	100.75[a]
		2006–2010			
Africa	Gambia, Benin	SAC	2018	42–64	157–318
Africa	Liberia	SAC	2011	321	244[a]
		2011–2015			
Africa	Ethiopia	SAC	2015	55	104
Asia	Afghanistan	SAC	2013	49	171.1
Asia	Afghanistan	WRA	2013	42	107.1
		2015–2017			
Africa	Madagascar	SAC	2015	63.2	46[a]
Africa	Niger	SAC	2015	95.7	101
Americas	Haiti	SAC	2018	84	77[a]

SAC school age children; *WRA* women of reproductive age; *PLW* pregnant and/or lactating women

[a] Negative health status change

28.3 Calcium and Vitamin D

Calcium and vitamin D are essential complementary nutrients for bone health. In nutritional deficiency diseases, withdrawal of key nutrients results in the occurrence of disease. A diet containing less than 50 mg of calcium/Kcal results in osteoporosis and various non-skeletal diseases. With an increasing deficiency of 25 hydroxy vitamin D and dietary calcium deficiency, the odds of developing rickets are very high. The dietary calcium intake to prevent nutritional rickets varies inversely with the vitamin D status of the individual [5]. In the background of low dietary calcium, the secondary hyperparathyroidism [elevated parathormone (PTH) levels] stimulates intracellular calcium influx and can trigger diseases like arteriosclerosis, hypertension, diabetes mellitus, degenerative joint diseases, neurodegenerative diseases, and malignancy coined 'calcium paradox diseases' [6].

The estimated average requirement (EAR) of calcium (mg/day) as per the FAO/WHO for different age groups are infants 240–300; children 440; adolescent (males & females) 1040; men and women and 50+ age 840; pregnancy 940 and lactation 1040 [7]. The dietary calcium status of various countries and regions is depicted in Table 28.2. Low calcium intake affects the population in low- and middle-income countries. Even though individuals in high-income countries do not meet the RDA, low calcium intake is linked to health outcomes like osteoporosis, pregnancy complications, cancer and cardiovascular diseases. The estimation of the prevalence of global calcium status and adverse health outcomes is limited by the lack of standard methods to assess such status in the population. This is a major setback for developing policies and interventions at a population level to improve calcium status [8].

The Recommended Daily Requirements (RDA) of vitamin D IU for various age groups as per the Institute of Medicine (IOM) guidelines are infants 0–1 year: 400; 1–8 years: 600; 9–18 years and adults of both genders: 600; >70 years: 800 [9]. Changing lifestyles—mechanization, urbanization and more indoor activities, and obesity are some of the risk factors for the increasing prevalence of vitamin D deficiency. The foetus depends on maternal vitamin D. Maternal vitamin D deficiency during pregnancy is a risk factor for preeclampsia, preterm birth and a high incidence of caesarean sections. Prenatal vitamin D affects neurodevelopment, cognitive deficit, intelligence quotient, psychomotor outcomes, attention deficit hyperactive disorders (ADHD) and autism spectrum disorders. Maternal vitamin D has an impact on foetal bone health. The various strategies to combat twin nutrient deficiency are listed in Box 28.2.

Box 28.2 Strategies to Combat the Twin Nutrient Deficiency

Government programs	1. Nutrition programs: The governments of each region have targeted nutrition programs to inform citizens about the importance and ways to consume calcium and vitamin D through food and food supplements [10]
	2. Nutrient-rich food for school children: The governments are providing calcium and vitamin D-rich food along with mid-day meals for school-going children. This will help in the proper growth and development of children [11]
	3. Implementing fortification policies: Governments build and deliver the guidelines for fortification in food and dairy products across the food chain. This helps maintain the nutrient requirements for different food products and makes it reachable to the citizens across the country [12]
	4. Guidelines for calcium supplementation: The government along with the industry bodies enforce guidelines for children, pregnant and lactating mothers, adults and the aged. This guideline can be a yardstick for the citizens to follow the intake levels of calcium and vitamin D [13]

Programs by independent organizations or industry bodies	1. Food fortification initiatives: Many organizations are working towards playing their part across the food supply chain to fortify the food to the appropriate amounts of calcium and vitamin D. Many firms are adhering to the fortification policies and ensuring that the food that they sell are fortified with right amount of nutrients [14]
	2. CSR activities to help the underserved: Some organizations in particular regions are providing free milk to children in government schools. For example, National Dairy Development Board (NDDB), through its 'NDDB Foundation for Nutrition' (NFN) has started a 'gift milk' program wherein the state milk unions or dairy cooperatives provide milk to children in government schools in 118 schools across Delhi, Gujarat, Jharkhand, Maharashtra, Tamil Nadu, Telangana in India [15]
	3. Development of Centres of Excellence: Reckitt Benckiser and Apollo Hospital Group have partnered to launch 'Arogya Rakshak—Protected by Dettol, Cared by Apollo' initiative which targets health outcomes of people as one of the focus areas. The two brands are planning to launch a Centre of Excellence(CoE) for community nutrition. This CoE will train the frontline health workers through virtual reality and gamification; the use of artificial intelligence to assist healthcare workers in detecting malnutrition [16]
	4. Increase in exposure to sunlight: Schools should promote sunshine hours to increase exposure to sunlight. Not only children, adults also be exposed to sunlight to improve their vitamin D levels of the individuals [17]

Table 28.2 The dietary calcium status of various countries and regions [18]

Region	Country	Intake mg/d	Population group	Age years	Gender	Number studies	Year	Calcium assessment method
Africa	Uganda	238	Adults	NA	Households	173	NA	Recall
	Burkina Faso	358	Adults	NA	Households	1005	2006	Recall
	Mali	444	Adolescent/adult	15–45	Women	108	2007	Recall
	Tanzania	471	Adults	35–74	Men and women	173	1987	Recall
	South Africa	479	Adults	15+	Men and women	3231	1983–2000	Recall
	Egypt	495	Adults	20–60	Women	1090	2004	Recall
	Botswana	558	Adults	18–79	Men and women	79	2007	Recall
	Algeria	616	Adult	Adult	Men and women	176	2009–10	Recall
	Nigeria	636	NA	NA	Households	13,142	2003–4	FFQ
	Ethiopia	664	Adults	18+	Men and women	356	2005	Recall
	Morocco	672	Adolescent/adult	16+	Men and women	691	2004	FFQ
	Cameron	760	Adults	NA	Households	557	2001	NA
Asia	Nepal	175	Adults	20+	Men and women	317	2003	Recall
	Thailand	313	Adults	20–85	Men and women	436	NA	Recall
	China	339	All	2–101	NA	68,962	2002	Recall
	Indonesia	342	NA	NA	NA	NA	1998	NA
	Vietnam	345	Adults	NA	Men and women	4080	2000	Recall
	Malaysia	399	Adults	18–59	Men and women	6886	2002–03	Recall
	India	429	Adults	18+	Men and women	306,329	2011–12	Recall
	South Korea	483	Adults	19+	Men and women	15,643	2012–12	Recall

Region	Country	Intake mg/d	Population group	Age years	Gender	Number studies	Year	Calcium assessment method
	Israel	492	Adults	25–64	Men and women	2782	1999–2001	Recall
	Myanmar	498	NA	NA	NA	NA	1998	NA
	Bangladesh	529	Children and adults	ALL	Men and women	31,066	2011	NA
	Japan	533	Adults	18–74	Men and women	22,712	2003–07	Food record
	Taiwan	587	Adults	19–64	Men and women	1942	2004–08	Recall
	Pakistan	642	Adults	18+	Women	200	2008	Recall
	Kuwait	695	Adults	19+	Men and women	1049	2008–9	Recall
	Iran	859	Adults	40+	Men and women	1922	2001	Recall
Americas	Colombia	297	Adults	20–60	NA	70	2003	Food record
	Ecuador	384	Adults	19–60	Men and women	10,592	2012	Recall
	Bolivia	458	Adults	Adults	Households	5746	2002	FFQ
	Argentina	472	Adults	18–49	Women	4189	2005–05	NA
	Brazil	508	Adults	20+	Men and women	21,003/4322	2009	Food record
	Costa Rica	673	Adults	20–65	Men and women	60	1996–98	Recall
	Chile	702	Adults	35+	Men and women	597/66	2012 and 2014	FFQ
	Canada	787	Adults	19+	Men and women	35,107	2004	Recall
	Mexico	805	Adults	20–59	Men and women	15,746	2006	FFQ
	United States	934	Adults	10+	Men and women	22,823	2001–10	Recall
Oceania	Australia	805	Adults	19+	Men and women	9339	2011–12	Assessment recall

(continued)

Table 28.2 (continued)

Region	Country	Intake mg/d	Population group	Age years	Gender	Number studies	Year	Calcium assessment method
	New Zealand	807	Adolescent/adult	15+	Men and women	4721	2009	Assessment recall
Europe	Norway	488	Adult	20–47	Men and women	18,914	1994–95	Assessment
	Hungary	673	Adult	19+	Men and women	3077	2009	Assessment recall
	Belgium	728	Adult	19+	Men and women	NA	2004	Recall
	Italy	765	Adult	18+	Men and women	2831	2005–06	Recall
	Austria	773	Elderly	55+	Men and women	641	NA	Recall
	Czech Republic	782	Adult	45–69	Men and women	7913	2005	Recall
	Russia	788	Adult	45–69	Men and women	9098	2005	FFQ
	Spain	789	Adult	19+	Men and women	1923	2002–02	Recall
	Poland	830	Adult	45–69	Men and women	9859/3862	2002–2005 and 2010–2011	FFQ
	Serbia	838	Adult	30–74	Men and women	1305	1998 and 2003	Assessment recall
	Latvia	865	Adult	19–64	NA	32	1997	Recall
	France	877	Adult	18–79	Men and women	1082	2005–07	Food record
	Portugal	923	Adult	19+	Men and women	2994	1999–2003	FFQ
	Greece	942	Adult	33–72 (95% of sample)	Men and women	1982	1992–2001	Assessment recall
	Denmark	958	Adult	18–75	Men and women	4479	2000–04	Food record
	Croatia	965	Adult	18–55	Men and women	161	NA	FFQ

Region	Country	Intake mg/d	Population group	Age years	Gender	Number studies	Year	Calcium assessment method
	Sweden	992	Adult	45–83	Men and women	61,443/48850	1997	FFQ
	United Kingdom	994	Adult	25–72 (94% of population)	Men and women	5885	1992–2004	Recall
	Germany	1068	Adult	19+	Men and women	13,959	2005–07	Assessment recall
	Ireland	1080	Adult	18–90	NA	1499	2010	Food record
	Finland	1098	Adult	25–64	Men and women	2007	2002	Assessment recall
	Iceland	1233	Adult	30–85	Men and women	944	2003	FFQ

Source: https://www.osteoporosis.foundation/educational-hub/topic/calcium/calcium-map

28.4 Role of Information Technology in Combating These Deficiencies

Information Technology (IT) plays an important role in addressing the challenges and delivering solutions to combat calcium and vitamin D deficiencies. While digitalization has led to advancements in the healthcare sector, there are many e-health and m-health approaches that have increased in use to help address nutrition deficiencies. The availability of mobile apps, analytics and artificial intelligence (AI) coupled with the availability of the internet has increased the adoption of m-health applications. With these applications being delivered through small-scale organizations, larger firms are focusing on delivering applications that help the larger audience. Microsoft has developed a Child Growth Monitor app to monitor children's growth and nutrition. The app scans children under 5 years for any signs of malnutrition using AI. Health workers were trained to use the app and were given a smartphone to collect the required data. This data was used to address the data sets where malnutrition was prevalent. [19] Bupa Healthcare is providing over-the-phone nutrition coaching with qualified dietitian to advice on general healthy eating, weight management, sports nutrition, etc., helping patients to eat healthy and lead a healthier lifestyle. [20] These are some of the many examples where IT has been a key enabler to deliver services specific to identifying nutrition deficiency and has helped address the larger problems of nutrition deficiency.

Nutrition deficiency is a global problem to combat using multiple approaches. Endocrine disorders have been prevalent and have a serious impact on the wellbeing of an individual. In addition to the adhering to guidelines on the daily nutrition intake, information technology acts as an enabler to enforce adherence to these guidelines using innovative methods. It is prudent to take advantage of such initiatives which help achieve some of UN Sustainable Development Goals.

References

1. Availability of Data on Health Status Before and After Mandatory Fortification—Global Fortification Data Exchange | GFDx. https://fortificationdata.org/availability-of-data-on-health-status-before-and-after-mandatory-fortification/. Accessed 25 Oct 2022.
2. Map: Population Coverage of Fortified Food Vehicle in Countries with Mandatory or Voluntary Fortification—Global Fortification Data Exchange | GFDx. https://fortificationdata.org/map-population-coverage-of-fortified-food-vehicle/. Accessed 25 Oct 2022.
3. Zimmermann MB, Andersson M. GLOBAL ENDOCRINOLOGY: global perspectives in endocrinology: coverage of iodized salt programs and iodine status in 2020. Eur J Endocrinol. 2021;185(1):R13–21. https://eje.bioscientifica.com/view/journals/eje/185/1/EJE-21-0171.xml. Accessed 25 Oct 2022.
4. Bhat S, Marklund M, Henry ME, Appel LJ, Croft KD. Neal B et al A systematic review of the sources of dietary salt around the world. Adv Nutr. 2020;11:677–86. https://doi.org/10.1093/advances/nmz134.
5. Sempos CT, Durazo-Arvizu RA, Fischer PR, et al. Serum 25-hydroxyvitamin D requirements to prevent nutritional rickets in Nigerian children on a low calcium diet—a multivariable reanalysis. Am J Clin Nutr. 2021;2021(114):231–7. https://doi.org/10.1093/ajcn/nqab048.
6. Fujita T, Palmieri GMA. Calcium paradox disease: calcium deficiency prompting secondary hyperparathyroidism and cellular calcium overload. J Bone Miner Metab. 2000;18:109–25. https://doi.org/10.1007/s007740050101.
7. Chapter 11. Calcium. www.fao.org/3/y2809e/y2809e0h.htm.
8. Shlisky J, Mandlik R, Askari S, Abrams S, Belizan JM, Bourassa MW, et al. Calcium deficiency worldwide: prevalence of inadequate intakes and associated health outcomes. Ann N Y Acad Sci. 2022;1512(1):10–28. https://doi.org/10.1111/nyas.14758. Epub 2022 Mar 5
9. Dietary Reference Intakes for Calcium and Vitamin D National Academies of Sciences, Engineering, and Medicine. 2011. Dietary Reference Intakes for Calcium and Vitamin D. Washington, DC: The National Academies Press. https://doi.org/10.17226/13050.
10. NHS. Calcium, vitamins and minerals. https://www.nhs.uk/conditions/vitamins-and-minerals/calcium/. Accessed 25 Oct 2022.
11. Harinarayan CV, Akhila H. Modern India and the tale of twin nutrient deficiency–calcium and vitamin D–nutrition trend data 50 years-retrospect, introspect and prospect. Front Endocrinol. 2019;10 https://doi.org/10.3389/fendo.2019.00493.
12. Niedermaier T, Gardner T, Kuznia S, et al. Vitamin D food fortification in European countries: the underused potential to prevent cancer deaths. Eur J Epidemiol. 2022;37:309–20. https://doi.org/10.1007/s10654-022-00867-4.
13. Ray A, National Guidelines for Calcium Supplementation During Pregnancy and Lactation, India. 2014. https://www.researchgate.net/publication/282337540_National_Guidelines_for_Calcium_Supplementation_During_Pregnancy_and_Lactation_India. Accessed 25 Oct 2022.
14. Kellogg's. Food Fortification in Focus. https://www.kelloggs.com/me/en/health-and-nutrition/food-fortification-definition-benefits.html.
15. Indian CSR. https://indiacsr.in/students-get-daily-dose-milk-nutrition-bokaro/. Accessed 29 Sept 2022.
16. Harinarayan CV, Akhila H, Shanthi sree E. Modern India and dietary calcium deficiency—half a century nutrition data—retrospect-introspect and the road ahead. Front Endocrinol. 2021;12:583654. https://doi.org/10.3389/fendo.2021.583654.
17. Harinarayan CV. How to treat Vitamin D deficiency in sun-drenched India—guidelines. J Clin Sci Res. 2018;7:131–40. https://www.jcsr.co.in/text.asp?2018/7/3/131/255663. Accessed 25 Oct 2022.
18. International Osteoporosis Foundation. Calcium map. https://www.osteoporosis.foundation/educational-hub/topic/calcium/calcium-map. Accessed 25 Oct 2022.
19. https://www.techradar.com/news/a-new-app-to-track-malnutrition-in-india-using-microsofts-ai-tech. Accessed 25 Sept 2022.
20. Bupa. Dietitian Health Coaching. https://www.bupa.com.au/health-programs/dietitianhealthcoaching. Accessed 25 Oct 2022.

29 Mental Health and Substance Abuse

Laura Jones and Daniel Vigo

Abstract

Mental illness causes 13% of the disease burden globally, including disability and mortality. The relative burden of mental illness compared to all other groups of illnesses is highest in settings with high sociodemographic index (21%), and lowest in countries with low sociodemographic index (nearly 7%), where all disorders are crowded out by the pervasive burden of infectious, maternal, and childhood disorders. The pattern of the burden of mental, neurological, substance use disorders and suicide (MNSS) varies substantially between men and women, as well as across the lifetime, which needs to be considered when planning for population level mental health services. Despite this burden, MNSS have been historically neglected by policy and decision-makers. In light of increased public awareness about the toll of mental illness, as well as availability of digital platforms that facilitate scale up, the global community has a unique opportunity to improve mental health outcomes at the population level.

L. Jones · D. Vigo (✉)
University of British Columbia, Vancouver, Canada
e-mail: laura.jones@ubc.ca;
vigo.daniel@mail.harvard.edu

Keywords

Mental health · Mental illness · Mental disorders · Substance abuse · Mental, neurological, substance use disorders and suicide (MNSS)

29.1 Introduction

Mental and substance use disorders are a group of highly prevalent conditions that impact mental health and have adverse socioeconomic consequences [1–4]. They are often comorbid with other mental and physical disorders and have substantial impacts on healthcare utilization [4, 5]. However, despite their widespread impact, these disorders have historically been neglected by policymakers and funders, with large degrees of imbalance between disease burden and health expenditure [6]. The reasons for this imbalance are varied and include factors such as stigma and discrimination towards people with mental disorders; insufficient knowledge about effective interventions; and systemic undercounting of the multiple burdens associated with mental illness [6–10].

M. C. B. Raviglione et al. (eds.), *Global Health Essentials*, Sustainable Development Goals Series,
https://doi.org/10.1007/978-3-031-33851-9_29

29.2 Methodological Considerations

The Global Burden of Disease (GBD) study is an international collaboration that estimates the impact of disease worldwide, providing comprehensive data for researchers, policymakers, and funders to study epidemiological trends and make evidence-based decisions [11, 12]. The project uses well-established metrics to measure burden of disease, such as the disability-adjusted life year (DALY), which is a composite measure calculated by the addition of years lived with disability (YLD) and years of life lost (YLL) [11]. As described in previous publications, we have developed a methodology to improve the estimation of the burden of mental illness reanalyzing raw GBD data [2, 13, 14]. This methodology involves the re-estimation of the GBD disease burden of an aggregate group of mental, neurological, substance use disorders and suicide (MNSS) which now includes suicide and self-harm, an estimate of somatic symptom disorder with prominent pain, specific high prevalence neurological disorders (such as neurocognitive disorders, epilepsy, and headache disorders), substance use disorders, and direct somatic consequences of alcohol use disorder.

29.3 An Overview: Global Burden of Disease

Our estimate indicates that 13.0% of the total burden of disease worldwide in 2019 was attributable to mental illness as measured by DALYs [13]. Our recent work shows that the disease burden of MNSS varies considerably across countries around the world, most notably across World Bank country income levels [15]. For the original analysis published here, we grouped countries by their sociodemographic index (SDI), which accounts for average educational attainment and fertility rates in addition to per capita income [16]. In high-SDI countries, the relative burden of MNSS is more than three times that of low-SDI countries (21.1% vs. 6.8%). The burden of disease attributed to MNSS in middle-SDI countries is in between the 2 at 13.6%. It is important to note that these differences in proportions are not caused by low absolute MNSS burden in low-SDI countries, but by the staggering burden of communicable, maternal, and neonatal disorders, which crowd out other disorder groupings: Fig. 29.1 shows that the relative burden of communicable, maternal, and neonatal disorders in low-SDI countries is 12.3 times the proportion in high-SDI countries.

29.4 Distribution of the MNSS Burden in Men and Women

An analysis of the age-standardized DALY burden of MNSS shows distinct patterns—with noteworthy similarities and differences—between the sexes and country SDI groupings. Overall, for both men and women the age-standardized burden of MNSS is lowest in middle-SDI countries. In men, the following four disorders are present in the top five globally and across SDI levels: alcohol use disorders, self-harm and suicide, depressive disorders, and somatic symptom disorder with prominent pain. Globally, and in low-SDI and middle-SDI countries headache disorders are also in the top five, whereas in high-SDI countries, drug use disorders are the top cause of disease burden in men. In women, the top five disorders globally and across SDI levels include the following four: headache disorders, depressive disorders, somatic symptom disorder with prominent pain and anxiety disorders. In high-SDI countries, drug use disorders are also a top five cause of burden in women, whereas globally, in low-SDI and middle-SDI countries Alzheimer's disease and other dementias are within the top five causes of burden. The full ranking of MNSS for men and women globally is shown in Table 29.1.

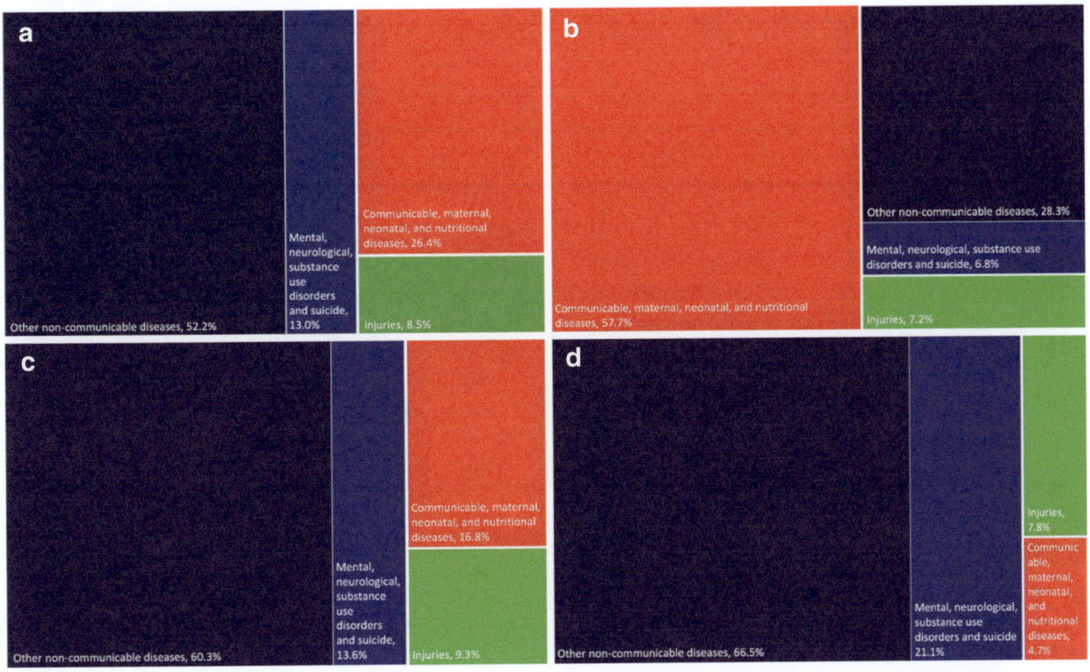

Fig. 29.1 Overall DALY disease burden distribution globally (**a**), and in low-SDI (**b**), middle-SDI (**c**), and high-SDI (**d**) countries

Table 29.1 Ranking of sex-specific burden (DALYs) of MNSS disorders globally. Values are age-standardized rates

Men		Women	
Disorder	DALYs per 100,000	Disorder	DALYs per 100,000
MNSS (all disorders)	4208	MNSS (all disorders)	4051
Alcohol use disorders	636	Headache disorders	725
Self-harm and suicide	577	Depressive disorders	702
Depressive disorders	452	Somatic symptom disorder with prominent pain	494
Headache disorders	440	Anxiety disorders	445
Somatic symptom disorder with prominent pain	365	Alzheimer's disease and other dementias	361
Alzheimer's disease and other dementias	304	Self-harm and suicide	274
Anxiety disorders	275	Drug use disorders	178
Drug use disorders	272	Schizophrenia	172
Schizophrenia	196	Alcohol use disorders	162
Idiopathic epilepsy	187	Idiopathic epilepsy	15
Other mental disorders	126	Bipolar disorder	109
Bipolar disorder	101	Other mental disorders	86
Conduct disorder	87	Idiopathic developmental intellectual disability	57
Autism spectrum disorder	85	Eating disorders	49
Idiopathic developmental intellectual disability	59	Conduct disorder	48
Eating disorders	25	Autism spectrum disorder	27
Attention-deficit/hyperactivity disorder	20	Attention-deficit/hyperactivity disorder	8

29.5 Political and Financial Considerations

From a policy standpoint, mental disorders have only recently begun emerging as a global priority. In May 2013, the World Health Assembly adopted WHO's Comprehensive Mental Health Action plan, which aims to address the growing burden of mental health disorders around the world [17]. In September 2015, mental health was included in the UN Sustainable Development Goals (SDGs), which include calls to reduce mortality from non-communicable diseases and promote mental health (target 3.4) and to prevent and treat substance use (target 3.5) [18]. While these are important developments, the inclusion of mental health in international policy is just the beginning, and substantial advocacy work will need to occur in order to make progress towards these goals. Another essential step will be increasing funding allocated towards mental health. The WHO recommends that health spending should be proportionate to burden [17, 19], but despite their enormous burden, MNSS disorders receive only a miniscule proportion of health expenditures. For example, the median ratio between MNSS disease burden and efficiently allocated government spending was found to be 32:1 in the Americas, with an imbalance that was inversely related to country GDP [6]. In addition to inadequate funding, this imbalance is due to inefficient spending practices such as allocating the majority of available funds to psychiatric hospitals. Cost-effective interventions should include integration of mental health treatment into the community and primary care [6, 17, 19].

29.6 Conclusion

Mental illness (including MNSS) is a leading cause of non-communicable disease morbidity and mortality around the world. By better understanding their burden, funders and policymakers are able to make more rational and evidence-based decisions. However, it is important to note that additional funding alone will not be enough to achieve global targets, and efficient use of resources through health system integration and mobilization of primary care will be essential. Increased awareness spurred by COVID19, as well as widespread availability of digital platforms for delivery present unique opportunities to improve mental health systems and scale up service delivery globally.

References

1. Prince M, Patel V, Saxena S, et al. No health without mental health. Lancet. 2007;370:19.
2. Vigo D, Thornicroft G, Atun R. Estimating the true global burden of mental illness. Lancet Psychiatry. 2016;3(2):171–8. https://doi.org/10.1016/S2215-0366(15)00505-2.
3. Trautmann S, Rehm J, Wittchen H. The economic costs of mental disorders. EMBO Rep. 2016;17(9):1245–9. https://doi.org/10.15252/embr.201642951.
4. Bloom DE, Cafiero ET, Jan-Llopis E, et al. The Global Economic Burden of Noncommunicable Diseases. In: World Economic Forum; 2011. https://ideas.repec.org/p/gdm/wpaper/8712.html.
5. Sporinova B, Manns B, Tonelli M, et al. Association of Mental Health Disorders with health care utilization and costs among adults with chronic disease. JAMA Netw Open. 2019;2(8):e199910. https://doi.org/10.1001/jamanetworkopen.2019.9910.
6. Vigo DV. Disease burden and government spending on mental, neurological, and substance use disorders, and self-harm: cross-sectional, ecological study of health system response in the Americas. Lancet Public Health. 2019;4:e89–96.
7. Thornicroft G, Brohan E, Rose D, Sartorius N, Leese M. Global pattern of experienced and anticipated discrimination against people with schizophrenia: a cross-sectional survey. Lancet. 2009;373(9661):408–15. https://doi.org/10.1016/S0140-6736(08)61817-6.
8. Lasalvia A, Zoppei S, Van Bortel T, et al. Global pattern of experienced and anticipated discrimination reported by people with major depressive disorder: a cross-sectional survey. Lancet. 2013;381(9860):55–62. https://doi.org/10.1016/S0140-6736(12)61379-8.
9. Henderson C, Noblett J, Parke H, et al. Mental health-related stigma in health care and mental health-care settings. Lancet Psychiatry. 2014;1(6):467–82. https://doi.org/10.1016/S2215-0366(14)00023-6.
10. Saxena S, Thornicroft G, Knapp M, Whiteford H. Resources for mental health: scarcity, inequity, and inefficiency. Lancet. 2007;370(9590):878–89. https://doi.org/10.1016/S0140-6736(07)61239-2.
11. Murray CJ, Ezzati M, Flaxman AD, et al. GBD 2010: design, definitions, and metrics. Lancet. 2012;380(9859):2063–6. https://doi.org/10.1016/S0140-6736(12)61899-6.

12. Protocol for the global burden of diseases, injuries, and risk factors study (GBD). 2018. https://www.healthdata.org/sites/default/files/files/Projects/GBD/GBD_Protocol.pdf.
13. Vigo D, Jones L, Atun R, Thornicroft G. The true global disease burden of mental illness: still elusive. Lancet Psychiatry. 2022;9(2):98–100. https://doi.org/10.1016/S2215-0366(22)00002-5.
14. Vigo D, Jones L, Thornicroft G, Atun R. Burden of mental, neurological, substance use disorders and self-harm in North America: a comparative epidemiology of Canada, Mexico, and the United States. Can J Psychiatry. 2020;65(2):87–98. https://doi.org/10.1177/0706743719890169.
15. Thornicroft G, Drake R, Gureje O, Mueser K, Szmukler G, editors. Oxford textbook of community mental health. 2nd ed. Oxford University Press; 2023.
16. Global Burden of Disease Collaborative Network. Global burden of disease study 2019 (GBD 2019) socio-demographic index (SDI) 1950–2019. Seattle: Institute for Health Metrics and Evaluation (IHME); 2020.
17. World Health Organization. Mental health action plan 2013–2020. World Health Organization; 2013. https://www.who.int/publications/i/item/9789241506021.
18. Votruba N, Thornicroft G. Sustainable development goals and mental health: learnings from the contribution of the FUNDAMENTALSDG global initiative. Global Mental Health. 2016;3:e26. https://doi.org/10.1017/gmh.2016.20.
19. World Health Organization. Comprehensive mental health action plan 2013–2030. World Health Organization; 2021. https://apps.who.int/iris/handle/10665/345301.

Violence Prevention

30

Alexander Butchart and Stephanie Burrows

Abstract

Violence affects billions of peoples' lives annually, through death, injury, and detrimental impacts on neurological, cardiovascular, immune, and other biological systems. High-risk behaviours such as unsafe sex, harmful alcohol and drug use, and smoking are more frequent among victims, among whom they contribute to lifelong ill health and premature mortality. Several Sustainable Development Goal targets call for ending or reducing violence. The science-based public health approach is used to: define the problem using descriptive epidemiology; conduct research within the framework of the social ecological model to identify risk and protective factors; use outcome evaluation studies to identify effective interventions; and scale up interventions shown to be effective. This chapter illustrates the operationalization of this approach in preventing violence against children in African countries, identifies challenges and opportunities for scaling up, and outlines the roles that multiple national-level government sectors and international agencies can play in advance the violence prevention agenda.

Keywords

Violence prevention and control · Public health · Monitoring and evaluation · Multisectoral collaboration · Social determinants · Social ecological model

30.1 Introduction

Violence is "the intentional use of physical force or power, threatened or actual, against oneself, another person, or against a group or community, that either results in or has a high likelihood of resulting in injury, death, psychological harm, maldevelopment or deprivation" [1]. It encompasses interpersonal violence, suicidal behaviour, and collective violence such as armed conflict.

30.2 Global Burden of Violence

Violence accounted for 1.3 million deaths, 73% of which were males, in 2019 [2]. Of these deaths, 56% were due to self-directed violence, 38% to interpersonal violence, and 6% to collective vio-

A. Butchart (✉) · S. Burrows
Prevention of Violence Unit, Social Determinants of Health Department, World Health Organization, Geneva, Switzerland
e-mail: butcharta@who.int; burrowss@who.int

M. C. B. Raviglione et al. (eds.), *Global Health Essentials*, Sustainable Development Goals Series,
https://doi.org/10.1007/978-3-031-33851-9_30

lence. Millions more people experience non-fatal violence. Globally, physical, sexual, or emotional violence affects one billion children aged 2–17 years each year [3], and one in three women suffer physical and/or sexual violence at least once from the age of 15 years, usually by an intimate partner [4].

In addition to causing injuries, exposure to violence impacts neurological, cardiovascular, immune, and other biological systems [1]. Consequently, high-risk behaviours such as unsafe sex, harmful alcohol and drug use, and smoking are more frequent among victims, among whom they contribute to lifelong ill health and premature mortality. Individuals maltreated in childhood are more likely to be involved in interpersonal violence as they grow up and to attempt suicide. Violence strains economies, with interpersonal and self-directed violence estimated to have had costs equivalent to 1.2 and 4% of gross domestic product in Brazil and Jamaica, respectively [5].

30.3 International Targets and Progress Towards Their Achievements

Several Sustainable Development Goals (SDGs) targets call for ending or reducing violence: Target 5.2 to eliminate all forms of violence against women and girls, Target 16.1 to significantly reduce all forms of violence and related death rates everywhere, and Target 16.2 to end abuse, exploitation, trafficking, and all forms of violence against children.

The United Nations 2021 annual SDGs Report indicates that while the global homicide rate is falling, the gap between regions with low levels of homicide and those with high levels keeps widening [6]. Trends in the prevalence of non-fatal violence are more difficult to ascertain since to do so requires periodic population-based surveys, and most countries still lack the data needed to track progress towards achieving the SDGs targets on ending violence against children and women.

30.4 Determinants and Risk Factors

Violence is rooted in individual biological and personal history factors, close relationships, community contexts, and societal factors, as shown in the social ecological model (see Fig. 30.1).

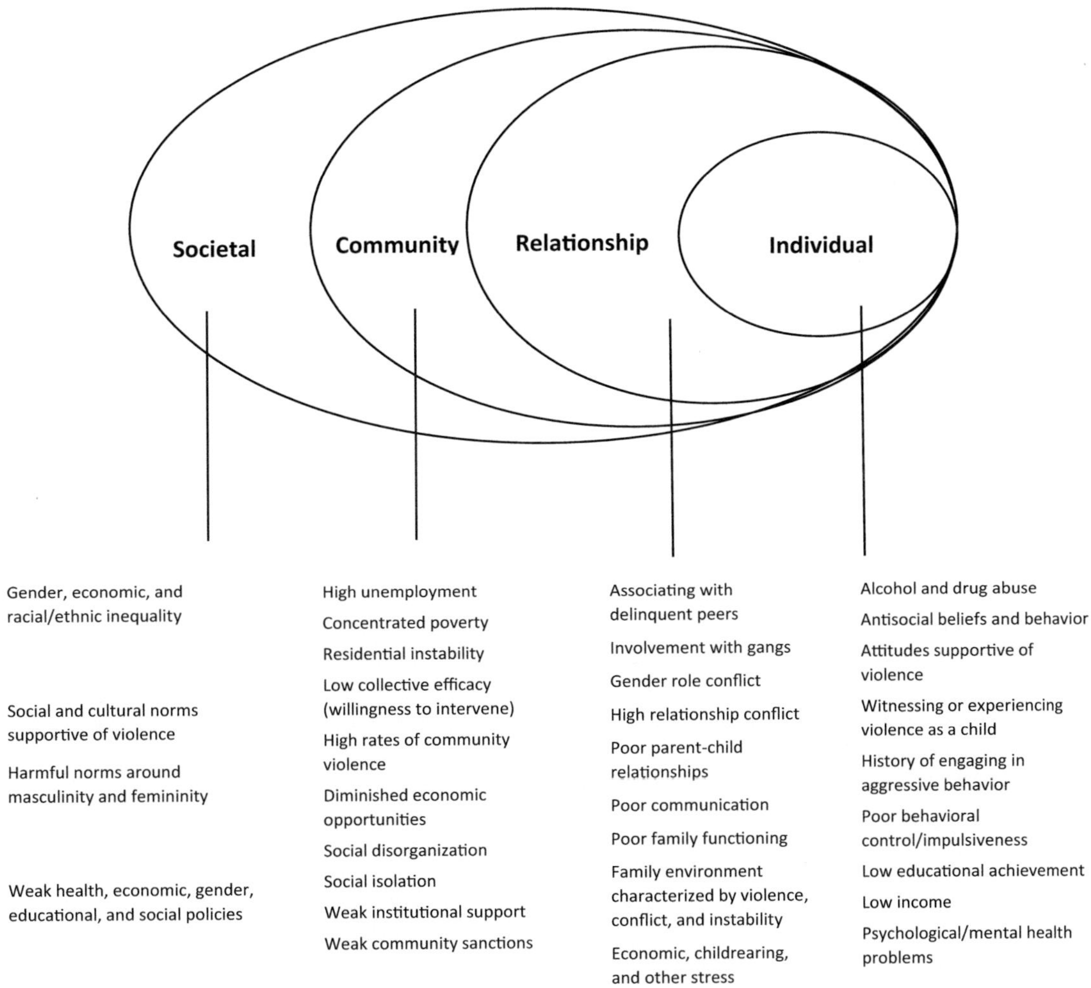

Fig. 30.1 Social ecological model for understanding and preventing violence. Reprinted with permission from World report on violence and health, Edited by Etienne G. Krug, Linda L. Dahlberg, James A. Mercy, Anthony B. Zwi, and Rafael Lozano, Chapter 1: Violence—a global public health problem, Page 12, Copyright World Health Organization (2002) [1]

30.5 Challenges Faced for Prevention and Control

Historically, violence has been addressed as a criminal justice problem and government emphasis has been on deterring violent offending through the enactment and enforcement of laws. This approach remains dominant in most low- and middle-income countries, where the challenge is to increase investment in data-driven, evidence-based approaches that address underlying causes. In high-income countries, there is increasing convergence between quantitative criminology and public health approaches, and a correspondingly greater investment in evidence-based prevention strategies.

The strong association between violence and societal level risk factors is also challenging. Violence occurs at substantially higher rates among the most economically and socially disadvantaged subgroups in societies characterized by high levels of economic and social inequity [1]. These inequities have widened in the wake of the COVID-19 pandemic [6], and sustainable population-wide reductions in violence will be difficult to achieve until they are reversed.

30.6 Approaches and Strategies for Prevention and Control

The public health approach to violence prevention aims to provide the maximum benefit for the largest number of people, while ensuring that individuals affected by the problem receive appropriate attention [1, 7]. The approach is science-based and anchored in evidence that violent behaviour and its consequences can be prevented. As shown in Fig. 30.2, it has four steps that provide a framework to organize prevention at all levels, from the community, through entire societies, to regional and global levels.

The process by which governments and international organizations are taking collective action to prevent violence against children in Africa illustrates the public health approach in action (see Box 30.1).

Box 30.1 Preventing Violence Against Children in Africa

Data on violence against children are obtained through supporting national census bureaus to administer the Violence against Children and Youth Survey (VACS) [8]. This nationally representative population-based survey of persons aged 13–24 years asks about violent victimization and perpetration prior to age 18 years, and risk and protective factors. As of 2022, VACS have been completed in some 15 African countries. Research on causes and risk factors involves analysing VACS questions on factors such as alcohol use, early marriage, being out of school, parental loss, harmful norms, and poverty. Support to countries in designing, implementing, and evaluating interventions is provided through the WHO-led *INSPIRE: Seven strategies for ending violence against children* technical package [9]. Step four of the public health approach begins when countries start to scale up INSPIRE programmes that show promise in their own settings. Repeat VACS will then be undertaken to monitor progress, as has already been done in Kenya, where the prevalence of lifetime sexual, physical, and emotional violence significantly declined in 2019 compared with 2010.

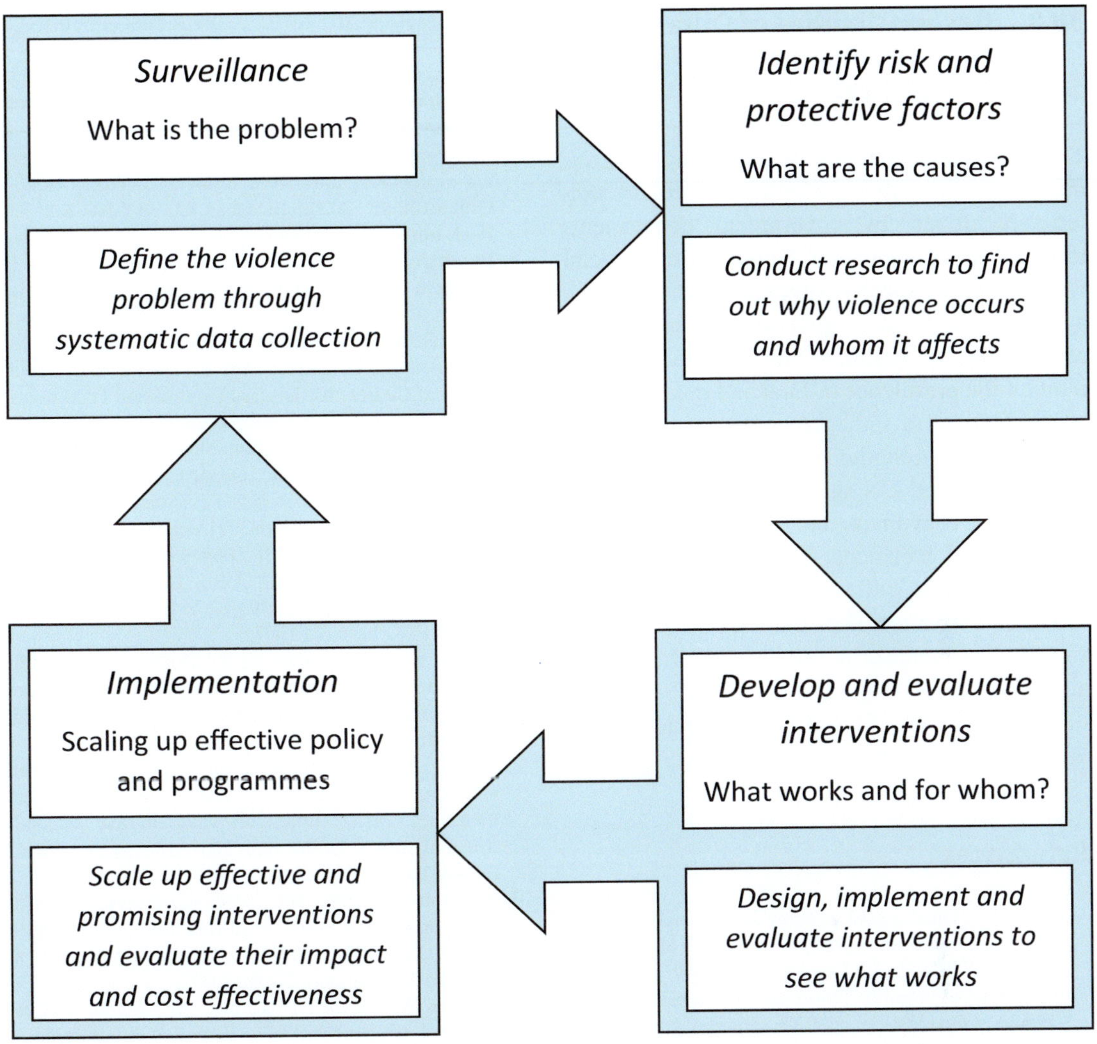

Fig. 30.2 Steps of the public health approach. (James A. Mercy, Mark L. Rosenberg, Kenneth E. Powell, Claire V. Broome, and William L. Roper. "Public health policy for preventing violence." Health Aff. 1993;12(4):7–29. https://doi.org/10.1377/hlthaff.12.4.7 [7]. Exhibit 4 Public Health Model Of A Scientific Approach To Prevention. Adapted with approval by Health Affairs)

30.7 Cost-Effectiveness and Financial Considerations

Cost-effectiveness studies of violence prevention find that most interventions yield good value for money in low-, middle-, and high-income countries [10]. For example, a South African programme to reduce parental violence against adolescents yielded savings per case averted of US$2644 for physical abuse and US$2804 for emotional abuse [11], and in Uganda a schools-based violence prevention programme saved US$148 per case averted [12].

30.8 Responsibilities of Different National and International Institutions

The multifaceted nature of violence and its determinants requires that prevention efforts are collectively driven by government departments responsible for education, health, justice, social welfare, civil society organizations, research agencies, and that government institutions responsible for national vital statistics should monitor the prevalence of fatal and non-fatal violence. Efforts to enhance violence prevention strategies are strengthened through international cooperation, and UN agencies such as UNICEF, UNODC, UN Women, and WHO all have mandates to develop evidence-based violence prevention guidance and support its uptake by countries.DisclaimerThe findings and conclusions in this manuscript are those of the authors and do not necessarily represent the official position or the views, decisions, or policies of the World Health Organization.

References

1. Krug EG, Dahlberg LL, Mercy JA, Zwi AB, Lozano R, editors. World report on violence and health. Geneva: World Health Organization; 2002. p. 346.
2. The Global Health Observatory. Geneva: World Health Organization; c2022. Summary tables of mortality estimates by cause, age and sex, globally and by region, 2000–2019, global summary estimates. 2020. https://www.who.int/data/gho/data/themes/mortality-and-global-health-estimates/ghe-leading-causes-of-death.
3. Hillis S, Mercy J, Amobi A, Kress H. Global prevalence of past-year violence against children: a systematic review and minimum estimates. Pediatrics. 2016;137(3):e20154079. https://doi.org/10.1542/peds.2015-4079.
4. Violence against women prevalence estimates, 2018: global, regional and national prevalence estimates for intimate partner violence against women and global and regional prevalence estimates for non-partner sexual violence against women. Geneva: World Health Organization; 2021. Licence: CC BY-NC-SA 3.0 IGO. https://srhr.org/vaw-data.
5. Butchart A, Brown D, Khanh-Huynh A, Corso P, Florquin N, Muggah R. Manual for estimating the economic costs of injuries due to interpersonal and self-directed violence. Geneva: World Health Organization & Department of Health and Social Services Centers for Disease Control and Prevention; 2008. https://apps.who.int/iris/handle/10665/43837
6. United Nations. The sustainable development goals report 2021. New York: Department of Economic and Social Affairs Statistics Division; 2021. https://unstats.un.org/sdgs/report/2021/extended-report/.
7. Mercy JA, Rosenberg ML, Powell KE, Broome CV, Roper WL. Public health policy for preventing violence. Health Aff. 1993;12(4):7–29. https://doi.org/10.1377/hlthaff.12.4.7.
8. Together for Girls. What are the violence against children and youth surveys? Washington, DC: Together for Girls; 2017. https://www.togetherforgirls.org/about-the-vacs/.
9. World Health Organization. INSPIRE: seven strategies for ending violence against children. Geneva; 2016. https://www.who.int/teams/social-determinants-of-health/violence-prevention/inspire-technical-package.
10. Peterson C, Kearns MC. Systematic review of violence prevention economic evaluations, 2000–2019. Am J Prev Med. 2021;60(4):552–62. https://doi.org/10.1016/j.amepre.2020.11.002.
11. Redfern A, Cluver LD, Casale M, Steinert JI. Cost and cost-effectiveness of a parenting programme to prevent violence against adolescents in South Africa. BMJ Glob Health. 2019;4(3):e001147. https://doi.org/10.1136/bmjgh-2018-001147.
12. Greco G, Knight L, Ssekadde W, Namy S, Naker D, Devries K. Economic evaluation of the good school toolkit: an intervention for reducing violence in primary schools in Uganda. BMJ Glob Health. 2018;3:e000526. https://doi.org/10.1136/bmjgh-2017-000526.

31 Blindness and Vision Impairment

Daniel Etya'ale

Abstract

Blindness is the ultimate stage of vision loss on both eyes and represents a major public health problem affecting at least 1.1 billion people worldwide. The major and leading causes of blindness and vision loss include uncorrected refractive errors, cataract, age-related macular degeneration, glaucoma, and diabetic retinopathy, with low- and middle-income countries (LMIC) disproportionately more affected. Blindness and visual loss have a significant human and social impact, often leading to reduced quality of life, social marginalization, and premature death among those affected. Similarly, their economic and financial impact are just as devastating, leading among others to huge productivity losses estimated at US$410 billion annually. While vision loss is still growing, and disproportionately much faster than existing service delivery can cope, especially in LMIC, solutions and cost-effective strategies to address that increase are available. What is urgently needed now is a renewed, upscaled, and coordinated efforts at global, regional, and country levels, using the new tools recently developed by WHO and its partners.

Keywords

Blindness · Vision loss · Causes · Burden · Control strategies

31.1 Introduction

Over the past two decades, there has been a progressive change of focus from blindness, a passive state, and an end point to vision impairment or vision loss. This is because both vision impairment or vision loss imply a process which, in the case of blinding diseases like cataract, glaucoma, or diabetic retinopathy, may take up to 25 years or more, and for which blindness is only the most extreme form. This new terminology also best explains why greater emphasis is placed today by WHO and its partners, not on the "fight against blindness", a strategy that is passive and seems to suggest waiting until people are blind, but on "the fight against vision loss", which is more proactive, promotes better eye health and enforces early detection and management of potentially blinding diseases across the entire life spectrum [1, 2].

D. Etya'ale (✉)
World Health Organisation, Geneva, Switzerland

M. C. B. Raviglione et al. (eds.), *Global Health Essentials*, Sustainable Development Goals Series,
https://doi.org/10.1007/978-3-031-33851-9_31

31.2 Definitions and Classification of Vision Impairment and Blindness

Vision is measured for both distance and near. Distance vision, measured at 6 m, informs on our ability to see far objects clearly; near-vision, tested at 40 cm, informs on our ability to see things up close, like reading or knitting for instance. The International Classification of Diseases (ICD11, 2019) defines and classifies both distance and near-vision impairment (VI) as shown in Table 31.1 below [3]:

Table 31.1 Definition and classification of distance and near-vision impairment

Type and level of vision impairment	Visual acuity in the better eye	
	Worse than	Equal to, or better than
Distance vision impairment (6 m)		
Mild	6/12	6/18
Moderate	6/18	6/60
Severe	6/60	3/60
Blindness	3/60	
Near-vision impairment (40 cm)	N6 or M.08	

31.3 The Global Burden of Vision Impairment

According to latest global prevalence studies (2020), there were at least 1.1 billion people worldwide living with vision loss [2]. Of these:

- 258 million people had mild vision impairment.
- 295 million people had moderate to severe vision impairment.
- 510 million people had near-vision impairment.
- 43 million people were irreversibly blind.

While vision loss may affect people of all ages, 73% of those with visual impairment and blindness are over the age of 50 years. This is because with increasing age, there is an increased prevalence of potentially blinding diseases like cataract, age-related macular degeneration, glaucoma, and diabetic retinopathy. Another major factor affecting the rate of vision loss is socioeconomic disadvantage. Thus, 90% of people with vision loss live in low- and middle-income countries (LMICs), with South Asia and Sub-Saharan Africa having the highest rates of vision loss among all the regions (Fig. 31.1).

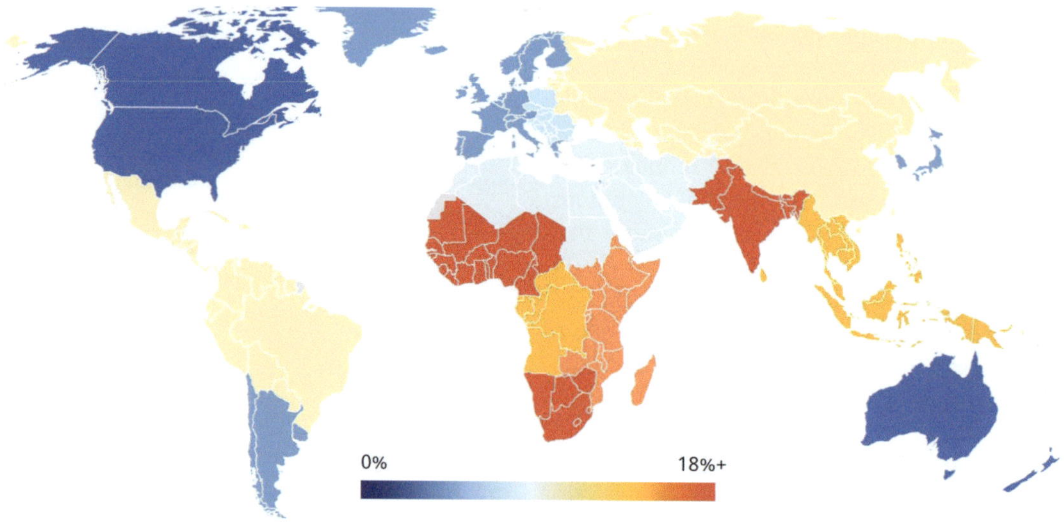

Source: https://www.iapb.org/learn/vision-atlas/inequality-in-vision-loss/

Fig. 31.1 Inequality of Vision Loss across various regions of the world. Source: https://www.iapb.org/learn/vision-atlas/inequality-in-vision-loss/

31.4 Causes of Vision Impairment

The causes of vision impairment vary from one region to another, within countries and by age. However, and overall, the leading causes of vision impairment are [4]:

- Uncorrected refractive errors, *161 million people* living with distance vision impairment or blindness, and *510 million people* with near-vision impairment.
- Cataract, *100 million people* affected, *17 million people* already blind, and *83 million* moderately or severely visually impaired.
- Age-related macular degeneration, *8.1 million people* affected, *1.9 million blind,* and *6.2 million* moderately or severely visually impaired.
- Glaucoma, at least *7.8 million people* affected, *3.6 million* blind, and *4.2 million* moderately or severely visually impaired.
- Diabetic retinopathy, with *4.4 million people* affected, *1 million* blind, and *3.3 million* moderately or severely visually impaired.
- Other causes, with *56 million people* affected. In this category are found causes of vision impairment that are either insufficiently documented or exist only in certain parts of the world. These include, corneal opacities (4.2 million), trachoma (2 million), onchocerciasis (1.15 million), xerophthalmia (0.5 million), retinopathy of prematurity (100,000), amblyopia, and ocular trauma.

31.5 Trends of Vision Impairment Over Time

Because of the projected demographic trends, including increased population ageing and growth (25%), and behavioural and lifestyle factors, and unless a major surge in current control efforts occurs, it is projected that vision loss is likely to increase by 55%, i.e., 600 million more people affected, by 2050 [4]. Given the limited scale and approach of existing service delivery to meet current population, it is hard to imagine how it could cope with the projected increases in vision loss by 2050.

31.6 Impact of Vision Impairment

31.6.1 Human and Social Impact

At the individual level, good vision improves health and well-being at all ages, and vision loss reduces the quality of life, increases the risk of marginalization in society, and often leads to premature death of affected adults. Similarly, and worse still, children with severe vision impairment in their early years of life are likely to lag behind their peers with respect to their motor, language, emotional, social, and cognitive development, and will often die prematurely, especially in LMICs. Older children with vision impairment and especially those with severe uncorrected refractive errors are likely to underperform at school and as a result, many may never go beyond primary school education [5]. The provision of appropriate glasses to these children will reduce their odds of failing at school by 44% recent studies have shown.

31.6.2 Economic Impact

Vision impairment poses an enormous global financial burden, leading to huge productivity losses estimated at US$410 billion annually. It also reduces employment rate by 32% in people with blindness or moderate to severe vision impairment. Similarly, and more specifically, the annual global costs of productivity losses associated with vision impairment from uncorrected myopia and presbyopia alone are estimated to be US$244 billion and US$25.4 billion, respectively, making every effort to fight uncorrected refractive errors a highly gratifying and worthwhile investment.

31.7 Solutions and Strategies to Address the Increasing Burden of Vision Impairment

As mentioned earlier, the scale and approach of existing service delivery in many regions are insufficient to meet current population needs, and worse still, to address the projected increases in vision loss by 2050. Fortunately, there are available today, effective and proven public health strategies and clinical interventions covering the entire spectrum of care—promotion, prevention, early detection, treatment, and rehabilitation, and some like cataract surgery to restore vision, or the provision of spectacles to correct refractive errors, are among the most cost-effective health care interventions available today [6], especially in LMICs. Moreover, concerted efforts to increase the coverage of some interventions during the past 30 years have already led to a substantial reduction in the number of children and adults blind from vitamin A deficiency and infectious causes, such as onchocerciasis and trachoma. The real and ongoing challenge remains how to quickly upscale and expand these control efforts, and make them work everywhere, especially for those who need them the most.

The consensus among experts today is that to address in an impactful manner, the scale of the growing problem of vision loss, a multi-faceted challenge, only a concerted, well-coordinated, multi-prong and multi-level approach—at global, regional, and country levels, will do. The key components of such a strategy, as recommended by WHO and its partners and summarized below, could be a real game changer in the fight against vision loss:

31.7.1 At the Global and International Level

- Coordinate and advocate for greater investment efforts (current estimates stand at US$24.8 billion), focusing initially on those highly cost-effective strategies such as cataract surgery, or the provision of spectacles to correct refractive errors.
- Promote and advocate for the use of the new tools developed by WHO and its partners to accelerate, upscale, and monitor future control interventions (see Box 31.1 below).

Box 31.1 List of New Set of Recent Tools/Documents Developed by WHO and Partners

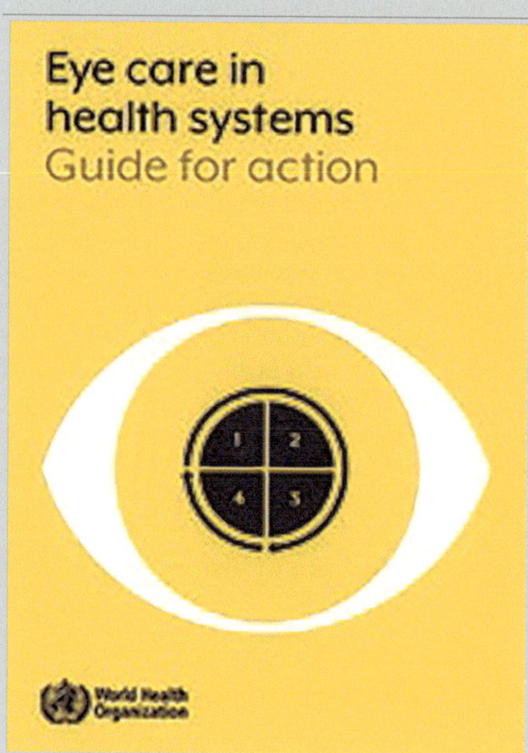

1. Eye care situation analysis tool (ECSAT)
Purpose: Questionnaire-based survey tool to comprehensively assess eye care in a country.

2. Eye care indicator menu (ECIM)
Purpose: List of recommended eye care indicators to be collected regularly.

3. Package of eye care interventions (PECI)
Purpose: Planning and budgeting for eye care at each level of the health system.

4. Eye care competency framework (ECCF)
Purpose: Planning tool for eye care human resources based on competencies.

31.7.2 At Regional Level

- Adapt the above strategies to best suit the specific needs and priorities of each region.

31.7.3 At Country Level

- Develop or update national eye care sector strategic plan that would accelerate the assessment of individual country needs and implement the recently developed WHO package of evidence-based and cost-effective eye care interventions (PECI), using the full range of additional tools developed alongside [7]. The package of eye care interventions, without doubt one of the most ambitious and comprehensive developed to date, provides detailed implementation guidelines (see Box 31.2 below).

Box 31.2 Areas Covered by the New WHO Eye Care Intervention Guidelines [7]

- Health promotion, education and prevention at primary, secondary and tertiary levels.
- Priority screening interventions in the field of eye care and how to go about them.
- Screening of high-risk population groups: neonatal period, children and adolescents, and people with diabetes.
- Essential clinical examinations for the diagnosis and monitoring of eye diseases.
- Priority, evidence-based treatment interventions in the field of eye care.
- Priority, evidence-based vision rehabilitation interventions.

Developed alongside and complementary to the PECI, as can be seen in Box 31.1 above, are the following tools:

1. The Eye Care Situation Analysis Tool (ECSAT), a questionnaire-based survey tool to comprehensively assess eye care in a country.
2. The Eye Care Indicator Menu (ECIM), a list of recommended eye care indicators to be collected regularly.
3. The Eye Care Competency Framework (ECCF), a planning tool for eye care human resources development based on competencies, an essential and highly needed tool in many LMIC.

31.8 Conclusion

Vision loss is still growing, disproportionately much faster than existing service delivery can cope, especially in LMIC. Thankfully, enough evidence exists today to build a strong case for a much-needed surge in funding efforts to control vision loss, starting with most cost-effective interventions. To that end, concerted efforts must continue at global, regional, and country levels. The new tools developed by WHO and its partners, if used adequately, can help revive and accelerate these efforts, especially at country level.

References

1. World Health Organization. World report on vision. Geneva; 2019. https://apps.who.int/iris/handle/10665/328717. Accessed 6 Mar 2022.
2. Burton MJ, Ramke J, Marques AP, Bourne RR, Congdon N, Jones I, et al. The Lancet Global Health commission on global eye health: vision beyond 2020. Lancet Glob Health. 2021;9(4):e489–551.
3. Adelson, J., Bourne, R. R. A., Briant, P. S., Flaxman, S., Taylor, H., Jonas, J. B., et al. Causes of blindness and vision impairment in 2020 and trends over 30 years, and prevalence of avoidable blindness in relation to VISION 2020: the right to sight: an analysis for the global burden of disease study Lancet Glob Health 2020. Accessed via the IAPB Vision Atlas. https://www.iapb.org/learn/vision-atlas.
4. WHO international classification of diseases, 11th revision (ICD-11). Geneva; 2018. https://www.who.int/classifications/icd/en/.
5. WEF EYElliance: eyeglasses for global development: bridging the visual divide; 2018. https://www3.weforum.org/docs/WEF_2016_EYElliance.pdf.
6. GBD 2017 Disease and Injury Incidence and Prevalence Collaborators. Global, regional, and national incidence, prevalence, and years lived with disability for 354 diseases and injuries for 195 countries and territories, 1990–2017: a systematic analysis for the Global Burden of Disease Study 2017. Lancet. 2018;392(10159):1789–858.
7. WHO Package of eye care interventions. Geneva; 2022. https://www.who.int/publications/i/item/9789240048959.

Global Oral Health

32

Sante Leandro Baldi, Gemma Bridge,
and Richard G. Watt

Abstract

Oral health is an essential component of good health and physical and mental well-being. Oral diseases are largely preventable; however, they remain a prominent public health concern affecting approximately 3.5 billion people globally (Global burden of disease study 2019 (GBD 2019), Institute of Health Metrics and Evaluation (IHME), Seattle, 2020). Evidence indicates that there are several shared risk factors between oral disease and NCDs (WHO, Oral Health Fact Sheet, https://www.who.int/news-room/fact-sheets/detail/oral-health) and that there is a correlation between socioeconomic status and the incidence and severity of oral disease. Poor oral health is costly, accounting for 4.6% (equivalent to US$356.80 billion) of health expenditure globally. Reducing the burden of oral disease will require upstream action, with a range of policies and implementations targeting the environments in which people live or work. Public health policies such as water fluoridation, taxing sugar sweetened beverages, and community-wide interventions to reduce free sugars consumption should be considered as they have the potential to promote both oral and general health.

Keywords

Oral health · Oral diseases · Caries · Periodontal diseases · Social Determinants of Health · Common risk factors approach · Universal health coverage · Public health · Global oral health · Universal oral health coverage

32.1 Introduction

Oral health is an "essential component of good health and physical and mental well-being and it includes the ability to speak, smile, smell, taste,

The original version of the chapter has been revised. The affiliation of Richard G. Watt has been corrected. A correction to this chapter can be found at https://doi.org/10.1007/978-3-031-33851-9_89

S. L. Baldi (✉)
Centre for Multidisciplinary Research in Health Science (MACH), University of Milan, Milano, Italy
e-mail: sante.baldi@unimi.it

G. Bridge
Leeds Beckett University, Leeds, UK
e-mail: g.bridge@yorksj.ac.uk

R. G. Watt
Department of Epidemiology and Public Health, University College London, WHO Collaborating Center for Oral Health Inequalities and Public Health, London, UK
e-mail: r.watt@ucl.ac.uk

M. C. B. Raviglione et al. (eds.), *Global Health Essentials*, Sustainable Development Goals Series,
https://doi.org/10.1007/978-3-031-33851-9_32

touch, chew, swallow and convey a range of emotions through facial expressions with confidence and without pain, discomfort and disease" [1]. Poor oral health is costly, accounting for 4.6% (equivalent to US$356.80 billion) of health expenditure globally [2], reduces productivity and increases absenteeism in school and work settings [3]. Oral and general health are linked, with shared modifiable risk factors such as tobacco use, unhealthy diet, and physical activity [4]. To ensure interventions are effective, they should target these common risk factors. It is also important to consider the broader social determinants of health (SDHs) and commercial determinants of health, which are the non-medical factors that influence health outcomes [5]. The SDHs are the root causes of oral diseases, with evidence indicating that factors such as poverty, educational attainment, and income impact on oral health outcomes [6].

32.2 Descriptive Epidemiology and Assessment of the Global Burden

Oral diseases affect approximately 3.5 billion people globally [7]. Dental caries is the most prevalent oral disease and the most prevalent non-communicable disease (NCD), with over two billion people suffering untreated caries of permanent teeth and over 520 million children suffering untreated caries in primary teeth [7]. Periodontitis affects approximately 14% of the global adult population, representing more than one billion cases worldwide [7]. Lip and oral cavity cancers ranked 16th between the most common cancers worldwide, with 177,757 deaths and 377,713 incident cases in 2020 [8]. Other prevalent oral diseases include oro-dental trauma, cleft lip and palate, noma and oral manifestation of HIV [4] (Box 32.1). Oral diseases are a major

Box 32.1 Oral Diseases

ORAL DISEASES	
	• **Ranked First and Third globally for prevalence and incidence in 2019**
	The global burden of oral diseases it is made up by 7 disorders that are:
	• *Dental caries*: when plaque forms on the surface of a tooth and converts the free sugars contained in foods and drinks into acids that destroy the tooth over time; caries are a chronic disease that can lead to pain, tooth loss, and infections.
	• *Periodontal gum diseases*: affect the tissues that both surround and support the tooth, causing teeth to become loose and sometimes fall out; the main causes of periodontal disease are poor oral hygiene and tobacco use.
	• *Oral cancers*: include cancers of the lip, other parts of the mouth and the oropharynx; tobacco and alcohol use are among the leading causes of oral cancer.
	• *Oro-dental trauma*: it results from injury to the teeth, mouth, and oral cavity; can even lead to tooth loss, resulting in complications for facial and psychological development and quality of life.
	• *Cleft lip and palate*: the most common craniofacial birth defects; genetic predisposition is a major cause but poor maternal nutrition, tobacco consumption, alcohol and obesity during pregnancy also play a role.
	• *Noma*: a severe gangrenous disease of the mouth and the face; it mostly affects children aged 1–6 years suffering from malnutrition, affected by infectious disease, living in extreme poverty with poor oral hygiene or with weakened immune systems, noma is fatal in 90% of cases if not treated.
	• *Oral manifestation of HIV*: include fungal, bacterial, or viral infections; the most frequent is oral candidiasis, which is generally the initial symptom.

cause of disability, with estimates from 2019 indicating that they caused 23.1 million (95% UI 13.6–37.4) Years Lived with Disability (YLD) [7]. Much of the poor health exists amongst those living in poverty, with a negative correlation between oral health and socioeconomic status (SES), resulting in health inequalities [5].

32.3 International Targets and Progress Towards Their Achievements

Oral diseases are largely preventable; however, they remain a prominent public health concern. Between 1990 and 2019, the burden of oral diseases increased [2, 7], rising from 2.5 billion cases to 3.5 billion cases across this period [7]. Many of the cases have been reported in low- and middle-income countries (LMICs) due to demographic changes such as population expansion, changes to dietary habits combined with limited access to affordable, high-quality dental care [4]. To reduce the burden of oral diseases globally, the World Health Organization (WHO) advocated for action to strengthen oral health promotion and oral health care within the primary care system. In May 2022, at the 75th World Health Assembly, WHO member states agreed to adopt a global strategy on oral health to inform the development of a new global action plan with targets to be achieved by 2030. The vision of the global strategy is to enable people to enjoy the highest attainable state of oral health living healthy and productive lives. To overcome barriers in accessing oral health care and make the vision concrete, there is a need to address the SDHs, target the shared risk factors of oral diseases and to include oral health within universal health coverage (UHC) (Fig. 32.1). In addition, the WHO strategy advocates for action on six strategic objectives, namely oral health governance, oral health promotion and oral disease prevention, the health workforce, oral health care, oral health information systems, and oral health research agendas [9].

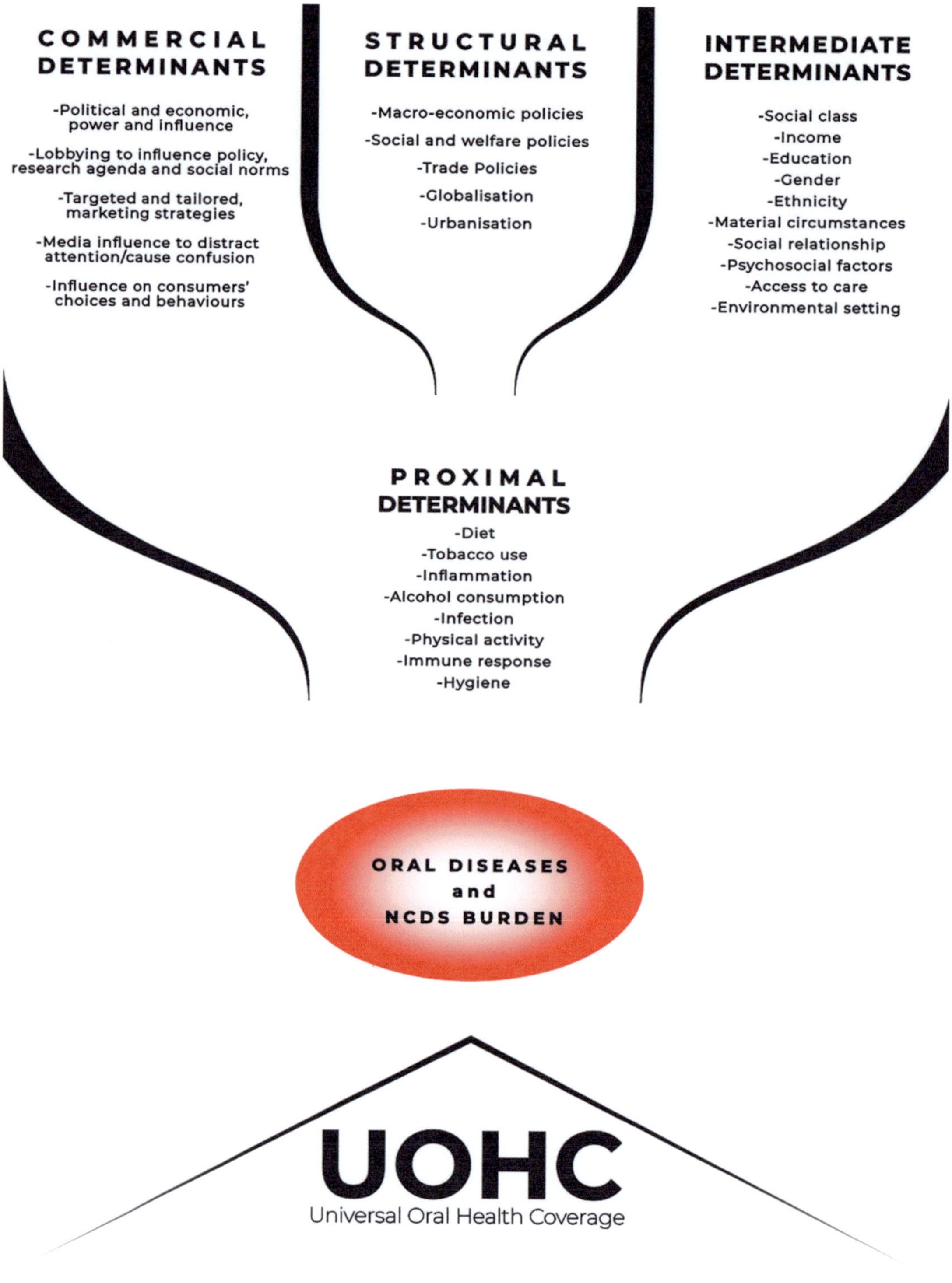

Fig. 32.1 "Social and commercial determinants of oral diseases and Universal Oral Health Coverage." (Used with permission of Elsevier from Peres et al. 2019 [5])

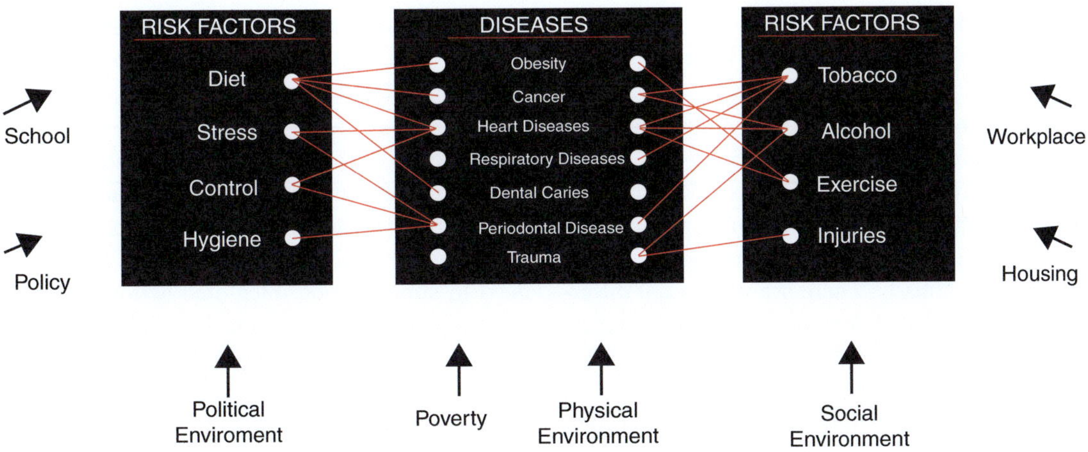

Fig. 32.2 Common risk factor approach and Social Determinant of Health. (Used with permission of John Wiley & Sons - Book from Sheiham and Watt 2000 [12])

32.4 Determinants and Risk Factors

Evidence indicates that there are several shared risk factors between oral diseases and NCDs including tobacco use, alcohol consumption, and a diet high in free sugars [4]. The SDHs also influence an individual's general health status. The most disadvantaged and vulnerable groups of the society experience the worst oral and general health outcomes with evidence suggesting that there is a correlation between SES and the incidence and severity of oral disease [5]. As such, addressing the SDHs is essential if improvements are to be made in improving health and reducing inequities in oral health globally (Fig. 32.2).

32.5 Challenges to Be Faced for Containment, Control and Elimination

The cost of oral health care is high, with most of the care provided by the private sector [10]. There is an unequal distribution of oral health professionals and health facilities, a lack of appropriate health policies, a lack of oral health literacy, and a lack of UOHC to meet population needs. Such challenges are limiting the effective prevention and treatment of oral health conditions [4]. Moreover, oral health care is still dominated by a treatment-focused and interventionist philosophy instead of a proactive and preventive approach. The separation of oral health care from other health services and care is the biggest challenge facing oral health improvement efforts [10].

32.6 Approaches and Strategies for Prevention and Control

Research suggests that there is a bidirectional relationship with oral diseases and NCDs [11]. Oral health care must be considered holistically, with efforts to promote actions towards a common risk factor approach alongside NCDs. Reducing the burden of oral disease will require upstream action, with a range of policies and implementations targeting the environments in which people live or work. Public health policies such as water fluoridation, taxing sugar sweetened beverages, and community-wide interventions such as school toothbrushing and other healthy public policies to reduce free sugars consumption should be considered as they have the potential to promote both oral and general health.

32.7 Cost-Effectiveness and Financial Considerations

In 2015, the global economic impact of oral health disorders amounted to US$544.41 billion between direct and indirect costs [2]. Over 80% of this expenditure occurred in high-income countries, demonstrating the inequities in oral health care globally. There are substantial differences in the costs of dental care and the recurrent use of Out-of-Pocket Payments (OOPs) within and between countries, which can limit access to and the use of care among people on low incomes. Individuals with low SES are prone to the direct and indirect costs of dental care and face a significantly higher risk of poor oral health when compared to those in higher SES [10].

32.8 Responsibilities of Different National and International Institutions

To improve oral and public health, national policy approaches targeting shared risk factors such as alcohol, tobacco, and sugar are needed. International institutions such as the WHO will need to support such integrated action and promote prevention-focused efforts. Implementation of the WHO Resolution on Oral Health, approved at the 74th World Health Assembly [9], should see a shift from the traditional downstream treatment approach towards an upstream health promotion one. The implementation of the resolution should also see oral health care integrated into existing health care systems to ensure inclusive and equal access to care and see oral health placed within the NCDs and UHC, and consequently on the Sustainable Development Goals agenda [9].

Global Oral Health Key facts	
	• *Oral diseases, despite largely preventable, have serious health and economic impacts on the society worldwide.*
	• *Oral diseases affect people during their life-course, disabling those affected with pain, discomfort, disfigurement, and even death and greatly reducing their quality of life.*
	• *Poor oral health is costly, accounting for 4.6% (equivalent to US$356.80 billion) of health expenditure globally.*
	• *Globally, there is a very strong and consistent association between SES and the prevalence and severity of oral diseases that disproportionally affect the poor and socially disadvantaged members of society.*
	• *Oral diseases are caused by a range of modifiable risk factors and their underlying social and commercial determinants of health, that are in common with the 4 leading NCDs.*
	• *Over two billion people are suffering from caries of permanent teeth and over 520 million children suffering from caries in primary teeth.*
	• *Severe gum diseases affect around 14% of the global adult population, representing more than one billion cases worldwide.*
	• *Lip and oral cavity cancers ranked 16th between the most common cancers worldwide, with 177,757 deaths and 377,713 incident cases in 2020 (Globocan).*
	• *Around 20% of people suffer from trauma to teeth at some point in their life.*
	• *Noma, according to latest estimates (from 1998) has an incidence of 140,000 new cases annually and without treatment is fatal in 90% of cases.*
	• *Oral diseases are a major cause of disability, with estimates from 2019 indicating that such diseases caused 23.1 million (95% UI 13.6–37.4) Years Lived with Disabilities (YLD).*

References

1. Glick M, Williams DM, Kleinman DV, Vujicic M, Watt RG, Weyant RJ. A new definition for oral health developed by the FDI world dental federation opens the door to a universal definition of oral health. J Am Dent Assoc. 2016;147(12):915–7. https://doi.org/10.1016/j.adaj.2016.10.001.
2. Righolt AJ, Jevdjevic M, Marcenes W, Listl S. Global-, regional-, and country-level economic impacts of dental diseases in 2015. J Dent Res. 2018;97(5):501–7. https://doi.org/10.1177/0022034517750572.
3. WHO. Oral Health. https://www.who.int/health-topics/oral-health#tab=tab_2. Accessed 11 May 2022.
4. WHO. Oral Health Fact Sheet. https://www.who.int/news-room/fact-sheets/detail/oral-health. Accessed 9 May 2022.
5. Peres MA, Macpherson L, Weyant RJ, Daly B, Venturelli R, Mathur MR, Listl S, Celeste RK, Guarnizo-Herreño CC, Kearns C, Benzian H, Allison P, Watt RG. Oral diseases: a global public health challenge. Lancet (London, England). 2019;394(10194):249–60. https://doi.org/10.1016/S0140-6736(19)31146-8.
6. Tellez M, Zini A, Estupiñan-Day S. Social determinants and Oral health: an update. Curr Oral Health Rep. 2014;1:148–52. https://doi.org/10.1007/s40496-014-0019-6.
7. Global Burden of Disease Collaborative Network. Global burden of disease study 2019 (GBD 2019). Seattle: Institute of Health Metrics and Evaluation (IHME); 2020. https://www.healthdata.org/results/gbd_summaries/2019/oral-disorders-level-3-cause. Accessed 11 May 2022.
8. WHO. The Global Health Observatory. https://gco.iarc.fr/today/data/factsheets/cancers/1-Lip-oral-cavity-fact-sheet.pdf. Accessed 11 June 2022.
9. WHO. https://www.who.int/news-room/feature-stories/detail/landmark-global-strategy-on-oral-health-adopted-at-world-health-assembly-75. Accessed 11 June 2022.
10. Watt RG, Daly B, Allison P, et al. Ending the neglect of global oral health: time for radical action. Lancet. 2019;394(10194):261–72. https://doi.org/10.1016/S0140-6736(19)31133-X.
11. Preshaw PM, Alba AL, Herrera D, et al. Periodontitis and diabetes: a two-way relationship. Diabetologia. 2012;55(1):21–31. https://doi.org/10.1007/s00125-011-2342-y.
12. Sheiham A, Watt RG. The common risk factor approach: a rational basis for promoting oral health. Community Dent Oral Epidemiol. 2000;28(6):399–406. https://doi.org/10.1034/j.1600-0528.2000.028006399.x.

Unintentional Injuries

33

Uzma Rahim Khan, Adnan A. Hyder, Umerdad Khudadad, and Nino Paichadze

Abstract

Unintentional injuries are responsible for almost three million deaths globally every year. There is striking disparity in the global burden of deaths due to unintentional injuries occurring in low- and middle-income countries (LMICs). Individual, socioeconomic, and environmental conditions all make a significant contribution to unintentional injuries. There are many proven interventions to prevent and control unintentional injuries, but they have primarily been implemented effectively in high-income countries. LMICs carry a significantly greater burden yet have not had the opportunity, or the resources, to effectively implement many of these interventions. Therefore, a major challenge for LMICs is to implement injury prevention policies at scale. State governments including health, transportation, and other sectors, international development organizations, academia and civil society must continue to work together to strengthen unintentional injury prevention globally.

Keywords

Unintentional injuries · Injury prevention · Global health · Low- and middle-income countries

33.1 Introduction

Injury is defined as body damage caused as a result of an abrupt transfer of energy (thermal, chemical, electrical, mechanical, or radiation) or the sudden absence of heat or oxygen [1]. Unintentional injuries are those that occur in the absence of predetermined intent and include road traffic injuries (RTIs), falls, drowning, poisoning, and burns [1].

Globally, unintentional injuries accounted for over three million deaths or about 71% of all injury deaths and RTIs contributed to 39% of unintentional injury deaths in 2019 [2]. This burden is disproportionately borne by low- and middle-income countries (LMICs) [3]. RTIs are the leading cause of unintentional injury deaths in LMICs followed by falls and drowning (Table 33.1).

Despite the huge burden of mortality and disability, unintentional injuries have received com-

U. R. Khan · U. Khudadad
Aga Khan University, Karachi, Pakistan
e-mail: uzma.khan@aku.edu; umerdad.khudadad.hpm53198@student.aku.edu

A. A. Hyder (✉) · N. Paichadze
Center on Commercial Determinants of Health and the Department of Global Health, Milken Institute School of Public Health, George Washington University, Washington, DC, USA
e-mail: hydera1@email.gwu.edu; npaichadze1@gwu.edu

M. C. B. Raviglione et al. (eds.), *Global Health Essentials*, Sustainable Development Goals Series,
https://doi.org/10.1007/978-3-031-33851-9_33

Table 33.1 Cause-specific death rates due to unintentional injuries globally and by income level, 2019[a]

Injury type	Global	High-income countries	Upper-middle-income countries	Lower-middle-income countries	Low-income countries
	Death rate (per 100,000 population)				
Road injuries	15	11	18	15	17
Falls	10	15	9	10	4
Drowning	3	2	3	3	3
Fire, heat, and hot substances	1	1	1	2	2
Poisonings	1	0.3	1	0.6	2

[a] Source: Global burden of diseases (GBD) data

paratively little attention as a global health concern, particularly in LMICs [1]. Emerging infectious diseases, such as the COVID-19 pandemic, have had a significant effect on the global health landscape and further threaten attention to unintentional injuries in the list of global health priorities.

33.2 Impact of Unintentional Injuries

Almost two-thirds of unintentional injury deaths occurred among males globally in 2019 [1]. The RTI death rates are higher than any other cause of injury in all age groups except falls in elderly aged 75 years or more (Fig. 33.1).

RTIs ranked seventh for all cause disability adjusted life years (DALYs) resulting in 7.1 million DALYs in high-income countries (HICs) compared to 26.6 in upper middle-income countries, 31.6 in lower middle-income countries and 7.6 in low-income countries [2]. The economic loss due to RTIs is lower in LMICs than in HICs with 46% of global economic loss in LMICs and 54% in HICs indicating high treatment costs in HICs [4].

The etiology of unintentional injuries is complex and multifactorial. Individual, socioeconomic, and environmental factors all play a role in unintentional injuries. Cognitive, behavioral, and audiovisual problems have all been individual factors associated with a higher risk of unintentional injuries [5]. High risk environments, infrastructure, speed, alcohol, lack of safety devices are some key risks [1]. The socioeconomic factors including low education and income levels increase the risk of unintentional injuries [3].

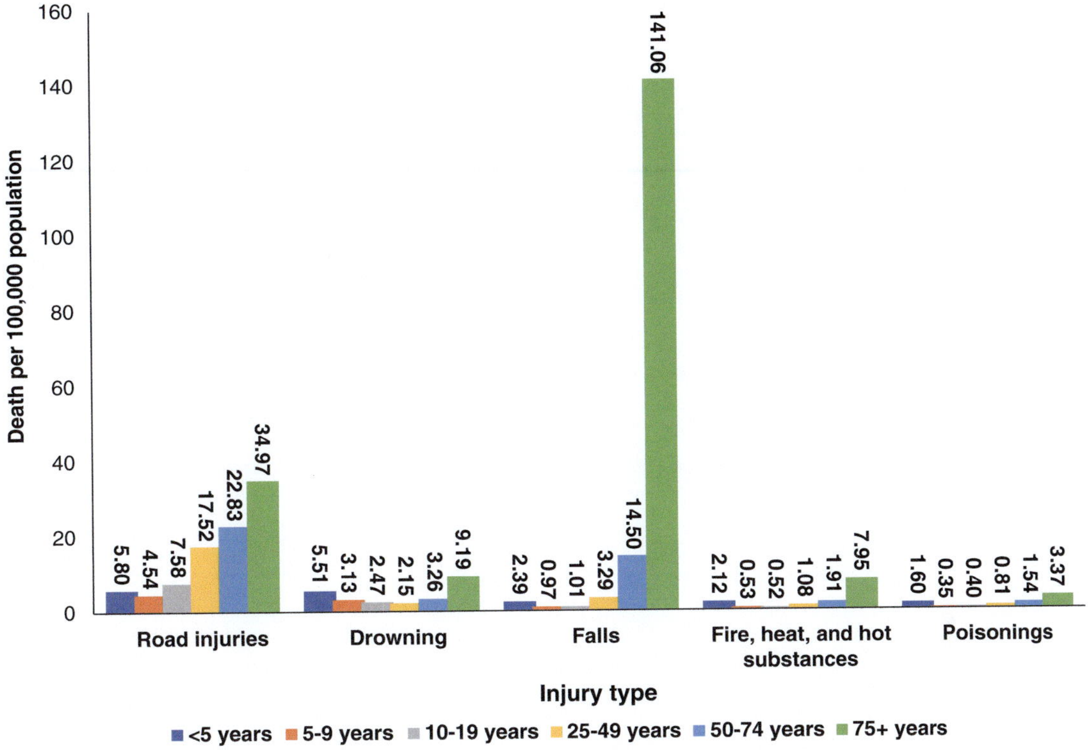

Fig. 33.1 Injury deaths per 100,000 population, by injury type and age group

33.3 Interventions

The conventional epidemiological paradigm of host, vector, and environment factors (all of which contribute to disease incidence) has been adapted and integrated in the Haddon matrix (that considers factors before, during, and after injury) to determine the causal pathway for injuries (Table 33.2) [1].

A systems approach is the underlying concept of a complete injury prevention program, which requires primary, secondary, and tertiary prevention to be offered at all levels of the health and transport systems [1]. While a list of the most widely proven and globally implemented interventions for unintentional injuries exists (Table 33.3), evidence on the effectiveness of these interventions in LMICs is relatively limited [1]. The strengthening of prehospital, hospital, and rehabilitative care systems could also help significantly decrease mortality, morbidity, and disability from unintentional injuries [1].

While the economic evaluation of interventions for unintentional injuries has been available from HICs, in recent decade, LMICs have made some progress in generating cost-effectiveness statistics on injuries. Drunk-driving laws, enforcement by random breath testing of drivers, speed limits, and motorcycle helmet use at 80% coverage have been shown to be very cost-effective interventions for prevention of RTIs in LMICs [8]. Social interventions and education programs for drowning prevention among children have also been shown to be cost-effective [9]. Despite this progress, a more comprehensive, cost-effectiveness analysis for various unintentional injury prevention interventions specific to LMICs remains a high research priority [10].

Over the last two decades, there have been some commendable achievements in the field of

Table 33.2 Examples of road traffic crash-related factors using Haddon Matrix

	Human (host)	Vector	Physical environment	Socioeconomic environment
Pre-event	Inadequate driving training	Faulty brakes and worn-out tires	Rain-slickened roads Poor lighting	Driving without driving license is socially acceptable
Event	Overspeeding	No airbag Shatterable mirrors	Sharp edges on the road	Ineffective enforcement of overspeeding laws
Post-event	Pre-existing co-morbidities		No prehospital care	Minimal assistance for re-integration of rehab patients into society

Table 33.3 Examples of effective interventions for unintentional injuries[a]

	Primary interventions	Secondary interventions	Tertiary interventions
Road traffic injuries	• Speed bumps • Transport planning • Drink-driving laws	• Seat belts • Child restraints	• First-responder training • Rehabilitation and physical therapy
Falls	• Exercise programs • Reduction of over prescription of sedative medications	• Protective padding • Nutrition and vitamin supplement • Exercise programs	• Spine precautions
Burns	• Public education • Hot water regulators • Smoke detectors	• Fire extinguishers • Safety zoning	• Specialized medical burn centers
Poisoning	• Public education • Blister packing and childproof containers of poisons and medicines • Safe containment of poisons • Appropriate labeling of poisons	• National poison control phone number	• Toxicology and in-patient poison control specialists
Drowning	• Drowning awareness • Learning swimming and water safety skills • Fencing domestic swimming pools • Covering drains	• Pool alarms	• Rescuer training

[a] Source: Adapted from WHO recommended interventions for selected unintentional injuries [6, 7]

unintentional injury prevention. The United Nations Sustainable Development Goals (SDGs) include two road safety-specific targets [11]: goal 3.6 that aims to halve the number of road traffic deaths and injuries by 2030; and goal 11.2 that calls for increased road safety and access to transportation systems, as well as the expansion of public transportation [12]. Progress made during the first Decade of Action for Road Safety 2011–2020 created the groundwork for more aggressive action during the current second decade in 2021–2030 [13]. Most recent analysis of RTIs indicates the potential for saving over half a million lives annually if evidence-based interventions were implemented globally; and over 200,000 lives could be potentially saved with improved emergency care systems [14].

33.4 Conclusion

National and international institutions (such as the World Health Organization), non-governmental organizations, academia, civil society, transportation and highway authorities, and lead government agencies must remain committed to working collaboratively in promoting unintentional injury prevention and implementing safety programs. However, the primary challenge for LMICs is to implement breakthroughs in injury research and implementation Future advances in the field of unintentional injury prevention will fundamentally depend on the delivery of evidence-based interventions globally resulting in reductions in deaths and disabilities.

References

1. Peek-Asa C, Hyder AA. Injury prevention and control: the public health approach. Oxford Textbook of Global Public Health: Oxford University Press; 2021.
2. Global burden of disease study 2019 (GBD 2019). Seattle: Institute for Health Metrics and Evaluation (IHME); 2022. https://doi.org/10.6069/1D4Y-YQ37.
3. Petridou E, Tursz A. Socio-economic differentials in injury risk. Inj Control Saf Promot. 2001;8(3):139–42.
4. Chen S, Kuhn M, Prettner K, Bloom DE. The global macroeconomic burden of road injuries: estimates and projections for 166 countries. Lancet Planet Health. 2019;3(9):e390–e8.
5. Zhang H, Wei F, Han M, Chen J, Peng S, Du Y. Risk factors for unintentional injuries among the rural elderly: a county-based cross-sectional survey. Sci Rep. 2017;7(1):1–9.
6. Peden MM, Khayesi M. Save LIVES technical package: 22 interventions that could make a difference. Inj Prev. 2018;24(5):381–3.
7. World Health Organization. A WHO plan for burn prevention and care. Geneva; 2008. https://www.who.int/publications/i/item/9789241596299.
8. Ralaidovy AH, Bachani AM, Lauer JA, Lai T, Chisholm D. Cost-effectiveness of strategies to prevent road traffic injuries in eastern sub-Saharan Africa and Southeast Asia: new results from WHO-CHOICE. Cost Eff Resour Alloc. 2018;16(1):1–10.
9. Rahman F, Bose S, Linnan M, Rahman A, Mashreky S, Haaland B, et al. Cost-effectiveness of an injury and drowning prevention program in Bangladesh. Pediatrics. 2012;130(6):e1621–8.
10. Bishai DM, Hyder AA. Modeling the cost effectiveness of injury interventions in lower and middle income countries: opportunities and challenges. Cost Eff Resour Alloc. 2006;4(1):1–11.
11. OECD/WHO, "Road safety", in Health at a Glance: Asia/Pacific 2020: Measuring Progress Towards Universal Health Coverage, OECD Publishing. Paris; 2020. https://doi.org/10.1787/65afc565-en.
12. Van den Berghe W, Fleiter J, Cliff D. Towards the 12 voluntary global targets for road safety. Guidance for countries on activities and measures to achieve the voluntary global road safety performance targets Vias Institute, Brussels and Global Road Safety Partnership. Geneva; 2020.
13. World Health Organization. Decade of action for road safety 2021-2030. Geneva, 2021. https://www.who.int/news/item/28-10-2021-who-kicks-off-a-decade-of-action-for-road-safety.
14. Hyder AA, Hoe C, Hijar M, Peden M. The political and social contexts of global road safety: challenges for the next decade. Lancet. 2022;400(10346):127–36.

Part VI

Social Determinants of Health

Poverty, Inequities, Inequalities, and Social Protection

34

Salla Atkins, Wanga Zembe-Mkabile, and Knut Lönnroth

Abstract

Poverty is one of the main drivers of health inequality and health inequity. While the objective measurement of poverty is complex, it colludes with other social determinants of health, such as access to services, education, and living conditions, to compound vulnerability, resulting in inequality and inequity, and negative health outcomes. The global outlook on poverty has improved over time, but inequality keeps increasing both across and within countries. The rising inequality is worsened by external shocks, such as COVID-19 and other recent crises. The main programme for mitigating the effects of poverty and inequality in health—social protection—is still globally inequitably distributed. This chapter describes global poverty, inequality and inequity and their effects on health and well-being. The chapter concludes with the evidence on social protection for health, and recent advances. Overall, social protection has great potential for improving health and well-being, but greater investments are still needed.

Keywords

Global poverty · Health inequality · Health inequity · Social protection · Health and wellbeing

34.1 Introduction to the Issue

Health inequalities and health inequities are often used interchangeably. Health inequalities are the "*differences, variations, and disparities in the health achievements of individuals and groups*" [1]. Health inequities are more difficult to measure and define, as they include a dimension of unfairness or injustice [1], stemming from normative judgements.

Poverty is an established driver of health inequality and health inequity, linked to several other social determinants of health. Poverty and other social determinants of health, such as gender, race, age, education and socioeconomic factors such as employment status, work and living environment, and access to health and social services, tend to be unfairly distributed and compound vul-

S. Atkins (✉)
Faculty of Social Sciences, Tampere University, Tampere, Finland

WHO Collaboration Centre on Tuberculosis and Social Medicine, Department of Global Public Health, Karolinska Institutet, Stockholm, Sweden
e-mail: salla.atkins@tuni.fi

W. Zembe-Mkabile
Health Systems Research Unit, South African Medical Research Council, Cape Town, South Africa
e-mail: wanga.zembe@mrc.ac.za

K. Lönnroth
WHO Collaboration Centre on Tuberculosis and Social Medicine, Department of Global Public Health, Karolinska Institutet, Stockholm, Sweden
e-mail: knut.lonnroth@ki.se

M. C. B. Raviglione et al. (eds.), *Global Health Essentials*, Sustainable Development Goals Series,
https://doi.org/10.1007/978-3-031-33851-9_34

nerability [2] and negative health outcomes. This chapter focuses on poverty and inequity, and the potential of social protection as a tool to mitigate their effects on health and well-being.

34.1.1 Poverty, Inequity, and Health

Poverty can be regarded as the lack of resources to obtain essential goods and services. There are a number of different definitions of poverty used, from absolute or extreme, relative, to non-monetary measures, driven by different understandings of what it means to be "poor". These definitions and poverty measurements in general are contested. Absolute poverty, a measure that captures those who are unable to meet basic daily needs, and thus fall below a minimum income threshold, is expressed in poverty lines such as the World Bank's 2.15 USD per person per day (updated September 2022, 1.90 USD per day per person for earlier estimates). The "absolute poverty" measure is criticised for being minimalist. Relative poverty, on the other hand, is benchmarked against median income levels in a country and therefore difficult to compare between countries. While appropriate measurements and definitions of poverty are key for developing effective, humane, and appropriate interventions and solutions for poverty and inequality [3], the existing contested measures can provide useful information about trends over time.

Extreme poverty is a measure of poverty defined according to an international poverty line. Latest World Bank estimates on extreme poverty (living on less than 2.15 USD per day) suggest that between 75 and 95 million were living in extreme poverty in 2022 [4]. While the global poverty rate has been consistently declining in the last 30 years, with about a quarter of the world's population rising above extreme poverty since 1990, poverty remains high in many countries [5]. The World Inequality Report 2022 shows that in the past two decades, inequality has increased in most countries, but inequalities between countries have declined. However, as a proportion of the share of the total world income, the poorest half of the world today captures half of the poor captured in 1820 [6].

Similar inequalities can be seen in health. As global health, and major mortality indicators and life expectancy have been improving in the past few decades, setbacks suggest that continued progress is not guaranteed [7]. Universal health coverage, also, increased from 1990 to 2019, though inequitably, due in part to health systems not keeping up with changing burden of disease and population change. Moreover, while health service coverage increased globally (with the exception for 2020–2021 due to the COVID-19 pandemic), incidence of catastrophic health expenditure increased, and large inequities persist both in service coverage and financial risk protection, especially in low-income countries [8].

The close connection between poverty, inequality, and health can be seen clearly through the impact of the COVID-19 pandemic on progress towards eradicating poverty. The global poverty rates were falling pre-Covid-19 in most of the world, besides for sub-Saharan African countries, which were expected to follow the global trend in due time. However, the pandemic could postpone expected declines until as far as 2030. For countries in the Global South already grappling with high levels of poverty, the COVID-19 pandemic and its linked economic crises [9], as well as conflicts and other crises, will leave long-lasting impacts.

Poverty and deprivation underlie many health problems, thus the health and well-being of populations largely depend on factors outside the health system. As such, the relationship between health, social, and economic factors has been cited as one of the greatest challenges facing health systems [10]. The interrelationship between poverty and health often results in a "vicious cycle", by which poverty predisposes to poor health and poor health predisposes to deepening poverty in the absence of measures to counteract and protect individuals. Key poverty-related diseases, such as tuberculosis, malaria, and malnutrition demonstrate this process well. Tuberculosis has an established socioeconomic gradient, and the long treatment course, as well as prolonged illness and disability preventing the ability to work, can result in high direct and indirect costs for the patient and their household, increasing poverty and thus putting the family at higher risk of TB. Moreover, these often catastrophic costs are predisposing to non-adherence and poor treatment outcomes [11].

Universal Health Coverage (UHC) has an indicator of catastrophic health expenditures, defined as direct out-of-pocket expenditure on health exceeding either 10 or 25% of total household consumption [8]. For tuberculosis, a similar indicator has been often used, defined as total direct and indirect costs (including income loss) exceeding 20% of household annual income [11]. While the cut-off for catastrophic costs is strict, the contributors to costs in the TB measure of catastrophic costs are more flexible, and include indirect costs such as transport and income loss, which are not included in the UHC financial risk protection indicator [8]. A linked condition, malnutrition, recognises underlying causes for the emergence and maintenance of the condition which are beyond direct healthcare. These include not only nutrition, but proximal and distal structural factors such as the environment in which food is produced, availed and accessed, adequate water and sanitation, housing and maternal educational attainment, all of which are linked to poverty.

For both conditions, while universal health coverage aims for reducing the direct costs of medical care, and providing quality, accessible healthcare for all, it does not address the indirect costs of care, including lost income, transport, and other costs during illness such as food and relocation [12]. Thus an additional layer of social policy beyond UHC is needed.

34.2 Social Protection as a Policy Instrument and Response to Counter Health Inequality and Poverty

Social protection is increasingly regarded as a critical policy instrument intrinsically linked to UHC as it can complement financial risk protection, enable access to care and address underlying social determinants of health. The most prominent definition of social protection is "*set of policies and programs designed to reduce and prevent poverty, vulnerability and social exclusion throughout the life cycle*" [13].

Stark inequities remain in social protection coverage across the world, with countries identified as low- or middle-income often having lower coverage of social protection [13]. For health outcomes, general cash transfers, disability benefits, and sickness benefits are key. Particularly sickness benefits are often lacking in low- and middle-income settings [14]. These would be key in protecting individuals during illness from losing income and therefore potential deepening of poverty for the individual and household. However, barriers remain in expanding social protection for health conditions, including country fiscal space, political will, dominance of an informal labour sector, poor institutional capacity including human resources, lack of data, and weak synergies between different government departments [15]. Countries also often prioritise pensions and cash transfers over disability and sickness protection for working age adults and the working poor. This means that in many countries social protection for the working age lag behind other programmes.

34.3 The Future: Towards Universal Social Protection

Evidence is mounting of the benefit of social protection for health, in terms of objective health outcomes, in health seeking and health behaviours, but also in less tangible outcomes of social protection such as empowerment and hope [16].

Social protection systems are developing rapidly, especially in sub-Saharan Africa. The COVID-19 pandemic has also increased the number of emergency relief programmes comprising different combinations of cash and in-kind transfers. However, whether these systems can be sustained in the long term and adopted into formal social protection programming remains to be seen. Expansion can be halted by crises and disasters [17] and requires sustained focus on outcomes, clear needs assessments and addressing the challenges noted above. There are some promising examples of extending coverage to specific vulnerable groups from low- and middle-income contexts, such as informal workers. Reaching all, including informal workers, people who are disabled or too ill to work, and covering them with social protection measures is key to ensuring equitable and fair systems.

Universal Basic Income Support (BIS) gained momentum during COVID-19 (e.g., [18]), as countries across the world considered some form of BIS. BIS aims for all individuals to be assured of a basic minimum that will keep them from falling below the poverty line. Sustaining such initiatives may help strengthen social protection systems that support low-income people.

34.4 Main Conclusions and Recommendations

While global poverty rates declined, the Covid-19 pandemic pushed back some of the advances made, particularly in the Global South. Concurrently, inequality within countries is increasing. Poverty, inequality, and inequity have powerful negative effects on health. Social protection is a potentially strong tool for addressing social determinants and consequences of poor health. Comprehensive social protection regimes that go beyond children and the elderly, including sickness benefits, disability benefits, maternity protection, and basic income support are needed to complement universal health coverage, to support the health of all populations throughout the life course.

References

1. Kawachi I, Subramanian SV, Almeida-Filho N. A glossary for health inequalities. J Epidemiol Community Health. 2002;56:647–52.
2. Gkiouleka A, Huijts T, Beckfield J, Bambra C. Understanding the micro and macro politics of health: inequalities, intersectionality & institutions—a research agenda. Soc Sci Med. 2018;200:92–8.
3. Haughton J, Khandker SR. The handbook on poverty and inequality. Washington, DC: The World Bank; 2009.
4. World Bank. Poverty. 2022. https://www.worldbank.org/en/topic/poverty/overview.
5. Development Initiatives. Poverty trends: global, regional and national. Fact sheet. 2021. https://devinit.org/documents/1100/Poverty_trends_-_global_regional_and_national_-_November_2021.pdf.
6. Chancel L, Piketty T, Saez E, Zucman G, et al. World inequality report 2022. World Inequality Lab; 2021. https://wir2022.wid.world/www-site/uploads/2021/12/WorldInequalityReport2022_Full_Report.pdf.
7. Vos T, Lim SS, Abbafati C, Abbas KM, Abbasi M, Abbasifard M, et al. Global burden of 369 diseases and injuries in 204 countries and territories, 1990–2019: a systematic analysis for the global burden of disease study 2019. Lancet. 2020;396(10258):1204–22.
8. World Health Organization and the International Bank for Reconstruction and Development/The World Bank. Tracking universal health coverage. 2021 global monitoring report—conference edition. Geneva; 2021. https://www.who.int/publications/i/item/9789240040618.
9. International Monetary Fund. World economic outlook: a long and difficult ascent. Washington, DC; 2020. https://www.imf.org/en/Publications/WEO/Issues/2020/09/30/world-economic-outlook-october-2020.
10. UNRISD. Health systems as social institutions: progress towards health in all policies. Social Policy and Development 2012–2013. 2013.
11. World Health Organization. The global tuberculosis report. Geneva; 2021. https://www.who.int/publications/i/item/9789240037021.
12. Lönnroth K, Glaziou P, Weil D, Floyd K, Uplekar M, Raviglione M. Beyond UHC: monitoring health and social protection coverage in the context of tuberculosis care and prevention. PLoS Med. 2014;11(9):e1001693.
13. International Labour Organization. World social protection report 2020–2022. Geneva; 2021. https://www.ilo.org/global/research/global-reports/world-social-security-report/2020-22/lang--en/index.htm.
14. Thorpe J, Viney K, Hensing G, Lönnroth K. Income security during periods of ill health: a scoping review of policies, practice and coverage in low-income and middle-income countries. BMJ Glob Health. 2020;5(6):e002425.
15. Atkins S, Tiitto J, Pajula J, Kervinen E, Miti JJ, Nhassengo P, et al. Social protection in Africa: a focus on gender equality and external shocks. Helsinki: Ministry for Foreign Affairs; 2022.
16. Yoshino CA, Sidney-Annerstedt K, Wingfield T, Kirubi B, Viney K, Boccia D, Atkins S. Experiences of conditional and unconditional cash transfers intended for improving health outcomes and health service use: a qualitative evidence synthesis. Cochrane Database of Systematic Reviews 2023, Issue 3. Art. No.: CD013635. https://doi.org/10.1002/14651858.CD013635.pub2. Accessed 19 June 2023.
17. Sojka B, Harvey P, Slater R. Ukraine—can social protection be sustained and support a humanitarian response? Wolverhampton: University of Wolverhampton; 2022.
18. Patel SB, Kariel J. Universal basic income and covid-19 pandemic. BMJ. 2021;372:n193.

35 Nutrition and Health

Francesco Branca

Abstract

Unhealthy diets and malnutrition are among the top risk factors for the Global Burden of Disease. Diets are unhealthy due to excess consumption of sodium, unhealthy fats, free sugars, red and processed meat, but also insufficient consumption of wholegrains, fruits, vegetables, nuts and seeds, and legumes.

The main forms of child malnutrition include Low Birth Weight, wasting, stunting, and overweight. For adults, the most common forms of malnutrition are overweight and obesity and micronutrient deficiencies, particularly iron deficiency. Addressing multiple forms of malnutrition requires actions in health, food and agriculture, social protection, education, trade, and the environment.

Keywords

Nutrition · Malnutrition · Unhealthy diets · Child malnutrition · Maternal malnutrition

35.1 Current Status and Trends

Good nutrition is defined as a physical growth aligned to the WHO growth standards and references, as well as adequate macronutrient, vitamin, and mineral intakes, aligned with WHO recommendations. Good nutrition supports optimal body functions and reduces disease risk. Conversely, deviations from those physiological ranges are leading to increased illness, disability, and death.

Altogether, unhealthy diets and malnutrition are among the top risk factors for the Global Burden of Disease (GBD). The Institute for Health Metrics and Evaluation (IHME) estimates that in 2019 approximately eight million deaths were accounted for by unhealthy diets, five million by overweight and obesity, and three million by maternal and child malnutrition. Altogether this represents over one fourth of all deaths [1].

The impact on disease and disability is even larger. Maternal and child malnutrition is the leading cause of disability, accounting for 295 million Disability-Adjusted Life Years (DALYs); unhealthy diet accounted for 188 million DALYs and high Body Mass Index (BMI) for 102 million DALYs. In total, unhealthy diets and malnutrition accounted for 22% of the total DALYs lost in 2019.

Diets are unhealthy not only due to excess consumption of sodium, unhealthy fats, free sugars, red and processed meat, but also insufficient consumption of wholegrains, fruits, vegetables,

F. Branca (✉)
Department of Nutrition and Food Safety, WHO, Geneva, Switzerland
e-mail: brancaf@who.int

M. C. B. Raviglione et al. (eds.), *Global Health Essentials*, Sustainable Development Goals Series,
https://doi.org/10.1007/978-3-031-33851-9_35

nuts and seeds, and legumes. Central Asia, Eastern Europe, and East Asia are the regions with the highest mortality due to unhealthy diet, to which the Pacific islands should be added when considering the DALYs scale [2].

The main forms of child malnutrition include Low Birth Weight (LBW), wasting, stunting, and overweight.

LBW, due to prematurity or intrauterine growth retardation, results largely from inadequate maternal nutrition. We estimate that in 2015 it affected 14.6% livebirths (20.5 million), 91% from low- and-middle income countries, mainly Southern Asia (accounting for 48% of all LBW live births) and sub-Saharan Africa (24% of LBW live births). In Southern Asia, one child in 4 (26.4%) is born with LBW [3].

Wasting is defined as a low weight-for-height (less than—2SD of the WHO child growth standards) in children under 5 years of age. It can occur acutely, such as in a food crisis, during seasonal food shortages or as a consequence of infectious diseases.

Stunting is defined as low height-for-age (less than—2SD of the WHO child growth standards) and is a condition that is progressively established as a result of chronically insufficient food intake, occurrence of infectious diseases (particularly, diarrhoeal, parasitic, and respiratory) and lack of care by caregivers or health services. Stunting is the most common form of child malnutrition.

Overweight in children under five is defined as a weight-for-height (more than +2SD of the WHO child growth standards), commonly resulting from an imbalance between calories consumed and calories expended, often due to an increased intake of energy-dense foods that are high in fat and sugars and a concurrent increase in sedentarism.

Globally in 2020, among children under 5 years of age, an estimated 149 million (22%) were stunted, 45 million (6.7%) were wasted, and 39 million (5.7%) were overweight [4]. It is also estimated that the epidemic of COVID-19 may have led to a 15% increase of wasting [5].

Vitamin and mineral deficiencies are also forms of malnutrition in children. The most common is iron deficiency (leading to anaemia), vitamin A (leading to impaired night vision and impaired immune response), folic acid (leading to neural tube defects and anaemia), iodine (leading to impaired neurodevelopment), and zinc (leading to impaired growth).

For adults, the most common forms of malnutrition are overweight and obesity and micronutrient deficiencies, iron deficiency occurring most often.

Adult obesity is on the rise in all regions, having increased worldwide from 11.8% in 2012 to 13.1% in 2016—the last year for which data are available.

For iron deficiency anaemia is used as a proxy. Globally in 2019, nearly one in three women aged 15–49 years (571 million) were affected by anaemia, with no progress since 2012.

Different forms of malnutrition coexist in the same country, in the same communities and in the same families, but also in the same individual simultaneously or at different times of the life course. Stunted children may be more frequently overweight, as observed in South America; micronutrient deficiencies can be present both in stunting and in overweight individuals. This phenomenon is known as the "Double Burden of Malnutrition" (DBM) and is increasingly present in low- and middle-income countries, mainly due to increases in overweight and obesity. Indonesia is the largest country with a severe DBM, but many other Asian and sub-Saharan African countries also face this problem. The DBM traps people in a lifelong status of poor nutrition and related consequences, which are more frequently infectious diseases in the younger ages and noncommunicable diseases in the adult age [6].

The Sustainable Development Goals (SDGs) framework has set the ambitious goal to end all forms of malnutrition by 2030 (SDG 2), linked to the six targets that the World Health Assembly (WHA) established through resolution WHA 65.6 (2012) (see Box 35.1) [7].

Box 35.1 The Six WHA Targets for 2025

1. 40% reduction of the global number of children under five who are stunted by 2025.
2. 50% reduction of anaemia in women of reproductive age by 2025.
3. 30% reduction of low birth weight by 2025.
4. No increase in childhood overweight by 2025.
5. Increase exclusive breastfeeding rates in the first 6 months up to at least 50% by 2025.
6. Reducing and maintaining childhood wasting to less than 5%.

Overall, there has been some progress in reducing stunting and improving breastfeeding, but the achievement of most global nutrition targets in 2025 is unlikely. For stunting in 2020, of the 155 countries with sufficient recent data to estimate progress, 53 were on track to reach the global target of 40% reduction in the number of stunted children by 2025 and 74 presented some progress towards that target. For anaemia in women of reproductive age, the 29.9% prevalence estimate of 2019 shows there has been no progress since 2012 (28.5%). For low birth weight, the 14.6% estimate of 2015 shows a minor decrease from 15.0% in 2012. For overweight in children under 5, there has been a modest increase at the global level in two decades—5.7% of all under-5-year-olds in 2020 compared with 5.4% in 2000. The increase has been persistent both in terms of prevalence and absolute numbers: there were 5.6 million more overweight children aged under 5 years in 2020 than in 2000.

For exclusive breastfeeding, 44% of infants under 6 months of age were exclusively breastfed in 2020—up from 37% in 2012. Based on the latest survey estimates for the period 2014–2020, 48 countries have exclusive breastfeeding rates higher than the 50% target and 87 countries have rates below it. Of 96 countries with sufficient data to estimate current trends, 35 are on track to reach the proposed target by 2025, 28% show insufficient progress and 33% show no improvement or are worsening. For wasting of the 100 countries with recent data, 57 have already reached or are on track to meet the 2025 target of reducing childhood wasting rates to below 5%, whereas 20 present show insufficient progress and 23 show no improvement or worsening trends.

35.2 Addressing Multiple Forms of Malnutrition: Cost-Effective Actions to Address Unhealthy Diets

Addressing multiple forms of malnutrition requires multi-sectoral actions in health, food and agriculture, social protection, education, trade, and the environment. The Second International Conference on Nutrition made 60 recommendations for action in the different sectors, based on proven cost-effective interventions [8].

In the health sector, WHO indicates a set of essential nutrition actions, including services to be provided across the life course to all people, such as iron and folic acid supplements during pregnancy, or promotion and support of breastfeeding, and dietary counselling [9].

In the food sector, WHO recommends actions aimed to shape the food environment and support the consumption of healthy diets, such as the provision of healthy food in schools and other public institutions, price and fiscal policies that discourage the consumption of unhealthy foods and encourage that of healthier foods, regulation of marketing of foods and beverages directed to children, front-of-the-pack interpretive nutrition labelling, and vitamin and mineral fortification of staple foods.

However, the food sector needs strong political will for a radical transformation that concerns both production and consumption. The actions and actors that are associated to the production, processing, and distribution of food as well as people consuming food are broadly described as "food systems". While food systems are meant to feed people and cover their nutrient needs, they do not function optimally. They are currently unable to provide sufficient food to over 800 million people and are not allowing three billion people to consume food of adequate quality, thus impacting on unhealthy diets and malnutrition described above. Food systems are also impacting health through unsafe food—leading to an estimated 420,000 deaths every year, through the spread of zoonotic pathogens—responsible for 2.7 million human deaths worldwide, antimicrobial resistance—responsible for at least 700,000 deaths per year globally, the contamination of the environment with fertilizers and pesticides, and impacts on the health of food workers [10]. Food systems need therefore to shift their priorities from a predominant commercial focus to the unique role of supporting nutrition and health for the whole world population.

References

1. IHME. GBD Compare. Data viewed on 22 August 2022.
2. GBD 2017 Diet Collaborators. Health effects of dietary risks in 195 countries, 1990–2017: a systematic analysis for the Global Burden of Disease Study 2017. Lancet. 2019;393:1958–72.
3. Blencowe H, Krasevec J, de Onis M, Black RE, An X, Stevens GA, Borghi E, Hayashi C, Estevez D, Cegolon L, Shiekh S, Ponce Hardy V, Lawn JE, Cousens S. National, regional, and worldwide estimates of low birthweight in 2015, with trends from 2000: a systematic analysis. Lancet Glob Health. 2019;7(7):e849–60.
4. FAO, IFAD, UNICEF, WFP and WHO. In brief to the state of food security and nutrition in the world 2022. Repurposing food and agricultural policies to make healthy diets more affordable. Rome: FAO; 2022. https://doi.org/10.4060/cc0640en.
5. Headey D, Heidkamp R, Osendarp S, Ruel M, Scott N, Black R, Shekar M, Bouis H, Flory A, Haddad L, Walker N. Standing together for nutrition consortium. Impacts of COVID-19 on childhood malnutrition and nutrition-related mortality. Lancet. 2020;396(10250):519–21.
6. Popkin BM, Corvalan C, Grummer-Strawn LM. Dynamics of the double burden of malnutrition and the changing nutrition reality. Lancet. 2020;395(10217):65–74.
7. WHO. Comprehensive implementation plan on maternal, infant and young child nutrition. Geneva; 2014. https://www.who.int/publications/i/item/WHO-NMH-NHD-14.1.
8. FAO/WHO. Second International Conference on Nutrition. Conference Outcome Document. Rome: Framework for Action; 2014. https://www.who.int/news-room/events/detail/2014/11/19/default-calendar/fao-who-second-international-conference-onnutrition-(icn2).
9. WHO. Essential nutrition actions: mainstreaming nutrition through the life-course. Geneva; 2019. https://www.who.int/publications/i/item/9789241515856.
10. WHO. Food systems delivering better health: executive summary. Geneva; 2021. https://www.who.int/publications/i/item/9789240031814.

36 Migration and Health

Santino Severoni, Rita Sá Machado, and Richard Alderslade

Abstract

Health matters associated with migration may be crucial public health challenges, with a possible impact on both the health and well-being of migrants and host populations.

Migrants may remain among the most vulnerable members of society when faced with xenophobia; discrimination; poor living, housing, and working conditions; and inadequate access to health services and other basic services.

To effectively protect people on the move and improve their health and well-being, a deep understanding of the drivers of migration, the contextual factors, normative, policy, and legal frameworks, as well as the main problems faced by migrants in accessing care, is vital. This will allow the implementation of responses which effectively address their needs. Evidence shows that an inclusive public health approach is the most appropriate regarding cost-effectiveness and health outcomes.

The purpose of this chapter is to reflect on the basic concepts of migration and health, highlighting its importance to the global health agenda.

S. Severoni (✉) · R. S. Machado · R. Alderslade
Health and Migration Programme, World Health Organization, Geneva, Switzerland
e-mail: severonis@who.int; samachador@who.int

Keywords

Migration and health · Migrants' health and wellbeing · Migration drivers · Migrants' access to care · Migrant-inclusive health systems and policies

36.1 Introduction and Background

The number of people on the move—within and outside borders—is increasing. In 2020, global estimates pointed out that around 281 million international migrants correspond to 3.6% of the worldwide population [1]. This total was 128 million more than in 1990 and over three times the estimated number in 1970 [2].

The correlation between health and migration is dynamic by nature and complex. Migration is recognized as a determinant of health, impacting the health systems of countries of origin and destination, and shaping access to healthcare and interactions with the health workforce [3, 4]. Not only migration may affect the health of refugees and migrants, but it may also affect the health of populations in countries along the migratory pathway. When not adequately supported by appropriate intersectoral policies, migration can expose the most vulnerable socioeconomic groups to inequity

M. C. B. Raviglione et al. (eds.), *Global Health Essentials*, Sustainable Development Goals Series,
https://doi.org/10.1007/978-3-031-33851-9_36

and difficulties in accessing health services, as well as other basic services.

Acting on the health needs of migrant populations is aligned and critical to public health principles, including the right to health for all. The right to health ought to be upheld irrespective of migration status and is applicable within all migration contexts, including population movements due to instability or humanitarian crises.

36.2 Aims of the Chapter

This chapter aims to contribute to the knowledge and understanding of the role of migration in the global health agenda and to allude to critical principles that should guide the essential work in the migration and health field.

36.3 Migration and Health

36.3.1 Defining "*Migration*" and "*Migrant*": The Spider Web

Migration is the movement of persons away from their place of usual residence, either across an international border–international migration or within a State–internal migration [5].

There is no universally accepted definition of *migrant*. The United Nations Department of Economic and Social Affairs defines an international migrant as "any person who changes his or her country of usual residence"[1] [6]. This includes any people who are moving or have moved across an international border, regardless of legal status, duration of the stay abroad and causes for migration.

The definition of the International Organization for Migration (IOM) includes persons who move away from their usual residence, whether within a country or across an international border, temporarily or permanently, and for various reasons" [5]. The IOM considers the term "migrant" as an umbrella term covering all forms of movement within and outside a State.

36.3.2 The Drivers of Migration: Why Are People Urged to Move?

Factors that compel people to migrate are usually referred as "drivers" of migration. These include movements which are expected or unexpected, voluntary or forced, permanent or temporary, and which take place at individual, household, or familial level. The migration decision-making may be associated with circumstances along the migration route in countries of origin, transit, and destination.

Drivers of migration can be economic, demographic, environmental, social, or political. People mostly migrate to improve the quality of life for themselves or their families, access a better financial situation or improve their labour or educational opportunities. They may be seeking to escape and flee from conflict and escalating violence brought about by war or complex emergencies; hunger, political, economic, and social instability; persecution; natural disasters or human-made crises. Some migrants move as they lack essential services, including health, shelter, water and sanitation, food or basic education, or due to poor or inadequate governance and security [7].

36.3.3 The Impact of Migration on Health: What Are the Main Health Issues Migrants May Face?

Patterns of morbidity and mortality in migrant population are influenced by the diversity of migrant groups (e.g., economic, labour or climate migrants, internal displaced, refugees, asylum seekers, undocumented migrants) and also by stressors linked to each stage of the migratory process (Box 36.1).

[1] For statistically purposes.

Box 36.1 Stressors: Migratory Process (Examples)

Existence of active conflict
Loss of relatives and friends
Urbanization
Stays in often overcrowded locations with poor sanitary conditions
Lack of access to health services
Existence of cultural and language barriers
Stigma and discrimination

Morbidity and mortality may be different in the beginning of the migratory process—more linked to the health epidemiology of the country of origin, whilst approaching the epidemiology of the host population in the destination country in due time. Some migrant populations may enjoy better health outcomes upon arrival than host populations; yet specific migrant groups (refugees, asylum seekers, and undocumented migrants) may be at a higher risk of poor health outcomes [8, 9].

The migration experience, which may involve inadequate transit conditions, restrictive entry and integration policies, exclusion, and acculturation stress, may also put at risk migrants of worse health outcomes (Table 36.1). Evidence suggests that many migrants will have experienced burdensome travels and stays in transit centres, during which they may have been exposed to poor living and working conditions, torture, and sexual and gender-based violence. The migration experience affects risk perception and risk behaviour, what can increase the vulnerability of migrants to specific communicable and non-communicable diseases [9]. Access to immunization and continuity of care are more difficult to ensure when people are on the move.

Evidence also suggests higher mental distress among migrant populations, exacerbated by lack of social support and increased stress after migration, and fear of detention or deportation. Structural features, such as insecure asylum status, financial difficulties, discrimination, and barriers to access healthcare can contribute to poor mental health outcomes.

Table 36.1 Most frequent health challenges and problems that specific vulnerable migrant groups may face

Health areas	Most frequent challenges and problems
Occupational health	• Workplace injury, death, musculoskeletal, respiratory, and mental health conditions, as well as other industry-specific hazards
Sexual and reproductive health	• Low awareness and use of services (including contraception and general sexual education) • Sexual and gender-based violence • Lower levels of knowledge of sexually transmitted infections
Maternal and child health	• Difficulties in accessing maternal and child health services • Higher risk of negative outcomes during pregnancy and delivery, including mortality • Higher rates of anaemia • Increased risk of both anaemia and malnutrition in some camp-based settings • Exposure to poor-quality substitutes for breast milk
Non-communicable diseases	• Interruption of care • Diabetes mellitus and hypertension may be left undiagnosed and uncontrolled, possibly leading to a higher risk of cardiovascular diseases • Cancer is often diagnosed at later stages
Mental health	• Higher prevalence of depression and anxiety • Higher levels of Post Traumatic Stress Disorder (PTSD) and other mental health issues • Higher incidence of psychoses
Communicable diseases	• Susceptibility to infection is increased by the environmental risk factors related to living and working conditions • Delayed HIV testing and diagnosis • Higher levels of multidrug-resistant TB and Latent TB Infection (LTBI)

Source: This table summarizes main key points on the health of migrants included in the WHO World Report on the health of refugees and migrants [9]

An impact on countries of origin is also seen as many health workers emigrate for economic or career opportunities, undermining the provision of adequate care locally.

36.3.4 Accessing Health Services: The Case of Migrants

Health[2] is an essential component of sustainable development; being and staying healthy is a fundamental precondition for migrants to work, to be productive and to contribute to the social and economic development of their communities of origin and destination.

According to international agreements and normative standards, migrants should have full access to high-quality care without discrimination based on gender, age, religion, nationality, or race, regardless of their legal status. However, they may experience formal and informal barriers in accessing health services. Examples include policies and legal frameworks that deny access to services (e.g., strict access to emergency care or exclusion from public health programmes that promote and protect the health of populations), lack of financial resources, unfamiliarity with the health system of the host country, low levels of health literacy, cultural and language differences, personal biases, stereotyped views, individual racism, lack of a culturally responsive health workforce, and inadequate use of interpreting services [8, 9].

36.3.5 International Initiatives to Improve the Health of and the Access to Care for Migrants

The global policy landscape on health and migration has advanced considerably in the last decade (Table 36.2).

[2]Health is defined as a state of complete physical, mental, and social well-being and not merely the absence of disease or infirmity (WHO, 2006)

Table 36.2 Main global policy frameworks—migration and health

United Nations
- 2030 Agenda for Sustainable Development, 2015
- New York Declaration for Refugees and Migrants, 2016
- Global Compact on Refugees, 2018
- Global Compact for Safe, Orderly, and Regular Migration, 2018
- Political Declaration of the High-level Meeting on Universal Health Coverage "Universal health coverage: moving together to build a healthier world", 2019
- Progress Declaration of the International Migration Review Forum 2022

World Health Organization
- Resolution on the Health of Migrants, WHA 61.17, 2008
- Promoting the health of refugees and migrants, WHA 70.15, 2017
- Framework of priorities and guiding principles to promote the health of refugees and migrants, WHA 70.24, 2017
- WHO Global Action Plan: Promoting the health of refugees and migrants: draft global action plan, 2019–2023 WHA A72/25 Rev.1 2019 and extended to 2030, WHA 76.14, 2023

The overarching framework is the United Nations 2030 Agenda for Sustainable Development, including not only through target 10.7 (Orderly and safe migration through well-managed migration policies), but also on target 3.8 (Achieve universal health coverage (UHC)).

The inclusion of migrants has also been reflected in the 2019 UN political declaration on UHC, that clearly states that "no one should be left behind" and calls states to address the needs and vulnerabilities of migrants (Box 36.2).

Also, of vital importance are the Global Compact on Refugees (GCR) and the Global Compact for Migration (GCM). The latter, in objective 15 asks that migrants have access to essential services, including health. Also, it aims to incorporate the health needs of migrants in national and local healthcare policies and plans.

In May 2019, the World Health Assembly acknowledged the health of refugees and migrants

Box 36.2 Universal Health Coverage: The Case of Migration

- Universal Health Coverage (UHC) means that all individuals and communities, including migrants, receive the health services they need without suffering financial hardship. It includes the full spectrum of essential, quality health services, from health promotion to prevention, treatment, rehabilitation, and palliative care across the life course.
- Countries that progress towards UHC will make progress towards the other targets, including the ones linked with migration (SDG 10.7).
- Moving towards UHC requires strengthening health systems, with primary health care and life course approaches. In the case of migration, this means that migrants can access services based on their needs, across all phases of life; multi-sectoral policies and actions are implemented to address the wider determinants of health; and engaging and empowering individuals, families, and communities, including migrants for increased participation and self-reliance in health.

as a global priority by noting the World Health Organization's Global Action Plan to promote the health of refugees and migrants (the WHO GAP). Within the WHO GAP, improvement of opportunities to support health of migrants, and better access to health services, are promoted [10].

36.3.6 Migrant-Sensitive Health Systems and Health Promotion

Strengthening the capacity of health systems to adapt to the health needs of all populations, including migrants, is an essential prerequisite for achieving UHC. Affordable and non-discriminatory access to health services should be facilitated by reducing communication barriers and developing a migrant-sensitive health workforce through educational provision, training, and continuous professional development [11].

Migrants in an irregular situation may not want to seek medical care due to fear of deportation or discrimination; hence, the introduction of effective firewalls between public health providers and immigration enforcement authorities is essential. Also, as migrants very often lack the economic capacity to be involved in health promotion, health protection, and medical care initiatives, they require effective financial protection mechanisms to be in place to enable them to access care.

Here the development of improved information systems allowing the identification and monitoring of standards for health service delivery, organizational management, and governance would also be an additional component to support the implementation of migrant-sensitive health systems. Intersectionality, fostering exchanges of information and good practice among all services working with migrants, and involving people and communities in the design of care and information about health and healthcare access are all also vital if the health needs of migrants are to be properly addressed.

36.4 Main Conclusions and Recommendations

To effectively protect people on the move, including their health, a deep understanding of the drivers of migration, contextual factors, and normative, policy and legal frameworks at global, regional, and country levels, is vital to coordinate tailored responses which respond effectively to their needs.

Migrant-inclusive health systems and policies are feasible and cost-effective. It will benefit host populations and migrants. Investing in migrants health makes a vital contribution to the overall improvement of global health, by committing to the development and well-being of societies [9].

References

1. World Migration Report 2022. International Organization for Migration (IOM), Geneva; 2021. https://publications.iom.int/books/world-migration-report-2022. Accessed 11 August 2023.
2. World Migration Report 2020. Geneva: International Organization for Migration; 2019. https://publi-

cations.iom.int/system/files/pdf/wmr_2020.pdf. Accessed 29 August 2022.
3. Castañeda H, Holmes SM, Madrigal DS, Young M-ED, Beyeler N, Quesada J. Immigration as a social determinant of health. Annu Rev Public Health. 2015;36:375–92.
4. Davies A, Basten A, Frattini C. Migration: a social determinant of migrants' health. Migr Health Eur Union. 2010;16:10–2.
5. Glossary on migration. Geneva: International Organization for Migration; 2019. https://publications.iom.int/system/files/pdf/iml_34_glossary.pdf. Accessed 22 June 2022.
6. Recommendations on statistics of international migration, revision 1 (1998). New York: United Nations Department of Economic and Social Affairs Statistics Division; 1998: para. 32. https://unstats.un.org/unsd/publication/seriesm/seriesm_58rev1e.pdf. Accessed 1 May 2021.
7. Addressing drivers of migration, including adverse effects of climate change, natural disasters and human-made crises, through protection and assistance, sustainable development, poverty eradication, conflict prevention and resolution. New York: United Nations; 2017. https://refugeesmigrants.un.org/sites/default/files/final_issue_brief_2.pdf. Accessed 29 Aug 2022.
8. Common health needs of refugees and migrants: literature review. Geneva: World Health Organization; 2021. https://www.who.int/publications/i/item/9789240033108. Accessed 11 August 2023.
9. World report on the health of refugees and migrants. Geneva: World Health Organization; 2022. https://www.who.int/publications/i/item/9789240054462. Accessed 11 August 2023.
10. World Health Assembly. Promoting the health of refugees and migrants—draft global action plan, 2019–2023 Report by the Director-General, A72.25 Rev1. 2019. https://apps.who.int/gb/ebwha/pdf_files/WHA72/A72_25Rev1-en.pdf.
11. Refugee and migrant health: global competency standards for health workers. Geneva: World Health Organization; 2021. https://www.who.int/publications/i/item/9789240030626. Accessed 11 August 2023.

37 Environmental Exposures and Health

Roberto Bertollini

Abstract

Environmental exposures are one of the main causes of ill health causing from 16 to 23% of all deaths and 22% of morbidity in the world. This is attributable to a wide range of chemical, biological and radiological substances which are associated to a number of diseases, from cancer to cardiovascular diseases, from developmental abnormalities to immunotoxicity. In this chapter, the main exposures and their pathways are reviewed, with special attention to air pollution and chemical substances, the latter occurring through contaminated air, soil, food and water. Reference to the main diseases associated to the environment will be made in connection to relevant exposures.

Knowledge of the role of environment on health has grown substantially over the recent decades and policies to reduce exposures are known and require an intersectoral, health in all policies approach. The adoption of this strategy will have a number of co-benefits for health and environment including the reduction of greenhouse gas emissions.

R. Bertollini (✉)
Ministry of Public Health, Doha, Qatar

Keywords

Environmental health · Chemicals · Air pollution · Environmental exposures · Water and sanitation

37.1 Background and Aim of the Chapter

Environmental exposures are responsible for a substantial proportion of deaths and disabilities at the global level ranging from 16% to 23% of deaths and 22% of Disability Adjusted Life Years.

In this chapter, an overview of the available data and evidence regarding major environmental exposures, (i.e. air pollution, chemicals, water and sanitation) and their impact on health is reviewed and the policy implications addressed.

37.2 Overall Impact on Environmental Hazards on Mortality and Morbidity

Environmental pollution includes contamination of air, water and soil by a number of biological, chemical and radioactive substances which have a negative effect on human health. In 2017, the Lancet Commission on pollution and health estimated that about nine million deaths in 2015 (16% of all deaths globally) were attributable to

M. C. B. Raviglione et al. (eds.), *Global Health Essentials*, Sustainable Development Goals Series,
https://doi.org/10.1007/978-3-031-33851-9_37

environmental exposures [1]. An update of this estimate carried out recently [2] using data from the Global Burden of Disease 2019 study [3], confirmed this figure. However, over the period 2015–2019, premature deaths due to modern hazardous environmental exposure (air pollution, lead and other chemicals) have increased while, on the contrary, fatalities due to traditional risk factors such as contaminated water and poor sanitation have decreased [2].

Other estimates conducted by WHO with a different methodology indicate that in 2012 environmental exposures were responsible for 23% of deaths and 22% of disability adjusted life years (DALYs). In this latter report, the fraction of a number of high prevalent diseases attributable to environmental exposure has been estimated (Fig. 37.1) [4].

In summary, both studies converge in indicating that a significant proportion of deaths and morbidity due to highly prevalent diseases, ranging from 16 to 23%, is attributable to known and preventable environmental exposures. However, these summary values hide a striking inequality whereas population in Low and Middle Income Countries (LMIC) are exposed to higher level of pollutants and are suffering from a larger impact on health than developed countries [2].

37.2.1 Air Pollution

Air pollution is one of the five main risk factors for chronic diseases together with smoking, lack of physical activity, unhealthy nutrition and alcohol consumption [5]. The Lancet Commission estimates that 4.5 million deaths per year are attributable to ambient air pollution and 2.3 million per year to indoor air pollution, the latter mainly associated to the use of fossil fuel in the household of LMICs for cooking and heating [2].

The health impacts of air pollution are mainly due to particulate matter, ozone, nitrogen oxides and sulphur dioxide. A myriad of other chemical substances such as VOCs are also associated to significant health effects.

Air pollution levels vary considerably in different countries of the world, reaching very high level in several megacities of LMICs.

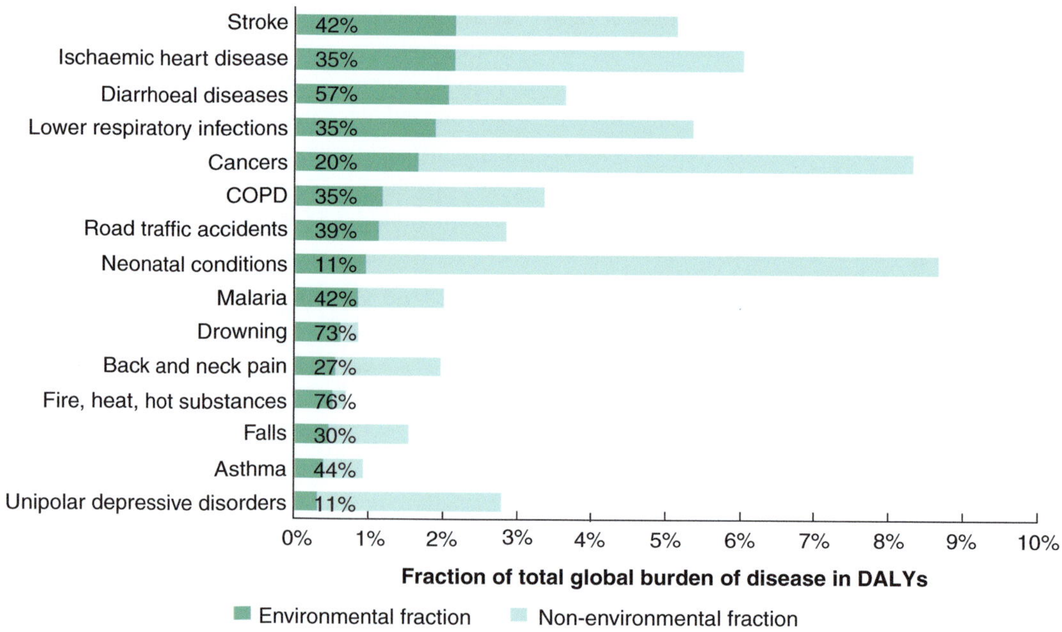

Fig. 37.1 Environmental fraction of burden of selected diseases (percentages relate to the environmental share of the respective diseases). Reproduced with permission from [4] under the terms of the Creative Commons Attribution 3.0 IGO License (http://creativecommons.org/licenses/by/4.0)

Levels of air pollution, and in particular of small particulate matter (PM2.5), beyond the WHO air quality guidelines [6] cause an increase of mortality and morbidity both for short-term and long-term exposures.

For short-term exposure, there is a 0.65% increase of daily non-accidental mortality for each 10 μg/m3 excess concentration of PM2.5 [7]. Days with high concentration of particulate matter are also associated with hospital admissions. An increase of 2.3% of hospital admissions for acute coronary syndrome, of 2.4% for congestive heart failure and of 2.8% for respiratory diseases, for any 10 μg/m3 increase concentration of PM2.5 has been observed [8].

As for long-term exposure to PM2.5, there is a 8% increase of non-accidental mortality for any 10 μg/m3 increase in the average yearly concentration of PM2.5 [9]. The impact is higher for specific causes of death: plus 11% for circulatory mortality, 10% for non-malignant respiratory mortality and 12% for lung cancer. In a number of European cities an overall decrease of the average life expectancy ranging from 0.4 months in Dublin to 22.1 months in Bucharest has been observed [10].

Small particles pass into the blood stream and are impacting several metabolic processes and inflammatory mechanisms, thus affecting a number of organ systems in the body. A joint statement of the American Thoracic Society and the European Respiratory Society [11] confirms that air pollution is associated to diseases of the respiratory, cardiovascular and reproductive systems, of the skin and also affects brain function and development. For example, a decrease of cognitive development among children exposed to high levels of traffic-related air pollutants has been observed [12]. This may cause long-term consequences for learning, school achievement and behaviour.

Finally, air pollution is also strictly related to climate change: its causes—mainly the emissions due the use of fossil fuel—are also the causes of greenhouse gases emissions. Actions against climate change translate in benefits for health through decreased air pollution, beyond those achievable by preventing a further increase on average temperature. [13],

37.2.2 Chemicals

Chemicals are widely disseminated in the environment. Over 350,000 chemicals and mixtures of chemicals have been registered for production and use with substantial differences across countries and regions [14]. Only a small fraction of this huge number of manufactured substances has been tested for safety and toxicity and the disease burden attributable to them is largely underestimated [15].

This is of particular concern for three specific consequences of chemical pollution, namely reproductive toxicity, immunotoxicity and developmental neurotoxicity. Reproductive toxicity is linked to a range of reproductive problems but also to increased incidence of disease of the reproductive system later in life, such as endometriosis, breast cancer, uterine and testicular cancer. Some chemicals such as perfluoroalkyl acids have been associated to reduced antibody response to vaccine and increased risk of children hospitalizations for infectious diseases. Of particular concern is the role of certain chemicals on developmental neurotoxicity, which includes autism spectrum disorders and attention-deficit hyperactivity. Out of 201 chemicals that are known to be neurotoxic in adults, only 11 have been demonstrated to be developmental neurotoxic [16]. It is possible that many more substances can affect the developing brain thus causing severe consequences on society and welfare including diminished quality of life, reduced academic achievement and behavioural disturbances.

One of these neurotoxic chemicals is lead which is both a public health success story and a persistent long-term problem. Lead has been removed from automotive fuel in every country due to the evidence collected and the pressure exercised by the public health community. Nevertheless, exposure to lead continues especially in LMICs through recycling of lead-acid batteries and e-waste, lead in paint, pottery and in other products. For example, in Senegal, a major mass lead intoxication causing children deaths and extensive clinical effects occurred through inhalation and ingestion of soil and dust heavily contaminated with lead as a result of informal and unsafe batteries recycling [17]. Lead is annually responsible for 0.9 million deaths [3]. Overall, around 800 million children are estimated to have blood lead concentrations that exceed 5 μg/dL. [1]. Children with this level of exposure could score 3–5 points lower on intelligence tests than children with lower concentration.

37.2.3 Water and Sanitation

Safe drinking-water, sanitation and hygiene are crucial to human health and well-being.

Contaminated water and poor sanitation are linked to transmission of diseases such as cholera, diarrhoea, dysentery, hepatitis A, typhoid and polio. Water can also be chemically polluted by toxic substances such as arsenic and fluoride. Globally, it has been estimated that 829,000 people die each year from diarrhoea as a result of unsafe drinking-water, sanitation and hand hygiene, including 297,000 under 5 children [18].

One of the growing concerns in urban areas is the scarcity of water. The term "dry cities" has been introduced to describe this condition which is due to become more common as a consequence of increased episodes of drought due to climate change. An estimated 150 million people live in cities which have perennial water shortage [19].

37.3 Main Conclusions and Recommendations

Addressing environmental health risks require strategies and policies in sectors beyond health through a multisectoral, health in all policies approach. Combating air pollution for instance, require actions and regulation involving the transport sector, energy production, urban development, industry and others. A multisectoral policy results in many health and non-health co-benefits: for example, less polluting vehicles, combined rapid transit with walking and cycling, and replacement of short urban motorized journeys by walking and cycling would increase physical activity, directly reduce a number of non-communicable diseases and mitigate climate change through reduced greenhouse gas emissions. Such co-benefits need to be accounted for in economic evaluations of environmental health action.

In this context, the health sector can play a significant role both by producing and updating the evidence on the health effects associated to environmental pollution and assessing the effectiveness on health of the actions and policies put in place to reduce the exposures. On the other hand, the health sector can directly implement actions to reduce emissions, control chemicals use and waste production, but also, at the same time, advocate with citizens and authorities for a proper understanding of the role of a polluted environment on health and of the actions required to introduce the necessary changes. "Be the change" and "Lead the change" should be the policy directions for the immediate future [20].

References

1. Landrigan PJ, Fuller R, Acosta NJR, et al. The Lancet Commission on pollution and health. Lancet. 2018;391:462–512.
2. Fuller R, Landrigan PJ, Balakrishnan K, et al. Pollution and health: a progress update. Lancet Planet Health. 2022;6:e535–47.
3. Murray CJL, Aravkin AY, Zheng P, et al. Global burden of 87 risk factors in 204 countries and territories, 1990-2019: a systematic analysis of the global burden of disease study 2019. Lancet. 2020;396:1223–49.
4. Prüss-Ustün A, Wolf J, Corvalan C, et al. Diseases due to unhealthy environments: an updated estimate of the global burden of disease attributable to environmental determinants of health. J Public Health. 2017;39(3):464–75.
5. United Nations. Political declaration of the third high-level meeting of the general assembly on the prevention and control of non-communicable diseases. Time to deliver: accelerating our response to address non-communicable diseases for the health and well-being of present and future generations. 2018. https://ncdalliance.org/sites/default/files/Political_Declaration_final_text_0.pdf

6. World Health Organization. WHO global air quality guidelines: particulate matter (PM2.5 and PM10), ozone, nitrogen dioxide, sulfur dioxide and carbon monoxide. World Health Organization. 2021. https://apps.who.int/iris/handle/10665/345329
7. Orellano P, Reynoso J, Quaranta N, Bardach A, Ciapponi A. Short-term exposure to particulate matter (PM10 and PM2.5), nitrogen dioxide (NO2), and ozone (O3) and all-cause and cause-specific mortality: systematic review and meta-analysis. Environ Int. 2020;142:105876. https://doi.org/10.1016/j.envint.2020.105876.
8. Belleudi V, Faustini A, Stafoggia M, Cattani G, Marconi A, Perucci CA, Forastiere F. Impact of fine and ultrafine particles on emergency hospital admissions for cardiac and respiratory diseases. Epidemiology. 2010;21:414–23.
9. Chen J, Hoek G. Long term exposure to PM and all-causes and cause-specific mortality: a systematic review and meta-analysis. Environ Int. 2020;143:105974. https://doi.org/10.1016/j.envint.2020.105974.
10. Pascal M, Corso M, Chanel O, et al. Assessing the public health impacts of urban air pollution in 25 European cities: results of the Aphekom project. Sci Total Environ. 2013;449:390–400. https://doi.org/10.1016/j.scitotenv.2013.01.077.
11. Thurston GD, Kipen H, Annesi-Maesano I, et al. A joint ERS/ATS policy statement: what constitutes an adverse health effect of air pollution? An analytical framework. Eur Respir J. 2017;49:1600419. https://doi.org/10.1183/13993003.00419-2016.
12. Sunyer J, Esnaola M, Alvarez-Pedrerol M, Forns J, Rivas I, López-Vicente M, et al. Association between traffic-related air pollution in schools and cognitive development in primary school children: a prospective cohort study. PLoS Med. 2015;12(3):e1001792. https://doi.org/10.1371/journal.pmed.1001792.
13. Haines A, Ebi K. The imperative for climate action to protect health. N Engl J Med. 2019;380:263–73. https://doi.org/10.1056/NEJMra1807873.
14. Wang Z, Walker GW, Muir DCG, Nagatani-Yoshida K. Toward a global understanding of chemical pollution: a first comprehensive analysis of national and regional chemical inventories. Environ Sci Technol. 2020;54(5):2575–84. https://doi.org/10.1021/acs.est.9b06379.
15. Prüss-Ustün A, Vickers C, Haefliger P, Bertollini R. Knowns and unknowns on burden of disease due to chemicals: a systematic review. Environ Health. 2011;10:9. https://ehjournal.biomedcentral.com/articles/10.1186/1476-069X-10-9.
16. Grandjean P, Landrigan PJ. Neurobehavioural effects of developmental toxicity. Lancet Neurol. 2014;13:330–8.
17. Haefliger P, Mathieu-Nolf M, Lociciro S, Ndiaye C, Coly M, Diouf BR, Neira M. Mass lead intoxication from informal used lead-acid battery recycling in Dakar, Senegal. Environ Health Perspect. 2009;117(10):1535–40.
18. https://www.who.int/news-room/fact-sheets/detail/drinking-water. Accessed 23 Oct 2022
19. Frumkin H, Bordia Das M, Negev M, Rogers BC, Bertollini R, Dora C, Desai S. Protecting health in dry cities: considerations for policy. BMJ. 2020;371(m2936) https://doi.org/10.1136/bmj.m2936.
20. https://2020.wish.org.qa/app/uploads/2020/09/IMPJ7849-01-Climate-Change-and-Health-WISH2020-201030-WEB.pdf

38 Power and Commercial Determinants of Health

Nino Paichadze and Adnan A. Hyder

Abstract

The global burden of non-communicable diseases (NCDs) is large and growing. Reversing this burden is a key global health and development challenge and requires addressing the threats to health stemming from private industry. The field of commercial determinants of health (CDoH) is rapidly evolving. Some of the existing definitions focus only on detrimental effects, while others highlight both positive and negative contributions of corporations to health and development. The current frameworks on CDoH also vary; some incorporate concepts of power, others integrate the principles of systems thinking, or analyze them as products of global economic system. The myriad tactics that corporations use to influence health policy and practice can be broadly categorized as political, financial, products and services, public relations, and advertising and legal tactics. While the need for addressing the health impacts of CDoH is evident, there are conflicting views on mechanisms for the governance of CDoH.

N. Paichadze (✉) · A. A. Hyder
Department of Global Health, Milken Institute School of Public Health, the George Washington University, Washington, DC, USA
e-mail: npaichadze1@gwu.edu; hydera1@email.gwu.edu

Keywords

NCD · Commercial determinants of health (CDoH) · Food · Drinks · Alcohol · Tobacco · Private sector · Corporation power

38.1 Introduction

Every year, 41 million people die from non-communicable diseases (NCDs) globally [1]. The burden is greatest among those of working age, 30 to 69 years. The effect is more pronounced in low- and middle-income countries (LMICs), where 77% of all NCD deaths and 85% of premature deaths occur [1].

The causation of NCDs is complex and multifactorial, influenced by a range of individual, social, environmental, political, cultural, economic, and commercial determinants [2]. The risk factors for major NCDs are strongly connected with the production, marketing, and consumption of commercially produced foods and drinks, alcohol, and tobacco [3]. In NCD prevention, lifestyle choices and personal responsibility usually receive the greatest attention, ignoring the limited control that many people have over their circumstances and the impact of strategies used by transnational corporations [4]. Reversing the global burden of NCDs is a key global health and development challenge and requires addressing the threats to health stemming from private industry.

M. C. B. Raviglione et al. (eds.), *Global Health Essentials*, Sustainable Development Goals Series,
https://doi.org/10.1007/978-3-031-33851-9_38

38.2 Definitions and Frameworks

The term "commercial determinants of health" (CDoH) defined as "factors that influence health which stem from profit motive" was first presented in the literature by West and Marteau in 2013 [5]. In 2016, Kickbush and colleagues, recognizing the overlaps among the domains of unhealthy commodities, industrial epidemics, profit-driven diseases, and corporate practices harmful to health, proposed uniting them under the term CDoH, which they defined as "strategies and approaches used by the private sector to promote products and choices that are detrimental to health" [6]. More recently, researchers and World Health Organization (WHO) have expanded on these definitions to highlight not only the negative impact of private industry activities, but more generally actions by corporate actors that affect health [7] (Table 38.1).

Table 38.1 Definitions of commercial determinants of health

Authors	Definitions
West and Marteau (2013) [5]	Factors that influence health which stem from the profit motive
Kickbusch et al. (2016) [6]	Strategies and approaches used by the private sector to promote products and choices that are detrimental to health
United Nations (2017) [8]	The commercial conditions, actions, and omissions that affect health. Commercial determinants arise in the context of the provision of goods or services for payment and include commercial activities, as well as the environment in which commerce takes place. Commercial determinants can have a beneficial and/or detrimental impact on health
Freudenberg et al. (2021) [9]	The social, political, and economic structures, norms, rules, and practices by which business activities designed to generate profits and increase market share influence patterns of health, disease, injury, disability, and death within and across populations
World Health Organization (2021) [7]	The conditions, actions, and omissions by corporate actors that affect health. Commercial determinants arise in the context of the provision of goods or services for payment and include commercial activities, as well as the environment in which commerce takes place. They can have beneficial or detrimental impacts on health.
Maani et al. (2022) [10]	Activities of the private sector that affect the health of populations

Existing frameworks on CDoH aim to analyze the influence of corporations and their practices on population health. The current rise in NCDs is partly a result of the global economic system as well as international trade, commerce, and investment policies that have traditionally prioritized wealth generation over health creation [6]. A framework proposed by Kickbush and colleagues outlines dynamics that constitute these CDoH with key drivers of power such as rising demand, expanding market coverage, and internalization of trade and capital that are channeled through marketing, lobbying, supply chain, and corporate social strategies. These drivers and channels work together to grow corporate influence and amplify the health impact of commercial operations. Corporate activities determine health outcomes by manipulating social determinants and environments where people live, which in turn impact individual consumers' choices [6].

Several frameworks on CDoH incorporate concepts of power [11, 12]. For example, a framework proposed by Lima and Galea is built around a three-dimensional view of power to better understand the practices through which corporations exercise power and influence population health [11]. Power over decision-making and control over the political agenda are the focus of the One-Dimensional View. The Two-Dimensional View centers on power to define what constitutes an issue and a potential issue. The Three-Dimensional View encompasses the power to avert observable conflict and power to keep the conflict between the interests of the powerful and those over whom power is exercised. Each of the dimensions of power are manifested through five "vehicles" (Political Environment, Preference Shaping, Knowledge Environment, Legal Environment, Extra Legal Environment) that are expressed through technical tools or "Practices of Power," that corporations use to implement their agenda. The exertion of power has two outcomes: distal that is an imbalance in macrosocial determinants of health which impacts the incidence of risk factors for disease, and proximal which is a deterioration of population health [11].

Knai and colleagues suggested using complex systems perspective to analyze the CDoH of NCDs and how unhealthy commodity industries influence health policy [2]. Baum and colleagues developed a draft framework that can guide a corporate health impact assessment within countries [13]. This framework focuses on both positive and negative effects of corporate activity and describes outcomes of these activities in broad range of social and environmental contexts [13]. Given the increasing need for more research and intervention in the field of CDoH, several frameworks on conducting research on CDoH have been proposed. Paichadze and colleagues proposed a research agenda that focuses on four conceptual domains (conceptual framework, governance, accountability, and transparency) and four pathways (marketing, lobbying, corporate social responsibility (CSR) strategies, and supply chains) by which corporations impact health [14].

38.3 Tactics of Corporations

Corporations use a plethora of strategies, often called tactics, to influence health policy and practice. These tactics can be categorized into five overlapping categories that can be used alone or in combination—political, finance, products and services, public relations, and advertising and legal tactics [15]. Political tactics are often operationalized through lobbying that aims to gain advantage over competitors and/or to prevent being disadvantaged, to increase government protections and subsidies. One of the most direct finance tactics is tax evasion which helps corporations increase their profits but puts higher burden on individuals and government agencies. Many corporations constantly change their operations, production processes, prices, or patent laws to avoid criticism or regulations and ensure their competitiveness on the market. For example, corporations often move their physical location to geographic areas where costs of operation are lowest, and labor and environmental regulations are weak or missing; and these are often located in LMICs. This allows corporations to avoid labor benefits including health, injury and disability insurance for employees, implementation of occupational health and safety practices at workplace, and escape meeting environmental standards—all of which has direct and indirect impact on individual and population health with high social costs. They also may change their product slightly to extend patent protections.

Corporations use public relations not only to directly promote the sales of their products and services, but more broadly to shape people's perception about corporation, its mission, goals, and operations. For example, corporations often use paid health professionals and experts to represent their interests. They describe the work of public health scientists whose research has shown the harmful effects of their products as "junk science." To influence health and health policy, corporations use a wide range of tactics within the judicial system such a liability, corporate trials, and unregulated activity. Corporations have been reported to even employ extra-legal tactics such as harassment, intimidation, bribing, or spying that falls outside of moral or ethical conventions of civil society to influence policy or governmental organizations [15].

38.4 Governance Models

In order to address the harmful practices of corporations, the public health community needs to refocus their research and education away from the model that focuses only on individual risk factor reduction and focus on the social, economic, and commercial determinants of health. The new approach needs to disconnect from corporate advertisements, sponsorships, and grants; and reframe the thinking about, and actions toward, corporation as an institution. The new focus has to recognize the corporation as an institution in order to address its global influence [15].

There are conflicting views on mechanisms for the governance of CDoH. Some consider public policy tools such as taxation and regulation of industry through trade and other policy mechanisms as more reliable strategies for reducing the impacts of CDoH. Others promote civil society engagement in policymaking, for accountability and advocacy. The three main models of CDoH governance include self-regulation by industry, regulation through partnership, and regulation of the private sector by the public sector [3]. Industry self-regulation which is the preferred approach of industry and the default approach of many governments and the United Nations relies on voluntary actions by private industry that includes responding to concerns of consumers, differentiating company from competitors, and preventing or delaying statutory regulations. Without robust accountability mechanisms or standards for self-regulation, it is an ineffective mechanism for CDoH governance [3].

Public, public-private, and civil-society partnerships focus on health issues around food supply, safety, and access to health care. The United Nations has also been promoting such partnerships at the highest level (Sustainable Development Goal 17). While some argue that industry representatives could be involved in multistakeholder platform aimed at mitigating the CDoH, others consider such involvement is a shield for their own corporate interests. The inadequacies of self-regulation and conflict of interest in co-regulation lead many experts to believe that public regulation is the only practical approach to addressing corporate practices that are harmful to health. The efforts to carry out public sector control over the private sector have met with resistance and the enforceable public authority over the private sector remains a major challenge [3]. Addressing the challenges stemming from the private sector requires robust governance infrastructure, accountability and transparency mechanisms, and policy coherence across different sectors.

38.5 Conclusion

To limit the power exerted by corporations, the public health community needs to challenge the dominant narrative and show how people's choices are shaped by forces not in their control, and how corporations have set these narratives over decades. There needs to be a redesign of the global health governance structure which will ensure accountability and provide oversight over the private sector. Addressing CDoH is critical to recognize the growing power of industry over health and important for sustainable development.

References

1. World Health Organization. Noncommunicable diseases: key facts Online: World Health Organization; 2021. https://www.who.int/news-room/fact-sheets/detail/noncommunicable-diseases
2. Knai C, Petticrew M, Mays N, Capewell S, Cassidy R, Cummins S, et al. Systems thinking as a framework for analyzing commercial determinants of health. Milbank Q. 2018;96(3):472–98.
3. Buse K, Tanaka S, Hawkes S. Healthy people and healthy profits? Elaborating a conceptual framework for governing the commercial determinants of non-communicable diseases and identifying options for reducing risk exposure. Glob Health. 2017;13(34)
4. Ireland R, Bunn C, Reith G, Philpott M, Capewell S, Boyland E, et al. Commercial determinants of health: advertising of alcohol and unhealthy foods during sporting events. Bull World Health Organ. 2019;97:290–5.
5. West R, Marteau T. Commentary on Casswell (2013): the commercial determinants of health. Addiction. 2013;108:686–7.
6. Kickbusch I, Allen L, Franz C. The commercial determinants of health. Lancet. 2016;4(12):895–6.
7. World Health Organization. Commercial determinants of health Online: World Health Organization; 2021. https://www.who.int/news-room/fact-sheets/detail/commercial-determinants-of-health
8. United Nations. Progress on the prevention and control of non-communicable diseases United Nations; 2017
9. Freudenberg N, Lee K, Buse K, Collin J, Crosbie E, Friel S, et al. Defining priorities for action and research on the commercial determinants of

health: a conceptual review. Am J Public Health. 2021;111(12):2202–11.
10. Maani N, Petticrew M, Galea S. Commercial determinants of health. Oxford; Forthcoming: Oxford University Press; 2022.
11. Lima JM, Galea S. Corporate practices and health: a framework and mechanisms. Glob Health. 2021;14(21)
12. Wood B, Baker P, Sacks G. Conceptualising the commercial determinants of health using a power lens: a review and synthesis of existing frameworks. Int J Health Policy Manag. 2021;11(8):1251–61.
13. Baum FE, Sanders DM, Fisher M, Anaf J, Freudenberg N, Friel S, et al. Assessing the health impact of transnational corporations: its importance and a framework. Glob Health. 2016;12(27):27.
14. Paichadze N, Werbick M, Ndebele P, Bari I, Hyder AA. Commercial determinants of health: a proposed research agenda. Int J Public Health. 2020;65:1147–9.
15. Wiist WH. The corporation: an overview of what it is, its tactics, and the what public health can do. In: Wiist WH, editor. The bottom line or public health. New York: Oxford University Press; 2010.

Part VII

Health Systems

39 Health Systems Frameworks

David H. Peters

Abstract

Health systems frameworks help to describe and analyze health systems, as well as frame interventions to strengthen health systems, while reflecting the agendas and biases of their authors. This chapter summarizes the uses and limitations of some widely used health systems frameworks, arguing that the choice of a framework should be fit-for-purpose. A comprehensive description of a health system framework is presented to fill some gaps by incorporating previously overlooked social and structural determinants of health, and as well incorporating broader population health services and health emergency and disaster risk management. We discuss how frameworks can support a systems thinking approach when they prompt how key stakeholders, functions, and outcomes are specifically related to each other and health system objectives, and outline considerations to help in selecting an appropriate framework.

D. H. Peters (✉)
Faculty of Health, York University, Toronto, ON, Canada

Department of International Health, Johns Hopkins Bloomberg School of Public Health, Baltimore, MD, USA
e-mail: dhpeters@yorku.ca

Keywords

Health systems framework · Health systems strengthening · Policy · Theory · Implementation · Systems thinking

39.1 Introduction to the Issue

It is broadly acknowledged that strengthening health systems is an important and ongoing challenge for all health systems around the world, and that frameworks can be very useful tools for strengthening health systems [1]. Frameworks can help us to understand health systems and provide a common language and organization for communication, planning, analysis, and action. But health systems frameworks can also mislead people when they are not well designed or are used for purposes other than those for which they were intended. At their best, health systems frameworks make explicit our assumptions, values, and objectives, point us in areas where inquiry or intervention are needed, or help to explain and anticipate changes. At their worst, they can reinforce the biases of those who developed them, neglect important stakeholders, components, or relationships in a health system, and distort understanding and undermine efforts to strengthen health systems.

M. C. B. Raviglione et al. (eds.), *Global Health Essentials*, Sustainable Development Goals Series,
https://doi.org/10.1007/978-3-031-33851-9_39

39.2 Background

Over the years, there have been many definitions of health systems that reflect various perspectives of how to improve people's health. The World Health Organization (WHO) uses a widely accepted definition of a health system as made up of *all the institutions, actors, and activities whose primary purpose is to promote, restore, or maintain health* [2]. One advantage of this definition is that it encompasses what comprises a system—a set of interconnected parts and their relationships that come together for a purpose, in this case related to people's health. Whereas this definition avoids many of the limitations and biases of other definitions, such as those that focus exclusively on health care, it can still be limiting since it can exclude actors and activities that strongly influence health but have other primary purposes. This may help to explain why people and communities have often been neglected, or why the importance of social and structural factors that affect people's health may be underestimated. In many contexts, the systems and practices that discriminate against some people or otherwise affect educational and work opportunities, incomes, clean water, nutrition, housing, and safety are critically important factors that affect people's health [3].

Defining the boundaries of a health systems framework may also be challenging. Health systems are not only dynamic and contain systems within systems they are also "open systems" that interact with their external environment and other systems. These include interactions with people, information, resources, policies, and many factors that influence people's health. Any boundary of a health system framework is arbitrary and contestable, and drawing the appropriate line around a health system may depend on how stakeholders understand the set of factors affecting health or their practical scope for interaction.

39.3 Aims of the Chapter

This chapter describes the main purposes of health systems frameworks and illustrates a range of health systems frameworks that can be best used when they fit a particular purpose. It also reviews some of the pitfalls of commonly used frameworks and presents a framework that can fill some of the gaps—by incorporating neglected components and pointing to a systems approach that shows the relationships of the components to each other and the overall objectives. It also provides guidance on how to select a health systems framework that is fit-for-purpose.

39.4 Description of the Issue

Health systems frameworks are used best when they are fit-for-purpose. Many frameworks are very useful, but it is better to be able to understand, critique, and adapt different frameworks than to pursue a one-size-fits-all model. In this chapter, we discuss different frameworks that include those described as theories or models [4] and involve both descriptive and explanatory elements with varying degrees of simplicity and focus.

Health system frameworks are simplifications of the various components, functions, and purposes of a health system. Every framework should be able to identify individual components and lend itself to some *description* or *analysis* of those components. This may help to better understand the extent to which each component fulfills its respective *function* within the whole system. A framework may also be used to organize a way to *monitor* the performance of individual components, subsystems, or the whole system, which can be used for problem identification and insights about potential remedial action. As described here, health systems frameworks have the potential to contribute to the full set of planning and evaluation, implementation, monitoring, and adaptation activities needed for a "learning health system," a critical capability of a strong health system [5].

Any framework has limitations, and in Table 39.1 we identify a number of common issues that can create negative consequences if not considered carefully. They highlight the issues of who is the author of the framework (and

Table 39.1 Factors contributing to the misapplication of health systems frameworks and their consequences

Issue	Assumptions	Consequences
Whose objectives are included in the framework?	Author's priorities take precedence, and are framed in ways that reflect their biases	Interests of powerful organizations get the attention and resources, which reinforces their ability to pursue their agendas. Those with relative power in global health include transnational organizations (e.g., WHO, World Bank, Bill and Melinda Gates Foundation) though there is also relatively more power held by national governments, researchers who publish in health journals, and funding organizations. Civil society, intended beneficiaries of a health system, and particularly marginalized communities are frequently neglected.
What is excluded in the framework?	Stakeholders, functions, causal pathways, and inter-dependencies of relevance that are not included are likely to be neglected	Excluded components of a health system framework will be relatively neglected and under-resourced, such as when people, communities, the private sector, social and structural determinants of health, and common goods for health like health emergency and disaster risk management and pandemic preparedness are not part of a framing of a health system. There is little progress in understanding and intervention in areas that are not part of the framework.
Does the framework try to explain a health system, or to describe it?	Assumptions about how components are connected and the causal pathways towards the system's objectives are not explicit.	Not informative for understanding root causes and the nature of how different components are related (e.g., feedback and non-linear relationships, inter-dependence and path dependency). This limits the ability to frame issues for identifying and prioritizing where to intervene, monitoring health system performance, or developing explanatory research questions and theories. Can serve to reinforce the status quo, or to focus on simplistic responses that address individual components in a system and contribute to unrealistic expectations of how a system should change.

therefore whose interests and biases are presented and whose are not); what components and linkages are excluded from a framework (including where the boundaries are drawn), and whether the application of the framework is intended to be purely descriptive or also explanatory (which can create a mismatch when applied for another purpose).

39.5 Approach to Solutions

In general, there have been many health frameworks published—Hoffman et al. [6] described 41 of them—but many fewer have been used in practice. There are also many more specific frameworks that focus on particular aspects of a health system and are highly relevant to efforts to strengthen health systems. These include frameworks around the continuum of barriers to effective health care coverage [7], the social and structural determinants towards health equity [3], or the more than 150 frameworks that are designed to support implementation research in health [8].

In Table 39.2, we review five of the more commonly used health systems frameworks. Each of them has a useful application and involves both descriptive and explanatory features. Yet each has excluded some key stakeholders and functions and are limited in how they support a systems thinking approach. A framework supports systems thinking when it shows how the components interact with each other in relation to their overall objectives.

We present another framework to address the gap of missing components of a health system in its wider context, and to better support a systems thinking approach (Fig. 39.1). This should be useful for health systems researchers, policy analysts, practitioners, and students, and is particularly relevant as shocks like pandemics and natural disasters force us to look at interdependencies and sources of inequities. Although lacking the simplicity of other frameworks, this comprehensive framework seeks to highlight how the main elements of a health system are related to each other and the system objectives. The boundaries of the health system are defined by the central blue box (identifying functions,

Table 39.2 Comparison of characteristics of selected health systems framework

Framework characteristics	Roemer health system model [9]	Kielmann health system model [10]	WHO building blocks [1]	Control Knobs framework [11]	High quality health systems [12]
Describes health systems actors, functions, and linkages	Partial (though fuller description in book)	Partial	Partial	Limited	Partial
Describes processes for health systems strengthening	Yes	Yes	No	Yes (focus on policy choices)	Yes (focus on health care delivery)
Explains health system through causal pathways	Partial	Partial	Limited	Partial	Partial
Main audiences for framework	Health professionals, students, and politicians interested in social and political development in health	Evaluators, health services managers, and professionals	Originally for government leaders outside the health sector (e.g., Prime Minister Offices and Ministries of Finance)	Those involved in health-sector reform (especially policymakers)	Academics, policymakers, health systems experts
Original application of the framework	Description and explanation for health professionals and students	Evaluation of health programs and improvements of health services to lead to improved results	Inform and persuade governments on where to invest in health systems. To offer an organizational structure for those organizations whose primary purpose is to improve health	Analytic framework for policy reforms in the health sector	Call to action to improve health care systems in LMICs
Health systems objectives	• Health results (health status included)	• Service outcomes (health status included). • Community engagement	• Improved health (level and equity) • Financial risk protection • Responsiveness • Improved efficiency	• Population health status • Customer satisfaction • Risk protection	• Better health • Confidence in system • Economic benefit
Main stakeholders identified in framework	• Implied: Management and service delivery	• Communities • "Management and organizations"	• Health workforce • Implied: "Leadership"	• "Target population" • Implied: Policymakers	• Population • "Non-health actors" • Workforce
Role of community involvement	No	Integral to the model	No	No	Implied
Main functions	Five functions (management; resources; economic support; organization; service delivery)	• Management and organization • Support systems	Six building blocks (service delivery; health workforce; information; medical products; financing; leadership and governance)	Five control knobs (financing; payment; organization; regulation; behavior)	• Processes of care • Governance (policy, insurance) • Learning and improvement
Social and structural factors included	No	Integral to the model	No	No	Limited

Table 39.2 (continued)

Framework characteristics	Roemer health system model [9]	Kielmann health system model [10]	WHO building blocks [1]	Control Knobs framework [11]	High quality health systems [12]
Uses a systems thinking approach (specifically linking components, functions, and objectives)	Yes (but very broadly defined components)	Yes (but very broadly defined components)	Partial	No	Partial
Main limitations	• Narrow focus on health care system Neglects: • External environment and community engagement (though book addresses political economy of reforms in detail)	• Little attention to role of policy, governance, and financing, and full set of actors involved in health system • Focus on health care system limits scope	Neglects: • Role of "people" and communities as part of health system • Theory and attention to causal pathways to outcomes • Explanations of dynamic connections between functions • Common goods for health • Social and structural determinants	• Largely supply side, limited set of actors Neglects: • Role of people and communities as change agents	• Focus on health care system limits scope • Limited specific connections between components and functions

stakeholders, and services and how they are related to each other) which is embedded in a larger grey box that includes a set of *Contextual Determinants* (social and structural factors) and their contribution to core objectives. **People** are identified (in green) as the main stakeholders within the health system, along with their key characteristics that affect other elements of the health system as well as the core objectives. Main actors are identified under *Input Management, Oversight, Financing,* and *Service Delivery* functions. Notably, *Service Delivery* incorporates population and prevention services, and health emergency and disaster risk management. Solid arrows highlight some of the most important direct connections between the different functions and stakeholders and as well as outcomes whereas the dotted arrows indicate more indirect influences. For example, there are linkages between services and people through a benefits package and demand (which are also influenced by *Oversight* and *Financing* functions and related stakeholders).

With so many frameworks to choose from, we suggest considering the following characteristics in selecting or adapting one to be better fit-for-purpose:

1. Assess the **purpose of the framework** (e.g., describing a health system, guiding a particular process in health systems strengthening, engaging with key health systems stakeholders, analyzing what influences health outcomes, informing or evaluating the efforts of health systems), and its relevance to the **audience** intending to use the framework (e.g., general public, policymaker, health workforce, researcher) [15].
2. Examine the **completeness of relevant key stakeholders** included within the framework and its development.

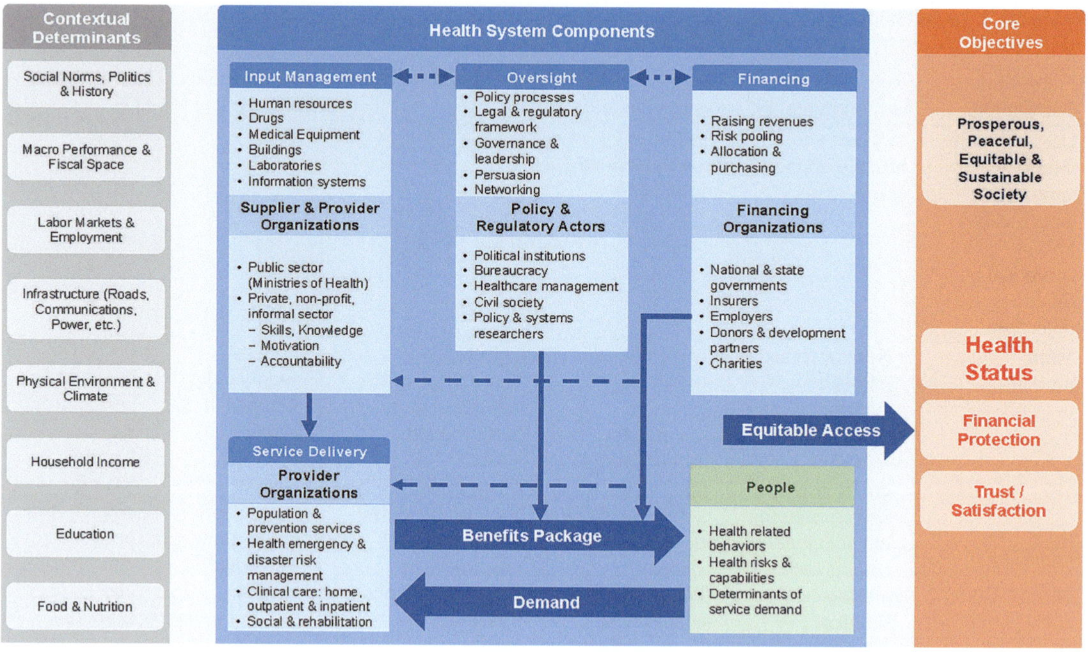

Fig. 39.1 A Comprehensive and Descriptive Health Systems Framework. (Sources: [2, 13]; Peters [14])

3. Identify the **boundaries** of the framework to see if there are critically **missing components, stakeholders, or functions** that can meaningfully influence the defined purposes of the system.
4. Assess the degree of **inclusion and depth of analysis of relevant health systems concepts**: types of health objectives, nature of the functions, types of determinants, identification of specific causal connections and theories of change, types of intervention strategies, and whether it supports a systems thinking approach by connecting the different components to each other and the objectives.

39.6 Main Conclusions and Recommendations

The chapter summarizes the uses and limitations of some widely used health systems frameworks. For policymakers and practitioners, they can provide shared language on how a health system is working, and a basis for practical tools for planning, implementing, and evaluating efforts to strengthen health systems. For researchers, they can guide the design and conduct of studies, inform the theoretical and empirical thinking of research teams, and aid interpretation of findings.

Superficial or inappropriate use of frameworks can lead to a distortion of which efforts are pursued and hinders the ability to learn from health systems strengthening. Health systems frameworks should be fit-for-purpose and carefully critiqued when using them to understand how they can be used, and what their limitations are. This chapter presents a comprehensive description of a health system that should aid in systems thinking analysis and recommends an approach to selecting an appropriate framework.

References

1. World Health Organization. Everybody business: strengthening health systems to improve health outcomes: WHO's framework for action. Geneva: World Health Organization; 2007.

2. World Health Organization. The World Health Report 2000. Health systems: improving performance. Geneva: World Health Organization; 2000.
3. Solar O, Irwin A. A conceptual framework for action on the social determinants of health. Social determinants of health discussion paper 2 (policy and practice). Geneva: World Health Organization; 2010.
4. Nilsen P. Making sense of implementation theories, models and frameworks. Implement Sci. 2015;10:53. https://doi.org/10.1186/s13012-015-0242-0.
5. Sheikh K, Abimbola S. Learning health systems: pathways to progress: a flagship report from the Alliance for Health Policy and Systems Research. Geneva: World Health Organization; 2021. https://apo.who.int/publications/i/item/learning-health-systems-pathways-to-progress. Accessed 15 June 2022
6. Hoffman S, Røttingen J-A, Bennett S, Lavis JN, Edge JS, Frenk J. A review of conceptual barriers and opportunities facing health systems research to inform a strategy from the World Health Organization. Geneva: Alliance for Health Policy and Systems Research; 2012. https://ahpsr.who.int/resources/meeting-report-item/a-review-of-conceptual-barriers-and-opportunities-facing-health-systems-research-to-inform-a-strategy-from-the-world-health-organization. Accessed 15 June 2022
7. Tanahashi T. Health service coverage and its evaluation. Bull World Health Organ. 1978;56(2):295–303.
8. Strifler L, Cardoso R, McGowan J, Cogo E, Nincic V, Khan PA, Scott A, Ghassemi M, MacDonald H, Lai Y, Treister V, Tricco AC, Straus SE. Scoping review identifies significant number of knowledge translation theories, models, and frameworks with limited use. J Clin Epidemiol. 2018;2018(100):92–102. https://doi.org/10.1016/j.jclinepi.2018.04.008.
9. Roemer MI. National Health Systems of the world. New York: Oxford University Press; 1991.
10. Kielmann AA, Neuvians D, Kipp W, et al. Quality, quantity and utilization of basic health services. In: Evaluation of the impact of health interventions. Belgium: Derouaux Ordina Editions; 1995.
11. Roberts MJ, Hsiao W, Berman P, Reich MR. Getting health reform right. A guide to improving performance and equity. New York: Oxford University Press; 2008.
12. Kruk ME, Gage AD, Arsenault C, et al. High-quality health systems in the sustainable development goals era: time for a revolution. Lancet Glob Health. 2018;6(11):e1196–252.
13. Baeza C, Packard TG. Beyond survival: protecting households from health shocks in Latin America. Washington DC/Stanford: World Bank/Stanford University Press; 2006.
14. Peters DH, El-Saharty S, Siadat B, Janovsky K, Vujicic M. Improving health services in developing countries: from evidence to action. Washington, DC: World Bank; 2009.
15. Siddiqi S, Peters DH, Mataria A. Introduction to health systems: setting the scene. In: Siddiqi S, Mataria A, Rouleau KD, Iqbal M, editors. Making health systems work. Cambridge: Cambridge University Press; 2023.

Global Health and Systems Change 40

Fabrizio Tediosi and Don de Savigny

Abstract

The emergent global health challenges make clear that we have so far failed to engage effectively with the intersections and interactions of health with the multitude of other complex systems and determinants. This chapter argues for the need for a systems-wide approach to these emerging global health challenges. This requires viewing these challenges through the various lenses of complexity science which include systems science, systems behavior, systems dynamics, and systems networks. The most important prerequisite can be found in the power of systems networks and partnerships. Major stakeholders and practitioners at all levels need the capability to at least understand the connections across their organizational silos. Connecting global health actors working in different spatial scales of the health system is critical to developing the pervasive systemic sensibility and literacy that is essential for systemic approaches to take root in global health.

Keywords

Systems thinking · Partnerships · Systems science · Systems dynamics · Systems networks

40.1 Emerging Global Health Challenges

As we enter the third decade of the twenty-first century, the trajectory of global health is pivoting away from 20 years of extraordinary and unprecedented improvement in health indicators. The rapid arrest and reversal of progress is a result of multiple, connected, existential, and systemic crises that are, in effect, a single syndemic [1] of intersecting climate change, ecologic disruption, and pandemic communicable disease coupled with the rapid transition to chronic non-communicable disease morbidities. New geopolitical frictions are creating faultlines and re-alignments in global affairs and economic markets that will add further negative ramifications for population health globally. The fracture in globalization and the discord in global markets and supply chains are predicted to accelerate demands for an "economy transition at the scale of the industrial revolution and the pace of the digital revolution" to respond to the underlying crises [2].

F. Tediosi (✉) · D. de Savigny
Department of Epidemiology and Public Health, Swiss Tropical and Public Health Institute Allschwill, Switzerland

University of Basel, Basel, Switzerland
e-mail: fabrizio.tediosi@swisstph.ch; d.desavigny@swisstph.ch

M. C. B. Raviglione et al. (eds.), *Global Health Essentials*, Sustainable Development Goals Series,
https://doi.org/10.1007/978-3-031-33851-9_40

The failures to prepare for the syndemic intersection of climate change, pandemic disease, health and demographic transitions are due in part to a lack of systems-wide conceptualization of these foreseen crises. Such preparation depends on a strong capacity for dealing with systems complexity. This lack of "systems thinking" is especially pronounced in global health, which still takes a largely vertical disease-by-disease approach based on technical fixes and over-medicalization while ignoring the systemic changes and delivering solutions equitably through effective health systems. More than 30 years after the landmark publication of the Commission on Health Research for Development [3], less than 2% of global health spending is on health systems strengthening and health policy and systems research [4]. Political and commercial determinants still dominate health policies and other intersectoral policies that affect population health [5, 6]. Finally, the colonial legacies of global health as currently configured impair the traction needed for supporting the necessary networks of actors and systemic reforms needed to affect change on the ground [7].

This chapter argues for the need for a systems-wide approach to these emerging global health challenges and suggests what could be done to accelerate the adoption of critical systems thinking and complexity science as part of the way forward.

40.2 The Missing Systems-Wide Approach

Health systems are porous systems open to and buffeted by exogenous factors. At the macro-level, health systems are embedded in a context of wider political, economic, and social systems. As such, they inherit diverse histories, cultures, and ideologies from societies of overlapping professional and community networks. The decision-making for health policies and systems involves trade-offs between investments in multiple sectors relevant to health that are often siloed from health policymakers. At the micro-level, health systems are currently framed by interacting sub-systems such as governance, finance, information systems, technologies, human resources, and service delivery [8]. Collectively this constitutes what is known as a complex adaptive system (Box 40.1). Such systems are dynamic architectures of interactions and synergies [9].

Box 40.1: System Dynamics Features of Complex Adaptive Systems

All complex adaptive systems are characterized by common systems dynamics features.

Self-organization: Systems dynamics and system behavior arise spontaneously from the internal structure of the system.

Constant change: Systems adjust and readjust at many interactive levels and time scales.

Tight-linkage: The high degree of systems connectivity means that change in one sub-system affects the others.

Governed by feedback: A positive or negative response may alter expected effects due to feedback loops.

Non-linearity: Relationships within a system cannot be arranged along a simple input-output line.

History dependence: Short-term effects of interventions or reforms may differ from lagged long-term effects.

Counter-intuitive: Cause and effect are often distant in time and space, defying solutions that pit causes close to the effects they seek to address.

Resistant to change: Seemingly obvious solutions may fail or worsen the situation.

Source: [10].

Since 2009, there has been an exponential surge in the health research literature referring to systems thinking, complexity theory, or complex adaptive systems [11]. Arising from this is greater clarity concerning what constitutes a systems thinking framework and methodological approach, along with a battery of over 35 systems thinking and systems dynamics tools and methodologic approaches [12] that can be applied for various purposes. Some of them can, for instance, facilitate recognizing and understanding interconnections and systems structure or identifying and understanding feedback. Others can be used to identify leverage points, understanding dynamic behavior, and dynamic simulation models can predict the impact of policies and suggest possible solutions.

Systems thinkers think in terms of "wholes" rather than "parts"; recognize and seek to understand interconnections and feedback; appreciate the concept of dynamic behavior; understand that the system is the cause of its own behavior and understand the way the system's architecture generates such behavior [13].

Yet, examples of the use of systems thinking and systems dynamics for addressing policy challenges at the governmental level are rare. An exception is the UK which has a tradition of engaging academic and managerial professionals with expertise in systems thinking [14]. This has led to extensive resources and practice guides to ground such approaches into the civil service and promoted throughout an "all-of-government" approach [15].

Examples of how systems thinking and systems dynamics approaches have been applied to health systems development and management outside of the research arena are also few. A notable exception is work done in Malaysia to analyze the successes and failures of health system development through a systems thinking lens [16]. Several lessons emerged. Due to the complexity of the system, key stewards and actors within the health system often do not have a fully comprehensive mental model of their health system, its boundaries, structure, stakeholders, and their influence pathways. They may have no organizing hypothesis or theoretical model for how feedback among the various sub-systems works. Without system insights, their understanding and decision-making are consequently overly simplistic.

Systems thinking and systems dynamics tools, methodologies, and approaches are well-developed and widely available to the health systems and other systems. But system problems cut across organizational boundaries both within the health system and beyond the health system. This makes systems analysis and intervention a very political enterprise. Convening power and ownership of the process of engineering change requires skills, engagement, communication, networks, and partnership. Not everyone needs to be a systems thinker or expert in systems dynamics. But health system experts need a basic capacity to understand interlinkages and manage feedback dynamics across organizational silos.

40.3 What is Needed to Accelerate a Systems-Wide Approach?

The emergent global health challenges make clear that we have so far failed to engage effectively with the intersections and interactions of health with the multitude of other complex systems and determinants. The pace and urgency with which the syndemic is unfolding suggest we need disruptive and radical systems-change rather than the usual incremental approach to "building back better." The complexity of the interacting systems requires a more prominent systems thinking approach. Rapid capacity for this needs to be built at various scales. We will need to move from external pushing to internal catalysis as this capacity grows.

Wider use of systems thinking for global health challenges requires viewing these challenges through the various lenses of complexity science which include systems science, systems behavior, systems dynamics, and systems networks. We believe that the most important prerequisite can be found in the power of systems networks and partnerships.

Systems Networks and Partnerships: Different stakeholders need different levels of understanding of complex adaptive systems. Major stakeholders and practitioners at all levels need the capability to at least understand the connections across their organizational silos. Connecting global health actors working in different spatial scales of the health system is critical [17]. For them, recognizing and understanding interconnections and systems structure is a key first step in systems thinking. There is a useful toolkit [12] for facilitators to assist with this, including stakeholder mapping, social network analysis, systems mapping, process mapping, logic maps, agent-based modeling, etc. Several of these tools are highly participatory and assist stakeholders to come together to better appreciate the whole system and not just their part of it. Through conversations, they help construct shared conceptual models and sense-making that help dissolve the theory/practice divide. Using the shared language of the systems thinking discipline leads to the co-production of solutions and collective action. However, this requires investment and convening power.

At the macro-level (global), the systems thinking capacity strengthening should initially focus on governance and funding bodies that need a UN Interagency approach to health systems change. This would include a radical reform in Development Assistance for Health and the many fragmented Global Health Initiatives that in the end should embrace more "Health in all Policies" approaches including One Health, Ecosystem, and Planetary Health. At the meso-level (national), such capacity strengthening should be directed to relevant national ministries, NGOs and academia with an initial focus on encouraging ownership and domestic investment in systems solutions. At the more micro-level (local governments and communities), orientation should be directed to systems learning from positive deviance and bottom-up efforts.

Leveraging the power of networks and partnerships for systems thinking, it is possible to develop the pervasive systemic sensibility and literacy that is essential for systemic approaches to take root in global health.

References

1. Horton R. Offline: COVID-19 is not a pandemic. Lancet. 2020;396(10255):874.
2. Simpson P. World Economic Forum. 2022. [cited 2022 14/11/2022]; https://www.weforum.org/agenda/risk-and-resilience/
3. Commission on Health Research for Development. Health Research: essential link to equity in development. Oxford: Oxford University Press; 1990.
4. Lin V, et al. Strengthening health systems globally: a lingering challenge of funding. Public Health Res Pract. 2021;31(4)
5. Becerra-Posada F, et al. Politics and political determinants of health policy and systems research funding in Latin America and the Caribbean. Public Health Res Pract. 2021;31(4)
6. Kickbusch I. Addressing the interface of the political and commercial determinants of health. Health Promot Int. 2012;27(4):427–8.
7. Kwete X, et al. Decolonizing global health: what should be the target of this movement and where does it lead us? Glob Health Res Policy. 2022;7(1):3.
8. World Health Organization. Everybody business: strengthening health systems to improve health outcomes: WHO's framework for action. Geneva: WHO; 2008.
9. Jackson MC, Sambo LG. Health systems research and critical systems thinking: the case for partnership. Syst Res Behav Sci. 2019;37:3–22.
10. de Savigny D, Adam T. Systems thinking for health systems strengthening. Geneva: World Health Organization; 2009.
11. Chughtai S, Blanchet K. Systems thinking in public health: a bibliographic contribution to a meta-narrative review. Health Policy Plan. 2017;32(4):585–94.
12. Applied systems thinking for health systems research: a methodological handbook. De Savigny D, Blanchet K, Adam T. editors. London: McGraw Hill; 2017
13. Stave K, Hopper M. What constitutes systems thinking? A proposed taxonomy. In 25th International

Conference of the Systems Dynamics Society. Boston; 2007

14. Seddon J. Systems thinking in the public sector: the failures of the reform regime and a manifesto for a better way. Axminster: Triarchy Press; 2008. p. 216.
15. UK Government Office for Science. Systems thinking for civil servants: How to use systems thinking to drive improved outcomes in complex situations. [Web Guidance] 2022 [cited 2022 31/05/2022]; https://www.gov.uk/government/publications/systems-thinking-for-civil-servants
16. Martins JM, et al. Systems thinking analyses for health policy and systems development: a Malaysian case study. Cambridge: Cambridge University Press; 2021.
17. Missioni E, Pacileo G, Tediosi F. Health systems in the global health landscape. In Global health governance and policy. London: Routledge; 2019. p. 246–57.

41 Primary Health Care and Global Health

Timothy G. Evans and Kumanan Rasanathan

Abstract

The Declaration of Alma-Ata in 1978 crystallized a global vision of justice in health, regardless of income, gender, ethnicity, or education, and called for "health for all by the year 2000" through primary health care (PHC). While much progress has been made since the declaration, more than 40 years later and in the midst of the global pandemic of COVID-19, much remains to be done to achieve health for all. This chapter outlines the important values and principles that underlie PHC, with attention to how global health policy has evolved and country trajectories have differed with respect to PHC since its historic debut in 1978. The chapter then identifies the current strategies for PHC in the global context of a pandemic and other challenges and opportunities, to outline an agenda for the renewal of primary health care allied to the movement to achieve universal health coverage.

T. G. Evans (✉)
McGill University, Montreal, QC, Canada
e-mail: timothy.evans@mcgill.ca

K. Rasanathan
World Health Organization, Geneva, Switzerland
e-mail: rasanthank@who.int

Keywords

Primary health care (PHC) · Alma-Ata declaration · Universal health coverage (UHC) · Policies · Community

41.1 Primary Health Care and Its Evolution over Four Decades in Global Health

The International Conference on Primary Health Care in Alma-Ata in 1978 represented through its declaration the first articulation of a unifying global vision and strategy for health. The shared outcome of "health for all by the year 2000" was fueled by the strategy of primary health care (PHC). The strategy's emphasis on primary care reflected widespread concern that recently independent low and middle-income countries were following an inequitable, high-tech, high-cost, hospital-based, urban-focused approach to their health systems as in many high-income countries. Importantly, the PHC strategy extended beyond personal health care services to identifying the importance of engaging other sectoral assets for health such as education, water and sanitation, mobilizing the participation of communities in health systems, and ensuring the development

M. C. B. Raviglione et al. (eds.), *Global Health Essentials*, Sustainable Development Goals Series,
https://doi.org/10.1007/978-3-031-33851-9_41

and use of technology that was appropriate in terms of setting and cost.

Progress was made in many low- and middle-income countries, however, the target of "health for all by the year 2000" was missed by a large margin. The reasons were complex but partly entailed a general failure to implement all aspects of the primary health care approach, particularly work across sectors to address social and economic factors that affect health and the mobilization of critical systems inputs including health workers and government financing. Furthermore, despite the consensus in Alma-Ata in 1978, the global health community rapidly became fractured in its commitment to the far-reaching measures called for by the declaration. Economic recession tempered enthusiasm for PHC, and momentum shifted to programs concentrating on a few priority measures for child survival such as growth monitoring, oral rehydration, breast-feeding and immunization leading to calls for more modest and focused efforts around "selective primary health care" [1].

Growing momentum with these initiatives supported the continued movement of health development efforts away from the comprehensive approach of PHC primary health care and toward programs that targeted specific public health priorities. By the 1990s, PHC had fallen out of favor in many global health policy circles reinforced by structural adjustment policies of multi-lateral development banks recommending cuts to public sector spending as a stimulus for economic growth [2]. Consequently, many low- and middle-income countries slashed public sector spending on health and were encouraged to get more health for the money by selecting a package of "best-buy services" [3].

Concerns about losing ground in child immunization and the emergence of the HIV/AIDS pandemic alongside longstanding scourges of tuberculosis and malaria, led to the establishment of the first-ever billion-dollar global funds (GAVI and GFATM) at the turn of the millennium and their inclusion as specific goals in the Millennium Development Goals (MDGs). Despite these focused priorities and unprecedented amounts of development assistance, slower than expected progress in equitable coverage of immunization and treatment for HIV, TB and malaria drew attention to dimensions of the health and social systems in countries that were holding back progress. This led WHO to re-direct global health policy towards PHC with the issuance of a triumvirate of publications on the 30th anniversary of Alma-Ata: (i) the report of the commission on the social determinants of health [4], (ii) a WHO framework to understand the core functions of health systems [5]; and (iii) a World Health Report titled "PHC: now more than ever" [6].

41.2 Primary Health Care in the Twenty-First Century

The renewal of PHC advocated four major reforms (see Fig. 41.1. WHR 2008) that would help to remediate three pervasive barriers to progress including: (i) shortfalls in systems performance; (ii) stratifying social conditions; and (iii) skews in science [7]. The first of these recommended reforms gave rise to renewed policy interest in Universal Health Coverage (UHC) [8] and its inclusion as a target under the health goal of Sustainable Development Goals (SDGs) in 2015. Subsequently, the global policy discourse has embraced the synergy between PHC and UHC in the mantra "no UHC without PHC". In 2018, at the Astana conference to celebrate the 40th anniversary of Alma-Ata, a Declaration reframed PHC as three components: (i) primary care and essential public health functions as the core of integrated health services; (ii) empowered people and communities; and (iii) multisectoral policy and action.

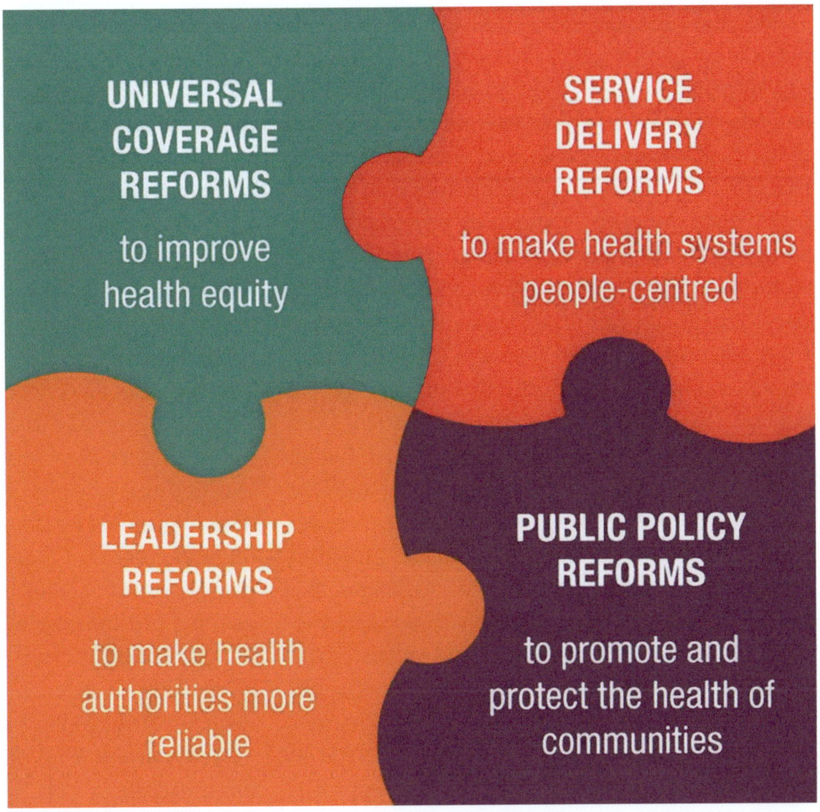
UNIVERSAL COVERAGE REFORMS
to improve health equity
SERVICE DELIVERY REFORMS
to make health systems people-centred
LEADERSHIP REFORMS
to make health authorities more reliable
PUBLIC POLICY REFORMS
to promote and protect the health of communities

Fig. 41.1 The four reforms of primary health care renewal. (Source: World Health Organization: Primary Health Care: Now More Than Ever. World Health Report 2008)

41.3 The Bumpy Road to Primary Health Care

Despite this array of global health policy convergence around PHC, the road ahead for all countries regardless of their levels of wealth looks anything but certain [9]. Traditional public financing systems for health and other social sectors are under extreme pressure not only in the wake of the pandemic and in the clutches of widespread inflation but also due to underlying trends towards a gig economy alongside persistently high levels of informal economic transactions that elude taxation. And while mobilization of development assistance and replenishments of global funds remain critical, the total envelope of development assistance ($37 Billion) represents such a small fraction of total health spending in LMICs ($2 trillion) that it must be more effectively deployed as a catalyst to greater domestic financing for health.

The organization and delivery of comprehensive, essential services from promotion to palliation with continuity and quality according to need faces daunting challenges from both the supply and demand sides. On the supply side many countries are seeing a dramatic shift in disease burden toward chronic diseases together with a rapidly growing menu of personalized and/or precision care services in the setting of pervasive health provider constraints manifested in their insufficient numbers, inequitable distribution, inadequate support and deteriorating morale and burnout. Recent estimates indicate a shortage of >18 million health workers globally, constituting a crisis that is greatly exacerbated by the migration of health workers from low- and middle-income countries to high-income countries. Sub-Saharan Africa carries 24% of the global disease burden but has only 3% of the health workforce [10].

On the demand-side, the expectations of patients for timely access to quality care are rising everywhere alongside growing skepticism and hesitancy with respect to trust in science and public health best buys like vaccines. At the same time, calls to decolonize and democratize global health are redefining the meaning of participation and community empowerment so central to the Alma-Ata declaration in 1978 and placing overdue demands on fair and accountable leadership for health nationally and globally. These demands on leadership are accentuated by the wider global context characterized by more frequent and severe infectious and climate-mediated health emergencies placing unprecedented pressures for coordinated multi-sectoral surge response capacity both within national boundaries and globally.

Despite this dizzying array of challenges that are both longstanding and new, there is ample evidence of remarkable progress and achievement with respect to PHC. Bangladesh, for example, has surged from one of the most impoverished nations on earth at the time of its independence in 1971 to achieve unprecedented health gains and improvements in health equity. The reasons include a society-wide mobilization around PHC inclusive of a focus on the empowerment of poor women through education, access to microcredit and primary care services made available by an army of community health workers [11]. Similar stories of PHC success through mass deployment of community health workers are found in Ethiopia, India and Niger. In middle-income countries like Brazil, Chile and Turkey in the setting of universal health care reforms, multi-disciplinary health teams have been dispatched to the front-lines together with social welfare benefits for disadvantaged groups resulting in accelerated improvements in health amongst those segments of the population previous left behind [12].

Further, recent breakthroughs in information and communication technologies like cell phones and drones are leading to innovative PHC applications that are transcending long standing PHC bottlenecks related to limited health providers and unreliable supply chains. While the primary health care approach has often been sidelined in the initial COVID-19 response, with a focus on hospitals and parallel delivery mechanisms, there have also been encouraging signs of the potential of PHC with dramatic increased uptake of the use of telemedicine and clinical support via digital means.

These and other examples of success, support Nobel Laureate Angus Deaton's prescient remarks in his World Institute for Development Economics Research annual lecture on September 29, 2006, "People in poor countries are sick not primarily because they are poor but because of other social organizational failures, including health delivery, which are not automatically ameliorated by higher income." Ensuring social organizational failures and successes are not dismissed as "outliers" and can inform reforms more widely requires re-directing global health policy efforts from the traditional centres of Geneva and Washington to the front-lines of health systems where the most exciting breakthroughs, in the face of overwhelming odds, abound. Primary health care's future is a bright one in this century provided policy and research move to the front-lines first!

The current COVID-19 pandemic has made the shortfalls in PHC more glaringly visible than ever, but has also mobilized awareness of its importance at the highest levels. Out of this crisis, then, lies an opportunity to recast global and national systems to enable an exciting new chapter to implement primary health care in all countries.

References

1. Walsh JA, Warren KS. Selective primary health care: an interim strategy for disease control in developing countries. N Engl J Med. 1979;301(18):967–74.
2. Kim JY. In: Kim JY, Millen JV, Irwin A, Greshman J, editors. Dying for growth: global inequality and the health of the poor. Monroe, ME: Common Courage Press; 2000. p. 604.
3. World Development Report 1993: Investing in Health. New York: World Bank; 1993. p. 348.
4. Closing the Gap in a Generation: health equity through action on the social determinants of health—Final report of the commission on social determinants of health. Geneva: World Health Organization; 2008. p. 33https://www.who.int/publications/i/item/WHO-IER-CSDH-08.1
5. Everybody's business—strengthening health systems to improve health outcomes: WHO's framework for

action. Geneva: World Health Organization; 2007. p. 44. https://apps.who.int/iris/handle/10665/43918
6. The World Health Report 2008: Primary Health Care Now More Than Ever. Geneva: World Health Organization; 2008. p. 119.
7. Evans T, Rasanathan K. Primary care and global health, Chapter 474. In: Harrison's principles of internal medicine. McGraw Hill; 2022.
8. Pablos A, Evans T. Universal health coverage and global health, Chapter 42 in this book. Springer Nature; 2023.
9. World Health Organization 2006 World Health Report 2006, Working Together for Health.
10. Rasanathan K, Evans TG. Primary health care, the Declaration of Astana and COVID-19. Bull World Health Organ. 2020;98:801–8.
11. Bangladesh: Innovation for Universal Health Coverage, Lancet Series; November 22, 2013.
12. Aquino R, de Oliveira NF, Barreto ML. Impact of the family health program on infant mortality in Brazilian municipalities. Am J Public Health. 2009;99(1):87–93. https://doi.org/10.2105/AJPH.2007.127480.

Universal Health Coverage (UHC): From Global Consensus to National Action

42

Ariel Pablos-Méndez and Timothy G. Evans

It is health that is real wealth and not pieces of gold and silver.

Mahatma Gandhi

Abstract

Universal health coverage (UHC) means access for all to *appropriate* health services without undue financial hardship to individuals and families. This aspiration requires organizing national health financing in pre-paid, cross-subsidized risk pools that minimize out-of-pocket spending. National leadership and technical capability are essential as health spending grows. Most services can be provided by public and private institutions building on strong primary health care. UHC is the new frontier for social justice, a central priority for WHO, and one of the targets for the UN Sustainable Development Goals. While half the countries of the world have nearly attained UHC, much needs to be done in Africa and South Asia to accelerate progress, and continued efforts are needed everywhere to sustain UHC.

Keywords

Health systems · Health financing · Health equity · Universal health coverage

A. Pablos-Méndez (✉)
Columbia University Medical Center, New York, NY, USA

T. G. Evans
McGill University, Montreal, QC, Canada
e-mail: timothy.evans@mcgill.ca

Universal health coverage (UHC) means access for all to *appropriate* health services without undue financial hardship to individuals and families [1]. The new millennium brought about unprecedented gains in health, development and democracy for much of the world. As extreme poverty receded and life expectancy surpassed 70 years, nations faced new challenges in the organization and financing of health services. As inequalities between rich and poor countries diminished, inequalities within countries became a growing challenge. This chapter summarizes historical developments behind the recent global movement for UHC, the moral and economic arguments underpinning these reforms, and the imperative of transforming health systems to foster the progressive and sustained realization of UHC.

42.1 A Global Movement for UHC

The UHC concept is not new. It originated in the nineteenth century with the introduction of employment-based social protection in Germany and further evolved with the tax-based national health system at the end of World War II in the UK. In the last 60 years, most OECD countries have adopted one or a combination of these approaches to insuring access to health services. The global movement for UHC, however, is more recent, finding inspiration in WHO's clarion call for "Health for All" in 1978. In 2008, the World Health Report on Primary Health

M. C. B. Raviglione et al. (eds.), *Global Health Essentials*, Sustainable Development Goals Series,
https://doi.org/10.1007/978-3-031-33851-9_42

Care identified Universal Health Coverage as one of four critical axes of reform towards the objective of health for all. Further mobilization catalyzed by the Rockefeller Foundation resulted in a World Health Report 2010 on financing for UHC, a Prince Mahidol Conference on UHC 2 years later and a UN resolution on UHC adopted by the General Assembly on November 12, 2012, a day that has since become designated as World UHC Day.

The global momentum has grown rapidly in the last decade. The World Bank Group adopted UHC as an apex objective for all health sectors globally in 2013 [2]. With the articulation of the Sustainable Development Goals (SDGs), UHC was embraced as a cornerstone for SDG #3 on health, anchoring a fragmented global health agenda around a common target across all countries poor and rich and as a critical contributor to the overall development objective of eliminating poverty (SDG #1). Japan's Prime Minister embraced UHC as a top priority for the G7 in 2016 and hosted a historic meeting of Ministers of Health and Finance at the G20 Summit in 2019. International health agencies including WHO, WB, OECD, EC, GAVI, GFTAM, GFF, ILO, and others have formed the International Partnership for UHC2030 [https://www.uhc2030.org].

42.2 The Moral and Economic Basis for UHC

There is widespread consensus on the fundamental right of every human being to enjoy the highest attainable standard of health. In addition, no family should have to sell the farm to pay for the care of a sick family member. The unfortunate reality is that without UHC, countries are more likely to fail in realizing these rights. Globally about half of the world's population lacks access to essential health interventions and every year 150 million households face catastrophic health care expenditures.

From an economic perspective, UHC also makes incredibly good sense despite misplaced concerns about growing health spending. The World Bank's recent focus on human capital recognizes that better health and education of a country's population are major drivers of economic growth. However, because the demand for health and wellbeing is seemingly infinite and health services are so labor-intensive, health spending is mistakenly seen by governments as an evil that can and should be controlled rather than harnessed for UHC.

The "first law" of health economics [3] states that health spending will grow with GDP and faster than inflation, accounting for an increasing proportion of the economy over time, as other sectoral needs are met with efficiency gains (e.g., food production or manufacturing) [4]. This tight relationship is seen across all countries, raising total health expenditures (THE) from 3% of GDP in the poorest countries to 10% or more in richer ones (see Fig. 42.1). Government reductions in public budgets are met with higher private spending and THE keeps growing (except during economic recessions). While health services expand, so does regressive and inefficient out-of-pocket spending unless public or private insurance is provided. Thus, UHC is "an affordable necessity" [5].

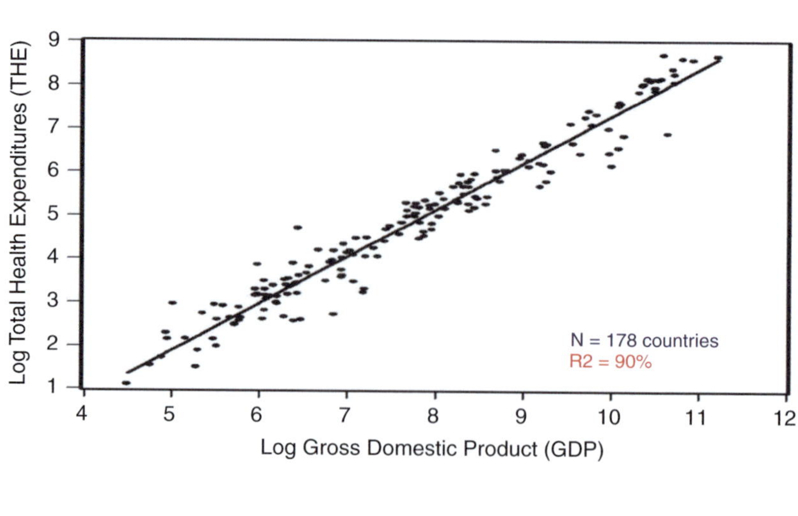

Fig. 42.1 First Law of Health Economics (2015): Economic growth drives health spending

42.3 Transforming Health Systems Towards UHC

UHC "implies a comprehensive scope of policy interventions, including the introduction of explicit ethical frameworks, the enhanced attention to financial arrangements, and the transformation of major dimensions of the organization of health systems" [6]. The breadth of reforms and the diversity of specific country contexts eschews a one-size-fits-all-approach to UHC [7]. Despite this complexity, there are common lessons emerging from the growing experience of countries in pursuing UHC reforms.

Political commitment at the highest level of government, not simply at the Ministry of Health, is critical [8]. The importance of UHC as a social investment makes it a whole of government priority. Bold commitments at the time of elections or following economic or health crises often get the UHC reform ball rolling [7]. The political road to reform is bumpy and must successfully traverse the inevitable schisms that are found across jurisdictional, sectoral, public-private, and provider-patient divides.

Technically, UHC involves reforms to all building blocks of the health system [9]. Foremost among them is financing. In low- and middle-income countries, there is a projected financing deficit for UHC by 2030, and this stresses the imperative for more effective strategies to mobilize domestic resources for health [2]. With close to two billion persons facing catastrophic or impoverishing health spending and as much as 40% of health spending wasted, the UHC challenge is both about more money for health and more health for the money. Addressing these challenges requires capacity and reforms for generating revenues, pooling risk, and purchasing services in specific contexts (see Fig. 42.2).

Reforms require considerations related to the breadth of services (promotive, preventive, curative, palliative) and level of delivery (self, primary, secondary, tertiary), and attention to the different combination of supply inputs like drugs or health workers and demand from patients and the public that influence "effective coverage" [10]. UHC reforms that are blind to inequity are insufficient: they must be able to monitor and adopt strategies to redress inequities [11].

Benefits packages are a logical construct to guide coverage in a way that is cost-effective and appropriate to local circumstances. In practice, UHC programs apply the concept in different ways, from "negative lists" (i.e., what they would not cover) to open-ended umbrellas limited by local resources and technical capabilities. There are some "verticals" services, like contraceptives, that may struggle for ideological/political rather than medical/economic rea-

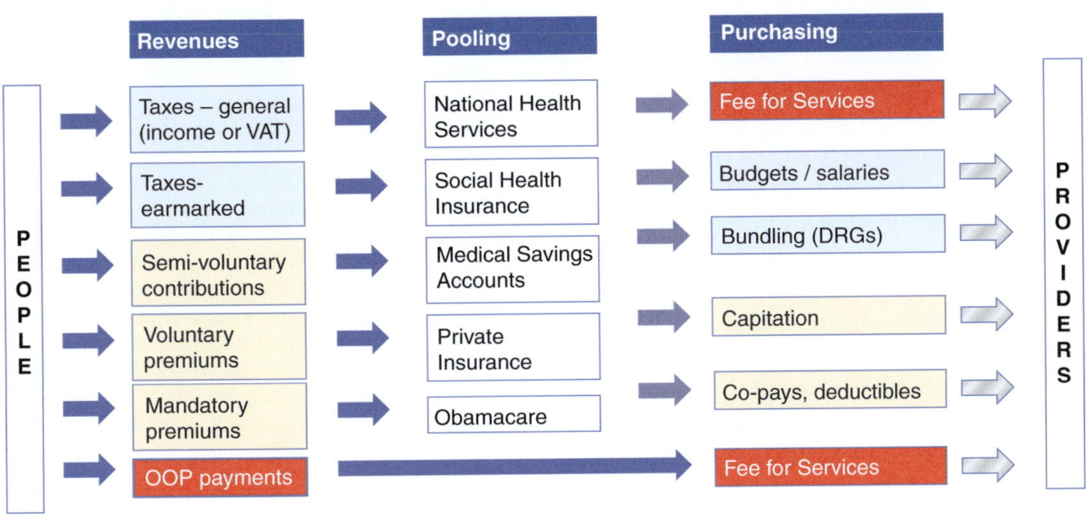

Fig. 42.2 Health financing functions and paths

sons. It is important to cover priority diseases like tuberculosis since half of patients and their families incur catastrophic expenditures as do 80% of patients treated for multi-drug-resistant disease. More importantly, patients may incur indirect, non-medical costs, stressing the need for broader systems of social protection beyond UHC [12].

Getting the right design and implementing UHC reforms places a high premium on appropriate technical capacity in core health systems functions. The Joint Learning Network for Universal Health Coverage (JLN) was formed in 2010 as a country-driven network of practitioners and policymakers from around the globe to share experience and products that help bridge the gap between theory and practice for UHC [13]. Monitoring progress relies on national Systems of Health Accounts and the two agreed SDG3 indicators for UHC. While coverage of essential services increased from 45% in 2000 to 65% in 2017, catastrophic health spending worsened from 9 to15% of the world's population as pre-paid, cross-subsidized health financing has lagged demand and economic growth.

42.4 Conclusions and Recommendations

While the case for UHC remains indisputable on moral and economic grounds, and roughly one third of countries enjoy near UHC, there remains a long road to travel to achieve global aspirations related to UHC. As per the latest reports from WHO and the WB on UHC, the modest progress in service coverage is tempered by the regressions in financial protection. With more than 2 years of the COVID-19 pandemic, UHC progress has likely stalled or reversed in many countries. Securing health systems that are better prepared to respond to infectious and other emergencies as well as sustaining equitable access to quality health services is a challenge faced by all countries. As the world approaches the mid-point on the road to the 2030 targets of the SDGs, recovering lost ground and accelerating progress towards UHC require unprecedented levels of health systems ingenuity that can be shared and scaled globally.

References

1. The World Health Report – Health systems financing: the path to universal coverage. Geneva, CH: World Health Organization 2010
2. Evans T, Pablos-Méndez A. Negotiating Universal Health Coverage into the global health mainstream: The promise and perils of multilateral consensus. Global Social Policy. 2020;20(2):220–4.
3. van der Gaag J, Stimac V. Toward a new paradigm for health sector development. Technical partner paper 3. Results for development. Washington, DC. September 2008
4. Pablos-Méndez A, Tabish H, de Ferranti D. The cost disease and global health. In: Baumol WJ, editor. The cost disease: why computers get cheaper and health care Doesn't. New Haven, CT: Yale University Press; 2012.
5. The Economist. Universal health care—An affordable necessity. The Economist Special report April 26th, 2018
6. Frenk J. Leading the way towards universal health coverage: a call to action. Lancet. 2015;385(9975):1352–8. https://doi.org/10.1016/S0140-6736(14)61467-7. Epub 2014 Oct 15
7. Tangcharoensathien V, Patcharanarumol W, Kulthanmanusorn A, Pablos-Mendez A. Paths towards universal health coverage: beyond political commitments. J Glob Health. 2021;11:16002. Published 2021 Nov 20. https://doi.org/10.7189/jogh.11.16002.
8. Hanson K, Brikci N, Erlangga D, et al. The Lancet Global Health Commission on financing primary health care: putting people at the Centre. Lancet Glob Health. 2022;10:e20.
9. World Health Organization (WHO). Everybody's business - strengthening health systems to improve health outcomes: WHO's framework for action. Geneva: WHO; 2007.
10. Marsh AD, Muzigaba M, Diaz T, et al. Effective coverage think tank group. Effective coverage measurement in maternal, newborn, child, and adolescent health and nutrition: progress, future prospects, and implications for quality health systems. Lancet Glob. Health. 2020;8(5):e730–6.

11. Paul E, Deville C, Bodson O, et al. How is equity approached in universal health coverage? An analysis of global and country policy documents in Benin and Senegal. Int J Equity Health. 2019;18:195.
12. Regan L, Wilson D, Chalkidou K, et al. The journey to UHC: how well are vertical programmes integrated in the health benefits package? A scoping review. BMJ Global Health. 2021;6:e005842. https://doi.org/10.1136/bmjgh-2021-005842.
13. Joint Learning Network for Universal Health Coverage Network. Secretariat at Management Sciences for Health in Arlington, VA. https://www.jointlearningnetwork.org/what-we-do/

Ariel Pablos-Mendez is Professor of Medicine, Division of General Medicine at Columbia University Medical Center, New York, NY. He is a former Director at WHO (Geneva), The Rockefeller Foundation (New York), and head of Global health at USAID (Washington, DC).

Timothy G. Evans is Inaugural Director and Associate Dean of the School of Population and Global Health (SPGH). Faculty of Medicine of McGill University, Montreal, Canada. He is a former Assistant Director General at WHO (Geneva) and *Global* Director for *Health* Nutrition and Population at *the World Bank (Washington, DC).*

Governance of Health Systems

43

Timothy G. Evans and Syed Masud Ahmed

Abstract

This chapter considers the governance of national health systems. In the context of the WHO building blocks on health systems, the governance building block is fundamental in setting the direction of the overall system, identifying how different actors engage with both authority and accountability, and monitoring performance. The chapter identifies the core governance functions found in all systems. It further considers governance as it relates to key actors, be it within government at national and sub-national levels or with other sectors, i.e., non-state actors. The convergence of core functions and diverse actors contributes to governance as a dynamic function of health systems. The chapter concludes by noting the growing scholarship on the governance of health systems that provides novel insights into how health systems can achieve their health goals more effectively and efficiently.

Keywords

Health systems · Governance · Transparency · Equity · Accountability · Strategic policy · Performance monitoring

43.1 Introduction

In the era of Millennium and Sustainable Development Goals, governance is often seen as a critical determinant of achieving specific targets, given its overall strong linkages to economic and social development. Accordingly, development institutions, including the United Nations Development Programme and the World Bank have made institution-wide efforts to promote good governance by articulating common principles, good practices, and monitoring tools to track progress. This broader discourse on governance has been drawn on to inform an awakening within the health sector to examine governance more directly.

43.2 Health Systems Governance: Towards a Definition

At the onset of the new millennium, the World Health Report on Health Systems Performance introduced the concept of stewardship, pointing to government's primary responsibility for the

T. G. Evans (✉)
School of Population and Global Health, McGill University, Montreal, QC, Canada
e-mail: timothy.evans@mcgill.ca

S. M. Ahmed
BRAC James P Grant School of Public Health, BRAC University, Dhaka, Bangladesh
e-mail: ahmed.sm@bracu.ac.bd

M. C. B. Raviglione et al. (eds.), *Global Health Essentials*, Sustainable Development Goals Series,
https://doi.org/10.1007/978-3-031-33851-9_43

health system's overall performance [1]. Several years later, the WHO released a further developed health systems framework based on six building blocks one of which was entitled governance and leadership. The governance and leadership building block attempted to capture the complexity of actors in a health system and was defined as "ensuring strategic policy frameworks exist and are combined with effective oversight, coalition-building, regulation, attention to system-design and accountability" [2].

More recent work has pointed out limitations of the building blocks framework noting that people-centered health systems need to more explicitly integrate community roles as critical constituents of governance and recognize both the formal and informal mechanisms by which governance is exercised [3]. Further work on health systems governance [4, 5] emphasizes that the notion of governance is in no way specific to the health system and draws on a diversity of theories that span political science, economics, social science, development studies, and international relations. These reviews note that amongst the frameworks put forward for health systems governance, there is significant heterogeneity in the underlying theories driving these frameworks [4]. This diversity reflects the complexity of this health systems function across its multiple parts as well as the broad range of national health systems contexts where governance and leadership are actioned in different ways.

43.3 Common Principles and Core Functions

While a single, unified definition of governance remains elusive many of the governance issues are common across health systems. Indeed, drawing on a framework of ten common governance principles for development [6], these have been applied to define the spectrum of governance principles more explicitly in the health sector to include: (1) strategic vision, (2) participation and consensus, (3) the rule of law, (4) transparency, (5) responsiveness, (6) equity and inclusiveness, (7) effectiveness and efficiency, (8) accountability, (9) intelligence and information, and (10) ethics.

These principles cut across many of the common issues that all countries must deal with in managing their health sectors. These include the role of the state and market in health, the role of the ministry of health and other ministries, the range of actors who participate in governance, and the need to be responsive to differential expectations and changing conditions such as emergencies or pandemics. As such, a set of discrete core functions can be further articulated as common components of the governance building block drawing on the WHO health systems framework [2].

The *strategic policy function* includes elements that embrace the vision and direction of the health system, often articulated through overarching health strategies for the sector, i.e., 5-year plans, and guided by values such as the universal right to health or health care. It has multiple levels that stretch from the articulation of policy to plans and operations at various levels of the system (central, sub-national, municipal as well as the engagement of other sectors) to their operationalization and implementation across institutions, inclusive of resources required to inform budgets.

The *participation and collaboration function* relates to who and how diverse actors, from individual citizens to health providers to institutions in public, private, non-governmental, and academic sectors engage in the design, implementation, and evaluation of the health sector. It also includes regional and global collaborative activities beyond national borders, such as with the World Health Organization or other bilateral or multi-lateral actors.

The *authority and accountability function* provides mandate to diverse health systems actors for specific activities, be it jurisdictional responsibility for policy, delivery of services, development of health products or training of health professionals. Accountability can be managed through self-regulation as is often seen in the case of health professionals or through purpose-specific institutional entities responsible for regulation such as in the accreditation of professional education programs or the approval of drugs, vaccines, and diagnostics.

The *performance monitoring function* recognizes the need for continuous assessment of the health challenges, the identification of knowledge gaps to direct research, and performance assessment of the health system in aggregate against various criteria such as equity, effectiveness, efficiency, and responsiveness.

43.4 Key Actors for Governance

A common theme running through the health systems governance literature is the need to avoid a static state-centric, top-down, hierarchical model of governance that fails to capture the dynamic diversity of actors who constitute the health systems and the many informal ways in which they shape the performance of health system [7]. From a health provider perspective, for example, in many countries governance may focus exclusively on formally trained allopathic health professionals when they constitute a minority of the de-facto health workforce as seen in Bangladesh (Fig. 43.1).

A simple but compelling approach to avoiding the state-centric governance trap can be found in a popular approach to health governance that has emerged in Thailand entitled "The triangle that moves mountains." In using the metaphor of the mountain to symbolize the size and complexity of the health system, a triumvirate of governance functions and their actors are identified on each corner of the triangle including the government or policy function, technical actors and knowledge, and non-state actors and social mobilization (Fig. 43.2). This has led to innovative efforts to engage the plurality of concerned actors in articulating health policy in Thailand through mechanisms such as the Thai National Health Assembly with many encouraging results [8].

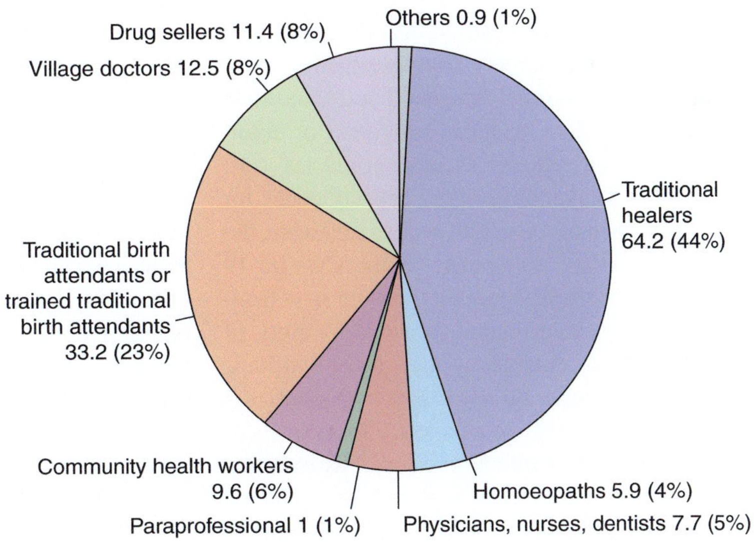

Fig. 43.1 Density of different types of health care providers per 10,000 population. Source [7]

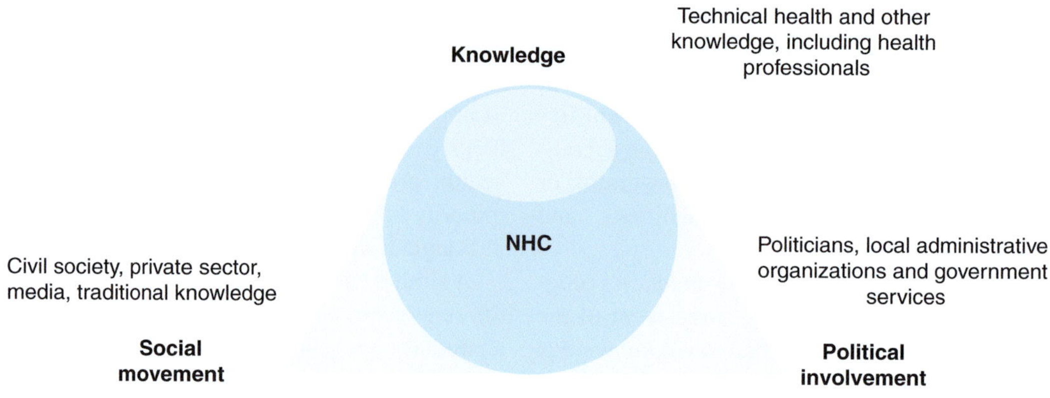

"The mountain means a big and very difficult problem, usually immovable. Combination of the 3 elements in the triangle is essential to overcome any difficulties." *(Prawase Wasi)* Thai health reform has been strongly influenced by this concept. In the National Health Assembly, the National Health Commission (NHC) acts as a coordinator, aiming to bring together the three elements of the triangle to achieve change.

Fig. 43.2 Creation of relevant knowledge. Source [8]

43.5 Governance Dynamics

The diverse functions and actors that constitute health system governance are most often in a constant state of flux. Newly elected governments often bring priorities to bear that shift governance arrangements fundamentally. For example, constitutional reforms that decentralize core functions like health to provinces or counties, as witnessed in several countries like Pakistan or Kenya, have major consequences for the governance of the health sector. Likewise, the need to mobilize a response to the COVID-19 pandemic has led governments to enter new frontiers in governance related to a wide variety of issues such as emergency use authorizations, advanced purchase agreements for vaccines not yet approved and whole-of-society lockdowns to stem the spread of infection as well as examine the speed at which response measures can be mounted [9]. Whether from within or beyond the health sector, these realities will inevitably shift governance arrangements including changes in rules or processes that determine authority and accountability for health policies, organizations, commercial products and health professionals, and the involvement of stakeholders in decision-making.

43.6 Governance: An Emerging Frontier in Health Systems Research

This example of assessing the impact of the Thai National Health Assembly mentioned above [7] raises the importance of studying governance more directly recognizing that the lessons related to the what and how of governance can be instructive in strengthening this complex but the central function of all health systems [5]. The global renewal of Primary Health Care, for example, has been the focus on several studies that have pointed to the importance of governance in supporting devolution and decentralization of health systems to deliver more effective primary care [3, 10]. Similarly, in an effort to understand better than expected outcomes in health given available resources, a number of studies have pointed to dimensions of governance such as effective engagement of other sectors, education of women, smart rebuilding after crises and strong primary care as engines of "good health at low cost" [11, 12]. A further study, trying to explain remarkable progress in health in Bangladesh in a setting of what is traditionally considered weak governance, raised important hypotheses that the pluralistic nature of the system may contribute disproportionately to rapid change and adoption of innovation [7].

More fundamentally, from a knowledge perspective, there is growing attention to strengthening the quality of research. This includes greater conceptual clarity [3, 4], robust methods including systematic review [13] and valid tools for understanding more deliberate approaches to governance practice. For example, a new Health Policymaking Governance Guidance Tool (HP-CGT) applied recently in Lebanon was found to be practical and useful to decision-makers in improving policy-making [14]. Further nurturing our understanding of health systems governance is part and parcel of the broader agenda to strengthen health systems research and generate knowledge and know-how that is vital to navigating and negotiating successful paths to achieve health objectives in the twenty-first century.

References

1. WHO. The world health report 2000. Health systems: improving performance. Geneva: WHO; 2000.
2. WHO. Everybody's business: strengthening health systems to improve health outcomes: WHOs framework for action. Geneva: WHO; 2007.
3. Abimbola S, Negin J, Jan S, Martiniuk A. Towards people-centred health systems: a multi-level framework for analyzing primary health care governance in low- and middle-income countries. Health Policy Plan. 2014;29 Suppl 2(Suppl 2):ii29–39. https://doi.org/10.1093/heapol/czu069.
4. Pyone T, Smith H, van den Broek N. Frameworks to assess healthy systems governance: a systematic review. Health Policy Plan. 2017;32(5):710–22. https://doi.org/10.1093/heapol/czx007.
5. Messen B. Health system governance: welcoming the reboot. BMJ Glob Health. 2020;5:e002404. https://doi.org/10.1136/bmjgh-2020-002404.
6. Siddiqi S, Masud TI, Nishtar S, Peters DH, Sabri B, Bile KM, Jama MA. Framework for assessing governance of the health system in developing countries: gateway to good governance. Health Policy. 2009;90(1):13–25. https://doi.org/10.1016/j.healthpol.2008.08.005.
7. Ahmed SM, Evans TG, Standing H, Mahmud S. Harnessing pluralism for better health in Bangladesh. Lancet. 2013;382(9906):1746–55. https://doi.org/10.1016/S0140-6736(13)62147-9.
8. Rajan D, Mathurapote N, Puttasri W, et al. The triangle that moves the mountain: nine years of Thailand's National Health Assembly (2008–2016). Geneva: World Health Organization; 2017. (WHO/UHC/HGF/HGS/2017.1)
9. Nagasivam A, Fryatt R, de Habich M, Johns B. Exploring the relationship between national governance indicators and speed of initial government response to COVID-19 in low- and middle-income countries. Public Health Pract (Oxf). 2022;4:100309. https://doi.org/10.1016/j.puhip.2022.100309.
10. Espinosa-González AB, Delaney BC, Marti J, Darzi A. The impact of governance in primary health care delivery: a systems thinking approach with a European panel. Health Res Policy Syst. 2019;17(1):65. https://doi.org/10.1186/s12961-019-0456-8.
11. Halstead B, Walsh JA, Warren KS. Good health at low cost. New York: Rockefeller Foundation; 1985.
12. Balabanova D, Mills A, Conteh L, Akkazieva B, Banteyerga H, Dash U, et al. Good health at low cost 25 years on: lessons for the future of health systems strengthening. Lancet. 2013;381(9883):2118–33. https://doi.org/10.1016/S0140-6736(12)62000-5.
13. Herrera CA, Lewin S, Paulsen E, Ciapponi A, Opiyo N, Pantoja T, et al. Governance arrangements for health systems in low-income countries: an overview of systematic reviews. Cochrane Database Syst Rev. 2017;9(9):CD011085. https://doi.org/10.1002/14651858.CD011085.pub2.
14. Hamra R, Siddiqi S, Carmel E, Ammar W. Assessing the governance of the health policy-making process using a new governance tool: the case of Lebanon. Health Res Policy Sys. 2020;18:66. https://doi.org/10.1186/s12961-020-00557-1.

Health System Financing

44

David B. Evans, Christoph Kurowski,
and Fabrizio Tediosi

Abstract

Health financing, one of the key building blocks of health systems, involves three interrelated functions—revenue mobilization, pooling funds, and purchasing health services. This chapter develops four key principles for high performance health financing across the three functions: (1) The predominant form of revenues for health should come from obligatory prepaid funds, not out-of-pocket health payments; (2) risk sharing works better when pools are large and health risk profiles diverse; (3) purchasing requires specifying a core set of health services guaranteed to all beneficiaries from pooled funds; (4) purchasing should use payment methods that ensure the universal availability of guaranteed services with quality, at the lowest possible cost. Additional principles will likely emerge in the future as health financing adapts to emerging and new threats: threats that increase the need to spend on health systems or that reduce country capacities to raise revenues.

Keywords

Health financing · Universal health coverage · High performance health financing · Resilience · Sustainability

44.1 Introduction to Health Financing

Health financing is one of the key building blocks of health systems, fundamental to achieving the targets associated with the Sustainable Development Goal for health including Universal Health Coverage (UHC). It involves three interrelated functions—**revenue mobilization**, **pooling** funds to allow access to needed health services and to spread the financial risks of ill-health and **purchasing** health services. Purchasing can be divided into what to purchase, and how to pay [1, 2].

Health financing **sustainability** is the capacity of health financing to adapt to predictable emerging threats such as aging populations or the growing burden of non-communicable diseases. Health financing **resilience** requires adapting to unanticipated shocks such as COVID-19 [3]. High performance health financing requires all

D. B. Evans (✉) · C. Kurowski
Health Financing Global Solutions Group, World Bank, Washington, DC, USA
e-mail: devans4@worldbank.org; ckurowski@worldbank.org

F. Tediosi
Department of Epidemiology and Public Health
Swiss Tropical and Public Health Institute
Allschwill, Switzerland
e-mail: fabrizio.tediosi@swisstph.ch

M. C. B. Raviglione et al. (eds.), *Global Health Essentials*, Sustainable Development Goals Series,
https://doi.org/10.1007/978-3-031-33851-9_44

three functions to perform well, while anticipating and adapting to emerging and new threats (Box 44.1).

Box 44.1: High Performance Health Financing

High performance health financing requires funding levels that are adequate, sustainable, and resilient to meet country health goals, pooling that is sufficient to spread the financial risks of ill-health across the population, and spending that is both efficient and equitable to assure the desired levels of health service coverage, quality, and financial protection for all people, as well as the range of public health and governance functions[a] that allow the system to function [3].

[a] Examples of public health functions are population-based health promotion, pandemic preparedness and response, development of norms and standards, health information systems and health research

44.2 Background

The vast gulfs across countries in health outcomes such as life expectancy are mirrored by rifts in their health financing capacities. The most obvious is the difference in per capita health spending: in 2019, the most recent year for which data are available, current per capita health expenditure averaged only $39 in low-income and $119 in lower middle-income countries (LICs and LMICs) compared to $472 in upper middle-income and $3191 in high-income countries (UMICs and HICs) [4]. Richer countries can, obviously, mobilize more resources than poorer countries, but some countries simply mobilize revenues more effectively than others at similar levels of national income.

There are also substantial differences across countries at similar levels of national income in the effectiveness of their pooling and purchasing arrangements [5]. The former contributes to differences in the incidence of financial hardship associated with paying out-of-pocket for needed health services, and the latter to differences in the efficiency and equity with which health resources are used. To address these issues, a set of well-known strategies spanning the three health financing functions can make a difference to health financing outcomes at any income level, accelerating progress towards the health-related SDGs [5].

44.3 Aims

This chapter summarizes key requirements for effective revenue mobilization, pooling and purchasing. It then uses these requirements to propose key **principles** related to the health financing functions.

44.4 The Objective of Health Financing

It is now widely accepted that the main objective of developing high performance health financing is to contribute to progress towards UHC, the goal that all people can use the health services they need, of sufficient quality to be effective, while also ensuring that the use of these services does not expose the user to financial hardship [6]. UHC in turn contributes to the broader social goal of increasing human welfare, through improvements in people's health and economic wellbeing.

44.5 Revenue Mobilization

Revenues for health come from government taxes and charges, and sometimes borrowing, health insurance premiums, private sector funds (for-profit and not-for-profit, domestic and external) and household out-of-pocket health payments (OOPs). These resources are frequently supplemented by development assistance for health in lower-income countries.

The need to pay out-of-pocket for health services, including medicines, is one of the reasons why some 840 million people do not receive the care they need [7]. In addition, 70 million are pushed into extreme poverty because of health OOPs, and 435 million are further into poverty [8]. Seeking to increase revenues by increasing OOPs would add to this problem.

The main alternative is prepayment in the form of government taxes and charges, some of which are allocated to health, and health insurance premiums. Government taxes and charges are, by definition, obligatory. Obligation is also required where governments decide to introduce social health insurance (SHI) as a financing mechanism. If it were voluntary, low-risk people and those who are rich enough to bear the costs of ill-health themselves would opt out, making it very difficult to finance the health care costs of the rest of the population from the remaining funds.

Voluntary health insurance, including community health insurance, might have a role to play to supplement obligatory funds, but its contribution has been very limited in terms of raising funds for health [2].

The two critical requirements for effective revenue mobilization in health are, therefore, **prepayment** and **obligation**. This drives the following revenue mobilization principle:

Principle 1. The predominant form of revenues for health should come from obligatory prepaid funds, not OOPs.

44.6 Pooling

Pooling requires combining the individual contributions to prepaid revenues, then using the funds to pay for a defined set of health services for the beneficiaries [1, 6, 9]. An effective pooling system lets people access the health services they need, when they need them, while protecting them from the risk of financial catastrophe or impoverishment associated with OOPs. There are two requirements for pooling to work effectively: **cross-subsidization** and **equalization**.

All people contribute to the pooled funds independent of their health status and risks, but only people who need to seek health care draw on the funds. People who are healthy pay, but do not use the funds, cross-subsidizing those who fall ill.

Pooling also implies equal benefits for equal needs for the guaranteed set of services covered from pooled funds. This contrasts with OOPs where people who can afford to pay obtain care, and those who cannot afford to pay do not obtain the services they need [2].

Cross-subsidization and equalization are compromised where the number of people participating to the health financing scheme is small. In this case, a few episodes of illness requiring high treatment costs can bankrupt the pool, meaning that most pools that cover a small number of people also define a small benefits package.

Principle 2. Risk sharing works better when pools are large and health risk profiles diverse.

44.7 Purchasing

Purchasing is the allocation of funds to: obtain personal health services (promotion, prevention, treatment, rehabilitation, palliation); develop population-based health services (e.g., information campaigns on the importance of vaccination); ensure health system governance; and operate a range of essential public health functions such as pandemic preparedness and response [2, 10].

44.7.1 To Do or to Make?

Ministries of health that operate health facilities use government revenues to purchase inputs to make the services they provide: they pay worker salaries, procure medicines and medical supplies, and invest in infrastructure.

In contrast, health insurance funds (and some governments) use pooled revenues to "buy" (i.e., pay for) the health services that people use. These services can come from public or private providers.

In the context of personal health services, the purchasing function comprises four core activities:

- Specification of benefits and beneficiaries.
- Identification, enrolment, and empowerment of beneficiaries.
- Identifying and contracting suppliers of the inputs used to provide services, including hiring the necessary health workers, or contracting and monitoring service providers from whom services are purchased.
- Paying health service providers for the services they deliver.

Both equity and efficiency are enhanced where these purchasing activities are performed well, regardless of the amount of funding available, ensuring more rapid progress towards the two pillars of UHC—coverage with health services and financial protection.

The first purchasing principle relates to the initial step of deciding what to purchase [11].

Principle 3. Purchasing requires specifying a core set of health services guaranteed to all beneficiaries from pooled funds. This includes a mix of personal and population-based services.

The second principle relates to the question of how to purchase. The way health providers are paid strongly influences their efficiency, the quality of care they provide and equity. Table 44.1 shows the incentives of three common health care provider payment methods [2, 12].

When providers are salaried employees, this payment mechanism does not encourage them to enroll more beneficiaries, see more patients, improve quality, or become more efficient. In contrast, reimbursing providers on a fee-for-service basis encourages multiple visits per episode, increased intensity of service provision, and a focus on high-cost patients. Capitation—when the provider is paid a fixed rate for each enrolled person in return for delivering a specified set of services—encourages enrolment of more beneficiaries, a careful assessment of the services patients need, and a reduction in the intensity of services per patient—sometimes leading to underservicing [13].

All methods have advantages and disadvantages, and the current consensus is that a mix of payment mechanisms works better than a single method [2].

Principle 4. Purchasing should use payment methods that ensure the universal availability of guaranteed services with quality, but at the lowest possible cost.

44.8 Conclusions

A set of key requirements determine if the health financing functions of revenue mobilization, pooling and purchasing are making the maximum possible contribution to progress towards UHC. These requirements lead to four key principles for high performance health financing, summarized in Box 44.2.

Table 44.1 Incentive effects of primary payment methods

Method	Beneficiary enrolment	Mix of service outputs	Volume of patient contacts[1]	Service intensity per contact	Attention to high-cost patients.
Salaries (e.g., through line-item budgets in a ministry of health)	0	0	0	0	0
Capitation	+	+	–	–	–
Fee for service	0	0	+	+	+

Note: + signifies increases or improves; o neutral; – decreases or deteriorates

Box 44.2: Four Key Principles for High-Performance Health Financing

1. The predominant form of revenues for health should come from obligatory prepaid funds, not out-of-pocket payments (OOPs).
2. Risk sharing works better when pools are large and health risk profiles diverse.
3. Purchasing requires specifying a core set of health services guaranteed to all beneficiaries from pooled funds. This includes a mix of personal and population-based services.
4. Purchasing should use payment methods that ensure the universal availability of guaranteed services with quality, but at the lowest possible cost.

More detailed breakdowns of the decisions that need to be made in each of the health financing functions lead to additional principles which can be found in Kurowski, Evans, and Irwin [2]. Recently, the COVID-19 pandemic has highlighted the need to consider new and emerging threats that increase the need to spend on health systems or that can reduce country capacities to raise revenues. As these threats and the responses are better understood, additional principles will emerge.

References

1. Mathauer I, Saksena P, Kutzin J. Pooling arrangements in health financing systems: a proposed classification. Int J Equity Health. 2019;18(1):1–1. https://doi.org/10.1186/s12939-019-1088-x.
2. Kurowski C, Evans DB, Irwin A. Scaling What Works: Convergence on Health Financing Policies for Universal Health Coverage in Low- and Middle-Income Countries. 2022 forthcoming
3. The World Bank. High-Performance Financing for Universal Health Coverage: Driving Sustainable, Inclusive Growth in the 21st Century; 2019. https://www.worldbank.org/en/topic/universalhealthcoverage/publication/high-performance-health-financing-for-universal-health-coverage-driving-sustainable-inclusive-growth-in-the-21st-century
4. Word Health Organization. Global health expenditure database. 2022. Global Health Expenditure Database (who.int). Accessed 29 June 2022
5. Kurowski C, Evans DB, Tandon A, et al. From double shock to double recovery. Implications and options for health financing in the time of COVID-19. The World Bank; 2021. https://openknowledge.worldbank.org/handle/10986/35298
6. World Health Organization. The World Health Report 2010: health systems financing: the path to universal coverage. Geneva: World Health Organization; 2010. https://apps.who.int/iris/handle/10665/44371
7. World Health Organization. Director General's opening address to the second plenary session of the 2022 World Health Assembly; 23 May 2022. Address by Dr Tedros Adhanom Ghebreyesus, Director-General (who.int). Accessed 29 June 2022
8. WHO and World Bank. Global monitoring report on financial protection in health 2021. Geneva: World Health Organization and International Bank for Reconstruction and Development / The World Bank; 2021. Global monitoring report on financial protection in health 2021 (who.int)
9. Smith PC, Witter SN. Risk pooling in health care financing: the implications for health system performance. Health Nutrition and Population Discussion Paper, World Bank, September 2004. Risk Pooling in Health Care Financing : The Implications for Health System Performance (worldbank.org)
10. Gottret P, Schieber G. Health financing revisited : a practitioner's guide. Washington, DC: World Bank; 2006. https://openknowledge.worldbank.org/handle/10986/7094
11. Benefit design: the perspective from health financing policy. Geneva: World Health Organization; 2022 (Health Financing Policy Brief, No. 8).
12. Mathauer I, Dale E, Jowett M, et al. Purchasing Health Services for Universal Health Coverage: How to Make it More Strategic? 2019. https://apps.who.int/iris/handle/10665/311387
13. Duckett S. Aligning policy objectives and payment design in palliative care. BMC Palliat Care. 2018;17(1):1.

Human Resources for Health: Health Workers, The Health System's Most Valuable Resource

45

Timothy G. Evans and Núria Casamitjana

Abstract

Human Resources for Health (HRH) are an essential resource to every health system, but there are chronic and growing challenges of harnessing this resource to meet the needs of the health systems. Training and education of health workforce, recruitment and retention, balancing supply and demand with needs are some of the key elements that demand attention at local, national, regional, and global level. Global Health has recognized the importance of the health workforce as a critical dimension of health systems requiring more concerted policy attention. However, the ability of countries to manage health workforce issues more optimally drawing on evidence informed policy is not a given in any setting. Attention to securing this capacity across health systems is critical to more successful stewardship of the health workforce, making sure health workers are catalysts rather than constraints to meeting health needs of the world population.

Keywords

Health workers · Health workforce · Training · Education · Health systems

T. G. Evans
School of Population and Global Health, McGill University, Montreal, QC, Canada
e-mail: timothy.evans@mcgill.ca

N. Casamitjana (✉)
Department of Medicine, Barcelona Institute for Global Health (ISGlobal), University of Barcelona, Barcelona, Spain
e-mail: nuria.casamitjana@isglobal.org

45.1 Introduction and Aims of the Chapter

Although it is widely recognized that health workers are an essential resource to every health system, there are chronic and growing challenges of harnessing this resource to meet the needs of the health systems. This chapter traces how over the last 20 years, global health has turned its attention to recognize the importance of the health workforce as a critical dimension of health systems that demands more concerted policy attention. Frameworks are presented that have been developed to guide focused attention to specific elements of the workforce such as training and education, recruitment and retention, balancing supply and demand with needs. It points to national, regional, and global drivers that are shaping both opportunities and challenges for the health workforce.

M. C. B. Raviglione et al. (eds.), *Global Health Essentials*, Sustainable Development Goals Series,
https://doi.org/10.1007/978-3-031-33851-9_45

45.2 Description of Key Points

45.2.1 Health Workers Matter

Beyond anecdotes of situations whereby a surgeon is unavailable for an emergency surgery and the patient dies, systematic evidence of the link of health workers to health improvements is in short supply. In 2006, the World Health Report [1] provided the first cross-country evidence that larger numbers of health workers are associated with better health outcomes (see Fig. 45.1). Further evidence on the link between health workers density and vaccination coverage for example, across countries showed how a greater density of nurse-midwives was associated with higher vaccination coverage [2]. More recently, evidence has been generated on the benefits and cost-effectiveness of community health workers [3].

45.2.2 A Chronic and Growing Crisis

Despite the growing evidence on the importance of health workers, there is a chronic and growing crisis. The WHR 2006 noted a shortfall of 4.6 million health workers required to meet the Millennium Development Goals (MDGs) targets by 2015 [1]. In the context of the Sustainable Development Goals (SDGs) 2030 and the target of Universal Health Coverage (UHC), the estimated shortfall has ballooned to 18 million! Beyond absolute numbers, their distribution continues to cluster in better off urban areas, leaving rural and remote communities underserved. Working conditions for health workers are too often characterized by inadequate supervision, shortages of key materials, lack of appropriate training, unsafe working conditions, insufficient and irregular remuneration. Across health systems, "burn out" is growing to epidemic proportions especially in the wake of the COVID-19 pandemic and is linked more generally to the "great resignation."

45.2.3 Putting HRH on the Global Health Agenda

Despite the major unmet needs across health systems, it is only recently that the health workforce has become an explicit and visible part of the global health agenda. In centuries past, in response to health crises there have been efforts to mobilize the health workforce, but primarily on a national level. During the great sanitary awakening in the UK in the nineteenth century, district public health officers and other cadres were established to mitigate the risks of epidemic disease among the laboring populations [4]. In the early twentieth century, three major reports written in the United States—the Flexner Report, the Goldmark Report, and the Rose-Welch Report—brought attention to the need for system-wide standards to guide the training of doctors,

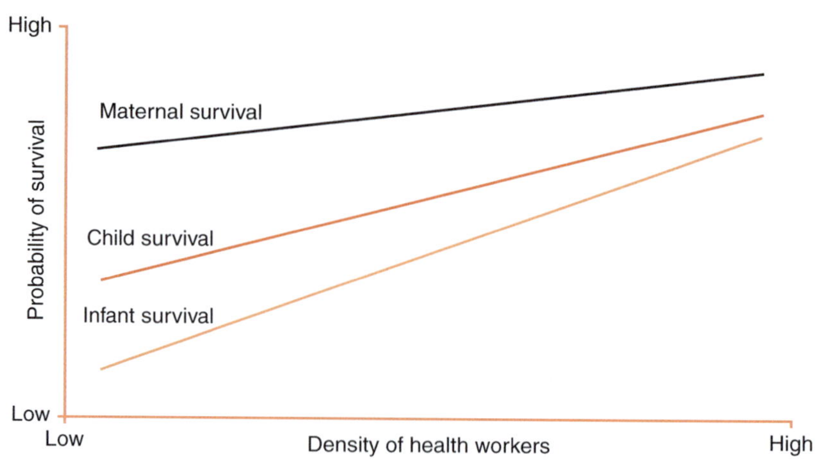

Fig. 45.1 Health workers save lives! (From 1. World Health Organization. (2006). The world health report: 2006: working together for health. World Health Organization. https://apps.who.int/iris/handle/10665/43432)

nurses, and public health workers, respectively. Later in the twentieth century, in the context of the Primary Health Care Declaration at Alma Ata 1978, the ideas of universal coverage of community health workers and barefoot doctors gained widespread currency. However, as the world entered the new Millennium there remained no concerted policy thinking at the global level to deal with the health workforce. The World Health Organization (WHO), for example, had a health workforce policy capacity that was limited to an office of medical education and a chief nursing officer!

With the advent of the MDGs, where three of the eight goals concerned health, there was a growing appreciation that achieving the targets by 2015 for the health of women, and those suffering from diseases such as HIV, tuberculosis, and malaria would require major attention to functioning of health systems. Lamentably, the WHO health systems framework of 2000 made no explicit mention of the health workforce [5]. This oversight was noted by the Rockefeller Foundation that in 2001 initiated a Joint Learning Initiative on Human Resources for Health (JLI HRH). They established working groups with global experts who focused on key elements of the health workforce like education or migration. The JLI report was issued in 2004 and called attention to the health workforce crisis [6]. In May 2004, South Africa introduced a resolution at the World Health Assembly—WHA [7] demanding reciprocity from countries that were recruiting health workers whose training was paid for by tax dollars from South Africa. The JLI report together with this resolution led to WHO creating for the first time ever a dedicated Department of Human Resources for Health, naming a special envoy to the Director General on HRH, the issuing of the WHR 2006 on the health workforce [1], and the establishment of the first-ever multilateral partnership—the Global Health Workforce Alliance.

In 2016, building on a proposal of the Board of the Global Health Workforce Alliance, the Global Health Workforce Network was established, and the adoption of the Global Strategy on Human Resources for Health: Workforce 2030 [8] and the recommendations of the High-Level Commission on Health Employment and Economic Growth [9] set the foundations for an ambitious, forward-looking health workforce agenda to progress towards UHC and the SDGs.

45.2.4 Framing the Health Workforce for Action

The WHR 2006 [1] provided a lifecycle framework to point to three critical dimensions of the health workforce linked to the entry, employment, and exit of a health worker. Within each of these areas, there is a web of policy entry points that demand attention.

In terms of preparing the health workforce, there are important issues related to having adequate numbers of appropriately qualified candidates for health professional training, their selection and admission criteria to ensure quality and diversity, and the range of professional training programs, their accreditation, and their performance in terms of rates of graduation/attrition and subsequent employment. In 2010, an independent global commission issued a vision for the education of health professionals for the twenty-first century that recommended an ambitious agenda of instructional and institutional reforms to accelerate achievement of health equity globally [10]. Key among its recommendations in terms of instruction was a recognition of the need to reform curricula for health professionals along the three dimensions of core competencies: informative, normative, and transformative (see Fig. 45.2). Institutionally, reframing the global market for health professional education around life-long acquisition of competencies is recognized as ripe for innovation [11].

Once trained, there are a wide set of issues related to enabling health workers to perform optimally according to the needs of the health system. Employment terms and conditions be they with the public, private, or not-for-profit sectors, along with the nature of the work environment (supportive, stimulating, and

Fig. 45.2 On three levels of learning. Reprinted from The Lancet, Vol. 376, Frenk, J. Chen, L. Bhutta, Z et al. Health professionals for a new century: transforming education to strengthen health systems in an interdependent world, Pages 1923–58, 2010, with permission from Elsevier. https://doi.org/10.1016/S0140-6736(10)61854-5

Level	Objectives	Outcome
Informative	• Information • Skills	Experts
Formative	• Socialization • Values	Professionals
Transformative	• Leadership attributes	Change agents

safe) and the medium-term prospects for career progression are among the critical factors that influence worker performance in terms of availability, responsiveness, and productivity.

The needs and demands for health workers far outweigh their supply, and as such these labor market imbalances lead to high levels of health workers movement within and between countries from lower paying to higher paying markets [12]. The scale and speed of these shifts are dramatic. Professional recruitment firms are retained by health or hospital systems to source large numbers of health professionals be it nurses, doctors, or laboratory technicians. Successful recruitment for the client is often associated with a critical loss of staff in a lower paying labor market with very few options for backfilling these shortages.

In the wake of these pressures, there have been important innovations. For example, under the banner of "task shifting," lower-level cadres in the health workforce (less likely to migrate) are taught and supervised to take on tasks normally performed by higher level cadres. The experiences of this in extending lifesaving care with respect to HIV have been encouraging [13, 14]. Similarly, health systems everywhere, especially after the lockdowns of the COVID-19 pandemic, are finding more ways to provide care online and promote self-care thus decreasing demands on scarce health care providers [15].

Last but not least, we should not forget the role of women in delivering health care. In 2019, the WHO Global Health Workforce Network's Gender Equity Hub produced a gender and equity analysis on the health workforce that calls for gender transformative policies and measures to be put in place if global targets such as UHC and SDGs are to be achieved [16].

45.3 Conclusions

The health workforce challenges within and across countries are critical dimensions of a new era of health systems knowledge and know-how in global health. All countries are facing similar pressures with respect to managing the myriad dimensions of the health workforce thereby raising the value of comparative analysis and joint learning. Given the robust movement of health workers across borders, there is an inextricable interdependence between health systems that would benefit from active monitoring and management rather than leaving it purely to market forces. The ability of countries to manage health workforce issues more optimally drawing on evidence informed policy is not a given in any setting. Attention to securing this capacity across all health systems will be critical to more successful stewardship of the health workforce and making sure health workers are catalysts rather than constraints to meeting health needs of the world population.

References

1. World Health Organization. The world health report: 2006: working together for health. World Health Organization; 2006. https://apps.who.int/iris/handle/10665/43432
2. Anand S, Bärnighausen T. Health workers and vaccination coverage in developing countries: an econometric analysis. Lancet. 2007;369:1277–85. https://doi.org/10.1016/S0140-6736(07)60599-6.
3. Kangovi S, Mitra N, Grande D, Long JA, Asch DA. Evidence-based community health worker program addresses unmet social needs and generates positive return on investment. Health Aff. 2020;39(2):207–13. https://doi.org/10.1377/hlthaff.2019.00981.
4. Chadwick E, Flinn MW. 1842 report on the sanitary condition of the Labouring population of Great Britain. Edinburgh: University Press; 1965.
5. World Health Organization. The World health report: 2000: health systems: improving performance. World Health Organization; 2000. https://apps.who.int/iris/handle/10665/42281
6. Chen L, Evans T, Anand S, Boufford JI, Brown H, Chowdhury M, Cueto M, Dare L, Dussault G, Elzinga G, Fee E, Habte D, Hanvoravongchai P, Jacobs M, Kurowski C, Michael S, Pablos-Mendez A, Sewankambo N, Solimano G, Stilwell B, De Waal A, Wibulpolpraser S. Human resources for health: overcoming the crisis. Lancet. 2004;364:1984–90. https://doi.org/10.1016/S0140-6736(04)17482-5.
7. World Health Assembly. Fifty-seventh World Health Assembly, Geneva, 17–22 May 2004: Resolutions and decisions, annexes. World Health Organization. 2004; 57: 52. https://apps.who.int/iris/handle/10665/20159
8. Global strategy on Human Resources for Health. Workforce 2030. Geneva: WHO; 2016. https://www.who.int/publications/i/item/9789241511131
9. Working for Health and Growth: Investing in the Health Workforce. Report of the high-level commission on health employment and economic growth. Geneva: WHO; 2016. https://www.who.int/publications/i/item/9789241511308
10. Frenk J, Chen L, Bhutta ZA, Cohen J, Crisp N, Evans T, Fineberg H, Garcia P, Ke Y, Kelley P, Kistnasamy B, Meleis A, Naylor D, Pablos-Mendez A, Reddy S, Scrimshaw S, Sepulveda J, Serwadda D, Zurayk H. Health professionals for a new century: transforming education to strengthen health systems in an interdependent world. Lancet. 2010;376:1923–58. https://doi.org/10.1016/S0140-6736(10)61854-5.
11. Darzi A, Evans T. The global shortage of health workers—an opportunity to transform care. Lancet. 2016;388:2576–7. https://doi.org/10.1016/S0140-6736(16)32235-8.
12. Liu JX, Goryakin Y, Akiko Maeda A, Bruckner T, Scheffler R. Global health workforce labor market projections for 2030. Hum Resour Health. 2017;15:11. https://doi.org/10.1186/s12960-017-0187-2.
13. Jones M, Cameron D. Evaluating 5 years' NIMART mentoring in South Africa's HIV treatment programme: successes, challenges and future needs. S Afr Med J. 2017;107(10):839–42. https://doi.org/10.7196/SAMJ.2017.v107i10.12392.
14. Seidman G, Atun R. Does task shifting yield cost savings and improve efficiency for health systems? A systematic review of evidence from low-income and middle-income countries. Hum Resour Health. 2017;15:29. https://doi.org/10.1186/s12960-017-0200-9.
15. World Health Organization. Health workforce policy and management in the context of the COVID-19 pandemic response. Geneva: WHO; 2020. https://www.who.int/publications/i/item/WHO-2019-nCoV-health_workforce-2020.1
16. Delivered by women, led by men: A gender and equity analysis of the global health and social workforce; 2019. https://www.who.int/publications/i/item/978-92-4-151546-7

46 Health Information Systems

What Are Global Health Estimates and Why Are They Needed?

Carla AbouZahr

Abstract

Countries report health-related indicators for monitoring progress towards agreed goals and targets such as the Sustainable Development Goals. However, national health information and statistical systems are not always able to produce data that meet quality standards, such as population coverage and completeness, representativeness, frequency, timeliness, and disaggregation. As a result, global reporting of progress towards international health goals depends to a great extent on statistical estimates produced by United Nations agencies and academic institutions. Health estimates are valuable for summarizing global health trends and enabling cross country comparisons. However, there is debate regarding their utility from a country perspective. Most global health estimates are developed in high-income settings. The statistical and mathematical methods used are frequently complex, lacking in transparency and hard to replicate at country level. The international community should direct resources to enhancing country capacities to produce and use reliable and complete health-related indicators.

Keywords

Monitoring heath · Statistical estimates · Country health information

46.1 Introduction

Since the start of the COVID-19 pandemic, the World Health Organization (WHO) has compiled daily counts of COVID-19 deaths officially reported by countries. By the end of 2021, a cumulative total of over 5.5 million COVID-related deaths had been reported. This is undoubtedly an underestimate of the true death toll of COVID; many COVID cases are never identified, and many deaths remain uncounted. A more realistic approximation can be obtained by monitoring *excess mortality*—the difference between observed and expected number of deaths compared with the same time period in previous years [1, 2]. Expert groups have developed statistical models to estimate excess mortality for 2020–21, with cumulative deaths totaling between 12 and almost 21 million, depending on the statistical modelling strategies employed (Fig. 46.1) [3, 4]. These examples provide a vivid illustration of the theme of this chapter—the benefits and risks of statistical modelling to generate country health estimates.

C. AbouZahr (✉)
Consultant, Vital Strategies, St. Légier, Switzerland

M. C. B. Raviglione et al. (eds.), *Global Health Essentials*, Sustainable Development Goals Series,
https://doi.org/10.1007/978-3-031-33851-9_46

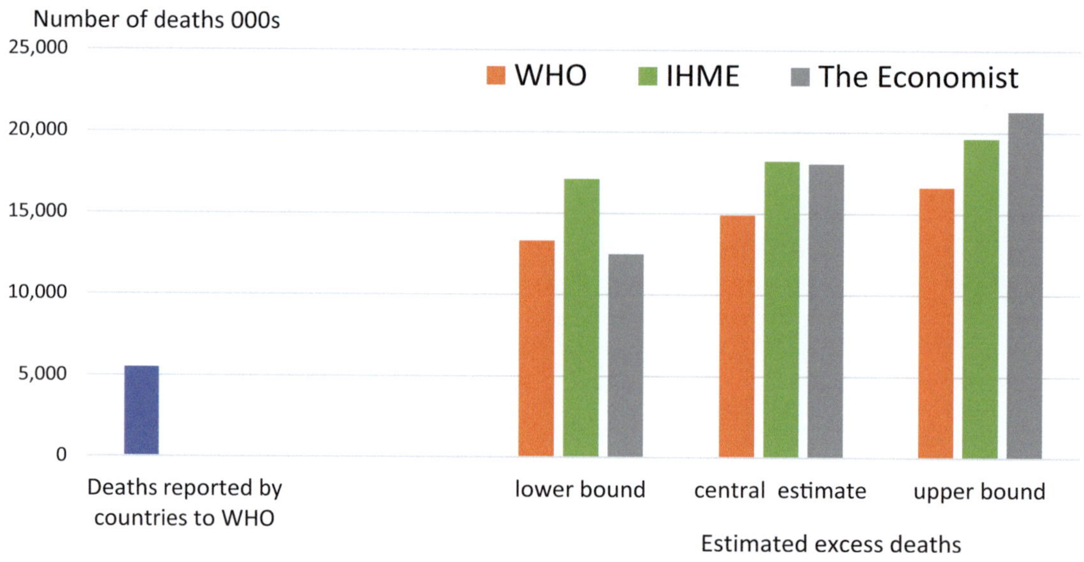

Fig. 46.1 Reported COVID-19 deaths compared with three estimations of excess mortality

46.2 Aims of the Chapter

We describe the demand for reliable health data and the limitations of data collection systems in many country health information systems. We explain the rationale for, and methods applied to modify and adjust available data and apply statistical modelling methods to generate estimates of health indicators and trends and fill information gaps. We examine the utility of these estimates from the perspectives of country data users and producers.

46.3 Background

Since the 1990s, governments have committed to reporting on progress towards goals and targets, of which the most recent are the 2030 Sustainable Development Goals (SDGs). However, country health information systems face challenges in generating data that meet the quality standards required to enable a realistic assessment of progress. Complete, timely, and comparable primary data for tracking health progress are not available everywhere. Fewer than half the deaths in the world are officially registered, counted, and have a defined cause. Population level data on incidence or prevalence of disease and injury are even less widely available. According to WHO, "50% of countries have limited or less capacity for systematic monitoring of health care quality, and only 59% of countries have good capacity to use data to drive policy and planning [5]."

Data challenges have increased with the expanding breadth and detail of the development goals and targets themselves. For example, SDG Goal 3 on health and wellbeing calls for data to monitor multiple indicators of maternal and child health, communicable and noncommunicable diseases, social determinants of health, and health system performance, including universal health coverage.

46.4 Country Health Information Systems

Health information is a core building block of the health system. Health Management Information Systems (HMIS) collect and use data at all administrative levels to support health system management and monitoring. Health data are also generated through the decennial census, population-based surveys, the civil registration of births and deaths, public health surveillance, independent research, analysis of secondary data, and harvesting big data [6]. The data generated through these diverse sources supports tracking of health status and health system performance and provides the basis for reporting on progress, including towards the SDGs.

In many settings, resources and capacities for collecting and evaluating data are limited and reported indicators of variable quality. In some instances, data from primary collection efforts are reported as direct tabulations of counts or transformed into indicators such as rates or ratios without any adjustments or corrections to account for bias or incompleteness. Differences in data definitions and measurement methods complicate trend assessment and comparisons between populations. Limitations in data quality include inconsistent case definitions; incomplete population-based surveillance or registration; and non-representative population bias.

46.5 Why Produce Statistical Estimates?

The rationale for global health estimates is summarized in Box 46.1. The utility of estimates and the relative importance of the various drivers will depend on the extent and quality of available country data. As noted by Mathers and colleagues, producers of estimates compensate for the limitations of available data by applying correction factors and adjustments and constructing mathematical and statistical models designed to:

- Synthesize data from multiple and overlapping sources of data
- Fill data gaps in time series and project to a common target year
- Improve accuracy and comparability over time or across populations
- Estimate quantities that cannot be directly measured, for example, by measuring intermediate outcomes and using a model to extrapolate to the outcome of interest
- Forecast indicators for a standard time frame (base year to latest target year) using a forward (and sometimes backward) projection [7].

There is value in such estimates for progress monitoring and prioritization of interventions [8]. The WHO annual World Health Statistics makes extensive use of comparable estimates to report on progress [9]. It notes, however, that such estimates "are subject to considerable uncertainty."

46.6 Who Generates Global Health Estimates?

The major producers of health estimates are several UN interagency estimation groups and academic institutions generally based in high-income settings, of which the most well-known is the Institute for Health Metrics and Evaluation (IHME).

The UN interagency groups bring together academic experts from around the world to provide methodological advice. Examples include the Child mortality Estimation Group, Maternal Mortality Expert Group, and interagency reference groups for malaria, AIDS, cancer, and adult mortality. The UN groups work with countries to gather available data and include a formal country consultation prior to finalization and publication. This is not a clearance process so estimates and country-reported values may diverge.

The IHME is an academic body based at the University of Washington. It collaborates with technical experts from around the world to develop statistical approaches to produce "timely, relevant, and scientifically valid evidence to improve health policy and practice." Estimates are not shared with country experts prior to publication which is usually done in a peer-reviewed journal such as The Lancet. Countries learn their own estimates if and when they read about them.

46.7 Limitations and Risks of Global Estimates

User confidence in the integrity of estimates is dependent on transparency, both about the use of and modification of all available input data and on clearly described methodological strategies. As Byass has observed, in some cases, the statistical and mathematical techniques for generating the estimates have become so complex that many users find them opaque and hard to understand [10]. The expansion of computing and storage capacity has increased technical complexity but reduced the ability of many country partners to replicate the findings for themselves.

Confidence in estimation methods is threatened when estimates change radically from year to year, when time series are retrospectively re-estimated, and when estimates generated by different producers yield significantly different results, as has occurred, for example, in relation to maternal mortality [11], malaria [12], and road traffic injuries [13].

Recent increases in global estimation have led to calls for more transparency and replicability of methods. WHO has formulated the GATHER Guidelines which define best practices for documenting studies that report global health estimates, thus facilitating the task of users seeking to better understand the basis of such estimates and to replicate them in situ when possible [14].

46.8 Main Conclusions and Recommendations

Health estimates are valuable for summarizing the global health situation and emerging trends but there is debate as to their utility from a country perspective. As pointed out by Pisani and Kok, most global health estimates are produced far from the local contexts where the data they are based on are collected, and where the results of estimation must be used if they are to make a difference to the health of individuals [15]. Externally generated values that differ substantially from country-reported data can have political and funding implications. Some policymakers question the need for estimates, preferring to use their national statistics, when possible.

Global health estimates cannot replace the responsibilities of countries to collect reliable, accurate, and regular empirical data. Nor should they absolve development partners and funders from providing financial and technical support to countries to collect and analyse their own data. Greater engagement of local actors would incentivize improved data collection and analysis in countries and increase the likelihood that data will be used by those able to translate them into health gains.

Box 46.1: Rationale for the Production of Global Health Estimates

Completeness
- To produce statistics for all countries for the same time period using standardized methods.
- To fill gaps, missing values in available data: reliable data are available only for some countries and/or time periods.

Comparability
- To deal with biases in the data; biases differ from place to place and may change over time within a country.
- To ensure temporal and international comparability using similar methodology and assumptions across countries.
- To reconcile differences between data sources and/or estimation method(s) for a specific data item and within sources over time.

Currency
- To produce data of immediate or current relevance.
- To respond quickly to demands for key indicators to meet demands for accountability and performance-based funding.

Cost
- To generate the needed estimates in an inexpensive and rapid way that is not dependent on long-term capacity development efforts.

Objectivity
- To ensure that country statistics are generated independently of political pressures.
- To underpin accountability for results.

Adapted from: AbouZahr C, Boerma T, Hogan D. Global estimates of country health indicators: useful, unnecessary, inevitable? Global Health Action 2017;10(supplement 1): 1290370, https://doi.org/10.1080/16549716.2017.1290370

References

1. Setel P, AbouZahr C, Atuheire EB, Bratschi M, Cercone EB, Chinganya O, et al. Mortality surveillance during the COVID-19 pandemic. Bull World Health Organ. 2020;98(6):374. https://doi.org/10.2471/BLT.20.263194.
2. Leon DA, Shkolnikov VM, Smeeth L, Magnus P, Pechholdová M, Jarvis CI. COVID-19: a need for real-time monitoring of weekly excess deaths. Lancet. 2020;395(10234):e81. https://doi.org/10.1016/S0140-6736(20)30933-8.
3. Karlinsky A, Kobak D. Tracking excess mortality across countries during the COVID-19 pandemic with the world mortality dataset. elife. 2021;10:e69336. https://doi.org/10.7554/eLife.69336. PMID:34190045
4. Wang H, Paulson K, Pease S, Watson S, Comfort H, Zheng P, et al. COVID-19 Excess Mortality Collaborators. Estimating excess mortality due to the COVID-19 pandemic: a systematic analysis of COVID-19-related mortality, 2020–21. Lancet. 2022;10(10334):1513–36. https://doi.org/10.1016/S0140-6736(21)02796-3.
5. World Health Organization. Global report on health data systems and capacity. 2021 ISBN 978-92-4-001870-9 (electronic version) ISBN 978-92-4-001871-6 (print version)
6. Macfarlane S, AbouZahr C, Tangcharoensathien V. National systems for generating and managing data for health. In: Macfarlane S, AbouZahr C, editors. The Palgrave handbook of global health data methods for policy and practice. London: Palgrave Macmillan; 2019. https://doi.org/10.1057/978-1-137-54984-6_1.
7. Mathers C, Hogan D, Stevens G. Global health estimates: modelling and predicting health outcomes. In: MacFarlane S, AbouZahr C, editors. The Palgrave handbook of global health data methods for policy and practice. London: Palgrave Macmillan; 2019. https://doi.org/10.1057/978-1-137-54984-6_21.
8. Boerma T, Mathers C. The World Health Organization and global health estimates: improving collaboration and capacity. BMC Med. 2015;13(1):50. https://doi.org/10.1186/s12916-015-0286-7.
9. World Health Statistics. Monitoring health for the SDGs. Geneva: World Health Organization; 2021. Licence: CC BY-NC-SA 3.0 IGO
10. Byass P. The imperfect world of global health estimates, e1001006. PLoS Med. 2010;7(11) https://doi.org/10.1371/journal.pmed.1001006.
11. Gerland P, Masquelier B, Helleringer S, Hogan D, Mathers C. Maternal mortality estimates. Lancet. 2014;384(9961):2211. https://doi.org/10.1016/S0140-6736(14)62424-7. PMID:25625396
12. Mathers C, Hogan D. Commentary: does the global burden of disease study substantially overestimate road traffic deaths in OECD countries? Int J Epidemiol. 2015;44(5):1657–9. https://doi.org/10.1093/ije/dyv162.
13. Mathers C. History of global burden of disease assessment at the World Health Organization. Arch Public Health. 2020;78(1):77. https://doi.org/10.1186/s13690-020-00458-3.
14. Stevens G, Alkema L, Black R, Boerma J, Collins G, Ezzati M, et al. GATHER Working Group. Guidelines for Accurate and Transparent Health Estimates Reporting: the GATHER statement. PLoS Med. 2016;13(6):e1002056. https://doi.org/10.1371/journal.pmed.1002056.
15. Pisani E, Kok M. In the eye of the beholder: to make global health estimates useful, make them more socially robust. Glob Health Action. 2017;10(sup1):1266180. https://doi.org/10.3402/gha.v9.32298.

47 Strengthening Health Service Delivery for Universal Health Coverage Through Synergistic Partnerships Between the Public and Private Health Sector

Hannah Monica Dias

Abstract

The COVID-19 pandemic coupled with ongoing crises such as armed conflicts, increasing food insecurity, political and economic instability, has halted progress made towards advancing universal health coverage (UHC), as reported by the World Health Organization (WHO) in 2021.

Getting UHC efforts back on track will require concerted action, not only through the public health sector, but also by strengthening engagement of the private health sector, which is often the first point of care in many settings. The pursuit of UHC requires countries to take ownership of healthcare, irrespective of where a person seeks care, in the public or private sector. The private health sector is a major provider of health services across regions and different socioeconomic groups including the poor.

The aim of this chapter is to highlight ongoing efforts and strategies to strengthen private health sector engagement for UHC, which includes showcasing ongoing efforts in this area to combat tuberculosis. Key challenges and opportunities are presented emphasizing the need to take private health sector engagement to scale in the quest to ensure health for all. WHO's Strategy "Engaging the private health service delivery sector through governance in mixed health systems" is shared alongside a case study on private sector engagement efforts to end tuberculosis.

Keywords

Universal health coverage (UHC) · Private services · Private providers · Public-private mix (PPM) · Tuberculosis

47.1 Introduction

Ensuring access to essential health services, including the ability to see a health worker, or safe, effective, and affordable medicines is core to achieving Universal Health Coverage (UHC) as targeted in the Sustainable Development Goals (SDGs) [1]. Unfortunately, approximately half the world's population lacks access to essential health services. Where accessible, these services are often fragmented, and continuity of care is hampered by poor coordination across providers and a lack of integration with other critical sectors such as social services. The COVID-19 pandemic coupled with ongoing crises such as armed conflicts, increasing food insecurity, political and economic instability, has halted progress made

H. M. Dias (✉)
World Health Organization, Geneva, Switzerland
e-mail: diash@who.int

M. C. B. Raviglione et al. (eds.), *Global Health Essentials*, Sustainable Development Goals Series,
https://doi.org/10.1007/978-3-031-33851-9_47

towards advancing UHC, as reported by the World Health Organization (WHO) in 2021 [2].

Getting UHC efforts back on track will require concerted efforts not only through the public health sector, but also by strengthening engagement of the private health sector, which is often the first point of care in many settings. The pursuit of UHC requires countries to take ownership of healthcare, irrespective of where a person seeks care, in the public or private sector [3].

The private health sector is a major provider of health services across regions and different socioeconomic groups including for the poor [4, 5]. Key factors contributing to the demand for private sector health services, include the perception that the public sector offers low-quality care compared to the private sector [6], a shortfall in public health facilities in some rural and peri-urban locations, and ease of access to private health facilities in terms of distance and timings (e.g. open after work hours). A large private sector thus exists in many countries spanning health service areas, including primary care, hospitals, diagnostics, specialist therapeutics and curative services, pharmaceutical supply chains as well as informal and traditional practice [7].

The aim of this chapter is to highlight ongoing efforts and strategies to strengthen private health sector engagement for UHC, including by showcasing advances in this area to combat tuberculosis. Key challenges and opportunities are presented emphasizing the need to take private health sector engagement to scale in the quest to ensure health for all.

47.2 Engaging the Private Health Service Delivery Sector

Private sector engagement is the meaningful inclusion of private providers for service delivery in mixed health systems. Private sector engagement requires that governments focus on governance of the whole health system—both private and public—to ensure quality of care and financial protection for patients, irrespective of where they seek care [8]. It requires that the private sector aligns with public sector health goals and commits to working to support the government agenda. WHO has recently launched a strategy, "Engaging the private health service delivery sector through governance in mixed health systems" [9]. Most health systems are mixed systems, where goods and services are provided both by the public and private sector, and health consumers are requesting these services from both sectors. The strategy redresses a critical health system governance gap for the effective engagement of the private sector in health in the context of UHC.

WHO's strategy outlines six governance behaviours critical to private sector health service delivery governance.

- Build understanding—Collection and analysis of data to align priorities for action.
- Foster relations—Working together to achieve shared objectives in a new way of doing business.
- Enable stakeholders—Institutional framework that empowers actors.
- Align structures—Organizational structures to align with policy objectives.
- Nurture trust—Mutual trust amongst all actors as reliable participants.
- Deliver strategy—Agreed sense of direction and articulation of roles and responsibilities (Fig. 47.1).

This strategy serves as a guide for WHO and Member States at various levels of engagement to promote a new way of doing business with the private sector. It builds upon WHO's mandate and normative work on health systems strengthening, governance, and financing.

WHO is working closely with countries to support the development of policy on private sector engagement for UHC, strengthen capacity to make informed decisions, and develop and implement suitable regulatory and financial tools for managing the private sector and public–private partnerships.

The strategy is well aligned with and builds upon other long-standing efforts led by WHO towards combatting infectious diseases like

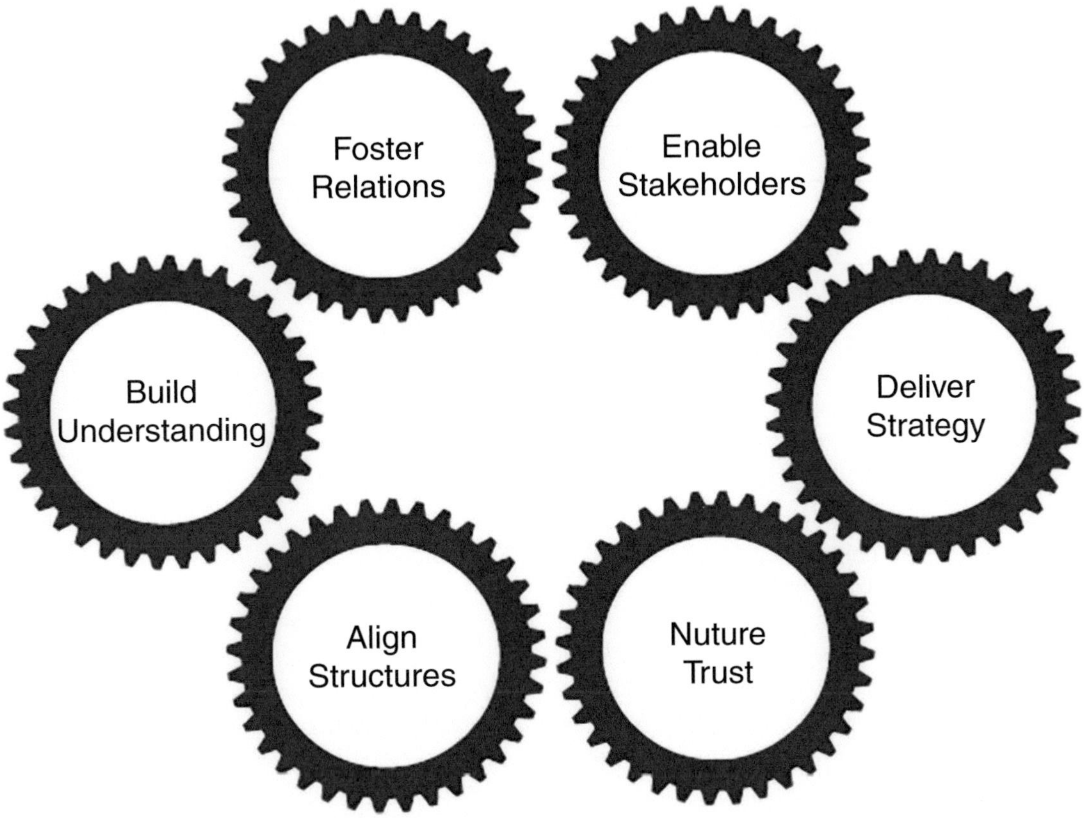

Fig. 47.1 WHO Strategic Framework on private sector engagement. Reference: World Health Organization 2020, Engaging the private health service delivery sector through governance in mixed health systems: strategy report of the WHO Advisory Group on the Governance of the Private Sector for Universal Health Coverage

tuberculosis (TB), malaria, and other non-communicable diseases. Private sector engagement towards ending TB is highlighted below as a case study to demonstrate the impact of public-private mix approaches in closing gaps in TB prevention and care on the road to UHC. Private sector engagement has been prioritized by WHO as part of efforts to end TB since the 1990s.

47.3 Public-Private Health Sector Engagement in the TB Response: A Case Study

TB remains one of the world's top infectious killers claiming over 4000 lives a day. This disease not only causes death and suffering but it also impacts financially on the lives of patients, their families as well as on the economy of countries and globally. Engaging all care providers both public and private in TB prevention and care is one of the most fundamental approaches to close gaps and reach all people who fall ill with TB. In 2021, of the 10.6 million people who fell ill with TB, 4.2 million people were missed by health systems [10]. It is estimated that a large proportion of these missed cases access and receive care of unknown quality from a wide array of health care providers not linked to public sector-based national TB programmes (non-state sector) [11]. COVID-19 disruptions have severely impacted access to essential TB services, with far fewer people being diagnosed and treated or provided with TB preventive treatment in 2020 and 2021 compared with 2019.

Data from countries (Fig. 47.2) and several project evaluations have shown that engaging all care providers through public-private mix (PPM)

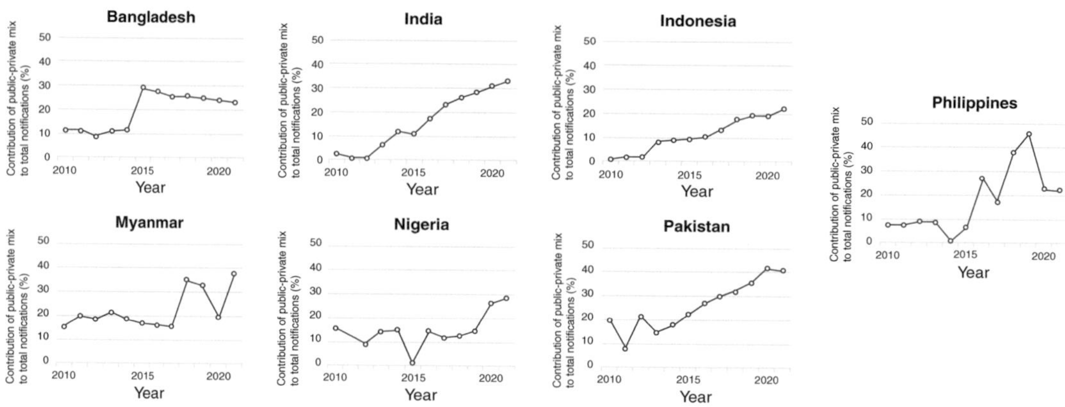

Fig. 47.2 Contribution of private sector engagement to national TB case notifications in the "Big Seven" PPM priority countries, 2010–2021, WHO Global TB Report 2022

approaches could help increase case detection (between 10% and 60%) and improve treatment outcomes (over 85%).

For the TB response, private sector engagement has been driven by a roadmap developed by WHO, the Public-Private Mix Working Group of the Stop TB Partnership, and global partners [12].

The roadmap recommends ten actions at national and global levels to scale up the engagement of all care providers towards universal access to care. National TB Programmes (NTPs) and their partners, in collaboration with the private sector, must:

(i) **Build** understanding about patient preferences, private sector dynamics and the rationale for engaging all providers.
(ii) **Set** appropriately ambitious PPM targets.
(iii) **Advocate** for political commitment, action, and investment in PPM.
(iv) **Allocate** adequate funding for engaging all providers, including by capitalizing on financing reforms for Universal Health Coverage.
(v) **Partner** with and build the capacity of intermediaries and key stakeholders.
(vi) **Establish** a supportive policy and regulatory framework.
(vii) **Adapt** flexible models of engagement applicable to local contexts.
(viii) **Harness** the power of digital technologies.
(ix) **Deliver** a range of financial and non-financial incentives and enablers.
(x) **Monitor** progress and build accountability.

The roadmap also contains a timeline with targets for 2020, 2022, 2025, and 2030, to showcase contribution to global end TB targets. Since 2018, over 20 countries are implementing the PPM roadmap with the support of WHO and partners.

47.4 Key Challenges and Opportunities

Despite the demonstrated importance and contribution of the private sector to health service delivery, challenges, and concerns remain. Many concerns are evidenced, such as the lack of regulation, the highly heterogeneous and fragmented nature of the private health sector and highly variable quality of care offered by the private sector [13, 14]. Monitoring of the private sector is also difficult due to differing information systems. Health services in the private sector can also pose a financial risk or burden for those affected due to high out-of-pocket costs, which is at odds with UHC objectives. There is also a lack of trust and concerns from the public sector on diversion of public resources for private use, or the undermining of primary care. These concerns need to be addressed as countries look at expanding private health sector engagement to ensure access to high-quality, equitable care free from catastrophic costs [15].

Lessons from private sector engagement during the COVID-19 pandemic also need to be leveraged. The pandemic presented an urgent need for health systems to work together and called for "all hands-on deck." WHO advised governments to take a whole-of-government and whole-of-society approach in their COVID-19 response by working along with the private health sector and civil society. While countries that had existing contracting mechanisms adapted quickly to engage the private health sector, others struggled to do so. Empanelment of private hospitals under national health insurance schemes, increased reimbursement for COVID-19 patients, price regulation and price capping for private service delivery, use of digital technologies for care and engaging private providers for non-COVID-19 treatment were some of the strategies adopted. These strategies and experiences need to be built into country efforts on UHC [11].

Several opportunities are emerging in the horizon where high level attention on UHC and on diseases like TB can be catalysed to expand private sector engagement for UHC. This includes the upcoming 2023 UN High Level Meetings on UHC and on ending TB that will bring together Heads of State to review progress and renew commitments. The digital revolution can also be utilized to overcome barriers of regulation and monitoring. For example, WHO is advancing efforts to develop enhanced private sector engagement TB data dashboards for countries to enhance monitoring and accountability of private sector collaboration in the TB response. Digital systems can enable additional innovations that further facilitate provider engagement at scale, such as digital vouchers for drugs and diagnostics, adherence monitoring technologies and digital payment of incentives and enablers to both patients and providers.

47.5 Conclusion

The advantages of private health sector engagement for UHC and clear strategies to facilitate this have been clearly elaborated in this chapter. However, to take this to scale, a mindset shift is required across countries to see the private sector as a co-creator and thought-partner in health service delivery. A more coherent and organised "whole of health sector" approach should be taken to private sector engagement building on WHO's Strategy on engaging the private health service delivery sector.

References

1. UN General Assembly, Transforming our world: the 2030 Agenda for Sustainable Development, 21 October 2015, A/RES/70/1. https://www.refworld.org/docid/57b6e3e44.html
2. Tracking Universal Health Coverage: 2021 global monitoring report. Geneva: World Health Organization and International Bank for Reconstruction and Development/The World Bank; 2021. https://www.who.int/publications/i/item/9789240040618. Accessed 7 Nov 2022
3. Hallo De Wolf A, Toebes B. Assessing Private Sector Involvement in Health Care and Universal health Coverage in light of the right to health. Health Hum Rights. 2016;18(2):79–92.
4. Grépin KA. Private sector an important but not dominant provider of key health Services in low- and middle-income countries. Health Aff (Millwood). 2016;35(7):1214–21. https://doi.org/10.1377/hlthaff.2015.0862.
5. Patouillard E, Goodman CA, Hanson KG, Mills AJ. Can working with the private for-profit sector improve utilization of quality health services by the poor? A systematic review of the literature. Int J Equity Health. 2007;6:17. https://doi.org/10.1186/1475-9276-6-17.
6. Das J, Hammer J, Leonard K. The quality of medical advice in low-income countries. J Econ Perspect. 2008;22(2):93–114. https://doi.org/10.1257/jep.22.2.93.
7. Hellowell M, O'Hanlon B. International organizations and the engagement of private healthcare providers: a background report for the advisory group on the governance of the private sector for UHC. Geneva: World Health Organization; 2020.
8. Clarke D, Doerr S, Hunter M, Schmets G, Soucat A, Paviza A. The private sector and universal health coverage. Bull World Health Organ. 2019;97(6):434–5. https://doi.org/10.2471/blt.18.225540.

9. Private sector landscape in mixed health systems. Geneva: World Health Organization; 2020. https://www.who.int/publications/i/item/9789240018303
10. Global tuberculosis report 2022. Geneva: World Health Organization; 2022. https://www.who.int/teams/global-tuberculosis-programme/tb-reports/global-tuberculosis-report-2022. Accessed 7 Nov 2022
11. Engaging private health care providers in TB care and prevention: a landscape analysis. Geneva: World Health Organization; 2021. https://apps.who.int/iris/handle/10665/333886. Accessed 7 Nov 2022
12. Public–private mix for TB prevention and care: a roadmap. Geneva: World Health Organization; 2018. https://www.who.int/publications/i/item/WHO-CDS-TB-2018.32. Accessed 7 Jan 2022
13. Mackintosh M, Channon A, Karan A, Selvaraj S, Cavagnero E, Zhao H. What is the private sector? Understanding private provision in the health systems of low-income and middle-income countries. Lancet. 2016;388(10044):596–605. https://doi.org/10.1016/S0140-6736(16)00342-1.
14. Hellowell M, O'Hanlon B. Managing Markets for Health (MM4H) Training Course; 2018. https://beam-exchange.org/community/events-training/details/803/
15. Towards better engagement of the private sector in health service delivery: a review of approaches to private sector engagement in Africa. Geneva: World Health Organization; 2022. https://www.who.int/publications/i/item/9789240047273. Accessed 7 Jan 2022

Community Engagement: Non-Governmental and Faith-based Organizations

48

Nicole Rose Nieman, Giovanni Putoto, and Andrea Atzori

Abstract

Non-Governmental and Faith-based Organizations (NGOs and FBOs, respectively) are a driving force in improving health and achieving equity in health for all people worldwide. Motivated by their values and invested in the social issues and lives of those they seek to improve, they often go where governments and large markets cannot or will not reach, including rural locations, conflict, and disaster areas. These organisations work closely within their local contexts, building an understanding of and relationships with the communities they serve, many of whom couldn't access or afford the essential services NGOs and FBOs step in to provide. Their knowledge and trust capital are essential elements in engaging communities, ensuring their participation in overcoming barriers to healthcare service delivery and quality of care. The kind of community engagement that is implemented by these organizations is a key factor both in routine circumstances and in emergency response, ensuring a continuum of care and delivery of effective services in states with fragile health systems.

Keywords

NGO · FBO · INGO · Continuum of care · Community engagement · Health equity

48.1 Aims of this Chapter

This chapter seeks to underscore the essentiality of non-governmental organisations (NGOs) and faith-based organisations (FBOs) within a global health response, demonstrating how they secure community engagement, a fundamental component required to grant continuum of care for those living in states with fragile health systems.

48.2 Introduction: Community Engagement as a Means to Grant Continuum of Care

Community engagement consists of involving the local population such as activists, trained staff, or community health workers, to play an active role in remediating for the lack of services, resources, or practical difficulties in accessing healthcare services [1]. The kind of community engagement implemented by NGOs and FBOs is a vital factor both in routine circumstances and in emergency responses.

N. R. Nieman (✉)
Missionary Sisters of the Sacred Heart, Rome, Italy

Missionary Sisters of the Sacred Heart, Chicago, IL, USA
e-mail: nrose@cabriniimpact.org

G. Putoto · A. Atzori
Doctors with Africa CUAMM, Padova, Italy
e-mail: g.putoto@cuamm.org; a.atzori@cuamm.org

M. C. B. Raviglione et al. (eds.), *Global Health Essentials*, Sustainable Development Goals Series,
https://doi.org/10.1007/978-3-031-33851-9_48

Continuum of care refers to an integrated approach providing health services to prevent, detect, treat, monitor, and refer patients to follow-up care in a comprehensive way [2]. It ultimately aims to support patients' medical care throughout their life. In already fragile healthcare systems, there are several problems hindering the successful implementation of the continuum of care and the quality of the services delivered, such as the lack of data related to patients, and the means to grant services to local communities [3]. In contexts where resources are lacking and numerous factors lead to the disruption of already vulnerable healthcare, the engagement of the local community becomes a necessary resource, filling the gap between patients and the healthcare system. To this end, NGOs and FBOs established in the community carrying out development projects play a pivotal role in fostering community engagement, thanks to the knowledge and trust they own among the local population. These elements are fundamental to grant continuum of care. The implementation of this model of care in fragile contexts must involve the beneficiaries' perspective as well as that of providers. The communities' active participation in the design and implementation of such services should be encouraged to improve and carry through affordable, accessible, and appropriate provision of services [4].

48.3 Background

NGOs and FBOs are a driving force in improving health and achieving equity in health globally. FBOs alone are major health providers in the developing world, providing an average of approximately 40 percent of services in sub-Saharan Africa [5]. The World Bank defines NGOs as "private organizations that pursue activities to relieve suffering, promote the interests of the poor, protect the environment, provide basic social services or undertake community development" (World Bank, 1995). Diverse in nature, NGOs and FBOs are shaped by the socio-economic, cultural, political, and legal situation of a country. Table 48.1 illustrates how CUAAM facilitates the continuum of care in the various contexts it serves.

Table 48.1 Overview of NGOs, FBOs, and International non-governmental organizations (INGOs) (Original table, free from copyright)

TABLE 1: OVERVIEW OF NGOS, FBOS, AND INGOS

SOME KEY FEATURES		NGO	FBO	INGO
Non-Profit	Any profits made are used as reserves for sustainability, or for expansion of operations / programs	✓	✓	✓
Values	Address a social, cultural, environmental, economic or political cause, and work towards the public good	✓	✓	✓
Faith-Based	Values and consequently the organization's mission are based on the values of a particular faith.	-	✓	(✓)
Private	Partially or entirely independent from government	✓	✓	✓
Legal Registration	It is mandatory in most countries for an NGO to be legally registered, however certain voluntary associations may be unregistered	(✓)	(✓)	✓
Geography	Operate locally or nationally	✓	✓	-
Geography	Operate internationally	-	-	✓
Engagement	Community engagement	✓	✓	(✓)
Engagement	Government engagement	(✓)	(✓)	✓

EXAMPLES OF HEALTH INGOS:

Broadly INGOs are divided into two categories: providers of humanitarian assistance, and of development assistance. Currently the International Federation of Red Cross and Red Crescent Societies (IFRC) is the world's largest humanitarian network, while Building Resources Across Communities (BRAC), which addresses social determinants of health, is the largest INGO in the world[1].

INGOs such as Médecins Sans Frontières (MSF), Project Hope, and Doctors of the World. offer emergency and long-term medical care in humanitarian situations[2]. There are several well-established international faith-based organizations with an extensive global reach, including Caritas (a confederation of 162 Catholic relief, development and social service organizations), The Joint (American Jewish Joint Distribution Committee), Islamic Relief Worldwide, and World Vision.[3]

[1] www.ifrc.org, www.brac.net

[2] www.msf.org, www.projecthope.org, https://doctorsoftheworld.org/

EXAMPLES OF POTENTIAL CHALLENGES	
Sustainability	May rely on volunteers and charitable giving (donations, grants, and in-kind gifts), which can be volatile and impact on an organizations projects, human resources, etc.
Hiring and Retaining Staff	NGOs / FBOs often pay less than profit-driven employees, and may lack appropriate systems to train and develop their employees. Additionally, employees maybe overworked or have to work in several different areas
Dependency	Over reliance on a funder(s) may impede an organization's ability to determine its direction or remain independent
Relevance	Several factors could impact on an organization's ability to remain relevant, for example, changes that may require additional finance (e.g., technology), refusal or inability to implement recognized good practice, or refusal or inability to adapt to changes within a community
Uncooperative	Possessiveness of an organization of a geographic area or project, viewing other NGOs/ FBOs as threatening or competing for the same funds or acknowledgment, instead of cooperating with one another and coordinating assistance

EXAMPLES OF POTENTIAL STRENGTHS:	
Mission Driven	Attract skilled, values-aligned individuals willing to be paid less for the satisfaction of working for a cause
Flexible and Responsive	Adapt to changes quickly and try innovative approaches as profit is not a motive, and closeness to the communities worked
Marginalized	Identify and respond to the needs of the most marginalized individuals and communities
Research	Contribute to research that shapes policy and strengthens health systems
Bridging devides	Inform government of local realities, and advocate for equitable service provision

[3] www.caritas.org, www.jdc.org, https://islamic-relief.org/, www.wvi.org

It was through its work with NGOs and FBOs that the WHO prepared for the Alma-Ata Declaration of 1978, to better understand healthcare in the developing world, and from this established the concept of primary healthcare [5]. Through implementation and holding governments to account, NGOs and FBOs continue to play an essential role in global health, moving the SDGs (and previously the MDGs) and universal health coverage from international commitment to concrete realisation. At a local level, given an institutional presence established in a territory, and large composition of community members, NGOs and FBOs are primed to understand the needs of the people and how to serve them.

48.4 Description of the Issue

From people living with chronic illness to expectant mothers, patients and their families have complex and changing needs, many of whom are additionally coping with the complications of poverty and discrimination. Patients require an effective continuum of care throughout their life cycle, and between places of caregiving, including households and outreach services [6]. Prime examples of challenges encountered in developing contexts which impede quality healthcare delivery include:

48.4.1 Lack of Data

Inequitable distribution of research efforts and funds directed towards populations suffering the world's greatest health problems is a major global health issue [7, 8]. At a country level, data gaps may arise due to inadequate national data collection and monitoring infrastructure, or in populations under-served by their national health system [9]. Accurate and timely data is required for treating individual patients, improving clinical care, and developing new ways of predicting or diagnosing illness.

48.4.2 Inequity and Impediments to Access

Fragile states have been defined as those where the government cannot or will not deliver basic services to the population, including vulnerable groups (DFID, 2005). For-profit health companies have little incentive to operate in marginated communities. In 2017, the World Bank and WHO produced a report detailing that at least half of the world's population cannot obtain essential health services, with millions of households pushed into poverty each year because they must pay for health care out of pocket [10]. Factors such as far travel distances, long wait times, and unaffordable services impede access, particularly in rural contexts.

48.4.3 Ignoring Culture and Tradition

Paramount to engaging communities is understanding the interplay of culture and tradition with beliefs and behaviours. This impacts on how, with whom and where to communicate messaging. If a service or intervention is not accepted within a community, it will likely fail, particularly in confronting stigmatised issues or communally accepted practices, for example, female genital mutilation. Acknowledging and working alongside decision-makers is foundational in unlocking patient participation.

48.5 Approach to Solutions

By design NGOs and FBOs can bridge these divides, connecting health seekers to services. Firstly, their bottom line is mission, not profit. Being values driven allows them to go where governments and large markets cannot, or won't reach, including rural locations and conflict and disaster areas. Secondly, their geographical establishment affords them knowledge of custom, tradition, and language, facilitating authentic and effective engagement. Through basic anthropological approaches they build relationship and ultimately trust, allowing them to tap into local resources, for example, youth mobilisers and local radio airtime, facilitating the distribution of health messaging. Thirdly, they have access to critical data. Through relevant and timely research in programme evaluation and health policy and advocacy, this data has the potential to enable improved health, reduced health inequities and strengthened health systems, particularly for marginalised groups and developing contexts [9]. Further, disease surveillance data collected by NGOs and FBOs provides an essential early warning system.

48.6 Illustrating the Power of Community Engagement

The examples below illustrate approaches used by two organisations in strengthening the continuum of care between communities and peripheral health centres in rural, developing contexts:

48.6.1 Improving Maternal and Child Health (MNCH) Outcomes [11]

In Ethiopia, the INGO Doctors with Africa CUAMM implemented a multifaceted MNCH project in three districts in South West Shoa Zone, Oromia region. The project aimed to improve access to and utilisation of MNCH services along the continuum of care focusing mainly on health centres and the community. In the districts, CUAMM focused on key determinants of maternal health service access and utilisation, including distance to health facilities, attitude towards and knowledge of maternal health care, perceived quality of services, birth preparedness, and involvement of the family members in decision-making on delivery place. CUAMM's interventions comprehensively addressed cultural, geographical, and financial barriers, including referrals. Between the pre-intervention period and the late intervention period, data evidenced that CUAMM's interventions subsequently resulted in both a substantial increase in the coverage of receipt of all three ante-natal care components, and skilled birth attendants at delivery. Figure 48.1 illustrates how CUAAM facilitates the continuum of care within the communities it serves.

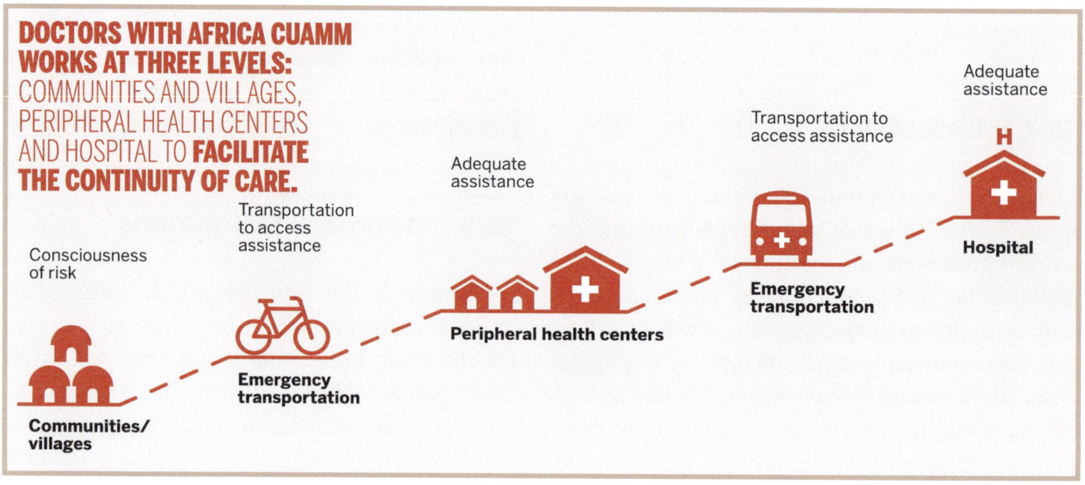

Fig. 48.1 Facilitation of continuity of care by an INGO. Figure courtesy of Doctors with Africa CUAMM www.doctorswithafrica.org

48.6.2 Provision of Culturally Sensitive Services

In eSwatini, the FBO Cabrini Ministries eSwatini has utilised its strong relationships within the Ngcampalala, Gamedze, and Mamba chiefdoms to deliver holistic, comprehensive, integrated care for over 50 years. Cabrini respects and works with traditional leadership, religious leaders, traditional healers, government officials, and community health workers among others. During the height of the HIV/AIDS pandemic in eSwatini, Cabrini provided palliative care. When ARVs were introduced and the community were hesitant in taking them, it leveraged trust capital, advocating within the community for the use of life-saving therapy. It further reduced loss to follow-up by actively calling, visiting home-to-home, running support groups, and placing clinical dispensing sites within remote areas. Today, Cabrini's community engagement model saw it attain UNAIDS's 90-90-90 strategy within its catchment area, and successful uptake of its other culturally sensitive services including cervical cancer screening and gender-based violence prevention initiatives.

48.7 Main Conclusions and Recommendations

Strengthening health systems at primary healthcare level with quality delivery of services to last-mile beneficiaries is the key to cope with current and future health crises, whatever their nature. Any action taken needs to be in solidarity with communities, supporting them to become protagonists and actors for change. In states with fragile health systems, engagement with local communities is a crucial factor in a global health response and is made possible by NGOs and FBOs, often the only service providers in those areas. Given the vital role that NGOs and FBOs play, strengthening their capacity and sustainability, and supporting them to coordinate with one another and collaborate with local government is essential. More needs to be done in creating enabling environments where these organisations can flourish, playing an increasingly intentional and active role in prevention, treatment, and care at grassroots level, and contributing to research which impacts on policy and health systems strengthening.

References

1. Tindana PO, Singh JA, Tracy CS, Upshur REG, Daar AS, Singer PA, et al. Grand challenges in Global Health: community engagement in research in developing countries. PLoS Med. 2007;4(9):e273. https://doi.org/10.1371/journal.pmed.0040273.
2. Evashwick C. Creating the continuum of care. Health Matrix. 1989;7(1):30–9.
3. World Health Organization, Global Health Cluster, Quality Improvement Task Team June 2020: Quality of Care in Humanitarian Settings. https://cdn.who.int/media/docs/default-source/quality-of-care/quality-of-care-in-humanitarian-settings-june-2020.pdf?sfvrsn=db78f8d4_1
4. World Health Organization, Declaration of Alma Ata, International Conference on Primary Health Care, Alma-Ata, USSR; 6–12 September 1978. https://cdn.who.int/media/docs/default-source/documents/almaata-declaration-en.pdf?sfvrsn=7b3c2167_2
5. World Health Organization. Building from common foundations: the World Health Organization and faith-based organizations in primary healthcare. Gary Bandy, Alan Crouch U' [et al]. Edited by Ted Karpf and Alex Ross; 2008. https://apps.who.int/iris/handle/10665/43884
6. World Health Organization. The World Health Report 2005. Make every mother and child count ISBN 92 4 156290 0 (NLM Classification: WA 540.1) ISSN 1020-3311. https://www.who.int/publications/i/item/9241562900
7. Delisle H, Roberts JH, Munro M, et al. The role of NGOs in global health research for development. Health Res Policy Sys. 2005;3:3. https://doi.org/10.1186/1478-4505-3-3.
8. Known as the "10/90 gap" where less than 10 percent of all health research funding is used to address 90 percent of the world's burden of disease. Global Forum for Health Research: The 10/90 report on health research 2000, c/o World Health Organization; April 2000. https://www.files.ethz.ch/isn/20413/10.90.FULLTEXT.pdf
9. Masefield SC, et al. Repurposing NGO data for better research outcomes: A scoping review of the use and secondary analysis of NGO data in health

policy and systems research. Health Res Policy Syst. 2020;18(1):1–22. https://doi.org/10.1186/s12961-020-00577-x.

10. World Bank and WHO: Half the world lacks access to essential health services, 100 million still pushed into extreme poverty because of health expenses; 13 December 2017. https://www.who.int/news/item/13-12-2017-world-bank-and-who-half-the-world-lacks-access-to-essential-health-services-100-million-still-pushed-into-extreme-poverty-because-of-health-expenses

11. Wilunda C, Tanaka S, Putoto G, et al. Evaluation of a maternal health care project in south west Shoa zone, Ethiopia: before-and-after comparison. Reprod Health. 2016;13:95. https://doi.org/10.1186/s12978-016-0213-1.

Selection and Use of Essential Medicines

49

Lorenzo Moja and Benedikt Huttner

Abstract

Essential medicines are those that satisfy the priority health care needs of a population. They are evaluated for efficacy and safety and comparative cost-effectiveness. They are intended to be available in functioning health systems at all times, in appropriate dosage forms, of assured quality and at prices individuals and health systems can afford. However, this is seldomly true. The World Health Organisation Model List of Essential Medicines and Model List of Essential Medicines for Children are updated and published every 2 years, intended as a guide for countries to adopt or adapt in accordance with local priorities and treatment guidelines for the development and updating of national essential medicines lists. Selection of a limited number of medicines as essential can lead to improved access through efficient procurement and distribution, support more appropriate prescribing and use, and lower costs for both health care systems and for patients.

Keywords

Essential medicines · Essential medicine list (EML) · Access · Medicine patent pools · AWaRe

49.1 Introduction

In the majority of countries thousands of medicines are available accounting for more than a trillion US Dollars per year in spending globally [1]. This amount is about a half of what is the annual global spending on food [2]. However, global spending on medicines is increasing more rapidly than spending on food.

There is a vicious circle of forces pushing the growth of the pharmaceutical market. In ideal world, new medicines represent an improvement over those previously available, which is used as justification to market the new products at higher prices. The promise of larger benefits then serves as an incentive to develop more new medicines which are then marketed at even higher prices.

In "real life" many medicines offer no, or at best only small, additional clinical benefit in comparison to older, available, alternatives. Furthermore, many medicines enter the market with insufficiently solid data supporting their efficacy and guiding clinical use as the requirements to obtain market approval by regulatory agencies are not too stringent. Post-marketing

L. Moja (✉) · B. Huttner
Secretariat of the Model List of Essential Medicines, Department of Health Products Policy and Standards, World Health Organization, Geneva, Switzerland
e-mail: mojal@who.int; bhuttner@who.int

M. C. B. Raviglione et al. (eds.), *Global Health Essentials*, Sustainable Development Goals Series,
https://doi.org/10.1007/978-3-031-33851-9_49

data might show lower treatment effects and benefits for patients than stipulated based on the trials used for approval. However, once a medicine enters the market it usually remains there (unless major safety concerns emerge). It is not too difficult to find a market niche for any given product resulting in low-value care and large real and opportunity costs for the health care system, societies, and patients. These are ubiquitous challenges.

49.2 WHO Model List of Essential Medicines

Since 1977, the World Health Organisation (WHO) has pioneered the concept that "some medicines are more important than others" through the Model List of Essential Medicines (WHO EML) [3]. There is now a global understanding among stakeholders that identifying essential medicines is an important element of strategies that aim at improving individual and public health and achieving universal health coverage, without dispersing resources. Another aim of the list is to provide guidance on appropriate use of essential medicines, often in complementarity with guidelines. If a medicine is listed as an essential medicine, it should be prioritized as part of guideline development. Ideally, the same evidence base should be both informing EML and guideline decisions.

WHO defines essential medicines as those that "satisfy the priority health care needs of the population, to which everyone should have access at all times, and that all governments should ensure are available, affordable and of assured quality for their populations [4]. They are selected with due regard to public health relevance, evidence on efficacy and safety (i.e., the magnitude of the net benefit must be relevant), and their selection take into consideration comparative costs and cost-effectiveness." Since 2001 the criteria for selection of essential medicines further state that "the absolute cost of a medicine is not a reason to exclude it from the WHO EML if it meets the stated selection criteria."

The first EML in 1977 listed about 200 medicines. Over the following four decades, the number of essential molecules has more than doubled to 479 medicines (350 of which are recommended for children) on the 2021 EML [5].

While covering a wide range of global health needs, the 479 essential medicines WHO recommends represent only a small proportion of the total number of medicines available.

49.3 Transparency on What Is Essential

A key characteristic of the WHO EML and other health product prioritization lists should be the transparency of the process and reporting of updating national EML (NEMLs) and reimbursement lists. Transparency helps to ensure trust in the decisions made. Updated NEMLs and reimbursement lists should be available in the public domain, such as on ministry of health websites.

Evidence synthesis and its critical appraisal have a central role in recognizing the value of a medicine. At WHO, changes or additions to the WHO Model List are made through the application process [6]. The WHO EML Expert Committee reviews applications and makes its decisions whether to include a medicine or not based on evidence presented in relation to disease burden, evidence of efficacy and safety, and cost and cost-effectiveness considerations. Applications for additions or changes to the Model List can be submitted by anyone: researchers, non-governmental organizations, academic institutions, patient groups or networks, pharmaceutical companies, or WHO technical departments. All applications, reviews, and comments will be posted on the WHO Essential Medicines Selection webpage, and a detailed report on decisions and recommendations by the Expert Committee, including the updated Model List, is released in the public domain. It is not expected that all countries will have the capacity or need to adopt exactly the same WHO processes, with full analysis of all dimensions (i.e., benefits, harms, cost and cost-effectiveness, feasibility, pharmacopeia), even at national level. Nevertheless, transparency is essential to assure an accountable medicines selection process.

49.4 One List with Broad Coverage

Essential medicines are used across the spectrum of patient care: from disease prevention (e.g., vaccines, pre-exposure prophylaxis of HIV), through treatment and management (e.g., medicines for chronic non-communicable diseases), to cure (e.g., antibiotics and some cancer medicines). It is important to note that the WHO EML also includes many medicines for rare diseases, as more value is placed in the absolute benefits associated with the use of a medicine than the incidence or prevalence of the disease per se.

Among all medicines on the WHO EML, about a half are recommended and used in the primary health care setting (referred as "core" medicines) while the other half targets secondary care facilities and hospitals (referred as "complementary" medicines, for which specialized diagnostic or monitoring facilities, and/or specialists are needed). Since the first WHO EML several medicines requiring specialized facilities with skilled health care professionals and sophisticated diagnostic capacities have been introduced, such as immunotherapies targeting cancers, lung surfactant for premature neonates or last-resort antibiotics.

49.5 Availability and Access Gaps

According to the WHO definition "Essential medicines of assured quality are intended to be available in functioning health systems at all times, in adequate amounts, in appropriate dosage forms; and at prices individuals and the community can afford." Access to essential medicines is heavily dependent on health system capacity to adequately diagnose and manage the diseases and on the availability and affordability of these medicines. During the period 2007–2014, the median availability (i.e., number of facilities with essential medicines in stock) of selected essential medicines in the public sector of all 78 low-income and lower-middle-income countries was 58% [7]. When specifically looking at essential medicines for non-communicable chronic diseases, this percentage was only 35% [8].

Using national EMLs as the basis for preferred procurement facilitates effective tendering processes. Focusing on high-volume purchasing of fewer medicines creates ideal conditions for competition. Priority lists of essential medicines can also be used at the subnational level, for example, at the regional or hospital level where drugs and therapeutics committees can develop procurement or reimbursement lists increasing the leverage to negotiate prices that are affordable at the community level.

49.6 International Strategies to Improve Access to Essential Medicines

In many countries, patients have to pay for most medicines out of pocket. Generics and biosimilars of essential medicines can be more affordable than originator brand molecules. The WHO EML takes this into account by being brand agnostic and specifically mentioning generics and biosimilars. However in recent surveys, generic availability was only 64% in public health facilities, and much less in private facilities [9].

Improving access to novel medicines can be facilitated through new strategies. One strategy is the use of patent pools, which enable third parties (i.e., generic manufacturers) to acquire nonexclusive licenses for the intellectual property that otherwise keeps them from marketing these medicines in many jurisdictions. Another strategy is the WHO's prequalification program, which helps low- and middle-income countries in manufacturing, regulating, and monitoring the quality of medicines considered important for public health. Be recommended by WHO as an essential medicine is a precondition to activate these strategies [3].

49.7 National Essential Medicines Lists

The WHO EML represents an international reference standard for what medicines—those that provide the best value in terms of benefits for individuals and communities—a capable and responsible health system should provide. It is intended to serve as a guide for countries to develop and maintain their own NEML as basis for public sector procurement and reimbursement of medicines according to national needs [6]. Some examples from countries illustrate how NEMLs can contribute for achieving universal health coverage.

India has implemented an NEML since 1996. Through the revision of the NEML India operationalizes coverage policies, determining which additional diseases and medicines will made available to its citizens. With the revision of the NEML in 2015 India has projected a 30% increase in its population's access to important medicines, improving or saving the life of 400 million additional people [10].

In China, the national EML became central in defining benefits under the insurance schemes since 1982, leading to large-scale increase in the number of people covered under formal insurance programs, which reached almost 100% coverage since 2003 [11]. Procurement of essential medicines is facilitated over non-essential medicines, and the former are reimbursed at higher rates than non-essential medicines.

It is important to note that the WHO EML is relevant for all countries and not merely for under-resourced health systems. Other countries not directly using the WHO EML often have reimbursement lists that act similarly to the WHO EML in prioritizing some medicines over others.

Canada has recently evaluated the potential impact of adopting a universal ambulatory list free of charge to patients [12]. Adopting a similar list in Canada would decrease financial burden on patients that are not covered by insurance mechanisms. A preliminary list of 125 medicines was shown to cover more than 90% of prescriptions and patients seen at city clinics and the suburban sites [13]. A randomized controlled trial tested free distribution of essential medicines against usual medicine access (e.g., involving co-payments and deductibles), showing improved medicine adherence and reduce total health care costs in patients receiving free distribution [14].

49.8 Medicine Monitoring

The WHO EML is also designed to deliver important messages on appropriate medicine use. Health professionals and policy makers need to be informed about medicine availability and prices so they can assess the impact of drug policies. This invariably includes some level of monitoring of prescription and price trends across medicines and diseases. Monitoring supports decision-making contrasting and selecting policy options for making medicines more affordable and available and to ensure system accountability. For example, in 2017, in response to the growing challenge of antimicrobial resistance, antibiotics on the WHO EML were reviewed and categorized into three groups: ACCESS, WATCH, and RESERVE—the WHO AWaRe categorization [15]—providing key guidance on when to use specific antibiotics and for which infections, in order to reduce the risk of antimicrobial resistance without restricting access to these vital medicines. The AWaRe categorization is considered a useful tool for monitoring antibiotic consumption, defining targets and monitoring the effects of stewardship policies that aim to optimize antibiotic use, privileging ACCESS over WATCH antibiotics, and curb antimicrobial resistance. The WHO released a country-level target of at least 60% of total antibiotic consumption being ACCESS group antibiotics for all countries.

Readers should be aware that essential medicines and related policies vary widely across countries, and, in some cases, both selection and use might be unsatisfactory in relation to what readers expect. However, the market of essential medicines is rapidly evolving: appropriate promotion of essential medicines is key to provide patients with better health care.

References

1. IQVIA Institute for Human Data Science. 2018 and Beyond: Outlook and Turning Points; 2018. https://www.iqvia.com/insights/the-iqvia-institute/reports/2018-and-beyond-outlook-and-turning-points
2. Hassoun-Kheir N, van Werkhoven CH, Dunning J, Jaenisch T, van Beek J, Bielicki J, et al. Perpetual observational studies: new strategies to support efficient implementation of observational studies and randomized trials in infectious diseases. Clin Microbiol Infect. 2022;28:1528–32. https://doi.org/10.1016/j.cmi.2022.07.024.
3. 't Hoen EF, Hogerzeil HV, Quick JD, Sillo HB. A quiet revolution in global public health: the world health organization's prequalification of medicines programme. J Public Health Policy. 2014;35(2):137–61. https://doi.org/10.1057/jphp.2013.53.
4. Executive Board 109/8. WHO medicines strategy Revised procedure for updating WHO's Model List of Essential Drugs. December 2001. https://apps.who.int/gb/e/e_eb109.html
5. World Health Organization Model List of Essential Medicines – 22nd List, 2021. Geneva: World Health Organization (WHO/MHP/HPS/EML/2021.02). Licence: CC BY-NC-SA 3.0 IGO; 2021. https://www.who.int/publications/i/item/WHO-MHP-HPS-EML-2021.02
6. Selection of essential medicines at country level: using the WHO model list of essential medicines to update a national essential medicines list. Geneva: World Health Organization. Licence: CC BY-NC-SA 3.0 IGO; 2020. https://apps.who.int/iris/bitstream/handle/10665/330898/9789241515443-eng.pdf
7. United nations. The millennium development goals report 2015. New York; 2015. https://www.un.org/millenniumgoals/2015_MDG_Report/pdf/MDG%202015%20rev%20(July%201).pdf
8. Mendis S, Fukino K, Cameron A, Laing R, Filipe A Jr, Khatib O, et al. The availability and affordability of selected essential medicines for chronic diseases in six low- and middle-income countries. Bull World Health Organ. 2007;85(4):279–88. https://doi.org/10.2471/blt.06.033647.
9. Bazargani YT, Ewen M, de Boer A, Leufkens HG, Mantel-Teeuwisse AK. Essential medicines are more available than other medicines around the globe. PLoS One. 2014;9(2):e87576. https://doi.org/10.1371/journal.pone.0087576.
10. Maiti R, Bhatia V, Padhy BM, Hota D. Essential medicines: an Indian perspective. Indian J Community Med. 2015;40(4):223–32. https://doi.org/10.4103/0970-0218.164382.
11. Barber SL, Huang B, Santoso B, Laing R, Paris V, Wu C. The reform of the essential medicines system in China: a comprehensive approach to universal coverage. J Glob Health. 2013;3(1):010303. https://doi.org/10.7189/jogh.03.010303.
12. Eom G, Grootendorst P, Duffin J. The case for an essential medicines list for Canada. CMAJ. 2016;188(17–18):E499–503. https://doi.org/10.1503/cmaj.160134.
13. Taglione MS, Ahmad H, Slater M, Aliarzadeh B, Glazier RH, Laupacis A, et al. Development of a preliminary essential medicines list for Canada. CMAJ Open. 2017;5(1):E137–E43. https://doi.org/10.9778/cmajo.20160122.
14. Persaud N, Bedard M, Boozary A, Glazier RH, Gomes T, Hwang SW, et al. Adherence at 2 years with distribution of essential medicines at no charge: the CLEAN meds randomized clinical trial. PLoS Med. 2021;18(5):e1003590. https://doi.org/10.1371/journal.pmed.1003590.
15. Sharland M, Pulcini C, Harbarth S, Zeng M, Gandra S, Mathur S, et al. Classifying antibiotics in the WHO essential medicines list for optimal use-be AWaRe. Lancet Infect Dis. 2018;18(1):18–20. https://doi.org/10.1016/S1473-3099(17)30724-7.

50 Equitable Access to Medicines, Vaccines, and Medical Devices

Tido von Schoen-Angerer
and James Packard Love

Abstract

This chapter provides an overview over the main initiatives to improve equitable access to health technologies in low- and middle-income countries. Improvements to access to medicines were made through medicine selection and better supply management, price reductions through generic competition, and not-for-profit development of medicines for neglected diseases. Vaccination coverage was successfully increased through international efforts, initially for basic vaccines and over the last two decades also for newer vaccines. Diagnostics remains the weakest link with insufficient laboratory infrastructure and tests missing for many diseases. High prices of new health technologies and lack of innovation for non-profitable diseases remain general challenges. New ways to coordinate and finance innovation have been developed and need more political support.

Unfortunately, access lessons from previous decades were ignored during the Covid-19 pandemic, with sobering results. Pandemic preparedness therefore needs to include guarantees for the equitable sharing of health technologies.

Keywords

Access · Medicines · Vaccines · Intellectual property · WTO · TRIPS agreement · Medicine patent pools · Pre-qualification

50.1 Access to Medicines

In 1977, the World Health Organisation (WHO) established its first essential medicines list, and in 1982 it began to support countries to establish reliable supply systems. This increased the number of people estimated to have access to essential medicines from 2.1 billion in 1977 to 3.8 billion in the late 1990s [1, 2].

50.1.1 Intellectual Property Protection of Health Technologies

Prior to the establishment of the World Trade Organization (WTO) in 1995, a handful of developing countries had robust patent exceptions for medicines, or sufficiently shorter terms, restrictive patentability criteria or lax enforcement to enable access to generic versions. The WTO's "Trade-Related Aspects of Intellectual Property Rights agreement" (TRIPS agreement) created new standards for patent protection including

T. von Schoen-Angerer (✉)
Fribourg University, Fribourg, Switzerland

J. P. Love
Knowledge Ecology International (KEI), Washington, DC, USA
e-mail: james.love@keionline.org

M. C. B. Raviglione et al. (eds.), *Global Health Essentials*, Sustainable Development Goals Series,
https://doi.org/10.1007/978-3-031-33851-9_50

mandatory 20-year terms and restrictions on exceptions. Some developing countries benefited from a 10-year transition period, and least developed countries continue to benefit from extensions of the transition period, set to expire in 2034. Over time, the introduction of TRIPS compliant patent laws and more aggressive enforcement practices have had a significant negative impact on affordability and access [3].

50.1.2 The AIDS Crisis and Access to Medicines

In 1997, life-saving antiretroviral triple therapy became available in high-income countries at over US$10,000 per person per year.

Faced with growing alarm over avoidable AIDS deaths in developing countries, outcry by patient and health advocacy groups, and a lawsuit by 39 drug companies over South Africa's patent law, a series of events unfolded in 2001 [3]:

- WTO adopted the Doha Declaration on TRIPS and Public Health, declaring that the TRIPS agreement would be "interpreted and implemented in a manner supportive of WTO members' right to protect public health and, in particular, to promote access to medicines for all."
- Generic combination treatments for HIV from India became available for a dollar per day (first-generation HIV medicines were not patented in India and several low- and middle-income countries—LMIC).
- The Global Fund for HIV, Tuberculosis, and Malaria was created.
- WHO began quality assessment of medicines through its pre-qualification program [4].

Since 2001, a number of compulsory licensing cases were pursued in Low and Middle Income countries (LMIC), for medicines to treat HIV, hepatitis C (HCV), cancer, heart disease, and influenza. A handful of these cases were successful, including in 2003, the settlement of the Hazel Tau case in South Africa that extended access to an important HIV cocktail throughout Sub-Saharan Africa, and notable cases in India, Indonesia, Malaysia, Thailand, Ukraine, Brazil, and Ecuador. Many other compulsory licensing cases were unsuccessful, due to a combination of restrictive national legal frameworks and political pressure from pharmaceutical companies and governments in the USA and Europe. By 2011, generic prices for first-line HIV treatment were reduced to $61 per year for many LMIC (see Fig. 50.1), including as 3-in-1 combination not available in high-income countries [5].

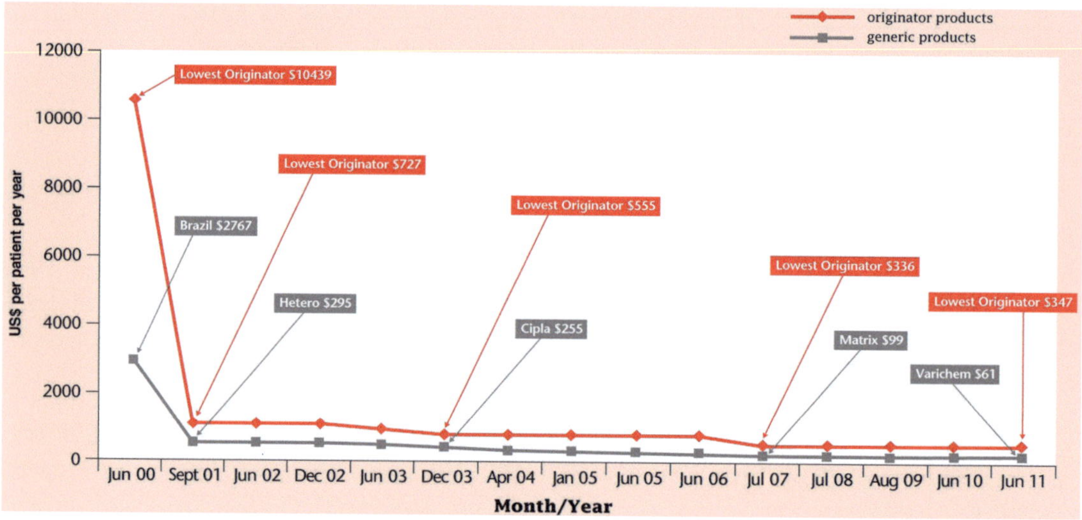

Fig. 50.1 Generic competition as a catalyst for price reduction. The fall in the price of first-line HIV treatment stavudine (d4T), lamivudine (3TC), and nevirapine (NVP) between 2000 and 2011. Courtesy of MSF Untangling the Web of Antiretroviral Price Reductions. 14th edition July 2011

For a group of roughly 115 developing countries, beginning in 2011, voluntary licensing of newer drugs for HIV, hepatitis B and C through the Medicines Patent Pool (MPP) have become common, enhancing affordability and access. For countries excluded from the geographic area of these licenses and for other diseases, most notably non-communicable diseases, new products are often available from a single supplier at high and restrictive prices.

Through these combined efforts (Table 50.1), access to HIV treatment increased from a few thousand in LMIC in 2000 to 28.2 million individuals as of 2021.

Table 50.1 Major international initiatives and policies affecting access to health technologies

Name of initiative	Category	Creation or starting date	Meaning for access
WHO essential medicines list	WHO program	1977	Prioritizes medicines that should be available at all times. Updated regularly
Expanded Program on immunization	WHO program	1974	First coordinated effort to expand immunization coverage
WHO pre-qualification	WHO program	1987 for vaccines 2001 for medicines 2010 for diagnostics and medical devices	Quality assessment of products. Supports regulatory and funding decisions
Gavi, the Vaccine Alliance	Multilateral funding organization	2000	Funds vaccination programs to increase access to new and underused vaccines
Doha Declaration on TRIPS and Public Health	Decision by the World Trade Organization ministerial conference	2001	Clarified the flexibilities enshrined in the TRIPS agreement to ensure access to health technologies, including strict patentability criteria and compulsory licensing
Global Fund to fight AIDS, TB and malaria	Multilateral funding organization	2001	Funds prevention and treatment in low- and middle-income countries
United States President's Emergency Plan for AIDS Relief (PEPFAR)	U.S. funding initiative	2003	Funds HIV/AIDS programs in more than 50 countries
Product Development Partnerships (PDPs)	Not-for-profit organizations	Examples: Medicines for Malaria Venture 1999, TB Alliance 2000, Drugs for Neglected Diseases initiative 2003, FIND 2003	Not-for-profit product developers, funded by governments and philanthropy
Unitaid	Multilateral funding organization	2006	Funds initiatives that reduce prices and that bring innovative products to low- and middle-income countries
Medicines Patent Pool	Foundation	2010	Negotiates agreements to allow generic production of medicines

50.2 Vaccines

WHO's Expanded Program on Immunization was created in 1974 to scale up basic vaccination. Vaccines were inexpensive and the main challenge was logistical, including establishing reliable cold chains. Through UNICEF's Universal Childhood Immunization Initiative, 62% of children in poorest countries had received three doses of diphtheria-tetanus-pertussis vaccination by 1990. However, LMIC were not yet benefiting from new and more expensive vaccines. To overcome this inequality, the Children's Vaccine Initiative was created in 1990, succeeded by the Vaccine Alliance Gavi in 2000. Gavi has driven the introduction and/or increased uptake of vaccines against hepatitis B, Hib, yellow fever, pneumococcus, rotavirus, inactivated polio, and papilloma virus [6]. Challenges remain. First, progress is uneven across countries. Second, countries lose Gavi support once their income rises even if they cannot afford the recently introduced vaccines—Gavi modified its criteria in 2021 so that children in vulnerable settings would still be supported. Third, price reductions through bulk purchasing and production in middle-income countries were successful for some vaccines but less so for others. The pneumococcal vaccine still costs $3.5 per dose, partially because of production complexity but also because Gavi's funding mechanism favored producers in high-income countries [7].

50.3 Diagnostics

Diagnosis is the weakest link in the care cascade with 47% of the world's population having little to no access to diagnostics [8]. For decades, the focus has been on clinical decision algorithms. Investment in laboratory staff and infrastructure as well as diagnostic development remains insufficient. A watershed moment was the widespread introduction of point-of-care tests for malaria, performed with a few blood drops. FIND (Foundation for Innovative New Diagnostics) was founded to develop simple and affordable diagnostics for the needs of LMIC. WHO began quality pre-qualification for diagnostics in 2010. The simplification of molecular diagnostics (PCR) remains a particular challenge, but new technology platforms have the potential to revolutionize diagnosis in LMIC.

50.4 Intellectual Property and Innovation

Intellectual property fails to stimulate innovation in areas that industry does not consider profitable. Only 0.3% of new chemical entities coming to market from 2000 to 2011 were for tropical diseases and tuberculosis although they represented 11% of the global disease burden [9].

In the early 2000s, several not-for-profit product development partnerships (PDPs) were created and funded by governments and philanthropy to address market failures in research and development (R&D). PDPs have shown that product development is cost-effective outside industry [10].

A wide range of needs not addressed through patent incentives or PDP's remains. For example, for the development of new antibiotics, repurposing existing off-patent medicines, identifying patients which do not benefit from products, and the innovation in areas where patent thickets require time consuming and costly efforts to obtain licenses, patents are either ineffective as an incentive or a barrier to innovation. Patents are also unhelpful in rewarding scientific advances that are pre-commercial.

50.4.1 Mechanisms to Stimulate Innovation that Do Not Lead to High Prices

Significant thinking and debate have gone into incentive mechanisms that could drive innovation towards agreed global health priorities without leading to high product prices.

The reform of the incentive mechanisms would involve the progressive migration from exclusive rights to a combination of monetary rewards for final products (market entry rewards) and upstream advances in useful science (open-source dividends, best progress, and milestone prizes). The reform of the international norms would progressively replace the reliance on exclusive rights in inventions and data with obligations to support biomedical R&D through a combination of incentives, subsidies, and direct funding [11].

Since 2003, the WHO created three expert groups and one intergovernmental working group on public health, innovation, and intellectual property rights to consider these reforms.

In 2016, the United Nations High Level Panel on Access to Medicines recommended a binding convention on coordination and financing of R&D [12]. Proposals to delink R&D from monopolies and high prices and to migrate global R&D norms from a sole focus on intellectual property to broader and more comprehensive and flexible obligations have met stiff opposition from the pharmaceutical industry and the Bill and Melinda Gates Foundation.

50.5 Covid-19

Expectations that access lessons could be applied to ensure rapid and equal access to Covid-19 technologies were disappointed. High-income countries quickly bought up available supplies of vaccines. The Covax Allocation Mechanism, established to channel vaccines into LMIC, secured less than half of the two billion doses projected for 2021 due to insufficient funds and donations. Vaccination coverage in October 2021 was only 4 doses per 100 people in low-income countries. The Covid-19 technology access pool was set up to share technology but received insufficient licenses. Despite early calls by LMIC to waive intellectual property rights for Covid-19, and the liberal use of compulsory licenses in the USA [13], it took countries two years to agree on a limited text that is unlikely to expand access to Covid-19 tools. Negotiations on an international pandemic treaty have started in 2022: success will depend on finding agreement that guarantees equitable access to technologies for any future pandemic [14].

50.6 Conclusions and Recommendations

Over the last 50 years, significant progress has been made towards access to medicines, vaccines, and diagnostics. However, the overreliance on the granting of exclusive rights to induce private sector investments in R&D has created access barriers and fails to stimulate innovation in several important areas. Efforts to compensate for these shortcomings have been successful in specific cases but cannot distract from the need for more systematic change (Box 50.1). Multilateral agreements are needed to coordinate and finance R&D in a way that delinks the cost of R&D from end prices. To better prepare for future pandemics, countries also need to make binding agreements to share both manufacturing knowledge and the production of health technologies to avoid the vaccine and medicines apartheid experienced during the Covid-19 pandemic.

Box 50.1: Intellectual Property and Access to Health Technologies

Benefits and limitations of an intellectual property driven innovation system:

- Profit-driven system that stimulates innovation by providing time-limited market monopoly to the innovator.
- Leads to high and often unaffordable prices of new medicines, vaccines, and diagnostics.
- Does not stimulate innovation where the market is not sufficiently profitable, for example, neglected diseases, antimicrobial resistance.

Example efforts to balance disadvantages of the intellectual property-driven innovation system:

- Strict patentability criteria, allowing only patenting of true innovations.
- Compulsory licenses to override patents in case of public health need.
- Limited duration of market exclusivity.
- Voluntary licenses such as those negotiated through the Medicines Patent Pool.
- Not-for-profit product development such as through the Drugs for Neglected Diseases initiative, Medicines for Malaria Venture, and others.

Alternative mechanisms to stimulate innovation not leading to access barriers:

- Public funding of product development with conditionality on price and access.
- Innovation prizes: cash rewards for successful product development in return for sharing of technology.
- Binding convention on coordination and financing of R&D that delinks the cost of R&D from end prices.

References

1. Quick JD, Hogerzeil HV, Velasquez G, Rago L. Twenty-five years of essential medicines. Bull World Health Organ. 2002;80(11):913–4.
2. Management Sciences for Health. MDS-3: managing access to medicines and health technologies. Arlington, VA: Management Sciences for Health; 2012.
3. 't Hoen EF. Private patents and public health: changing intellectual property rules for access to medicines. Amsterdam: Health Action International; 2016.
4. 't Hoen EF, Hogerzeil HV, Quick JD, Sillo HB. A quiet revolution in global public health: the World Health Organization's prequalification of medicines programme. J Public Health Policy. 2014;35(2):137–61.
5. Moon S, Jambert E, Childs M, von Schoen-Angerer T. A win-win solution?: a critical analysis of tiered pricing to improve access to medicines in developing countries. Glob Health. 2011;7:39.
6. Lindstrand A, Cherian T, Chang-Blanc D, Feikin D, O'Brien KL. The world of immunization: achievements, challenges, and strategic vision for the next decade. J Infect Dis. 2021;224(Suppl 4):S452–S67.
7. Medecins Sans Frontieres. Analysis and critique of the advance market commitment (AMC) for pneumococcal conjugate vaccines (PCVs) and impact on access. MSF Briefing Document; 2020. https://msfaccess.org/analysis-and-critique-advance-market-commitment-amc-pneumococcal-conjugate-vaccines. Accessed 6 Oct 2022
8. Fleming KA, Horton S, Wilson ML, Atun R, DeStigter K, Flanigan J, et al. The Lancet Commission on diagnostics: transforming access to diagnostics. Lancet. 2021;398(10315):1997–2050.
9. Pedrique B, Strub-Wourgaft N, Some C, Olliaro P, Trouiller P, Ford N, et al. The drug and vaccine landscape for neglected diseases (2000–11): a systematic assessment. Lancet Glob Health. 2013;1(6):e371–e9.
10. Viera M, Moon S. Research synthesis: costs of Pharmaceutical R&D. Knowledge portal on innovation and access to medicines. Geneva: Graduate Institute; 2020. https://www.knowledgeportalia.org/cost-of-r-d. Accessed 6 Oct 2022
11. Love J. Alternatives to the patent system that are used to support R&D efforts, including both push and pull mechanisms, with a special focus on innovation-inducement prizes and open source development models. World Intellectual Property Organization CDIP/14/INF/12; 2014. https://www.wipo.int/meetings/en/doc_details.jsp?doc_id=287218. Accessed 6 Oct 2022
12. United Nations Secretary-General's High-Level Panel On Access To Medicines. Promoting Innovation and Access To Health Technologies. United Nations; 2016. http://www.unsgaccessmeds.org/final-report/. Accessed 6 Oct 2022
13. Knowledge Ecology International. Selected U.S. Government COVID Contracts with Authorization and Consent to Non-Voluntary Use of Third Party Patents. KEI Briefing Note 2022:1; 2022. https://www.keionline.org/bn-2022-1. Accessed 6 Oct 2022
14. Perehudoff K, Et H, Mara K, Balasubramaniam T, Abbott F, Baker B, et al. A pandemic treaty for equitable global access to medical countermeasures: seven recommendations for sharing intellectual property, know-how and technology. BMJ Glob Health. 2022;7(7):e009709. https://doi.org/10.1136/bmjgh-2022-009709.

Essentials of Global Surgery

51

Paolo Rodi, Kiki Maoate, Viliami T. Tangi, and Kathryn M. Chu

Abstract

Five billion people worldwide lack timely access to safe and affordable surgical care, the majority of whom live in low-middle-income countries (LMICs). Only 3.5% of the 266 million needed operations are performed there with large inequity between high income (HICs) and LMICs. Successful efforts to improve surgical care have included political achievements such as The Lancet Commission on Global Surgery, World Health Assembly resolution 68.15, and the creation of National Surgical, Obstetric and Anaesthesia Plans in several countries. In addition, there have been new surveillance and standardisation of procedures, innovative funding mechanisms and the creation of global surgery advocacy organisations and networks. Further coordination between stakeholders is needed to ensure that surgery is an essential component of universal health care.

Keywords

Surgery · Access · Universal health coverage (UHC) · Lancet Commission · NSOAP

P. Rodi (✉)
University Hospital Zürich, Zürich, Switzerland
e-mail: paolo.rodi@usz.ch

K. Maoate
Christchurch Hospital/University of Otago, Christchurch, New Zealand
e-mail: kiki@healthspecialists.co.nz

V. T. Tangi
Vaiola Hospital, Nukualofa, Tonga

K. M. Chu
Stellenbosch University, Stellenbosch, South Africa
e-mail: kchu@sun.ac.za

51.1 Aims of the Chapter

This chapter provides a definition of global surgery (GS), discusses its relationship to universal health coverage (UHC) and political prioritisation, outlines the barriers to surgical access in low- and middle-income countries (LMIC), and highlights some of the ways global surgery could become a more effective global health network.

51.2 Introduction and Background

GS is the academic discipline of improving health and well-being by expanding universal access to timely, quality, and affordable surgical care. It includes the study of the clinical and public health issues related to surgical, anaesthesia, and obstetric care, as well as transnational themes thereby making it a global health (GH) field.

M. C. B. Raviglione et al. (eds.), *Global Health Essentials*, Sustainable Development Goals Series,
https://doi.org/10.1007/978-3-031-33851-9_51

Unlike some other GH issues that might focus on vertical conditions, surgical care is cross-cutting and linked to health system strengthening. Indeed, GS encompasses the studies of socio-economic structures, human resource needs, finances, policy, and investment in follow-up systems [1].

GS is an important GH discipline: worldwide 5 billion people lack timely access to safe and affordable surgical care, the majority of whom live in LMICs. Conditions treatable with surgery are responsible for 16.9 million deaths annually, a death toll that outweighs that of HIV, tuberculosis, and malaria combined. Of the 266 million surgical operations performed annually, only 3.5% take place in LMICs, [1] a struggle intensified by a small workforce, poor governance, and fragile health systems. Consequently, there are bigger unmet surgical needs and higher health and socio-economic burdens in LMICs, which produce a significant inequity compared to HICs [2].

Equitable surgical access is an essential component of UHC and shares the same core pillars such as universal access for a comprehensive range of services for the entire population, a range of provided services, and low financial risk. The 2019 UNGA Political Declaration on UHC stated: "address the growing burden of injuries and deaths, [...] including essential surgery capacities, as an essential part of integrated health-care delivery" [3]. Moreover, surgery is a treatment option in all WHO disease subcategories, from cancer to cardiovascular diseases, injuries, infections, reproductive, maternal, and child health. Therefore, universal surgical and anaesthesia care is essential to reaching several Sustainable Development Goals [4] (Fig. 51.1).

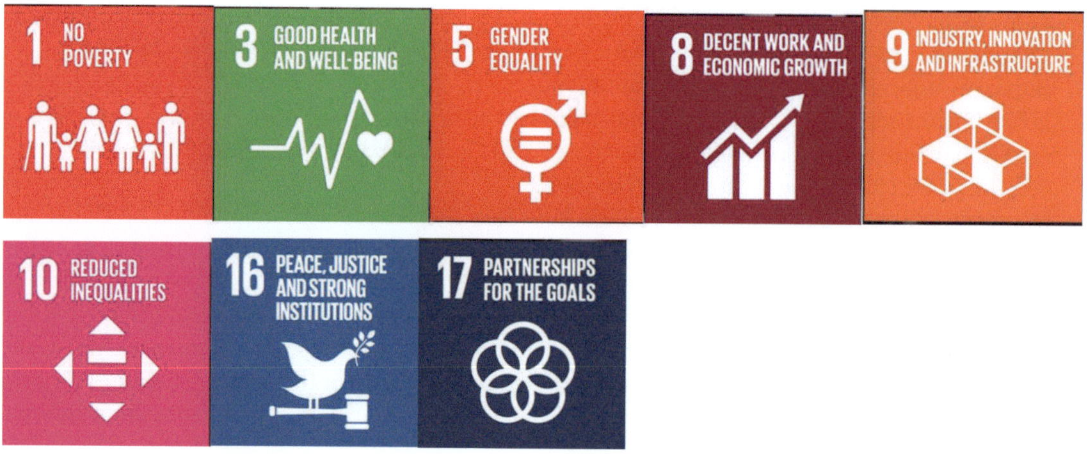

Fig. 51.1 Sustainable Development Goals that can be improved through universal surgical and anaesthetic care (www.un.org/sustainabledevelopment). *The content of this publication has not been approved by the United Nations and does not reflect the views of the United Nations or its officials or Member States*

51.3 Barriers to Surgical Care

Surgical access is not yet equitable within or between countries. The Four Delays framework can be used to examine barriers to access to surgical care. These four delays include the delay to (1) seek, (2) reach, (3) receive, and (4) remain in care:

Delay 1. Once an individual recognises they have a health problem, this delay describes barriers to seeking health care. Individuals may await to seek care because of fear of incomplete health insurance coverage or loss of earnings, poor health education and recognition of injury, perceived distance from health care, or preference toward traditional healers, this latter involving 80% of LMICs population.

Delay 2. Once an individual has made the decision to seek care, this delay describes barriers to reaching a health facility. Often, physical barriers impede access to care, for example, because of poor infrastructure quality, non-available ambulances, and transport costs. For instance, average distance to hospital, a proxy for healthcare facility density, differentiates enormously between HICs, <5 km, and LMICs, ca. 30 km.

Delay 3. Once a patient has reached a health facility, this delay describes barriers to receiving definitive surgical care. Facilities may fail to perform essential surgical services, mostly due to capacity gaps of district hospitals and the inability to provide adequate supplies, spaces, staff, and systems. Solutions have been proposed, for example, blood supply delivery by drones in Uganda or mid-level providers in South Africa and Vietnam. However, more development is still needed.

Delay 4. This delay describes barriers to staying in care including returning for follow-up and rehabilitation. This can include economic and educational barriers, i.e. direct and indirect costs of attending follow-ups, lack of information, and poor services [2, 5].

51.4 Political Commitment

Despite international recognition that GS is a valuable GH network, GS remains isolated and does not have the same political momentum and effectiveness of other networks such as HIV/AIDS or TB. While the GS network has made great strides in the past few years, there are still areas that can be improved. Strategically, GS needs to develop its niche within the global framework of the MDGs or in the SDGs like all other health conditions. Additionally, GS's intrinsic horizontal and multi-faceted nature makes a unified message and consolidated actor power more challenging [6].

Nevertheless, given the role of equitable surgical care access to achieving UHC, some political initiatives have been commenced in the last few decades. In 2005, WHO launched the Global Initiative for Emergency and Essential Surgical Care, a biennial meeting with the purpose of encouraging collaboration and discuss progress. In 2015, the Lancet Commission on Global Surgery (LCoGS) was started and WHA approved Resolution 68.15 on "Strengthening emergency and essential surgical care and anaesthesia as a component of UHC" [7]. In 2019, GS returned to WHA with Resolution 70.38 in form of progress report, where some—although insufficient—international effort was acknowledged [8]. As of 2019, 24/82 LMICs had committed to introduce surgical services in their national plans [9]. In 2021, USAID Administrator publicly promised increased funds inflow in GS-related projects [10] although never disclosing the intended amount. Embedding surgical, obstetric, and anaesthesia care within the National Health Policy framework of 22 Pacific countries (see Box 51.1) is one of the strategic enablers to have access to political support and dedicated governmental and international funding. Continued advocacy in other regions of the world is still needed to make GS a GH priority.

Box 51.1: The Virtuous Example of Surgical Advocacy in Western Pacific

The Western Pacific Region is a virtuous example of how GS can be endorsed at the highest political level, with the consequent improvement of surgical policies. In this Box, we present key events that fostered surgical advocacy in the Western Pacific Region and brought to the rapid implementation of National Surgical, Obstetrics and Anaesthesia Plans.

In 2012, the third International Development Symposium organised by the Royal Australasian College of Surgeons, held together with the Alliance for Surgery and Anaesthesia Presence, set the political momentum of surgical care of the Pacific. In the following years, the concept and monitoring of perioperative mortality rate was introduced in Tonga, Fiji, Tuvalu, PNG, Vanuatu, Samoa, Cook Islands, and the Solomon Island's through their National Health Information Systems. In 2015, the LCoGS and WHA Resolution 68/15 were published, among others; thanks to Pacific figures in key positions, who strongly advocated the need of those reports and declarations. By 2016, 12 Pacific countries had reported the first four of the six LCoGS proposed metrics. Efforts culminated in 2019, when Tonga, Fiji, and Palau successfully sponsored a side-event on surgical care. It was probably fortuitous that these three countries had surgeons as health ministers. Following momentum generated, Pacific Health Ministers jointly published a resolution in their 13th Pacific Health Ministers Meeting promoting the introduction of NSOAPs in their country's health plans, along with the Healthy Islands vision of expanding UHC in the Pacific. Already in 2020 Cook Islands, Fiji, Tonga, Vanuatu, and Palau had the implementation process started.

51.5 Approach to Solutions

51.5.1 National Surgical, Obstetric and Anaesthesia Planning Manual (NSOAP)

In 2020, WHO and the United Nations Institute for Training and Research published the National Surgical, Obstetric and Anaesthesia Planning Manual (NSOAP), a framework for countries to embed strong and cost-effective surgical systems in national health plans and to finance them equitably. The approach covers six domains, namely, infrastructure, service delivery, workforce, information management, financing, and governance. Its development follows eight steps: analysis of baseline indicators, partnership with local champions, broad stakeholder engagement, consensus building and synthesis of ideas, language refinement, costing, dissemination, and implementation.

As for all governmental policies, adequate funding is a priority to ensure successful implementation. Generally, LMICs rely strongly on external resources such as the Development Assistance for Health (DAH) for their national programs, as domestic financing is often insufficient. However, DAH destined to surgical diseases—mostly non-communicable diseases—only make up 2% of total DAH, and despite an increase in the last decades, this is insufficient to ensure universal surgical care [11].

The NSOAP Manual proposes various methods to financially expand national health system strengthening plans to also include surgical plans. General economic growth, reprioritisation of government budgets, increase of health-specific resources, improved efficiency of existing resources and spending review, and increased access to external resources are all traditional methods. In addition, the concept of "innovative financing" is introduced as a viable option, which involves novel financial approaches to expand budget, such as the use of financial levering mechanisms, for example, partnerships with large global brands, voluntary contributions, voluntary solidarity levy, and "Vaccine bonds," secured by long-term commitments with governments [12].

51.5.2 Surveillance and Standardisation of Procedures

Building on 2009 WHO Safe Surgery Save Lives metrics, the LCoGS introduced in 2015 a set of 3 groups of 2 core indicators to monitor global progress that were admitted into the WHO's 100 Basic Global Health Indicators and the World Bank's World Development Indicators [13]:

1. "Preparedness to care," including population accessibility and workforce availability of a country.
2. "Delivery of care," including annual surgical volumes and perioperative mortality.
3. "Effect of care," including financial indicators on impoverishing and catastrophic expenditures [2].

Although partly used in the Pacific area, all the indicators have not been widely implemented due to challenges in data collection [14]. By 2021 no country had produced data on the financial indicators ("effect of care") leaving a knowledge gap of the global status. A 2021 Utstein study revised these indicators, as shown in detail in Table 51.1 [13].

In addition, a set of essential surgical conditions and operations has been outlined in the third edition of Disease Control Priorities (DCP) by the World Bank, as presented in Table 51.2. They represent operations defined to be essential and necessary, which vary according to hospital level [15]. Other lists have been proposed (see Box 51.2).

Box 51.2: Standardisation of Procedures and Monitoring Across Countries and Health Systems

Lists similar to the DCP of the World Bank have been introduced although for a different purpose. While the DCP list aims at describing essential operations that a hospital should provide, other lists have been proposed to ensure appropriate evaluation and comparison of surgical capacities across facilities, countries, and health systems. For instance, the Bellwether procedures (Laparotomy, C-section, and open fractures treatment) serve as a proxy indicator of hospitals that, in terms of human resources, supplies, and infrastructure, yield sufficient resources to provide most primary surgery procedures. To further allow standardisation and monitoring across countries, as well as uniforming national data collection, a 2021 Delphi study proposed a basket of 32 surgical procedures representative of the health system's capacity to provide surgical care. The list is shown below [14]:

- Trauma laparotomy
- C-section
- Cataract surgery
- Inguinal hernia repair
- Stoma formation
- Tracheostomy
- Open appendectomy
- Partial colectomy
- Modified radical mastectomy
- Trauma thoracotomy
- Extremity amputation
- Small bowel resection
- Hysterectomy
- External fixation femur
- Uterine evacuation
- Partial mastectomy
- Splenectomy
- Trauma craniotomy
- External fixation tibia
- Tube thoracostomy
- Laparoscopic cholecystectomy
- Obstetric fistula repair
- Internal fixation femur
- Laparoscopic appendectomy
- Paediatric colostomy
- Salpingectomy
- Imperforate anus repair
- Open cholecystectomy
- Coronary artery bypass graft
- Percutaneous coronary angioplasty
- Cleft lip/palate repair
- Thyroidectomy

Table 51.1 Revised core indicators to monitor global progress on GS goals

Indicator	Definition	Summary of data elements
Geospatial access	Proportion of a country's population with geographic access (<2 h) to a facility capable of providing surgical and anaesthesia care for the Bellwether procedures (caesarean section, laparotomy, and surgical management of open long bone fracture)	• Population estimates • Facility locations • Capacity of health facilities to do Bellwether procedures • Distance and travel time of population to facilities
Workforce	Number of each surgery, obstetric, or anaesthesia providers who are actively practicing, per 100,000 population	• Number of providers (a precise definition has not been provided and its definition left to the countries) • Total country population
Volume	Number of surgical procedures done in an operating theatre using any form of anaesthesia, per 100,000 population per year	• Number of procedures per year • Total country population
Perioperative mortality rate	Deaths from all causes, before discharge (up to 30 days), in all patients who have received any anaesthesia for a procedure done in an operating theatre, divided by the total number of procedures, per year, expressed as a percentage	• Number of patients undergoing a surgical procedure in an operating theatre using any form of anaesthesia who died before hospital discharge (up to 30 days), per year • Number of procedures done in an operating theatre, using any anaesthesia, per year
Financial risk protection	Percentage of the population at risk of catastrophic expenditure if they were to require a surgical procedure	• Out-of-pocket expenditure (OOP) • Household expenditure • Catastrophic expenditure threshold, which is crossed when OOP is >10% of household expenditure

Table 51.2 Set of essential surgical conditions and operations outlined by the third edition of Disease Control Priorities by the World Bank [15]

Procedure	Primary health centre	First-level hospital	Second- and third-level hospital
Dental procedures	Extraction Drainage of dental abscess Treatment for caries		
Obstetrics and gynaecology	Normal delivery	Caesarean birth Vacuum extraction/forceps delivery Ectopic pregnancy Manual vacuum aspiration and dilation and curettage Tubal ligation Vasectomy Hysterectomy for uterine rupture or intractable postpartum haemorrhage Visual inspection with acetic acid and cryotherapy for precancerous cervical lesions	Repair obstetric fistula

Table 51.2 (continued)

Procedure	Primary health centre	First-level hospital	Second- and third-level hospital
General surgery	Drainage of superficial abscesses Male circumcision	Repair of perforations: For example, perforated peptic ulcer, typhoid ileal perforation Appendectomy Bowel obstruction Colostomy Gallbladder disease, including emergency surgery Hernia, including incarceration Hydrocelectomy Relief of urinary obstruction: catheterisation or suprapubic cystostomy	
Injury	Resuscitation with basic life support measures Suturing lacerations Management of non-displaced fractures	Resuscitation with advanced life support Basic life support Measures, including surgical airway Measures Tube thoracostomy (chest drain) Trauma laparotomy Fracture reduction Irrigation and debridement of open fractures Placement of external fixator; use of traction Escharotomy/fasciotomy (cutting of constricting tissue to relieve pressure from swelling) Trauma-related amputations Skin grafting Burr hole	
Congenital			Repair of cleft lip and palate Repair of club foot—Shunt for hydrocephalus Repair of anorectal malformations and Hirschsprung's disease
Non-trauma orthopaedics		Drainage of septic arthritis Debridement of osteomyelitis	Cataract extraction and insertion of intraocular lens Eyelid surgery for trachoma

51.6 Conclusions

Between HICs and LMICs there is substantial inequity in the delivery of surgical and anaesthesia care. Scarce surgical volumes, small workforce, poor infrastructures, inadequate funding, and a general weakness of the health system represent relevant barriers to the universal availability and accessibility of surgical care. In turn, this poses a significant burden on people and society in LMICs.

Since 2015, unprecedented interest has been generated in the field of GS. The topic reached international fora and significant achievements have been reached. However, many obstacles still impede adequate generation of political priorities and mobilisation of funding. Therefore, much effort is still required to ensure universal access to affordable and safe surgical, obstetric, and anaesthesia care.

References

1. Bath M, Bashford T, Fitzgerald JE. What is 'global surgery'? Defining the multidisciplinary interface between surgery, anaesthesia and public health. BMJ Glob Heal. 2019;4:1–9. https://doi.org/10.1136/bmjgh-2019-001808.
2. Meara JG, Leather AJM, Hagander L, Alkire BC, Alonso N, Ameh EA, et al. Global surgery 2030: evidence and solutions for achieving health, welfare, and economic development. Lancet. 2015;386:569–624. https://doi.org/10.1016/S0140-6736(15)60160-X.
3. UN. General Assembly. (74th sess. : 2019–2020). Political Declaration of the High-Level Plenary Meeting on Universal Health Coverage: resolution/adopted by the General Assembly. A/RES/74/2 2019. https://doi.org/10.1017/s0020818300030393
4. Roa L, Jumbam DT, Makasa E, Meara JG. Global surgery and the sustainable development goals. Br J Surg. 2019;106:e44–52. https://doi.org/10.1002/bjs.11044.
5. Odland ML, Whitaker J, Nepogodiev D, Aling' CA, Bagahirwa I, Dushime T, et al. Identifying, prioritizing and visually mapping barriers to injury Care in Rwanda: a multi-disciplinary stakeholder exercise. World J Surg. 2020;44:2903–18. https://doi.org/10.1007/s00268-020-05571-6.
6. Shawar YR, Shiffman J, Spiegel DA. Generation of political priority for global surgery: a qualitative policy analysis. Lancet Glob Health. 2015;3:e487–95. https://doi.org/10.1016/S2214-109X(15)00098-4.
7. World Health Organization. Sixty-eighth World Health Assembly. Strength Emerg Essent Surg Care Anaesth as a Compon Univers Heal Cover Rep by Secr 2015:16–18
8. WHO. Progress reports. Report by the Secreteriat 2019;12:1–5
9. Jumbam DT, Reddy CL, Roa L, Meara JG. How much does it cost to scale up surgical systems in low-income and middleincome countries? BMJ Glob Health. 2019;4:1–4. https://doi.org/10.1136/bmjgh-2019-001779.
10. Explanatory statement for department of state, foreign operations, and related programs appropriations Bill, 2021. p. 2021 2021;000
11. Rodi P, Obermeyer W, Pablos-Mendez A, Gori A, Raviglione MC. Political rationale, aims, and outcomes of health-related high-level meetings and special sessions at the UN General Assembly: a policy research observational study. PLoS Med. 2022;19:1–18. https://doi.org/10.1371/journal.pmed.1003873.
12. Reddy CL, Reddy CL, Peters AW, Peters AW, Jumbam DT, Jumbam DT, et al. Innovative financing to fund surgical systems and expand surgical care in low-income and middle-income countries. BMJ Glob Health. 2020;5:1–10. https://doi.org/10.1136/bmjgh-2020-002375.
13. Davies JI, Gelb AW, Gore-Booth J, Mellin- Olsen J, Martin J, Åkerman C, et al. Global surgery, obstetric, and anaesthesia indicator definitions and reporting: an Utstein consensus report. PLoS Med. 2021;18:1–13. https://doi.org/10.1371/journal.pmed.1003749.
14. Odland ML, Nepogodiev D, Morton D, Martin J, Bekele A, Ghosh D, et al. Identifying a basket of surgical procedures to standardize global surgical metrics: an international Delphi study. Ann Surg. 2021;274:1107–14. https://doi.org/10.1097/SLA.0000000000004611.
15. Debas H, Donkor P, Gawande A, Jamison D, Kruk M, Mock C. Volume 1: Essential Surgery. Disease Control Priorities, 3rd Ed 2015;1:1–4. This is an adaptation of an original work by the World Bank. Views and opinions expressed in the adaptation are the sole responsibility of the author or authors of the adaptation and are not endorsed by The World Bank

52 Health Conversations Through Personal Communication Networks

Daniel Low-Beer, Dereck Mpofu, Beat Stoll, and Albert Nyathi

Abstract

Health communication is increasingly seen as a two-way conversation, involving listening, learning, and adjustment to cultural context as well as promoting health. It is therefore important to ensure the balance of communication channels recommended by the 2017 World Health Organization Strategic Communications Framework for effective communications.—mass media, organization and community, and personal communication. This section shows the importance of health conversations through personal networks, between a health care practitioner and patient and at the population level, in catalysing health outcomes.

A continuous personal relationship between health provider and patient can independently improve adherence to medication, reduce emergency admissions, and improve mortality by 25% over 15 years. Similarly, at the population level, personal communication networks enhance or reduce the uptake of interventions, behavioural engagement, and outcomes. They can be catalysed or switched off to health issues like HIV, tobacco, sexual violence, or mental health. Health conversations are primary to communications and health care delivery, and the evidence for their impact on a wide range of health areas is summarised.

Keywords

Health communications · Behaviours · Conversations · Health promotion · Prevention · Outcomes · Role of music and dance · Community prevention · Mental health · Stigma · HIV · Healthy lives · Continuity of care · Communication networks · Digital communication

52.1 Introduction

Health communication is defined as "the process of informing, discussing and dialoguing, influencing, and motivating individual, institutional, private and public organisations and audiences about relevant health issues" [1]. It contributes to the overall goals of health promotion as "the process of enabling people to increase control over, and to improve their health" [2].

D. Low-Beer (✉)
World Health Organization, Geneva, Switzerland
e-mail: lowbeerd@who.int

D. Mpofu
Conversations, Harare, Zimbabwe

B. Stoll
Geneva University, Geneva, Switzerland

A. Nyathi
Midlands State University, Bulawayo, Zimbabwe

M. C. B. Raviglione et al. (eds.), *Global Health Essentials*, Sustainable Development Goals Series,
https://doi.org/10.1007/978-3-031-33851-9_52

Health communication is often seen as a strategy to disseminate information, inform and influence individual and community decisions to enhance health. Yet it is increasingly recognised as a two-way conversation, involving listening, learning, adjustment to cultural context as well as promoting health. Health conversations are an important diagnostic approach in the clinical setting and on how we adjust public health interventions to context and demand.

The World Health Organization (WHO) Strategic Communications Framework highlights the balance of communication channels needed to address health issues [3]:

- **Mass media**. These channels have broad reach and include television, radio, newspapers, magazines, outdoor and transit advertising, direct mail, social media, and websites.
- **Organisation and community**. These channels reach specific groups of individuals based on geography (e.g. a specific village) or a common interest, such as occupational status. Channels may include community-based media, such as local radio talk shows, organization newsletters; community-based activities, such as health fairs; and meetings at schools, workplaces, and houses of worship.
- **Interpersonal.** People seeking advice or sharing information about health risks often turn to family, friends, health care practitioners, co-workers, teachers, counsellors, and faith leaders. These one-on-one discussions are often the most trusted channels for health information.

This section introduces the importance of the basic health conversation in clinical settings and for population health. Health communication is not just delivered as messaging but increasingly involves two-way engagement and uses the technologies of music, dance, science, with modern electronic forms and social media, to engage in contemporary health conversations in cultural contexts.

52.2 Background

A continuous relationship and conversation between doctor and patient is an important health diagnostic ("as all good doctors know their medicines, they also know their conversations") [4, 5]. There is evidence of the health benefits of this interpersonal relationship and conversation over time, including greater patient satisfaction, closer adherence to medical advice and medication, better uptake of vaccines, reduced use of out of hours services, lower referral rates, better job satisfaction and retention of doctors and fewer Accident and Emergency admissions [5, 6].

According to a large-scale study from Norway, the longer the interpersonal relationship between doctor and patient, the lower the mortality rate, 25% after 15 or more years, with a dose response relationship suggesting causation [7]. The chair of the Royal College of General Practitioners commented "If relationships were a drug, guideline developers would mandate their use" [5].

Similarly, at the population level, a community conversation on a health issue can switch on or off the uptake of interventions, behavioural engagement, and the hundreds of adjustments which precede and exceed public health interventions in different cultural contexts.

The importance of person-to-person conversations in addition to vertical messaging was shown in the HIV response, which provides an example of their role in detail. In the early 1990s, there were the first signs of declines in HIV incidence in Africa [8]. A WHO team investigated communities where HIV incidence was declining by 50–75%, and explained they were working on AIDS. There followed a stream of opinions, stories and questions, personal about families and communities, with some stigma and plenty of care. Communication networks were mobilised or switched on to HIV.

When the team went to communities where HIV had not declined, in Kenya or South Africa, the response was different. They explained they were working on AIDS, and there would be silence or a change of subject. As the team left, people would sometimes ask what could be done about a relative who was ill, with pneumonia or tuberculosis. Despite similar interventions and mortality, there was a different health conversation.

These observations were confirmed when communication networks were analysed, published in the journal *Science* [8]. The major source of knowledge of AIDS was horizontal personal networks of friends and family where HIV declined. Where there was no impact, the major source was vertical channels from official sources, and there had not been a shift from vertical to personal communication networks. The information and disease were similar, but the health conversation was different. In one community, it was switched on, in the other switched off.

52.3 Personal Communications

The HIV response was the result of direct public health programs, communication was delivered as a two-way conversation with communities and social networks, going beyond the delivery of messages, media campaigns, or transferring knowledge. The opening of conversations on a health issue allows the response to precede formal interventions and often exceed them, to get ahead of the epidemic.

The communication networks behind successful community responses illustrated several characteristics [9]. First, alongside formal vertical channels for information, horizontal person to person networks were mobilised. Second, there was greater openness in communication networks, which allowed health conversations to spread. This was the outcome of direct public health policy, AIDS was notifiable and discussed in health care, patient and family settings, every public official visiting a community had to address a village meeting on AIDS, and NGOs like The AIDS Support Organisation (TASO) combined care, communication, and prevention. There was still stigma in 10–20% of respondents yet the majority showed attitudes of care [9].

Finally, there was a series of secondary, personal health conversations, which far exceeded the information and behavioural content of health promotion campaigns. They communicated trust, engagement, and engaged behaviours by age and gender in the cultural context in which they were negotiated. Behaviour change was not communicated vertically (A, B, or C) but was the outcome of catalysing personal communication networks on AIDS (a conversation rather than a prescription). There was "a clear policy implemented with local conviction … crucially, health policy was converted into social communications working through local networks of chiefs, musicians and village meetings" [9].

When communication and HIV epidemic networks were modelled, communication networks were more multiplicative (Fig. 52.1). Where communication networks were open, over 75% of the population had personal knowledge of the epidemic before incidence peaked. Conversely if personal communication networks are restricted, less than 20% will know someone with AIDS before peak HIV incidence. Due to the multiplicative effect of communication networks, the community response can be catalysed or switched off and is sensitive to misinformation or silence on a health issue. It requires a direct public health policy of two-way conversation and engagement. These findings had wider relevance for health.

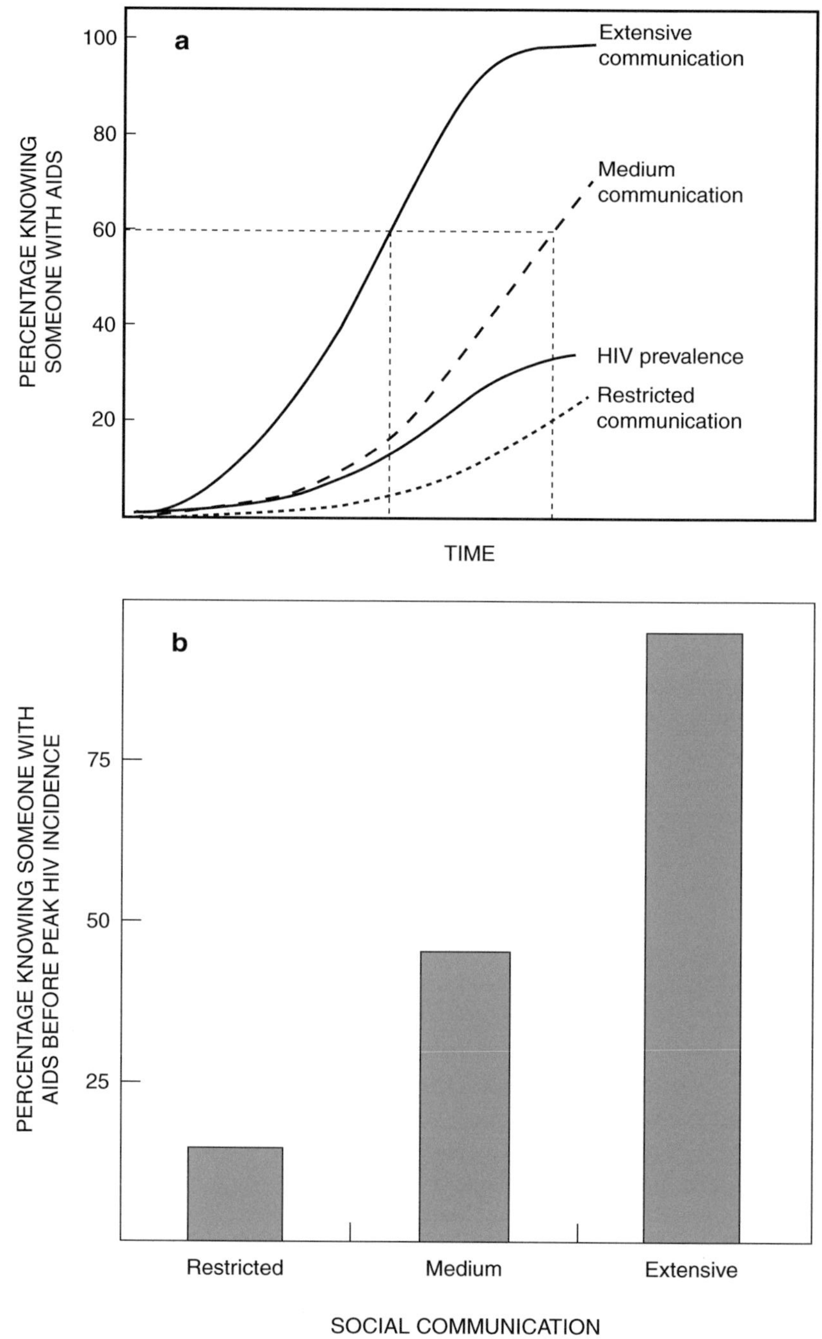

Fig. 52.1 The impact of personal communications on the number of people who know someone with AIDS at different stages of the epidemic (**a**) Over time with extensive, medium, and restricted social communications (**b**) Before peak HIV incidence, % knowing someone with AIDS [6]

52.4 Culture-Sensitive Conversations Across Health Areas

Health communication often uses a written communication model that can be delivered as a vertical intervention with information provision, leaflets, posters, and promotion. Yet health conversations require horizontal personal engagement and depend on a much older oral communication technology, renewed with digital media. They are also prone to misinformation, and it is important that health conversations are supported through trusted networks of public health leaders, health workers, and individuals. Case surveillance and community data is catalytic, so disease is officially recognised and discussed in clinical settings and public meetings. Community data is necessary to link a population response to the reality of health events in a community.

In addition, public health diplomacy should include oral communication technology through music, poetry, theatre, and the arts. They are often seen as entertainment. Yet how have communities traditionally discussed sensitive issues? For centuries they were the primary technology of culture-sensitive behavioural communication and the conversation on health within communities [10, 11]. Studies show people forget 80% of information within 24 h (the curve of forgetting). Yet 75% of information is retained when presented as part of a story, song or conversation and linked to emotions and behaviours [9, 12–14]. After two decades of improved clinical services, the major declines in HIV incidence in Africa have been preceded by songs: Philip Lutaaya with AIDS touring Uganda, Oliver Mtudkudzi with "What shall we do?" in Zimbabwe, or Attention Na Sida by Franco in West Africa. They were only limited parts of direct public health community programs but extended their reach into personal communications.

A recent comprehensive WHO review of over 900 publications assessed the role of the arts in improving communication, health, and well-being [10]. The evidence showed the catalytic role of music, theatre, and the arts across a wide range of health areas from communicable diseases, maternal and child health, mental health, caregiving, trauma, surgery, cancer, diabetes, and non-communicable diseases, as summarised in Table 52.1.

Table 52.1 Evidence of the role of arts in improving communication, health, and well-being alongside other interventions, extracted from the scoping review by WHO [10]

Heath area	Evidence
Healthier lives, eating healthily, physically active and value of effort into food	Observational studies of engagement in arts show improved outcomes irrespective of socioeconomic status and social capital. Improved body mass index, blood biomarkers, and musculoskeletal function with dance activities greater than regular exercise interventions. Effects in both overweight and people with a healthy weight.
Substance abuse disorders	Song-writing workshops reduce cravings and plays and improve participation in substance abuse prevention. Arts events are more effective than sports in promoting antismoking.
Health communication	Artists mediate between public health professionals and public in different cultural contexts, meta-analysis shows improvements in knowledge, attitude, and behaviours from projects involving performing arts and visual arts. Impact only when artists hold status of opinion leaders and agents of change.
Engagement with health care	Arts projects are linked to improvements in medication and treatment adherence: Storytelling improves hypertension and medication adherence; arts and music improve management of diabetes in children and sickle cell disease in adolescents. Well-selected songs enhance self-efficacy in those with HIV, improving adherence and decreasing viral loads.
Health-related stigma and engagement of marginalised groups	Arts in schools improve mental health literacy. Arts and fiction disrupt stereotypes about HIV among young, understanding of dementia and disrupt stigma. Arts build trust between children in foster care and social care with an increase in self-esteem, resilience, and skills. Singing engages military veterans in mental health and addiction treatment and dance in rehabilitation.
Isolation and loneliness, complex and long-term conditions, chronic pain and well-being	Arts on prescription are used for two decades in United Kingdom to tackle isolation and loneliness (which is the case in 20–30% of all visits to UK doctors). Local evaluations show benefits for mental health, chronic pain, and well-being. Evaluations show a return of investment 2.3 times.
Cognitive decline	Playing music, dance, and theatre slow cognitive decline and partly slow progression of dementia and frailty.
Clinical skills	Musical experience linked with surgical skills, and arts classes linked with visual diagnostic skills for doctors and nurses improve verbal and nonverbal communication skills. Theatre training of doctors was linked to improved case presentations to clinical teams and the reduced use of medical jargon with patients.

(continued)

Table 52.1 (continued)

Heath area	Evidence
Perinatal health	Music and singing during pregnancy can decrease maternal blood pressure and increase foetal heart rate, improve bonding and reducing postnatal depression.
Mental health	Research shows music and dance can modulate serotonin, reduce stress hormones such as cortisol, and decrease inflammatory immune responses. Music therapy reduces depression, affective symptoms, and negative syndrome symptoms in schizophrenia. Though large-scale studies have had mixed findings with severe mental health.
Trauma and post-traumatic stress disorder (PTSD)	Music and diaries can reduce the incidence of PTSD through reducing depression and improving pleasure, and dance can help people with PTSD build healthy relationship with body. Specific beats can help manage cardiovascular reactivity in military personnel with post-deployment stress.
Premature infants	Music has benefits for heart rate, respiration rate, oxygen saturation, feeding ability, and behavioural state as well as is linked to overall reduction of stay in intensive care.
Intensive care	Music can reduce anxiety, heart rate, blood pressure and respiratory rate in patients who are mechanically ventilated, reducing the time spent on a ventilator and in intensive care.
Stroke and neurological function	Music has been shown to help develop new neural pathways and enhance structural neuroplasticity following a stroke and improve recovery of verbal memory. Music and dance can improve motor rehabilitation and some studies show improved memory. Dance has repeatedly shown clinically meaningful improvements in motor scores for people with Parkinson's disease. Music has been shown to support cognition in people with dementia, particularly vis a vis Alzheimer's where brain areas associated with musical memory are well preserved even in later stages of disease.
Cancer	Music and participation in arts shown benefits for children and adults, to reduce anxiety, distress, loss of appetite, nausea, and reduced need for anti-sickness medication during cancer treatment. Music listening shown to reduce length of hospital stay following surgery for cancer. Drawing used to identify symptoms among young children.
Diabetes	Music found to help control blood glucose levels and glycated haemoglobin during ordinary and stressful situations in both those with diabetes and those without.

52.5 Conclusions

Health communication is increasingly seen as a two-way conversation, involving listening, learning, adjustment to age, gender, and cultural contexts as well as promoting health. It is therefore important to ensure the balance of communication channels recommended by WHO—mass media, organization and community, and personal communications [3]. This section has shown the importance of personal communications and a basic conversation on health, between a health care practitioner and patient and at the population level, in catalysing health outcomes.

With the shift to digital communication, personal communications have a renewed importance at global scale, with new possibilities as well as risks of disinformation and moral panics. The communication theory behind the term "global village" is that it is as much village as global, with the return of horizontal person-to-person communications at the global scale alongside vertical, written communication [15]. Health communication will increasingly need to combine traditional public health dissemination with the renewed importance and characteristics of personal communications, as seen with the information and disinformation regarding COVID-19. To do so, it will need to combine the technologies of the arts, science, with modern electronic forms, to engage in contemporary health conversations in context. There are critiques, and improved observation, hypotheses and testing of the mix of interventions are always required [16].

The resulting skills of health diplomacy and communication should reach into cultural settings often outside the comfort zone of health professionals "health diplomacy, not diplomat to diplomat, but diplomacy that can form common actions with the private sector, communities, reach out to private foundations, and most importantly those affected by health issues ...a health diplomacy of diversity, recognising different constituents of health, and able to reach into village meetings, company board meetings, engage most at risk populations as much as health assemblies" [17]. The health conversation remains a basic model of communication for health personnel and public health programs.

References

1. Porta M, Last JM. A dictionary of public health. Oxford: Oxford University Press; 2018.
2. World Health Organization. Health promotion glossary. Geneva: WHO; 1998.
3. World Health Organization. WHO strategic communications framework for effective communications. Geneva: WHO; 2017.
4. Nyathi A, Low-Beer D. Ten Conversations for Health. 2019. https://www.10conversations.net. Accessed 20 Aug 2022
5. Morland P. A fortunate woman – a country doctor's story. London: Picador; 2022.
6. Pereira Gray D, Sidaway-Lee K, White E, Thorne A, Evans P. Continuity of care with doctors – a matter of life and death? A systematic review of continuity of care and mortality. BMJ Open. 2018;8:e021161. https://doi.org/10.1136/bmjopen-2017-021161.
7. Sandvik H, Hetlevik O, Blinkenberg J, Hunskaar S. Continuity in general practice as predictor of mortality, acute hospitalization, and use of out-of-hours care. Br J Gen Pract. 2022;72(715):e84–90. https://doi.org/10.3399/BJGP.2021.0340.
8. Stoneburner RL, Low-Beer D. Population-level HIV declines and behavioural risk avoidance in Uganda, Science 2004;304(5671):714–718. https://doi.org/10.1126/science.1093166. Erratum in: Science 2004 Nov 26;306(5701):1477
9. Low-Beer D, Stoneburner RL. AIDS communications through social networks: catalyst for behaviour changes in Uganda. Afr J AIDS Res. 2004;3(1):1–13. https://doi.org/10.2989/16085900409490313.
10. Fancourt D, Finn S. What is the evidence on the role of the arts in improving health and well-being? A scoping review. 2019 World Health Organization. Regional Office for Europe https://apps.who.int/iris/handle/10665/329834
11. Barber EW. Women's work: the first 20,000 years. New York: Norton; 1994.
12. Schacter DL. The seven sins of memory: how the mind forgets and remembers. Boston, MA: Mariner Books; 2001.
13. Baddeley A, Eysenck M, Anderson M. Memory. 3rd ed. Abingdon: Routledge; 2020.
14. Sacks O. Musicophilia: Tales of music and the brain. London: Picador; 2007.
15. McLuhan M, Powers B. The Global Village: transformations in world life and media in the 21st century. Oxford: Oxford University Press; 1989.
16. Clift S, Philips K, Pritchard S. The need for robust critique of research on social and health impacts of the arts, Cultural Trends 2021;30(5):442–459.
17. Low-Beer D. Innovative health partnerships: the diplomacy of diversity. Singapore: World Scientific Press; 2011.

53 The Private Sector in Global Health: Roles and Opportunities

Sebastien Mazzuri, Srividya Prakash, and Farhad Riahi

Abstract

The *private sector* is the part of the economy that is run by individuals and companies *for profit* and is not state controlled. In healthcare, the private sector comprises a wide range of actors and already plays a major role in global health by virtue of its range, size, and capabilities. Conversely, global health is of great and increasing relevance to the private sector, for example, because health itself is a multiplier of economic growth. The private sector will continue to play an essential role in national health systems and the global health environment, given the range of healthcare system needs and the private sector's potential for innovation. Maximizing its impact requires answering two questions: where and how can the private sector contribute positively to improve health system performance; and how to get that contribution in ways that recognize the different incentives and constraints of private, public, and non-profit actors?

Keywords

Private sector · Public-private partnership · Corporate social responsibility (CSR) · Novartis · Private actors

53.1 What Is the Private Sector, and How Is it Relevant to Global Health?

The *private sector* is the part of the economy that is run by individuals and companies *for profit* and is not state controlled. It encompasses all for-profit businesses that are not owned or operated by the government, as distinct from companies and corporations that are government run (public sector), and from charities and other nonprofit organizations (voluntary sector, addressed in Chap. 48) [1].

This definition encompasses a wide range of actors, in terms of both activities and scale:

- Private sector activities range from "traditional" ones (e.g., providing direct patient care, managing healthcare facilities, and creating new diagnostics and therapies), through activities directly supporting healthcare (e.g., communications, analytics, investment), to

S. Mazzuri
FSG, Geneva, Switzerland

S. Prakash
Antara International, Santa Clara, CA, USA

F. Riahi (✉)
Global Innovative Commercial Partnerships, Novartis Innovative Medicines International, Basel, Switzerland

Faculty of Medicine, McGill University, Montreal, QC, Canada
e-mail: farhad.riahinejad@mcgill.ca

M. C. B. Raviglione et al. (eds.), *Global Health Essentials*, Sustainable Development Goals Series,
https://doi.org/10.1007/978-3-031-33851-9_53

broader activities that have an impact on health (e.g., healthcare-focused corporate social responsibility (CSR), nutrition, new technologies such as wearables).
- The scale of private sector activities ranges from single individuals (e.g., single-practice physicians) through local-, regional-, and national-scale companies (e.g., most hospitals and health insurers), to multinational actors (e.g., life sciences, medical device, and health technology companies).

The private sector plays a major role in global health by virtue of its range, size, and capabilities:

- It is already part of all elements of healthcare, from frontline delivery to public-private partnerships to engagement on global health architecture.
- It is material in size, with potential for leverage for system improvement at all levels, for example[2].
  - At national level: the private health sector in India is at least a $56 billion market. It accounts for three times the amount spent by the public sector on health. Even in countries where public sector utilization is high, drugs are often procured in the private sector.
  - At global level: while the precise level of private sector health services is not well defined, there are estimates that between 50 and 70% of all health expenditures are within the private sector. Recent estimates show that the private sector, including informal providers, administer more than half of health care services in Africa specifically.
- It has capabilities and capacity relevant to solving global health challenges, which are often not present in the public and nonprofit sectors, for example, product and service innovation, large-scale manufacturing, distribution and marketing, and complex implementation.

Conversely, global health is of great and increasing relevance to the private sector:

- With the paradigm shift from shareholder to stakeholder returns, the private sector is shifting from reactive and CSR-oriented activities towards participation in sustainable business models in new multi-sectoral ecosystems of stakeholders.
- Health is a multiplier of economic growth, and healthy populations and economies are necessary for private sector to thrive in the long run.
- The confluence of global health challenges and new technologies presents new business opportunities for the private sector, e.g., exploring the role of telehealth and wearables in areas such as obesity, chronic disease management, and mental health.

53.2 Who Are Private Sector Actors and What Roles Do They Play?

The private sector comprises a wide range of actors, both in the traditional health sector and beyond.

Actors in the traditional health sector conduct many of the core activities in a healthcare system, e.g., (see also Table 53.1):

Table 53.1 Private sector activities in the traditional health sector

Healthcare provision (e.g., outpatient and inpatient care, telemedicine)
Healthcare products (diagnostics, therapeutics)
Healthcare-related services (e.g., infrastructure management, training healthcare professionals)
Payor services (e.g., private insurers)
Technological enablers (e.g., communications, data, analytics)
Investment activities (e.g., resource mobilization to tackle the COVID-19 pandemic, investment fund for the development of drugs and diagnostics to combat antimicrobial resistance)
Advisory (e.g., management consulting)

- Healthcare provision: in India, the private sector, including private medical practice by physicians in individual and group practice, provides an estimated 70% of outpatient care for noncommunicable diseases (NCDs) such as diabetes and hypertension, and even for infectious diseases such as tuberculosis, which are traditionally managed through public sector driven programs[ii].
- Healthcare products and services:
  - Small and medium sized businesses provide a range of services including cold storage, supply chain management, and hospital and clinic groups.
  - Product innovation is increasingly globalizing, e.g., India's biotech industry had US$12 billion in revenues in 2021 [3].

These actors each decide for themselves in what ways to contribute to global health, based on their own goals, strategy, and history. There are currently three main categories of role:

- *Honoring the social contract*: not only complying with laws and regulations, but also participating in relevant industry benchmarks (e.g., Access to Medicine Index [4]) and reporting standards (e.g., Integrated Reporting Framework and SASB Standards [5]), and conducting environmental, social, and governance (ESG) activities.
- *Innovating the "what"*: developing new products, services, and solutions to improve access to essential products and services for underserved populations, e.g.:
  - "Frugal innovation" products, e.g., GE's Lullaby baby warmer, initially developed to reduce infant mortality in India [6], and services, e.g., $30 cataract surgery at Aravind Eye Hospital and $2000 heart surgery at Narayana Health [7]
  - Product development partnerships, e.g., for malaria (Medicines for Malaria Venture [8]) and for neglected tropical diseases (Drugs for Neglected Diseases initiative [9]).
- *Innovating the "how"*: conducting business to better meet the needs of the underserved, e.g.:
  - Research & Development (R&D): increasing diversity in clinical trials; building clinical trial capacity in low- and middle-income countries (LMICs).
  - Voluntary licensing, e.g., through the United Nations' Medicines Patent Pool [10].
  - Go-to-market model, e.g., franchise and cooperative models of pharmacy chains in Latin America [11].

Some companies with a longstanding involvement in global health have evolved their activities towards increasingly innovative and holistic approaches. Novartis' engagement with global health, for example, has evolved over the past 20 years, from being the sole donor to the World Health Organization (WHO) of multidrug therapy for leprosy, through the creation of local brands for innovative medicines in Low and Middle Countries (LMICs), to integrating its different business units into a single entity focused on sub-Saharan Africa, launching a sustainability-linked bond to improve access to innovative therapies in LMICs, and building an R&D pipeline focused on the needs of underserved populations. Novartis' Africa Sickle Cell Disease program is a holistic collaboration with partners to develop a comprehensive approach to accessible and affordable screening, diagnosis, and treatment, and to promote scientific research, training, and education [12].

Others, such as digital native healthcare actors with disruptive business models, start directly in the innovative categories.

Looking beyond the traditional health sector, other private actors also play four critical roles that affect global health. Of course, traditional healthcare actors can also play these roles:

- *Employee health coverage or provision*: the private sector provides around 90% of jobs in developing countries [13], and in some cases also healthcare benefits to employees. E.g., the South African mining industry employs over 500,000 workers [14] and is the primary provider of healthcare in mining townships to workers and their families.

- *Corporate social responsibility funding for health*: e.g., in 2020-21, the healthcare and nutrition sector received 26% of all India's CSR funds (and 55% of the state of Gujarat's), behind only education [15].
- *Adapting product portfolios to better address health concerns*: e.g., food and beverage companies reformulating products to increase their nutritional value or decrease their potential for harm.
- *Creating disruptive or new technologies*: e.g., the use of wearables and smartphones for healthcare purposes.

53.3 Future Directions

With very few exceptions, the private sector will continue to play an essential role in national health systems and the global health environment.

The range of health systems' needs is broad, as are the existing and potential contributions that the private sector can offer in response. In coming years, it is likely that experimentation will continue, and more and more efficient models will solidify, not only in the explicit form of public-private and public-nonprofit-private partnerships, but also more transactional relationships, for example between public payors and private providers.

At the same time, the operating environment for private sector actors is becoming increasingly challenging, with raising public scrutiny over profit-making in the health care space, and a domestic and international policy landscape growing in complexity.

All around the world, there are multiple examples of good practice for the private sector to contribute positively to health outcomes, with a shared sense of urgency among stakeholders, clarity on a common purpose and goals, effective governance mechanisms, and mutually reinforcing activities. Those examples will need to crystallize around a set of consistent approaches that would fit a variety of settings.

A critical component of this evolution for the private sector and those looking to engage with it will be to align economic and health outcomes. All too often, despite pledges to advance health system performance and setting ambitious targets, private sector efforts to improve health outcomes for marginalized groups remain peripheral for lack of short-term profitability. Health outcomes targets remain disconnected from companies' financial projections communicated with investors, creating potential for miss-alignment on expectations. And company executives are increasingly under pressure and face a dilemma of managing capital.

As the trend towards cross-sector collaborations will continue towards creating new ecosystems that can tackle in a coordinated way the multiple systems barriers standing in the way of absorbing innovation, two fundamental questions need to be considered: (i) where and how can the private sector contribute positively to improve health system performance, and (ii) how to get that contribution in ways that recognize the different incentives and constraints of private, public, and non-profit actors?

The "where to play" question is one that should be answered by health care services decision-makers, who have the responsibility to shape the overall architecture of their system.

The "how to play" question will benefit from new approaches to measurement that can help companies manage the economics of impact for global health activities, and systemically, actively, and transparently connect and reconcile their financial and societal objectives by linking financial and societal outcomes, understanding the outcome-profit relationship and the factors driving the status quo, and surfacing trade-offs and their underlying dimensions.

With those new tools in place, the next frontier for positive impact in global health will be to confront the internal and external causes of inequities, focus innovation resources, and create a stronger basis for collaboration to advance access and health equity—building trust, relationships, and solutions with all system partners, from regulators to marginalized communities that do not currently fully benefit from private sector innovations.

References

1. Brock T, Reeves M. What is the private sector? Definition and Business Examples https://www.investopedia.com/terms/p/private-sector.asp. Accessed 26 June 2022
2. World Health Organization. Private Sector Landscape in Mixed Health Systems. https://www.who.int/publications/i/item/9789240018303. Accessed 26 June 2022
3. India Brand Equity Foundation. Biotechnology Industry in India. https://www.ibef.org/industry/biotechnology-india. Accessed 26 June 2022
4. Access to Medicine Foundation. 2022. Ranking: Company Report Cards and Comparison. https://accesstomedicinefoundation.org/access-to-medicine-index. Accessed 26 June 2022
5. Value Reporting Foundation. https://www.valuereportingfoundation.org. Accessed 26 June 2022
6. Denecker J. How Healthcare Hacks Help Doctors Innovate https://www.ge.com/news/taxonomy/term/5630. Accessed 26 June 2022
7. Bhatti Y, Taylor A, Harris M, Wadge H, Escobar E, Prime M, et al. Global lessons in frugal innovation to improve healthcare delivery in the United States. Health Affairs. 2017. https://www.healthaffairs.org/doi/10.1377/hlthaff.2017.0480
8. Medicines for Malaria Venture. https://www.mmv.org. Accessed 26 June 2022
9. Drugs for Neglected Diseases Initiative. https://dndi.org/. Accessed 26 June 2022
10. Medicines Patent Pool. https://medicinespatentpool.org. Accessed 26 June 2022
11. Shops Plus Project. Understanding the Growth of Pharmacy Chains in Latin America. https://shopsplusproject.org/sites/default/files/resources/SP_Brief_LAC_060820_v08f-print_red2.pdf accessed 2022.08.31
12. Novartis Sickle Cell Disease. https://www.novartis.com/diseases/sickle-cell-disease. Accessed 26 June 2022
13. International Finance Corporation. IFC Jobs Study: Assessing Private Sector Contributions to Job Creation and Poverty Reduction. https://openknowledge.worldbank.org/handle/10986/16979. Accessed 26 June 2022
14. Statistics South Africa. Four facts about the mining industry. 2019. https://www.statssa.gov.za/?p=14682. Accessed 26 June 2022
15. Shah M. Top 5 healthcare CSR trends to look out for in 2022. https://indiacsr.in/top-5-healthcare-csr-trends-to-look-out-for-in-2022/#:~:text=In%20FY%202020%2D21%2C%20healthcare,resources%20towards%20healthcare%20CSR%20initiatives. Accessed 26 June 2022

Health Systems Resilience

54

Dell D Saulnier, Karl Blanchet, and Fabrizio Tediosi

Abstract

Health systems need to continue functioning and providing essential health services, even when they experience challenges that threaten their ability to do so. Resilience describes the ability for health systems to manage change when they are shocked, so that essential functions are maintained. The capacity to change ranges from absorbing the shock using existing resources to fundamentally reorganizing the system. Resilience is needed proactively to prepare and plan for shocks, during a shock to respond to the event, and to learn from a shock after it ends. Strengthening the whole system can help to build resilience, such as strengthening the ways that actors and groups in the system interact. Understanding the processes that support change in a system will help us understand how to build resilience.

Keywords

Resilience · Health systems · Shocks · Capacity

54.1 Introduction

We rely on health systems to keep populations healthy. We expect health systems to function and provide health services to the population to improve health outcomes, being responsive to emerging needs while ensuring financial and social protection. Yet health systems are constantly facing challenges that threaten their ability to function: climate change, conflict and civil unrest, financial crises, outbreaks and pandemics, and mass migration are all potential threats to health systems. What happens when a crisis changes the demands placed on the system or changes the way the system needs to adapt to deliver healthcare? What does the health system need to do to continue functioning and maintain essential health services?

Over the last decade, the global health community has been trying to address those questions using the concept of health system resilience, broadly defined as the ability of a system to manage change when it is shocked, to maintain essential functions [1]. Resilient health systems are stronger health systems that deliver equitable health services and outcomes in periods of stabil-

D. D Saulnier (✉)
Lund University, Malmö, Sweden
e-mail: dell.saulnier@med.lu.se

K. Blanchet
University of Geneva, Geneva, Switzerland
e-mail: karl.blanchet@unige.ch

F. Tediosi
Department of Epidemiology and Public Health
Swiss Tropical and Public Health Institute
Allschwill, Switzerland
e-mail: fabrizio.tediosi@swisstph.ch

M. C. B. Raviglione et al. (eds.), *Global Health Essentials*, Sustainable Development Goals Series,
https://doi.org/10.1007/978-3-031-33851-9_54

ity and in periods of turbulence. Health system resilience gained global attention and became mainstream following the outbreak of the Ebola Virus Disease in West Africa (2014–2016), when it became clear that health systems were struggling to contain the outbreak and that they could potentially collapse because of the scope and scale of the event. This experience demonstrated the need for health systems to anticipate and prepare for acute shocks and to continue addressing the health needs of the population in the face of these shocks [2]. Beyond acute events health systems also face a range of day-to-day challenges (chronic stressors) that themselves demand what has been termed 'everyday resilience' [3].

Building on resilience thinking from other disciplines like disaster risk reduction or ecology, theories of health system resilience have helped us to identify some common characteristics and capacities of resilient health systems [4]. This chapter aims to first describe the basic concepts of health system resilience and then to summarize different approaches and theories for building the capacity for resilience in health systems.

54.2 Description of the Issue

Health systems adopt different strategies when reacting to shock and stress (Table 54.1). Absorptive strategies resist challenges and enable continued system functionality without changes in system configuration. Higher intensity challenges however may exhaust the system's ability to absorb shock/stress and require adaptations which involve incremental adjustments that facilitate continued performance. Transformative strategies entail significant functional or structural changes that transform the system to an entirely new state that is better able to deliver equitable healthcare services and outcomes, implying preferential benefits for the poorest and most vulnerable population groups. Absorptive capacity requires the least degree of change, and a system may be able to cope with a minor shock using only absorptive capacity. Adaptation can protect the system's functions and services, but the system may no longer be able to operate at the same quality or quantity. Transforming the system requires a radical degree of change and may occur with the most severe shocks. These three capacities can all transpire at once, or occur linearly, or at different times, or among different parts of the system.

Resilience is about more than the response to a shock. Health systems can have the capacity for resilience without experiencing a shock. This makes resilience equally important before a shock happens (*proactive resilience*) and after a shock (*recovery resilience*), as well as the *reactive resilience* that is on display in a middle of a response. Health systems that are proactively resilient can identify and reduce their own vulnerabilities and plan how to respond if a shock does occur. For instance, staff may recognize that there is a substantial delay in sharing information about suspected cases of an outbreak-prone disease. If it takes too long to identify new cases, responders may not be able to react quickly enough to contain an outbreak. Shortening such a delay before an outbreak occurs would mitigate the spread of the disease and improve the performance of the surveillance system overall.

Table 54.1 Absorptive, adaptive, and transformative capacity

Capacity	Definition	Examples from COVID-19
Absorb	Ability to use existing reserves, resources, and strategies in the short term to absorb the impact of a shock on the system's functions and services	Hospitals operating at 80% bed capacity before the pandemic to ensure surge capacity
Adapt	Ability to make organizational changes to use fewer or different resources and strategies in the short- or long term to manage a shock	Task shifting COVID-19 vaccination to trained members of the UK public
Transform	Ability to fundamentally change the system's structure or functions when its current form becomes unbearable during a shock	Creating telehealth structures to replace and supplement facility-based services

Once a shock ends, recovery resilience helps the health system learn from the experience, identify the processes that supported the system's functioning and those that hindered good performance. Learning from the response can improve the system's ability to respond to shocks in the future. The system will also need to deal with any lasting consequences from the shock on its structure or performance. For example, as the COVID-19 pandemic wanes and emergency funding is reduced, health systems will need to adjust to operating within smaller budgets.

54.3 Approaches to Building Health System Resilience

So, what can be done to build the capacity for resilience in health systems? There is no 'one size fits all' approach to building resilience because every health system is complex, structured differently, and embedded in its own context. However, conceptual frameworks developed from research evidence describe some of the attributes, abilities, and processes that may build resilience [1, 2, 5–7]. From these, certain common threads can be identified. For instance, systems must have stability and redundancy so that minor shocks do not overwhelm their functions yet be flexible enough to adjust their decision-making processes and resource use when needed. Systems that have a sufficient supply of well-organized resources are at an advantage. Systems must be able to interact with the other systems, groups, and organizations like other government ministries and international partners, because the health system will be affected by their response to the shock as well. Individuals, groups, and organizations must be able to easily share information with each other, which can help with decision-making, planning, and monitoring. Community trust and engagement are essential to both inform and support the system's response to a shock and to create a system that the population can trust.

Health systems strengthening is at the heart of transformation to build resilience. Simple strategies for building resilience or strategies that have worked in another system may have no effect at all in another system, may lead to worse performance, or may have unintended and unexpected consequences. Strengthening health systems aims to permanently improve the function of the system at the system level. Focusing on the system as whole, rather than individual parts, means looking beyond short-term strategies, immediate outcomes, and stop-gap interventions. Instead, long-term, well-designed, and contextually relevant reforms transform the system and can reduce its risk to similar shocks in the future.

Looking beyond the inputs and immediate outcomes of the system also means considering the social aspects like values, norms, and power. This system 'software' helps to explain why health systems behave the way they do (particularly when we expect it to behave in another way). Software also affects the system's performance and the success of its policies and reforms [8]. As resilience is about the capacity of the system to manage change, then software becomes a key determinant for understanding how to create the capacity for resilience in each system. Building and managing resilience of health systems requires being able to involve and manage actors, networks and institutions that have an influence on the health systems [9]. Strengthening health system governance—the implicit and explicit rules and institutions that shape power, relationships between actors, and the actions of these actors—is therefore key to promote the ability of health systems to be resilient [10, 11] (Box 54.1).

Box 54.1: Governance Strategies for Building Resilience from the COVID-19 Pandemic [9, 12]

The COVID-19 pandemic has been a catalyst for learning about what works to create health system resilience, in what contexts, and under what conditions. Although many lessons are yet unknown, some resilience strategies have been identified by comparing the ways that health systems across the world have responded to the shock of COVID-19.

Governance is crucial to building resilience, as governance is what steers the preparedness, response, and learning of the health system. Two rapid reviews of European countries and of fragile or conflict-affected states (FCAS) identified numerous strategies and capacities that supported governance during the early stages of the pandemic. In both reviews, a key set of strategies involved utilizing effective structures to coordinate the response across the health system, the government, and other national and international stakeholders beyond government, like civil society and communities. Having sufficient human and financial resources and a strong monitoring and surveillance system assisted coordination, together with the appropriate skills, such as technical expertise and effective political leadership. Clear and regular communication with stakeholders and populations supported leadership and transparency in the response and helped translate new evidence into appropriate policy. In the FCAS, development agencies needed to be better integrated into coordination structures.

54.4 Conclusions and Recommendations

The growing field of health system resilience is a useful way to understand how health systems manage shocks. To understand it, we need to understand the processes and actions that support the system in planning for shocks, responding to them, and learning from them. Ultimately, these lessons can be used to strengthen health systems for resilience during times of calm and of crisis.

References

1. Blanchet K, Nam SL, Ramalingam B, Pozo-Martin F. Governance and capacity to manage resilience of health systems: towards a new conceptual framework. Int J Health Policy Manag. 2017;6(8):431–5. https://doi.org/10.15171/ijhpm.2017.36.
2. Kruk ME, Myers M, Varpilah ST, Dahn BT. What is a resilient health system? Lessons from Ebola Lancet. 2015;385(9980):1910–2. https://doi.org/10.1016/S0140-6736(15)60755-3.
3. Gilson L, Barasa E, Nxumalo N, Cleary S, Goudge J, Molyneux S, et al. Everyday resilience in district health systems: emerging insights from the front lines in Kenya and South Africa. BMJ Glob Health. 2017;2(2):e000224. https://doi.org/10.1136/bmjgh-2016-000224.
4. Biddle L, Wahedi K, Bozorgmehr K. Health system resilience: a literature review of empirical research. Health Policy Plan. 2020;35(8):1084–109. https://doi.org/10.1093/heapol/czaa032.
5. Barasa E, Boga M, Kagwanja N, Kinyanjui S, Molyneux C, Nyikuri M, et al. Learning sites for health system governance in Kenya and South Africa: reflecting on our experience. Health Res Policy Syst. 2020;18(1):44. https://doi.org/10.1186/s12961-020-00552-6.
6. Haldane V, De Foo C, Abdalla SM, Jung AS, Tan M, Wu S, et al. Health systems resilience in managing the COVID-19 pandemic: lessons from 28 countries. Nat Med. 2021;27(6):964–80. https://doi.org/10.1038/s41591-021-01381-y.
7. Hanefeld J, Mayhew S, Legido-Quigley H, Martineau F, Karanikolos M, Blanchet K, et al. Towards an understanding of resilience: responding to health systems shocks. Health Policy Plan. 2018;33(3):355–67. https://doi.org/10.1093/heapol/czx183.
8. Sheikh K, Gilson L, Agyepong IA, Hanson K, Ssengooba F, Bennett S. Building the field of health policy and systems research: framing the questions. PLoS Med. 2011;8(8):e1001073. https://doi.org/10.1371/journal.pmed.1001073.
9. European Observatory on Health Systems and Policies. Health systems resilience during COVID-19: lessons for building back better. Copenhagen: The European Observatory on Health Systems and Policies; 2021.
10. Saulnier DD, Blanchet K, Canila C, Cobos Muñoz D, Dal Zennaro L, de Savigny D, et al. A health systems resilience research agenda: moving from concept to practice. BMJ Glob Health. 2021;6(8):e006779. https://doi.org/10.1136/bmjgh-2021-006779.
11. Thomas S, Sagan A, Larkin J, Cylus J, Figueras J, Karanikolos M. Strengthening health systems resilience: key concepts and strategies. Copenhagen: European Observatory on Health Systems and Policies; 2020.
12. Gooding K, Bertone M, Loffreda G, Witter S. Strengthening coordination for shock preparedness and response: lessons for health system resilience (working paper). Oxford: Oxford Policy Management; 2022.

55 Epidemic Preparedness and Response

Antoni Plasència and Jaime Sepúlveda

Abstract

Effective epidemic preparedness and response (EPR) involve the capabilities of public health and health care systems, together with people and communities, to prevent, respond and recover from health emergencies, particularly those which can overwhelm routine capacities. A health systems approach can be useful to outline the basic architecture of the main functions involving EPR actions and their interactions, reinforcing the need for collaborative and integrated schemes. EPR is largely the duty of governments and multilateral agencies, with a cross-sectoral approach. The many lessons learned from the Covid-19 pandemic need to be actively implemented, from global instruments for transnational response to multidisciplinary capacities at all levels along the continuum of prevention, surveillance, case detection, diagnostics, treatment and prophylaxis and community control, as well as resilience and recovery actions. Finally, the unacceptable impact of epidemics and pandemics on vulnerable populations world-wide requires that equity-oriented policies and programmes be embedded into EPR actions.

Keywords

Epidemic preparedness and response (EPR) · Preparedness · Health systems · BARDA · HERA · Africa CDC · ACPHEED · ECDC · Pandemics · Epidemics

55.1 Introduction and Aims

Effective epidemic preparedness and response (EPR) to emerging diseases is one of the key global health challenges of our times, as shown by the recent Covid-19 pandemic experience. In an intensely interconnected and increasingly interdependent world, the rapid spread of infectious agents can become a global threat with formidable negative consequences, not only on health but also on the economy, trade, social cohesion and security, among others. Despite early warnings from the scientific community, from advisory panels and the World Health Organization (WHO), the world is still largely unprepared to prevent and respond to such challenges [1].

This chapter briefly covers some of the main definitions of EPR, their most relevant components from a health systems' thinking perspective and the main functions involved. It also delves

A. Plasència (✉)
Barcelona Institute for Global Health (ISGlobal), Hospital Clínic and Universitat de Barcelona (UB), Barcelona, Spain
e-mail: antoni.plasencia@isglobal.org

J. Sepúlveda
Institute for Global Health Sciences, University of California, San Francisco (UCSF), San Francisco, CA, USA
e-mail: jaime.sepulveda@ucsf.edu

M. C. B. Raviglione et al. (eds.), *Global Health Essentials*, Sustainable Development Goals Series,
https://doi.org/10.1007/978-3-031-33851-9_55

into some of the lessons learned from the SARS-Cov-2 crisis and proposes some key actions to ensure that the world is better prepared to prevent and manage upcoming epidemics and pandemics. Failing to do so entails the real risk that pandemics will emerge more often and from anywhere in the world, spread more rapidly, cause more damage to economy and society at large, killing more people than COVID-19.

55.2 Some Definitions, Functions and Models

The European Centre for Disease Control (ECDC) has formulated the core competencies

for preparedness for public health emergencies [2], defined as "the capability of the public health and health care systems, communities, and individuals, to prevent, protect against, quickly respond to, and recover from health emergencies, particularly those whose scale, timing, or unpredictability threatens to overwhelm routine capabilities". It includes: a) the detection and assessment of health risks (especially through epidemic intelligence); b) risk management, largely through the prevention and control roles of health services; and c) the communication of risks, both between the agents involved and the general population, as defined by the US Centers for Disease Control (CDC [3]).

EPR is largely the duty of governments and multilateral agencies, with a cross-sectoral approach, involving not only health and social systems, but also research and innovation stakeholders, together with businesses and communities and citizens, to ensure the necessary "glocal" (global and local) capacities and resources.

Different models have been proposed to conceptualize the main components of EPR planning, implementation and evaluation [4–7]. Some of them make more emphasis on specific aspects like financial needs, security systems, and health systems, including primary health care, community-risk reduction strategies or urban settings, while some include outcomes like recovery and resilience, as part of the continuum of EPR.

55.3 A Health Systems Approach

A systems approach can be useful to outline the basic architecture of the main health systems components and functions and their interactions, reinforcing the need for collaborative and integrated schemes, using the WHO "building blocks" [8] framework, which has also been applied to the evaluation of the response to Covid-19 at country level [9, 10]. Such components, namely: a) Leadership and governance; b) Financing; c) Procurement; d) Information; e) Service delivery; f) Workforce; g) People and communities; h) Communication; i) Research and innovation and j) Equity and sustainability vision are summarized in Table 55.1, including a selection of their main functions adapted to the implementation of EPR capabilities. Note that components h), i) and j) are an addition to the initial a) to g) components in the original scheme. This approach is relevant not only at national level, but also, with some adaptations, to the supranational (regional) and subnational (local) levels.

Table 55.1 The Health Systems Framework: implications for EPR activities

Health systems building blocks[a]	Selected EPR functions
1. Leadership and governance	• Horizon scanning of major infectious threats to health • Whole-government and multisectoral strategy, policies and plans, with strong evidence-based and data-driven decision-making processes • Approved supporting legal instruments • Executive agency-driven organizations • Resource allocation • Dissemination of monitoring and evaluation results • Accountability and flexibility to adapt to evolving needs • Management of bureaucracy and corruption • Adaptation to conflict and migration areas • Transnational and global cooperation and solidarity

Table 55.1 (continued)

Health systems building blocks[a]	Selected EPR functions
2. Financing	• Specific funding schemes for health and other social needs • Special effort for vulnerable populations and communities to prevent financial hardship and catastrophic expenditure • Funding (public and private) for research and innovation
3. Procurement	• Regulatory system for marketing authorization and safety monitoring • Access to (rapid) testing procedures and facilities • Supply, stockpiling and distribution systems for access to essential medical countermeasures, including treatment and prophylaxis procedures and facilities, medical equipment and Personal Protection Equipment (PPE) • Manufacturing capacity • Public-private purchase agreements
4. Information	• Surveillance systems with a broad One-health perspective (human, animal, environmental and climatic factors) • Availability of digitalized (big) data bases—including vital registrations, record linkage and data science capabilities • Epidemic intelligence systems with early warning procedures, risk assessment and transmission modelling capabilities, predictive scenarios building and intervention evaluation • Case identification, contact tracing and outbreak analysis tools • Information on broader health issues, including the performance of the health system, financial trends, access to quality health care and workforce • Information in other relevant areas: Mobility, equity, migration, urbanization
5. Service delivery	• People-centred and integrated models of prevention, treatment and care • Primary and community care services and networks, with a comprehensive range of clinical and public health interventions, responding to the full range of epidemic threats, with the coordinated back-up of specialized and hospital services, responsible for defined populations • Special focus on immunization strategies and services • Standards, norms and guidance to ensure access and essential dimensions of service quality: safety, effectiveness, integration, continuity and people-centredness • Mechanisms to hold health providers accountable for access and quality and to ensure patients' and communities' voices
6. Workforce	• Responsive to the needs and expectations of people, fair and efficient, to achieve the best individual and collective outcomes possible given available resources and circumstances • Mapping and measurement of occupations delivering EPR functions • Adequate competency-based recruitment, education, training and distribution programmes, enhancing performance and improving retention
7. People and communities	• Engagement and training for leadership and empowerment, prevention, early detection and response, and citizens' science • Understand and strengthen community resilience factors, including risk communication and management, as well as linkage with services • Involvement of civil society organizations, in partnership with local governments and private stakeholders
8. Communication	• Expertise in objective, timely and transparent risk communication, both internally to involved organizations and externally to relevant stakeholders and the public • Use of digital platforms and social networks • Strategies, tools and procedures to handle infodemia and misinformation • Health education and literacy
9. Research and Innovation	• Prioritization of knowledge areas, including evidence generation, intervention development, modelling and evaluation • Funding programmes including basic, clinical and population-based interdisciplinary research • Behavioural, social and organizational components • International networks and partnerships, involving local, regional and global levels • Independent integrated advisory models and interaction with political and technical levels

(continued)

Table 55.1 (continued)

Health systems building blocks[a]	Selected EPR functions
10. Equity and sustainability vision	• Comprehensive approach to social, environmental and climatic determinants of health, across infectious diseases • One-health/planetary health, as well as SDGs frameworks for transformation • Health as a human right and a global public good challenge, facing the impact of neocolonialism in LMICs • Focus on poorest, most affected and most vulnerable and marginalized groups, ensuring within and between-country equity by gender, ethnicity, socioeconomic status, education and urbanization

[a] Adapted and expanded by the authors from: World Health Organization. Monitoring the building blocks of health systems: a handbook of indicators and their measurement strategies (2010) (Ref. [8])

55.4 Lessons Learned: From Context to Systems

Many reports, including regional and country case studies have attempted to summarize some of the lessons learned about preparedness during the Covid-19 pandemic [11], including low- and-middle-income countries (LMICs)[12] (see also Box 55.1 on country case studies prepared for the Independent Panel for Pandemic Preparedness and Response). Country preparedness levels, as measured by different indices, failed to predict the performance of health systems and their ability to reduce the negative impact of the pandemic [1].

Box 55.1: The Experience of the Panel for Pandemic Preparedness and Response [1]

The Independent Panel for Pandemic Preparedness and Response (IPPPR) was formally initiated on May 2020, by petition of the head of the WHO, and with distinguished leaders as members. The new coronavirus outbreak in China had been declared a pandemic just 2 months before, with COVID-19 already present in most countries of the world. The goal of IPPPR was to evaluate the international response to the pandemic. After 8 months of hard work, IPPPR issued in May 2021, a harsh report calling for transformational changes to make this the last pandemic.

Recommendations of IPPPR in their report include seriously strengthening WHO both financially and politically; the creation of a Global Health Threats Council with heads of state as members; and the establishment of a new global fund with the ability to disburse up to $50–100 billion at short notice. More than a year after the thoughtful IPPPR report, it is unfortunate to attest that the recommendations have not been implemented, and that the world is still unprepared for the next pandemic.

Selected Countries Case Studies

The Independent Panel identified a number of best-performing and worst-performing countries. Among the latter, the United States, the United Kingdom, Brazil, and Mexico were included [27]. Interestingly, several of the best-performing countries had a woman as head of government.

Not all regions of the world have been similarly affected. Some countries have performed much better than others. Understanding what elements made a difference and what lessons can be derived is most important. In a case study about the United States' response—invited by IPPPR—a group of scholars from UCSF [27] found that there are four areas of particular importance: First is good governance, which includes institutional strength and effective leadership. The second is good communication. This means communication from leaders that is clear, accurate and honest and builds trust between the government and its people. The third lesson is that, as a global community, we can trust science. With COVID-19, science has once again come to the rescue, delivering innovative vaccines, diagnostics and drugs in record time.

Good governance implies the formulation and enforcement of policies to benefit the public. This is premised on institutional strength and effective leadership. Countries that had both conditions like New Zealand and Norway, fared well. Poor leadership and lack of institutional strength are of course a bad combination—Mexico being a case in point. But even in places with solid institutions, like the United States, bad leadership led to disastrous consequences in 2020. Therefore, some level of political accountability for poor leadership and performance needs to be instituted. There are many lessons learned from this pandemic response that need to be incorporated into future pandemic preparedness. This will require more than just a plan; it will require the public health infrastructure, trained personnel, financial resources, and competent leadership that were so painfully lacking in the terrible Covid-19 pandemic.

Perhaps the most important lesson from this pandemic is that "no country will be safe until all countries are safe". Global immunologic equity should not only be a humanitarian desire, but a national security concern. To ensure that the world is prepared for the next pandemic, we will require more than just a plan; we will require global and national public health institutions to be well funded, with the authority and the ability to move nimbly and forcefully in the face of uncertainty.

The following aspects summarize some of the most recurrent recommendations for which reasonable evidence is available:

(a) Smarter surveillance systems, including high-tech tracking genomics in high-risk populations and other innovative early warning tools, building open-source quality data platforms with safe shared access [13] and interoperable statistical modelling [14], adapted to policy-making decisions [15].
(b) Faster and more equitable diagnostics, vaccine and therapeutics production and distribution around the world [16].
(c) Combat infodemia (both disinformation and misinformation), with the engagement of social networks and communication stakeholders, to reinforce transparency, credibility and trust—both interpersonal and in governments [17], as well as collective self-efficacy [18].
(d) Strengthen public health capabilities, including agencies and other executive technical bodies in charge of EPR measures, ensuring their independence from political pressure, and develop resilient health security systems, involving global, national and local levels, periodically informed by dynamic preparedness metrics [19].
(e) Ensure dedicated personnel who have no other job except to improve readiness for active response, as well as primary care nursing and community worker staffing, as part of an adequate health coverage [20].
(f) Promote global pandemic governance agreements in support of collaboration among countries [21], as well as of ambitious financial commitments to ensure adequate EPR capabilities.
(g) Expand multi- and interdisciplinary research in support of EPR goals, through One-health and planetary health approaches, as well as strengthen research and innovation systems with global financial support [22], including discovery, pre-clinical and clinical research, manufacturing, early clinical testing of candidate products and implementation research [23].

(h) Emphasize the need for an equity approach, from transmission modelling [24] to post-pandemic global economy [25], so as to leave no one behind.

Specific executive bodies, like the Biomedical Advanced Research and Development Authority (BARDA) in the United States, the Health Emergencies and Response Authority (HERA) in the European Union [26], the Africa Centers for Disease Control and Prevention (Africa CDC https://africacdc.org/) or the **ASEAN Centre for Public Health Emergencies and Emerging Diseases** (ACPHEED) are strengthening or newly implementing many of these lessons at the regional and national levels.

55.5 Conclusions

Health as a global public good requires adequate harmonized EPR measures. Despite the growing likelihood and impact of global health threats related to infectious agents, EPR activities have been largely inadequate or insufficiently deployed, both globally, regionally and locally. EPR effectiveness is inconsistently related with the quality of public health and acute care health systems and services. Science, technology and innovation have proven to be game changers in the management of the Covid-19 pandemic response. Leadership and governance, as well as communication and social engagement are also indispensable components of a strengthened health systems response. The latter components failed in most countries, with catastrophic consequences.

Before the waning of the political momentum and of social awareness on the importance of EPR, the many lessons learned from the Covid-19 pandemic need to be actively implemented, from global transnational legal instruments—including the possibility of a global pandemic treaty—to multidisciplinary capacities at all levels, along the continuum of prevention, surveillance, case detection, diagnostics, treatment and prophylaxis and community control, as well as resilience and recovery actions, with dynamic indices to regularly assess and improve the status of EPR capacities. Moreover, the unacceptable impact of epidemics and pandemics on vulnerable populations world-wide requires that equity-oriented policies and programmes be embedded into all EPR actions.

References

1. The Independent Panel for Pandemic Preparedness and Response. Making it the last pandemic. 2021. https://theindependentpanel.org/mainreport/
2. European Centre for Disease Prevention and Control. Public health emergency preparedness – Core competencies for EU Member States. Stockholm: ECDC; 2017. https://www.ecdc.europa.eu/sites/default/files/documents/public-health-emergency-preparedness-core-competencies-eu-member-states.pdf
3. Centers for Disease Control and Prevention (CDC). Public health emergency preparedness and response capabilities. Atlanta, GA: U.S. Department of Health and Human Services; 2018. https://www.cdc.gov/cpr/readiness/capabilities.htm
4. Oppenheim B, Gallivan M, Madhav NK, et al. Assessing global preparedness for the next pandemic: development and application of an Epidemic Preparedness Index. BMJ Glob Health. 2019;4(1):e001157. https://doi.org/10.1136/bmjgh-2018-001157.
5. Haldane V, Jung A, Neill R, et al. From response to transformation: how countries can strengthen national pandemic preparedness and response systems. BMJ. 2021;375:e067507. https://doi.org/10.1136/bmj-2021-067507.
6. Nguyen L, et al. Global health security preparedness and response: an analysis of the relationship between joint external evaluation scores and COVID-19 response performance. BMJ Open. 2021;11:e050052. https://doi.org/10.1136/bmjopen-2021-050052.
7. Haider N, et al. The Global Health Security index and Joint External Evaluation score for health preparedness are not correlated with countries' COVID-19 detection response time and mortality outcome. Epidemiol Infect. 2020;148:e210. https://doi.org/10.1017/S0950268820002046.
8. World Health Organization. Monitoring the building blocks of health systems: a handbook of indicators and their measurement strategies. 2010. https://apps.who.int/iris/handle/10665/258734
9. Haldane V, De Foo C, Abdalla SM, et al. Health systems resilience in managing the COVID-19 pandemic: lessons from 28 countries. Nat Med. 2021;27(6):964–80. https://doi.org/10.1038/s41591-021-01381-y. Epub 2021 May 17

10. Balqis-Ali NZ, Fun WH, Ismail M, et al. Addressing gaps for health systems strengthening: a public perspective on health systems' response towards COVID-19. Int J Environ Res Public Health. 2021;18:9047. https://doi.org/10.3390/ijerph18179047.
11. Maxmen A. Has covid taught us anything about preparedness? https://media.nature.com/original/magazine-assets/d41586-021-02217-y/d41586-021-02217-y.pdf
12. Bwire G, Ario AR, Eyu P, Ocom F, Wamala JF, Kusi KA, Ndeketa L, Jambo KC, Wanyenze RK, Talisuna AO. The COVID-19 pandemic in the African continent. BMC Med. 2022;20(1):167. https://doi.org/10.1186/s12916-022-02367-4.
13. Kucharski AJ, Hodcroft EB, Kraemer MUG. Sharing, synthesis and sustainability of data analysis for epidemic preparedness in Europe. Lancet Reg Health Eur. 2021;9:100215. https://doi.org/10.1016/j.lanepe.2021.100215.
14. Nicholson G, Blangiardo M, Briers M, et al. Interoperability of statistical models in pandemic preparedness: principles and reality. Stat Sci. 2022;37(2):183–206. https://doi.org/10.1214/22-STS854.
15. Mandal S, Parchani K, Arinaminpathy N, Sarkar S, Bhargava B, Panda S. 'Imperfect but useful': pandemic response in the Global South can benefit from greater use of mathematical modelling. BMJ Glob Health. 2022;7(5):e008710. https://doi.org/10.1136/bmjgh-2022-008710.
16. Ramchandani R, Kazatchkine M, Liu J, et al. Vaccines, therapeutics, and diagnostics for covid-19: redesigning systems to improve pandemic response. BMJ. 2021;375:e067488. https://doi.org/10.1136/bmj-2021-067488. Published 2021 Nov 28
17. COVID-19 National Preparedness Collaborators. Pandemic preparedness and COVID-19: an exploratory analysis of infection and fatality rates, and contextual factors associated with preparedness in 177 countries, from Jan 1, 2020, to Sept 30, 2021. Lancet. 2022;399(10334):1489–512. https://doi.org/10.1016/S0140-6736(22)00172-6.
18. Cordova-Pozo KL, Korzilius HPLM, Rouwette EAJ, et al. Using systems dynamics for capturing the multicausality of factors affecting health system capacity in Latin America while responding to the COVID-19 pandemic. Int J Environ Res Public Health. 2021;18(19):10002. https://doi.org/10.3390/ijerph181910002.
19. Kandel N, Chungong S. WHO Technical Working Group of the Dynamic Preparedness Metric and Health Security Preparedness Department. Dynamic preparedness metric: a paradigm shift to measure and act on preparedness. Lancet Glob Health. 2022;10(5):e615–6. https://doi.org/10.1016/S2214-109X(22)00097-3.
20. Okeahalam C, Williams V, Otwombe K. Factors associated with COVID-19 infections and mortality in Africa: a cross- sectional study using publicly available data. BMJ Open. 2020;10:e042750. https://doi.org/10.1136/bmjopen-2020-042750.
21. Duff JH, Liu A, Saavedra J, et al. A global public health convention for the 21st century. Lancet Public Health. 2021;6(6):e428–33. Final del formulario. https://doi.org/10.1016/S2468-2667(21)00070-0.
22. Lurie N, Keusch GT, Dzau VJ. Urgent lessons from COVID 19: why the world needs a standing, coordinated system and sustainable financing for global research and development. Lancet. 2021;397(10280):1229–36. https://doi.org/10.1016/S0140-6736(21)00503-1.
23. Means AR, Wagner AD, Kern E, Newman LP, Weiner BJ. Implementation science to respond to the COVID-19 pandemic. Front Public Health. 2020;8:462. https://doi.org/10.3389/fpubh.2020.00462.
24. Zelner J, Masters NB, Naraharisetti R, Mojola SA, Chowkwanyun M, Malosh R. There are no equal opportunity infectors: Epidemiological modelers must rethink our approach to inequality in infection risk. PLoS Comput Biol. 2022;18(2):e1009795. https://doi.org/10.1371/journal.pcbi.1009795.
25. Labonté R. Ensuring global health equity in a post-pandemic economy. Int J Health Policy Manag. 2022;11(8):1246–50. https://doi.org/10.34172/ijhpm.2022.7212.
26. Villa S, van Leeuwen R, Gray CC, et al. HERA: a new era for health emergency preparedness in Europe? Lancet. 2021;397(10290):2145–7.
27. UCSF Institute for Global Health Sciences: The United States' and Mexico's Responses to Covid-19. IPPR; 2021. https://globalhealthsciences.ucsf.edu/news/united-states-and-mexicos-response-covid-19

Precision Global Health and Epidemic Forecasting

56

Antoine Flahault

Abstract

With more billions of Internet users across the globe and the accelerating power of Artificial Intelligence, our capacity to collect, integrate, analyse and visualise large volumes of data is unprecedented. However, to overcome the challenges of past applications of technology-driven global health strategies and the fragmentation of historically distinct health science disciplines, we need a more comprehensive approach to global health. Building on precision medicine, and more recently precision public health, we propose Precision Global Health as a strategic, innovative, multi-level and transdisciplinary approach that aims at equitably improving human health by addressing complex global health challenges, and working with and for targeted populations, their specific needs, and the delivery of sustainable and impactful tailored health interventions. The COVID-19 crisis burst into a digitalised interconnected world we may take huge benefits from. The use of real-time quality data was extremely useful to allow precision epidemic forecasting and improving our response to the crisis. The mathematical theory of infectious diseases allowed for guiding public policies in this pandemic to an extent which has never been seen before. The concept of reproductive rate with its threshold theorem had implications in terms of preventive measures, screening methods and herd immunity.

Keywords

Precision health · Epidemic forecasting · Artificial Intelligence · Data science · Infectious disease dynamics

56.1 Background

We have seen major achievements in global health in the past decades. Life expectancy has doubled in every single country since 1870, child mortality has halved in the world since 1990, smallpox has been eradicated (1980), poliomyelitis was on the verge of eradication just before the COVID-19 pandemic. However, despite these extraordinary results, pandemics and emerging infectious diseases remain a major threat for humanity which reveals to be unprepared or poorly prepared. This is not a totally unexpected situation since Bill Gates wrote prior to the pandemic that “there is a significant probability that a large and lethal modern-day pandemic will occur in our lifetime” [1]. We are confronted with an unprecedented pandemic risk which is concomitant with an unprecedented digital revolu-

A. Flahault (✉)
Faculty of Medicine, Institute of Global Health, University of Geneva, Geneva, Switzerland
e-mail: antoine.flahault@unige.ch

M. C. B. Raviglione et al. (eds.), *Global Health Essentials*, Sustainable Development Goals Series,
https://doi.org/10.1007/978-3-031-33851-9_56

tion. People are more equipped with smartphones; they are more intensively connected to the internet and social networks. Data sciences are infiltrating much more our daily lives than ever, allowing for delivering more appropriate health services with greater precision to those who need them the most. This is what we could name "Precision Global Health". However, taking action in due time requires that decision-makers are timely informed, precise and reliable nowcasting and forecasting. Predicting outbreaks of emerging infectious diseases is indeed key to take decisions in the right place at the right time. This chapter will review reasons for failures and conditions for successes in epidemic forecasting and will discuss why deeper integration of life, social, engineering and data sciences are needed to allow for better performing models.

56.2 Aims of the Chapter

The aim of this chapter is to review existing achievements in Precision Global Health and to see to what extent epidemic forecasting can benefit from better accuracy and reliability.

56.3 Description of the Issue

Epidemic nowcasting and forecasting often failed to deliver in the recent past. Nowcasting addresses the question of estimating current epidemiological situations in near real time. It aims to estimate the number of cases or deaths. For achieving such an objective in the domain of influenza, Google Flu Trends was created. When collecting a couple of relevant search terms, Google search engine was able to accurately estimate the level of influenza virus circulation on the territory it addressed, and to confront it with official statistics on influenza activity. The US Centers for Disease Control and Prevention (US-CDC) relies on sentinel physicians who collect data on influenza-like-illnesses as diagnosed from their own practices, send them electronically to the federal agency which has to check received data, consolidate their analyses and post them on their website. It takes between one and 2 weeks before the US-CDC publicly deliver their data, which could be a while when addressing the highly evolving situation during seasonal outbreaks. In the years 2010s, all eyes were therefore turned towards Google Flu Trends which instantaneously delivered their data from almost everywhere the company was acting. When for New York City, in January 2013, Google Flu Trends reported flu levels which were higher than during the 2009 swine flu pandemic, Michael Bloomberg, the mayor at that time, declared the state of emergency which probably led to increase searches on influenza on Google and the epidemic curve continued its exponential growth. However, 2 weeks later the US-CDC published their field data which did not confirm any abnormal signal. It seems Google algorithms were not able to control the overamplification signal which was due to the rumour of a large influenza outbreak occurring in New York City at that period [2]. Nowcasting models from Google went wrong and the IT company eventually decided to shut down its service all over the world. In September 2014, when an Ebola outbreak did emerge in Western Africa, modelers working for the US-CDC produced forecasts for Liberia, predicting more than 1.2 million cases in less than 6 months [3]. In total, there were less than 30,000 cases of Ebola reported all over Western Africa, exhibiting large overestimation of Ebola cases by the US models endorsed by the World Health Organization [4].

Models drive most of public health policies when outbreaks of emerging infectious diseases do occur. Based on a mathematical formula, the reproductive rate is the product of probability of transmission, contact number and generation interval [5]. Policy makers are invited to take action to decrease the value of these three parameters, in order to keep the reproductive rate as low as possible, knowing that below 1, it would avoid any epidemic growth. Applied to COVID-19, this formula justified implementation of non-pharmaceutical measures such as face masks, which decreased probability of transmission and reproductive rate by 19% [6], and lockdown measures, which decreased contact numbers. Vaccine immunity is expected to decrease probability of transmission and generation interval.

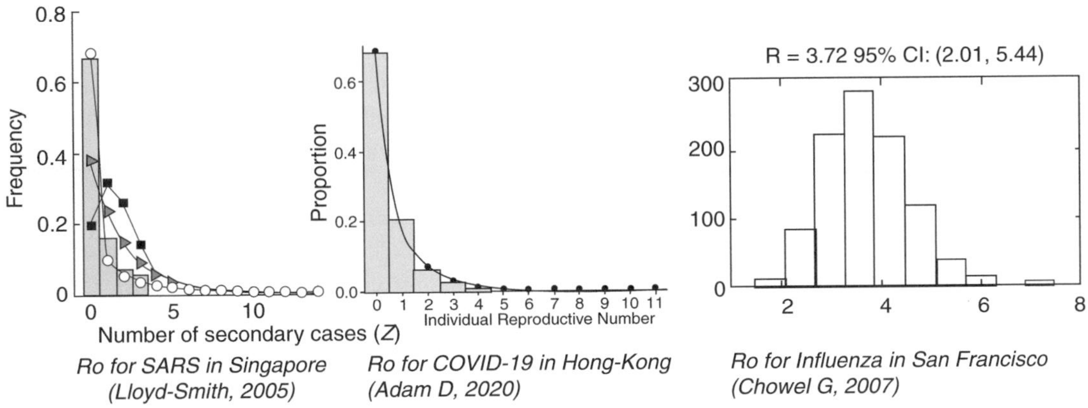

Fig. 56.1 SARS-CoV and SARS-CoV-2 are overdispersed, Influenza is not

Existing models which were initially developed for influenza were applied to COVID-19 and they resulted to be wrong in predicting at long and even mid-term [7, 8]. They led to debatable actions too, such as opting for mitigation strategies instead of suppression or elimination in the beginning of the pandemic, when no vaccine was available. Because COVID-19 was not influenza, as shown by the distribution of the reproductive rate which is well shaped for influenza, but over dispersed for SARS-CoV-2 as it was for SARS-CoV (see Fig. 56.1). Incubation period was much shorter for influenza than coronaviruses, and severity was too much higher with COVID-19.

One of the biggest challenges with epidemic forecasting is that epidemics have so many dimensions which are not taken into account. There are also new challenges that are definitely coming into effects and which are not yet considered by most models, but they need to be, for example, public policies, human behaviours, genetic mutations of the viruses and/or the vectors, climate change, air pollution, decline in biodiversity, demography, the One Health dimension, acquired immunity, and vaccines.

56.4 Approach to Solutions

To refine models and to deliver more precise predictions, we need to build a multi-layered network where each layer represents a particular strand of knowledge (see Box 56.1). Each of them needs to be fed with accurate and reliable real-time data. Here are examples of some of these layers:

- *Disease incidence*, which should be precisely estimated, for example, as it is by the UK Office for National Statistics, by random sampling of the population [9].
- Disease vector model, which is not applicable with diseases like Influenza or COVID-19, but needed for Malaria, Zika, Dengue Fever of Chikungunya which are transmitted by mosquitoes.
- *Economic factors*, which can play a leading role. It has been shown during the COVID-19 pandemics that financial compensation mechanisms for covering, for example, sick leaves or isolation were strong determinants for success of the response, since they are highly effective interventions for helping population in their adhesion to isolation and quarantine measures.
- *Biological factors*, which drive molecular epidemiology. Intensive sequencing programs are needed to ascertain which variants or subvariants of the viruses are emerging, circulating and eventually prevailing. When mutations do occur and when new variants are replacing older strains is key for predicting risks of new waves. Biological factors include data on immunity too. Immunity levels of the population, when documented through well-designed

serosurveys, can be very useful to include in models.

- *Environmental conditions*, since they can dramatically influence spread of infectious diseases. For example, flooding, heat waves and draught are linked with development of vectors and microbes; air pollution with fine particles is known to favour respiratory diseases and has been linked with more frequent and more severe outbreaks of respiratory viruses such as influenza and COVID-19 [10]. Indoor air quality is key in the transmission of respiratory viruses too [11]. We include here animal health interface, the One Health approach.
- *Climatic conditions*, as mentioned above with precipitations and temperatures, or also seasonal effect, and other climatic variability like El Niño Southern Oscillation, which is a key driver for climate all over the world and has been linked with many infectious diseases [12].
- *Satellite imagery*, which can prove useful for spotting health care facility, roads and urban settings, helping to deliver appropriate services with more precision. Sometimes, mapping from satellites can be complemented with other sources of field data such as cell phone data for specifying with more accuracy where people are living and moving.

Box 56.1 A Multi-Layered Approach for Better Precision Epidemic Forecasting

- Disease incidence
- Disease vector model
- Economic factors
- Biological factors
- Environmental conditions
- Climatic conditions
- Satellite imagery

56.5 Main Conclusions and Recommendations

Precision Global Health is about "using the power of data to improve health and achieve social justice, equity, social inclusion, and empowerment. It should not be feared. It should be embraced" [13]. We desperately need more precision in epidemic forecasting to allow for better intervention and finally for better health outcomes [14]. We were not good in predicting influenza or Ebola. We have not been better in predicting COVID-19 or Monkeypox. Precision epidemic forecasting needs higher investment in capturing accurate data, not only epidemiological data, but additional contextual data, coming from different disciplines and domains. Only this multi-layered acquisition of data can allow for better reflecting complexity of epidemic procaesses. The human, animal and environmental interfaces are key in understanding the dynamics of infectious diseases [15].

References

1. Gates B. Innovation for pandemics. N Engl J Med. 2018;378:2057–60. https://doi.org/10.1056/nejmp1806283.
2. Butler D. When Google got flu wrong. Nature. 2013;494:155–6. https://doi.org/10.1038/494155a.
3. Meltzer MI, Atkins CY, Santibanez S, Knust B, Petersen BW, Ervin ED, Nichol ST, Damon IK, Washington ML. Centers for Disease Control and Prevention (CDC). Estimating the future number of cases in the Ebola epidemic–Liberia and Sierra Leone, 2014-2015. MMWR Suppl. 2014;63(3):1–14. https://www.cdc.gov/mmwr/preview/mmwrhtml/su6303a1.htm
4. Butler D. Models overestimate Ebola cases. Nature. 2014;515:18. https://doi.org/10.1038/515018a.
5. HealthKnowledge. Epidemic theory (effective & basic reproduction numbers, epidemic thresholds) & techniques for analysis of infectious disease data (construction & use of epidemic curves, generation numbers, exceptional reporting & identification of significant clusters. The UK Faculty of Public Health. 2022. https://www.healthknowledge.org.uk/public-

health-textbook/research-methods/1a-epidemiology/epidemic-theory. Accessed 21 Dec 2022
6. Leech G, Rogers-Smith C, Monrad JT, Sandbrink JB, Snodin B, Zinkov R, Rader B, Brownstein JS, Gal Y, Bhatt S, Sharma M, Mindermann S, Brauner JM, Aitchison L. Mask wearing in community settings reduces SARS-CoV-2 transmission. Proc Natl Acad Sci U S A. 2022;119(23):e2119266119. https://doi.org/10.1073/pnas.2119266119.
7. Moran KR, Fairchild G, Generous N, Hickmann K, Osthus D, Priedhorsky R, Hyman J, Del Valle SY. Epidemic forecasting is messier than weather forecasting: the role of human behavior and internet data streams in epidemic forecast. J Infect Dis. 2016;214(Suppl 4):S404–8. https://doi.org/10.1093/infdis/jiw375.
8. Ioannidis JPA, Cripps S, Tanner MA. Forecasting for COVID-19 has failed. Int J Forecast. 2022;38(2):423–38. https://doi.org/10.1016/j.ijforecast.2020.08.004.
9. Dean N. Tracking COVID-19 infections: time for change. Nature. 2022;602(7896):185. https://doi.org/10.1038/d41586-022-00336-8.
10. Rohrer M, Flahault A, Stoffel M. Peaks of fine particulate matter may modulate the spreading and virulence of COVID-19. Earth Syst Environ. 2020;4:789–96. https://doi.org/10.1007/s41748-020-00184-4.
11. Leung NHL. Transmissibility and transmission of respiratory viruses. Nat Rev Microbiol. 2021;19:528–45. https://doi.org/10.1038/s41579-021-00535-6.
12. McGregor GR, Ebi K. El Niño southern oscillation (ENSO) and health: an overview for climate and health researchers. Atmosfera. 2018;9(7):282. https://doi.org/10.3390/atmos9070282.
13. Horton R. Offline: in defence of precision public health. Lancet. 2018;392(10157):1504. https://doi.org/10.1016/S0140-6736(18)32741-7.
14. Sheath DJ, Ruiz de Castañeda R, Bempong NE, Raviglione M, Machalaba C, et al. Precision global health: a roadmap for augmented action. J Public Health Emerg. 2020;4:5. https://doi.org/10.21037/jphe.2020.01.01.
15. Krymova E, Béjar B, Thanou D, Sun T, Manetti E, Lee G, Namigai K, Choirat C, Flahault A, Obozinski G. Trend estimation and short-term forecasting of COVID-19 cases and deaths worldwide. Proc Natl Acad Sci U S A. 2022;119(32):e2112656119. https://doi.org/10.1073/pnas.2112656119.

Part VIII

Innovations in Global Health

Genomics and the "-Omics" 57

Francesca Saluzzo, Andrea Spitaleri, and Daniela Maria Cirillo

Abstract

The progresses in the "omics" field have revolutionized the approach to diagnosis and treatment for several communicable and non-communicable diseases. The application of these new technologies allows a more precise diagnosis that can be followed by the most appropriate therapeutic course. Through the integration of different omics data, from genomics and proteomics to metabolomics and phenomics, multi-omics aim to tackle global health challenges delivering precision and personalized medicine solutions. Nonetheless, several gaps still exist in the implementation of new technologies in low- and middle-income countries, associated with the risk of furthering increasing inequalities in global access to health. In this chapter, we revise the main contributions of the different "omics" technologies in improving global health, we discuss the current achievements and limitations and possible solutions to ensure accessibility and availability at global level of these breaking through technologies.

Keywords

Omics technologies · Whole genome sequencing · Proteomics · Genomics · Precision medicine

57.1 Definition of "Omics"

The suffix "-omics" is used to refer to a field in life science able to generate and analyze a large amount of data or information to better understand the biological processes [1].

The era of omics was started with the fields of genomics and proteomics. Since then, with the advancement of life science supported by continuously evolving technologies has led to the development of other "omics" to detects targets in a specific biological sample and in a non-targeted manner [1]. Among those we have epigenomics, transcriptomics and spatial transcriptomics, metabolomics including lipidomics and glycomics and finally microbiomics.

The integration of these techniques is called "systems biology". The system biology approach responds to the basic concept that integration of different technologies allows a better understanding of a complex system [2].

F. Saluzzo · A. Spitaleri
IRCCS San Raffaele Scientific Institute, Milan, Italy

Università Vita Salute San Raffaele, Milan, Italy
e-mail: saluzzo.francesca@hsr.it; spitaleri.andrea@hsr.it

D. M. Cirillo (✉)
IRCCS San Raffaele Scientific Institute, Milan, Italy
e-mail: cirillo.daniela@hsr.it

M. C. B. Raviglione et al. (eds.), *Global Health Essentials*, Sustainable Development Goals Series,
https://doi.org/10.1007/978-3-031-33851-9_57

In this chapter, we will briefly describe how the advancement of technology has provided essential contribution in the field of global health and what are the existing challenges that needs to be overcome to implement these technologies in low resources settings.

57.2 Technologies Adopted for the "Omics" Studies

The omics field has been powered essentially by technological improvements leading to new cost-efficient, high-throughput analysis of biologic molecules [3]. The main omics and related techniques are summarized in Table 57.1. Whole Genome Sequencing (WGS) and mass spectrometry (MS) are basic experimental tools in the omics sciences. WGS-based approaches are feasible for studies on genome and transcriptome, whereas MS-based techniques can be exploited to characterize proteins and metabolites that do not involve DNA/RNA.

57.2.1 Genomics

Genomics is the study of the structure, function, and expression of all the genes in an organism. It allows to detect polymorphisms, single nucleotide variations that may reflects or not in difference at the protein level and on the regulation of activation or shut down of selected genes (epigenetic) [4].

Genomic techniques investigate the genomic variations via WGS. Next-Generation Sequencing has increased the speed and throughput of genome sequencing in the last 10 years. Illumina, short-read technology, is the sole company dominating this field, with the MiSeq, HiSeq, and NextSeq series. Importantly, these short-read approaches have limits in capturing structural variants (SVs) repetitive elements, or sequences with multiple homologous elements in the genome. To overcome these limitations in the last 10 years, PacBio and Oxford Nanopore Technologies (ONT) focused their effort in developing long-read sequencing [5]. Moreover,

Table 57.1 Summary table of the Omics Sciences described in the chapter

Omics sciences	Target	Analysis	Technique	Importance
Genomics	DNA	Mutations screening; DNA copy number	WGS	Genetic disorders
Epigenomics	DNA	Epigenetic modification	WGS	Genetic disorders, diagnostic biomarkers
Transcriptomics	RNA	Gene-expression profile; microRNA	RNA-seq, microarray	Diagnostic biomarkers, therapeutics target, cell heterogeneity
Proteomics	Proteins	Protein profile: Identification, quantification, characterization	NMR, X-ray, ESI/MS, HPLC/MS, MALDI/MS	Proteomic landscape, therapeutics target
Metabolomics	Metabolite (amino acids, nucleotides, hormones, signaling molecules)	Small molecules profile	LC/MS, GC/MS, NMR, IR	Identifying candidate genes and metabolites, revealing metabolic mechanism of the therapeutic efficacy
Glycomics	Carbohydrate	Glycan profile: Structures and pathways	LC/MS, GC/MS, NMR	Metabolic mechanism
Lipidomics	Lipids	Lipid profile	MALDI/MS, ESI/MS, DESI/MS	Metabolic mechanism
Microbiomics	Microorganisms	Bacteria, protozoa, fungi, viruses	WGS metagenomics, WGS 16S	Insights into human diseases

ONT sequencers are also available in pocket-size, highly portable, and need a little sophisticated laboratory setup. Those characteristics make the technology attractive for clinical routine implementation and for use in resources limited settings.

57.2.2 Epigenomics

Epigenomics is an "omics" analyzing epigenetic changes across many genes in a cell or entire organism [6]. It studies the alterations in the regulation of gene activities without modifying genetic sequences. High-throughput chromosome conformation (Hi-C) is a comprehensive technique developed to characterize the 3D genome organization. Whole genome bisulfite sequencing represents a standard approach for methylated Cytosine base detection. Long-read sequencing technologies such as PacBio and Oxford nanopore sequencing techniques have been adapted for epigenome interrogation.

57.2.3 Transcriptomics

Transcriptomics is the study of the transcriptome defined as all RNA transcripts coded by the genome of an organisms. The study of transcriptomes allows to identify genes that are differentially expressed in response to a specific stimulus. Transcriptomics techniques aim to detect and quantify RNA molecules transcribed, from a particular genome at a given time. RNA microarrays can be exploited to profile differentially expressed genes, identifying markers able of discriminate cells between the normal and cancer states. Recently, a new omic, namely spatial transcriptomics, has arisen. This technique uses specific technologies to measure gene expression in a tridimensional manner in order to identify where specific activities occurs [7].

57.2.4 Proteomics

Proteomics refers to all proteins in an organism (proteome) and how they interact (interactome). It represents the systematic large-scale analysis of the entire protein complements of a cell, tissue, or organism under a specific, defined set of conditions. Proteomics provides a robust and representative picture of the functioning cell. The proteome is a complex and dynamic entity that can be defined in terms of the sequence, structure, abundance, localization, modification, interaction, and biochemical function of each of its components [8]. The analysis of the diverse properties of the proteome requires an equally diverse range of technologies as well as methods for data integration and mining. MS plays a crucial role in enabling the analysis of proteome and is typically the method of choice for identifying proteins present in biological systems [5]. One significant advance brought by MS to the omics field is the rate at which it identifies proteins in an entirely discovery-driven way.

We can identify three kinds of proteomics: expressional (MS, Electrophoresis, SAGE), functional (functional assays, ligand chips, deletion, and motif analysis), and structural (X-Ray, Nuclear Magnetic Resonance, modeling) proteomics.

57.2.5 Metabolomics

Metabolomics studies, on a qualitative and quantitative matter, all metabolites and low-molecular-weight molecules. Metabolites—small molecules with <1500 Da[1]—participate in cell metabolism, function as energy sources, signaling molecules, and metabolic intermediates with protein modulatory roles. Methods for metabolome interrogation include Fourier transform-infrared (FT-IR)

[1] Dalton (or Da) is a unit of mass, widely used in physics and chemistry, expressing the weight of molecules.

spectroscopy, Raman spectroscopy, NMR spectroscopy, and MS-based approaches [9].

Evolving technology makes metabolomics a very promising tool for the precision medicine [9]. Two subfields of metabolomics are lipidomics and glycomics. The former is the "full characterization of lipid molecular species and of their biological roles with respect to expression of proteins involved in lipid metabolism and function, including gene regulation" [10]. The latter is defined as the study of carbohydrate polymers (glycans) structure and their cellular function [11].

57.2.6 Microbiomics

Finally, microbiomics is a new emerging field in which all the microorganisms of a given community (a "microbiota") are investigated together [12]. Microbiomics investigates the composition of a particular microbial community, and it aims to investigate host-microbiome interactions to understand the role of the microbiome and host responses in health and disease. This is typically done using ribosomal RNAs and metagenomic profiling.

57.3 Contribution of Omics to Global Health

The proper integration of data collected from individual omics technologies can inform several basic bioscience or clinical biology investigations and multi-omics is frequently reported as a pivotal step to delivering modern, personalized, precision medicine [13].

In particular, the implementation of a systems biology approach, as described in Fig. 57.1, can contribute to the improvement of both individual and population health. From the individual point of view, it can allow accurate diagnosis and personalized treatment of a diverse range of diseases.

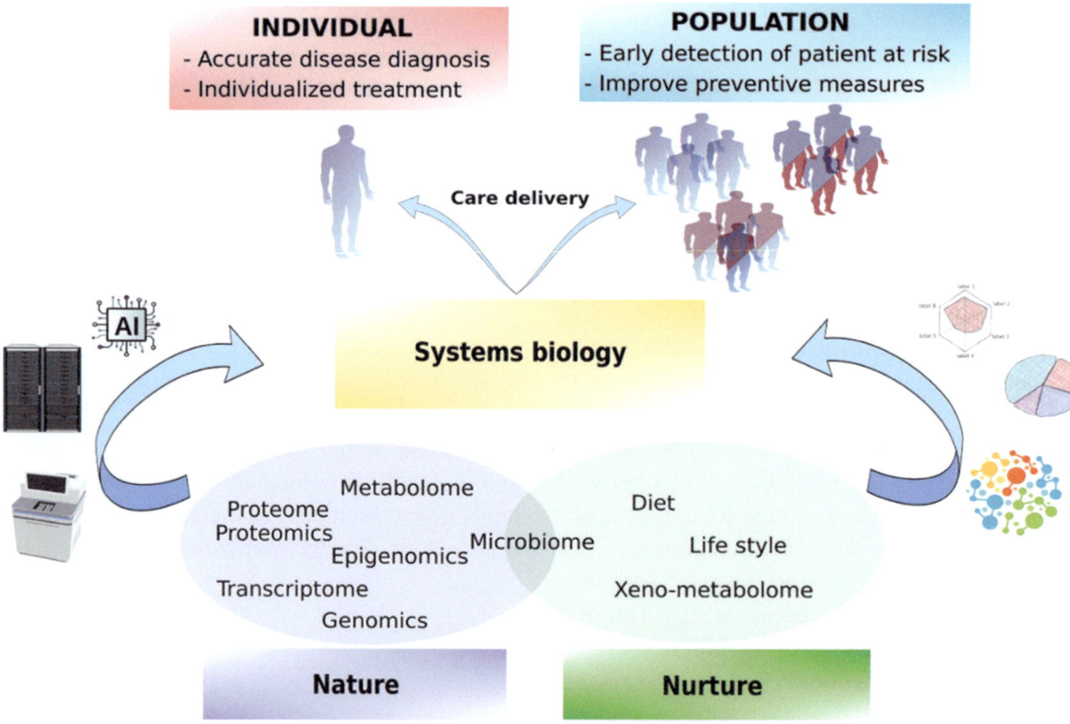

Fig. 57.1 Omics and systems biology applications at the individual and population level. (The vectorial icons are from https://bioicons.com/ under CC0 license and the image assembled using Inkscape-1.2 program)

Whereas, from the population side, it can contribute to early detection of individuals at risk of developing chronic or acute pathologies, thus, improving the possible preventive measures (e.g., precise screening, preventive therapies, modification to the lifestyle).

The application of omics technologies contributes to speed up the development of new drugs by guiding the selection of therapeutical targets and driving the allocation of participants in the best promising treatment arms of clinical trials.

Genomics has been the first of the omics sciences to have had an impact on precision medicine, followed by the "other -omics," first of all in the oncology field. In this branch of medicine, a multi-omics approach is contributing to the development of sophisticated markers able to predict treatment response [14, 15]. This process has increased the survival rate of populations affected and decreased the costs associated to improper use of expensive therapies.

There is an increasing number of examples of how "omics" have contributed to improve cancer diagnosis and treatment, such as for acute myeloid leukemia [16], prostate cancer, and gastric and other cancers [15].

Cardiovascular diseases (CVDs), one of the leading causes of death and disability worldwide, are just another example of how omics technologies have contributed to increase our understanding of the mechanisms underlined these illnesses. Among the different omics techniques, genome-wide association studies along with NGS could lead to new approaches in early diagnosis and possible treatments of CVDs. Besides genomics, regulation of gene expression by transcriptomics approaches can provide new insights on cellular damage mechanisms and metabolomics may be the endpoint on the downstream of multi-omics approaches to confront CVDs from the early onset [17].

In infectious diseases, omics have contributed to study pathogens' evolution and transmission as well as to identify and monitor virulence determinants. Molecular epidemiology is a new way to investigate transmission of both viruses and bacteria. It can be used to detect clusters and to investigate transmission of pathogens of public health interest. Genomic sequencing, for example, is now considered by the European Center of Disease Control the standard to investigate the dynamic of transmission of *M. tuberculosis* [18]. Next-generation sequencing technology-based diagnostics are essential to detect both bacteria and virus resistance to antimicrobics [19]. A recent example of the value of genomics in the field of infectious diseases is how the massive effort to sequence SARS-CoV-2 virus has allowed to monitor the Covid-19 pandemic and to spot the emergence of variants of concern [20].

All emerging data have shown that the strategy "do not let anybody behind" is key to anticipate uncontrolled emergence and spreading of highly virulent variants [21].

57.4 Challenges to Implement Omics in Low- and Middle-Income Countries (LMICs)

The decrease in the cost of the technology has led to an increase in the use of omics for research and for clinical purposes. Nonetheless, the uneven distribution of infrastructures and human capacity, coupled with the increase of reagents' cost, in settings with limited resources may increase the gap between the Global North and the Global South, preventing the access to personalized medicine to many people.

The main barriers to the implementation of omics technologies are:

- Lack of data in global database on specific populations leading to a poor applicability of results to underrepresented populations [22].
- Ethical issues linked to consent model for data sharing and specimen collection including country-specific regulatory framework challenging large collaboration and preventing sharing of metadata [22].
- Poor infrastructures to promote omics research linked to both lack of sustainable financial support and logistical challenges such as unstable power, limited connectivity, and access to proper maintenance of equipment [23].

- Unavailability of biorepositories to store biological material. Progresses are ongoing and biorepositories across Africa have been established with the support of H3Africa [24, 25].
- Unavailability of data storage facilities [22].
- Lack of trained human resources in the different professional profiles required for both research implementation of omics and their translation in routine practice. Drainage of formed human resources [26].
- Existing barriers to data sharing including concern about intellectual properties, lack of guidelines or poor knowledge of guidelines among scientists [22].

Moreover, the major implementation of genomics is linked to the decreasing costs of reagents and platforms. In LMICs, reagents and equipment are purchased through intermediary companies inflating the costs: as a result, genome sequencing is more expensive in resource-limited settings than it is in North America or Europe, creating a further barrier for implementation.

The response to Covid-19 has mobilized funds to implement sequencing as technology to monitor the emergence of variants in the African continent as well as in other LMICs, it is now crucial that what has been established is further sustained and utilized beyond SARS-CoV-2 sequencing [24].

In conclusion, the realization of the infrastructures and capacity needed for the implementation of omics technologies are a key step in the development of personalized and precision medicine. This represents a pivotal step in the evolution of the current approach to patients and illnesses, finally improving and guaranteeing high quality care.

Nevertheless, the risk of an uneven global implementation of omics technologies is a harsh reality that could contribute to further increasing the gap already existing between countries in patients' care.

References

1. Yadav SP. The wholeness in suffix -omics, -omes, and the word om. J Biomol Tech. 2007;18(5):277. /pmc/articles/PMC2392988/
2. Spivey A. Systems biology: the big picture. Environmental health perspectives. 2004:112(16), A938–A943. https://doi.org/10.1289/ehp.112-a938.
3. Hasin Y, Seldin M, Lusis A. Multi-omics approaches to disease. Genome Biol. 2017;18(1):1–15. https://doi.org/10.1186/S13059-017-1215-1.
4. Kuska B. Beer, Bethesda, and biology: how "genomics" came into being. J Natl Cancer Inst. 1998;90(2):93. https://doi.org/10.1093/JNCI/90.2.93.
5. Logsdon GA, Vollger MR, Eichler EE. Long-read human genome sequencing and its applications. Nat Rev Genet. 2020;21(10):597–614. https://doi.org/10.1038/s41576-020-0236-x.
6. Wang KC, Chang HY. Epigenomics—technologies and applications. Circ Res. 2018;122(9):1191. https://doi.org/10.1161/CIRCRESAHA.118.310998.
7. Marx V. Method of the year: spatially resolved transcriptomics. Nat Methods. 2021;18(1):9–14. https://doi.org/10.1038/s41592-020-01033-y.
8. Aslam B, Basit M, Nisar MA, Khurshid M, Rasool MH. Proteomics: technologies and their applications. J Chromatogr Sci. 2017;55(2):182–96. https://doi.org/10.1093/CHROMSCI/BMW167.
9. Clish CB. Metabolomics: an emerging but powerful tool for precision medicine. Cold Spring Harb Mol Case Stud. 2015;1(1):a000588. https://doi.org/10.1101/MCS.A000588.
10. Naudí A, Cabré R, Jové M, Ayala V, Gonzalo H, Portero-Otín M, Ferrer I, Pamplona R. Lipidomics of human brain aging and Alzheimer's disease pathology. Int Rev Neurobiol. 2015;122:133–89. https://doi.org/10.1016/bs.irn.2015.05.008.
11. Krishnamoorthy L, Mahal LK. Glycomic analysis: an array of technologies. ACS Chem Biol. 2009;4(9):715. https://doi.org/10.1021/CB900103N.
12. Berg G, Rybakova D, Fischer D, Cernava T, Vergès MCC, Charles T, Chen X, Cocolin L, Eversole K, Corral GH, Kazou M, Kinkel L, Lange L, Lima N, Loy A, Macklin JA, Maguin E, Mauchline T, McClure R, et al. Microbiome definition re-visited: old concepts and new challenges. Microbiome. 2020;8(1):1–22. https://doi.org/10.1186/S40168-020-00875-0/FIGURES/7.
13. Ahmed Z. Multi-omics strategies for personalized and predictive medicine: past, current, and future translational opportunities. Emerg Top Life Sci. 2022;6(2):215–25. https://doi.org/10.1042/ETLS20210244.

14. Lin VTG, Yang ES. The pros and cons of incorporating transcriptomics in the age of precision oncology. J Natl Cancer Inst. 2019;111(10):1016. https://doi.org/10.1093/JNCI/DJZ114.
15. Nam AS, Chaligne R, Landau DA. Integrating genetic and non-genetic determinants of cancer evolution by single-cell multi-omics. Nat Rev Genet. 2021;22(1):3. https://doi.org/10.1038/S41576-020-0265-5.
16. Haferlach T, Schmidts I. The power and potential of integrated diagnostics in acute myeloid leukaemia. Br J Haematol. 2020;188(1):36–48. https://doi.org/10.1111/BJH.16360.
17. Sohag MMH, Raqib SM, Akhmad SA. OMICS approaches in cardiovascular diseases: a mini review. Genomics Inform. 2021;19(2):e13. https://doi.org/10.5808/GI.21002.
18. Tagliani E, Anthony R, Kohl TA, de Neeling A, Nikolayevskyy V, Ködmön C, Maurer FP, Niemann S, van Soolingen D, van der Werf MJ, Cirillo DM. Use of a whole genome sequencing-based approach for mycobacterium tuberculosis surveillance in Europe in 2017–2019: an ECDC pilot study. Eur Respir J. 2020;57(1):2002272. https://doi.org/10.1183/13993003.02272-2020.
19. Gwinn M, Maccannell D, Armstrong GL. Next generation sequencing of infectious pathogens. JAMA. 2019;321(9):893. https://doi.org/10.1001/JAMA.2018.21669.
20. Cyranoski D. Alarming COVID variants show vital role of genomic surveillance. Nature. 2021;589(7842):337–8. https://doi.org/10.1038/D41586-021-00065-4.
21. Wilkinson E, Giovanetti M, Tegally H, San JE, Lessells R, Cuadros D, Martin DP, Rasmussen DA, Zekri ARN, Sangare AK, Ouedraogo AS, Sesay AK, Priscilla A, Kemi AS, Olubusuyi AM, Oluwapelumi AOO, Hammami A, Amuri AA, Sayed A, et al. A year of genomic surveillance reveals how the SARS-CoV-2 pandemic unfolded in Africa. Science. 2021;374(6566):423–31. https://doi.org/10.1126/SCIENCE.ABJ4336.
22. Hamdi Y, Zass L, Othman H, Radouani F, Allali I, Hanachi M, Okeke CJ, Chaouch M, Tendwa MB, Samtal C, Mohamed Sallam R, Alsayed N, Turkson M, Ahmed S, Benkahla A, Romdhane L, Souiai O, Tastan Bishop Ö, Ghedira K, et al. Human OMICs and computational biology research in Africa: current challenges and prospects. OMICS J Integr Biol. 2021;25(4):213–33.
23. Laurance WF, Sloan S, Weng L, Sayer JA. Estimating the environmental costs of Africa's massive development corridors. Curr Biol. 2015;25(24):3202–8. https://doi.org/10.1016/J.CUB.2015.10.046.
24. Inzaule SC, Ondoa P, Loembe MM, Tebeje YK, Ogwell Ouma AE, Nkengasong JN. COVID-19 and indirect health implications in Africa: impact, mitigation measures, and lessons learned for improved disease control. PLoS Med. 2021;18(6):e1003666. https://doi.org/10.1371/JOURNAL.PMED.1003666.
25. Rotimi CN, Bentley AR, Doumatey AP, Chen G, Shriner D, Adeyemo A. The genomic landscape of African populations in health and disease. Hum Mol Genet. 2017;26(R2):R225–36. https://doi.org/10.1093/HMG/DDX253.
26. Zimbudzi E. Stemming the impact of health professional brain drain from Africa: a systemic review of policy options. J Public Health Africa. 2013;4(1):19–23. https://doi.org/10.4081/JPHIA.2013.E4.

58 Digital Technology for Global Health

Dennis Falzon, Zelalem Temesgen,
and Alistair Story

Abstract

The rapid expansion and confluence of digital technologies, including advances in hardware, software, and mobile technologies has a significant impact on daily life. These technologies have begun to play a substantial role in health care and their potential utility to improve the health of populations is an area of great interest. We provide a brief discussion of the application of digital technologies in global health, including the rational for their use, their classification into thematic categories, and principles to guide sound investment in digital development.

Keywords

Digital health · eHealth · mHealth · Digital technologies · eLearning

D. Falzon
WHO Global TB Programme, Geneva, Switzerland
e-mail: falzond@who.int

Z. Temesgen (✉)
Mayo Clinic, Rochester, MN, USA
e-mail: temesgen.zelalem@mayo.edu

A. Story
University College London, London, UK

58.1 Introduction

The term "digital technology" encompasses all electronic tools, automatic systems, technological devices, and resources that generate, process, or store data. Digital technologies provide opportunities to overcome health system challenges and to enhance the coverage and quality of health services. Digital health refers to the use of digital technologies for health (Box 58.1). While the notion of employing information and communications technology (ICT) to address health needs is not new, recent years have seen a rapid transformation in digital health. This chapter provides a brief overview of the ever-expanding scope of old, new, and nascent digital technologies across the health spectrum of both low- and high-income settings, for the management of communicable diseases, health risks and non-communicable conditions alike. It also underlines how technological advances and contemporary challenges are helping to shape the role of digital technologies in the health sector.

Box 58.1 Definitions of Common Terms [1–4]
eHealth (or "electronic health"): The use of ICT in support of health and health-related fields, including healthcare services, health surveillance, health literature,

M. C. B. Raviglione et al. (eds.), *Global Health Essentials*, Sustainable Development Goals Series,
https://doi.org/10.1007/978-3-031-33851-9_58

and health education, knowledge, and research.

mHealth (or "mobile health"): The use of mobile and wireless technologies to support health objectives. mHealth is a component of eHealth.

Digital health: An overarching term that comprises eHealth (which includes mHealth), and emerging areas, such as the use of computing sciences in the fields of artificial intelligence, big data, and genomics.

Interoperability: The ability of multiple ICT systems and software applications to communicate with one another, exchange data, and use the information that has been exchanged.

58.2 Why Digital Health?

The basic argument in support of a greater role of digitization in health care is rooted in the capture and transfer of information. Communication between key actors of a healthcare system—be it patient, caregiver, or machine—is critical to quality, timely integrated care and to the improved functioning of health systems. Enhanced management of data (e.g., speed, completeness, integrity, security, low cost) is conducive to better decision-making, better performance, and lower costs. The computerization of health care over the last decades has indisputably revolutionized data transfer processes. These basic premises underpin the drive to scale up global access to equipment, software, and connectivity with the expectation of improving health system performance and quality (effectiveness) or reducing costs (efficiency), or ideally, both.

58.3 Digital Health and Global Commitments

In 2015, the United Nations launched its Sustainable Development Goals (SDGs) as global targets towards which countries should work to maximize development in the years post-2015 [5]. On publication of the SDGs (Chap. 71), it was acknowledged that digital technologies will be important for their attainment [6]. The SDG9 on investment in ICT and in research by the public and private sectors relates directly to digital health. Strategic and innovative use of cutting-edge digital technologies is also considered central by the World Health Organization (WHO) to achieving the triple billion targets of its 13th General Programme of Work, 2019–2023: 1 billion more people to benefit from universal health coverage; 1 billion more people to be better protected from health emergencies; and 1 billion more people to enjoy better health [7]. WHO has developed a global strategy for digital health unto 2025, to encourage international collaboration and garner support for national health programs on research, evidence collection, and information sharing [8].

58.4 Recent Developments

The increasing global reach of affordable hardware, open-source or free software, and mobile internet in recent years has facilitated the extension of digital technologies worldwide. Mobile subscription is increasing and is expected to reach 5.7 billion (70% of the world's population) by 2025 [9]. While these increases are expected across all regions, stark inequities in mobile broadband coverage and affordability persist across the rich and poor world, with about half of the world's population remaining without access to the internet [10]. The gulf in access to computers and the internet is due to wide variation in mobile broadband coverage and affordability, internet literacy, [1] lack of public conviction in its relevance to their needs, and concerns about safety and internet security. This digital divide impacts women more than men. The COVID-19 pandemic has propelled the adoption and trans-

[1] Internet literacy is the ability to use devices, such as smartphones or laptops, to access and navigate websites and apps, with the intent to seek out information and communicate with others.

formation of digital technologies across their diversity. Public health measures to mitigate transmission including "stay-at-home" orders rapidly shifted healthcare services to online platforms and telemedicine. While the pandemic enabled many millions of people to continue to access health care and support, for those without ready access to the internet, it also fueled the digital divide.

58.5 What Role for Digital Technologies in Global Health?

Much has been written and speculated about the transformative potential of digital technologies, but practitioners are interested in the evidence to support digital health. In 2019, WHO issued recommendations for the use of digital technologies in health following an assessment of the evidence for the benefits, harms, acceptability, feasibility, resource use, and equity [1]. This guideline examined the extent to which digital health interventions can address health system challenges along the pathway to universal health.

There are different ways to categorize the way digital technologies can be applied in global health. One pragmatic approach is to classify products into one or more thematic categories, aligned to the most common applications in programmatic work. A recent example of this has been WHO's digital health agenda for action for the End TB Strategy, which organizes the role of digital technologies into four functions: patient care, surveillance, program management, and eLearning (Fig. 58.1) [11, 12]. Some digital prod-

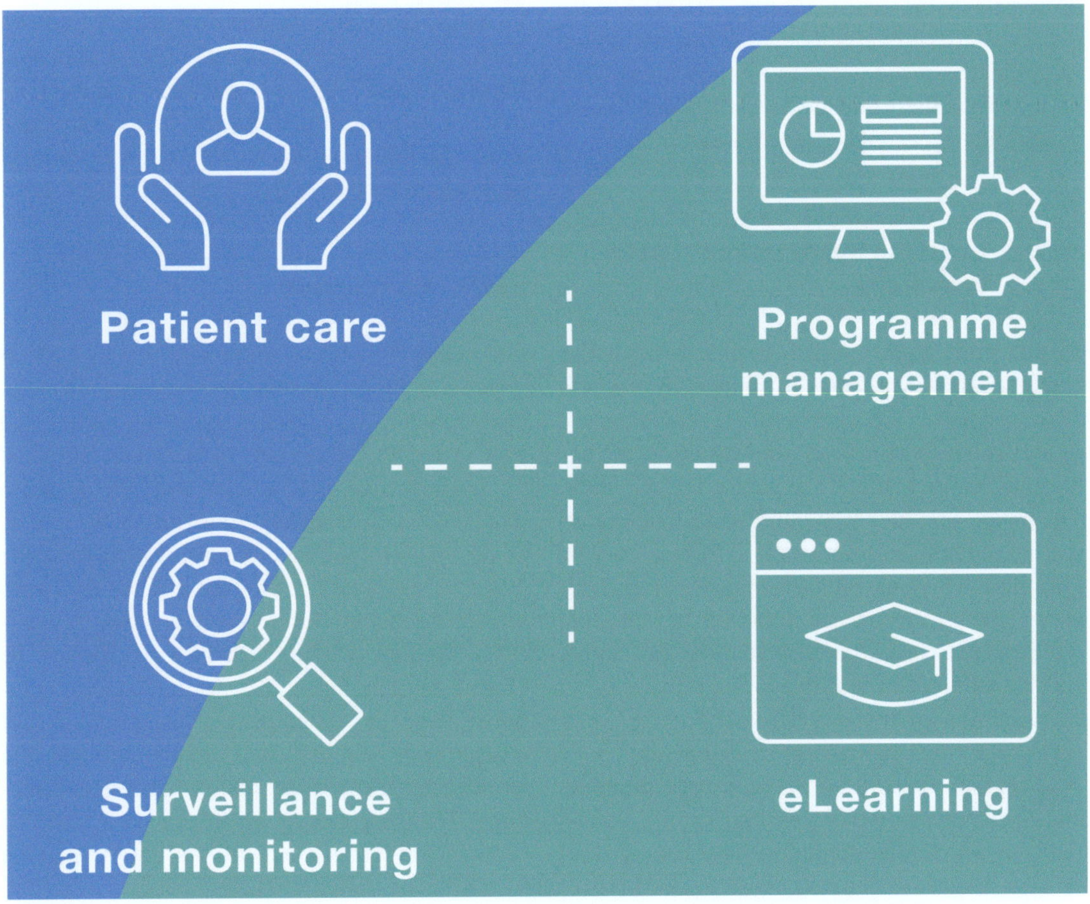

Fig. 58.1 Conceptual framework to classify the role of digital technologies in tuberculosis care

ucts can perform multiple functions, for example, electronic health records can serve both patient care and surveillance and monitoring while digital adherence technologies, like video-support, can enable both patient care and program management. The digitization of programmatic processes, such as electronic records, has a long history in tuberculosis care [13]. Many of the digital technologies evaluated and employed in tuberculosis prevention and care have had a direct application to the COVID-19 response, such as video-conferencing capacity for patient support, telemedicine, and eLearning techniques [14].

The 2019 WHO recommendations on digital health are organized along critical points when the healthcare system interacts with individuals seeking care—such as notification of births and deaths, and remote consultations—or when healthcare workers provide service, such as stock management, provider-to-provider tele-medicine, decision-support, and eLearning [1]. The same guideline also provides a detailed taxonomy that distinguishes different interventions under four groupings, namely clients, health workers, health system managers, and data services.

58.6 Creating Systems that Last: Principles

Health practitioners today face a bewildering choice of digital products to support their work. This array of choices, the highly technical nature of the products themselves, and variations in digital literacy are some of the barriers to adoption. The health provider lack confidence when making investment decisions, even in the presence of guidance. There is typically much uncertainty around the operability and durability of a product within a landscape of rapid technological change. Can the tool service multiple programmatic functions simultaneously and achieve economies of scale? How to maximize the interoperability of systems (see Box 58.1)? What are the practical and legal implications of certain license conditions? A set of nine principles have been articulated to guide sound investment in digital development [15] (see Box 58.2).

Box 58.2 Principles for Digital Development [15]

1. Design with the user
2. Understand the existing ecosystem
3. Design for scale
4. Build for sustainability
5. Be data driven
6. Use open standards, open data, open source, and open innovation
7. Reuse and improve
8. Address privacy and security
9. Be collaborative

Effective stewardship to maximize the potential contribution of digital health for all requires visionary leadership and creativity [16]. In 2020, WHO released an investment guide for decision-makers, describing a systematic process to develop costed digital health plans integrated across health program areas, within a national digital architecture [17].

58.7 Conclusion

Digital health systems are powerful tools without which it is difficult to conceive progress in human development. Managers in both the public and private health sectors are increasingly attracted by leading-edge innovations with the promise that they will swiftly transform their work. Digital health products increasingly harness the power of artificial intelligence and big data analytics in both their development and routine operation. Digital health technologies should be viewed as tools rather than comprehensive solutions: they are intended to complement not replace core health system components like the workforce, leadership, and governance structures. Decision-makers in health care must be cognizant of the notion of "digital equity" and the potential for differential access to technologies to widen and exacerbate inequalities among vulnerable populations [18]. Despite multiple challenges and complexities, evidence-based digital health innovations need to be evaluated and implemented carefully along sound principles of investment. Evidence for the impact of emerging technologies needs to be strengthened and implementation research mounted alongside all innovation to better understand contextual factors that hinder or facilitate effective scale-up [19].

References

1. WHO. WHO guideline: recommendations on digital interventions for health system strengthening. Geneva: World Health Organization; 2019. https://apps.who.int/iris/bitstream/handle/10665/311941/9789241550505-eng.pdf
2. WHO. mHealth: new horizons for health through mobile technologies (Global Observatory for eHealth series, Volume 3). Geneva: World Health Organization; 2011. http://www.who.int/goe/publications/goe_mhealth_web.pdf.
3. WHO. Resolution WHA71.20. mHealth: use of appropriate digital technologies for public health: report by the Director-General. In: Seventy-first World Health Assembly, vol. 26. Geneva: World Health Organization; 2018. https://apps.who.int/gb/ebwha/pdf_files/WHA71/A71_20-en.pdf.
4. WHO. Resolution WHA71.7. Digital health. In: Seventy-first World Health Assembly, vol. 26. Geneva: World Health Organization; 2018. https://apps.who.int/gb/ebwha/pdf_files/WHA71/A71_R7-en.pdf.
5. United Nations Department Of Economic And Social Affairs. Sustainable development goals. 2015. New York, USA. https://sustainabledevelopment.un.org/sdgs.
6. WHO. Health in 2015: from MDGs, millennium development goals to SDGs, sustainable development goal. Geneva: World Health Organization; 2015. http://apps.who.int/iris/bitstream/10665/200009/1/9789241565110_eng.pdf?ua=1.
7. WHO. The Thirteenth General Programme of Work, 2019–2023, as approved by the 71st World Health Assembly in Resolution WHA71.1. on 25 May 2018 (WHO/PRP/18.1), vol. 2019. Geneva: World Health Organization. https://www.who.int/about/what-we-do/thirteenth-general-programme-of-work-2019%2D%2D-2023
8. WHO. Global strategy for digital health 2020–2025. Geneva: World Health Organization; 2021. https://www.who.int/docs/default-source/documents/gs4dh-daa2a9f352b0445bafbc79ca799dce4d.pdf.
9. GSM Association. The mobile economy 2021. GSM Association; 2021. https://data.gsmaintelligence.com/api-web/v2/research-file-download?id=60621126&file=250621-Mobile-Economy-2021.pdf
10. GSM Association. The state of mobile internet connectivity 2021. GSM Association; 2021. https://www.gsma.com/r/wp-content/uploads/2021/09/The-State-of-Mobile-Internet-Connectivity-Report-2021.pdf
11. WHO/ERS. Digital health for the End TB Strategy: an agenda for action. (WHO/HTM/TB/2015.21). Geneva: World Health Organization; 2015. http://apps.who.int/iris/bitstream/10665/205222/1/WHO_HTM_TB_2015.21_eng.pdf.
12. Falzon D, Timimi H, Kurosinski P, Migliori GB, Van Gemert W, Denkinger C, et al. Digital health for the end TB strategy: developing priority products and making them work. Eur Respir J. 2016;48(1):29–45.
13. Doy RW. A simple computerised tuberculosis register with data collection in the field (suitable for a developing country). Cent Afr J Med. 1973;19(6):120–8.
14. WHO. Second round of the national pulse survey on continuity of essential health services during the COVID-19 pandemic: January–March 2021. Geneva: World Health Organization; 2021. https://www.who.int/publications-detail-redirect/WHO-2019-nCoV-EHS-continuity-survey-2021.1.
15. Principles for Digital Development. (2015). http://digitalprinciples.org/
16. Frost MJ, Tran JB, Khatun F, Friberg IK, Rodríguez DC. What does it take to be an effective National Steward of digital health integration for health systems strengthening in low- and middle-income countries? Glob Health Sci Pract. 2018;6(Supplement 1):S18–28.
17. WHO. Digital implementation investment guide (DIIG): integrating digital interventions into health programmes. Geneva: World Health Organization; 2020. https://www.who.int/publications/i/item/9789240010567
18. World Bank. World development report 2016: digital dividends [Internet]. 2016. http://www.worldbank.org/en/publication/wdr2016. Accessed 1 Feb 2016.
19. IR4DTB Implementation research for digital technologies and TB (IR4DTB) [Internet]. https://www.ir4dtb.org/.

59 Data Science for Global Health

Karen Meagher, Dennis Falzon, and Zelalem Temesgen

Abstract

Data science promises to revolutionize healthcare, providing insight into disease mechanisms, enabling a more personalized approach to care, improving public health surveillance and the ability to predict trends. However, there are challenges and barriers to its application and implementation, requiring careful attention to data governance and ethics. In this chapter, we present examples of the application of data science in global health and briefly discuss the challenges that should be addressed for its equitable implementation.

Keywords

Data science · Big data · Equitable data science · Data sharing · Data transparency

K. Meagher · Z. Temesgen (✉)
Mayo Clinic, Rochester, MN, USA
e-mail: Meagher.Karen@mayo.edu; temesgen.zelalem@mayo.edu

D. Falzon
WHO Global TB Programme, Geneva, Switzerland
e-mail: falzond@who.int

59.1 Introduction

Data science is the field of study that develops and uses scientific methods, processes, algorithms, and systems to extract meaningful knowledge and insights from large volumes of structured and unstructured data. Just as data science is being used to improve manufacturing, product design and marketing there is good reason to believe that it could improve analogous processes in healthcare. The health sector is well positioned to benefit from data science as it generates a large amount of clinical and non-clinical information (e.g., payer records, drug cost, research output), the effective and accurate interpretation of which can help in better decision-making and improve both efficiency in management and quality of care. While the utilization of data science in the health sector is rapidly evolving in high-income countries, there is interest in its application to lower resource settings that concentrate the burden of several global challenges to health, both communicable and non-communicable [1]. In this chapter, we provide examples of how data science is already being implemented in global health and briefly discuss the challenges it faces in realizing its full potential in this context.

M. C. B. Raviglione et al. (eds.), *Global Health Essentials*, Sustainable Development Goals Series,
https://doi.org/10.1007/978-3-031-33851-9_59

59.2 Examples of Data Science for Global Health

Data science is beginning to demonstrate its potential in different areas of health and disease. Coronavirus disease 2019 (COVID-19), because of its rapid and wide-reaching impact on global health and economies, has made a stronger case for data science. It has highlighted the critical need for timely and accurate data and has provided opportunities for data science to contribute to its surveillance and control [2]. Examples of data science use in the response to COVID-19 include epidemiological modeling [3] contact tracing [4], diagnosis [5], vaccine design [6], and disease course prediction [7].

The use of data to predict events in the field pre-dates the pandemic and is being studied in other areas of health and disease. Artificial neural network, applied to data sets with information from people with presumptive tuberculosis, was able to predict tuberculosis disease with high accuracy in Pakistan [8]. Computer-aided detection of tuberculosis on chest radiography is in use in several low-resource settings. Analysis of person-generated health data has been used to predict the risk of developing diabetes or obesity, with the potential to allow for risk mitigation/behavioral intervention before disease onset [9]. In oncology, data science has been used to predict colorectal cancer recurrence and survival in a population-based study in South Africa [10] and to predict risk of breast cancer in African women [11]. A standard data set of cases with built-in training and validation sets has been proposed to facilitate the development of biomedical informatics tools in accelerating research into antineoplastic therapeutic response [12]. Machine learning and predictive tools have been used to predict cardiovascular and stroke risk [13]. Data science has also been applied in efforts to understand and combat antimicrobial resistance, an ever-increasing threat to global health. Antimicrobial susceptibility testing has been augmented by artificial intelligence tools, resulting in faster and more accurate results. Machine learning techniques have been used to identify predictors of antimicrobial exposure and resistance, understand antimicrobial usage patterns, predict synergistic drug combinations, and predict drug–drug interactions [14, 15].

59.3 Opportunities and Challenges of Data Science for Global Health

Despite its undeniable promise of a transformational impact on the future of global health, data science faces a number of formidable challenges in its implementation. The requisite infrastructure requirement—electronic health records, information and communication technologies, web connectivity—is not uniformly available, and where available, may not be sufficiently advanced to enable data science activities. The knowledgebase may not be sufficiently large or representative; social determinants of health that are relevant to low resource settings, such as undernutrition, may not be accounted for. A real potential for creating and/or exacerbating inequities exists; thus, ethical considerations in the design, application, and governance of data science assume critical importance.

Data science for global health draws from the long tradition of population health sciences, including epidemiology and demography [16]. This tradition generates objectives, methods, and results driven by an ethos of service and policy formation. The data science agenda, therefore, ought to be shaped by priority consideration of population health, such as morbidity, mortality, quality of life, and health inequities.

59.3.1 Equitable Data Science

While the era of "big data"[1] is new, data science is not. Lessons from genomics and HIV/AIDS research reflect how disparities in healthcare and

[1] Big data refers to a large volume or quantity of information. In addition to its size, big data is also characterized by its diversity (various formats and types, structured and unstructured) as well as the speed with which it accumulates.

historical forces of oppression and marginalization influence data collection efforts. The most convenient and available data are less likely to come from the most affected communities. Data collection efforts must attend to these structural root causes from inception, or else risk accentuating health inequities [17]. Equitable data collection efforts are likely to require more community engagement to earn trust and take longer time.

59.3.2 Data Sharing

Data science relies on information collected from non-traditional sources, enabling statistical inferences that were previously not possible. Global health collaborations must attend to the differential capacity and stakes of researchers and populations from high- vs. low- and middle-income settings [18]. Global health collaborations should seek to actively counter power inequities reflective of the legacy of colonialism. One way is to build research or clinical capacity in under-resourced settings; another way is to mentor early career talent from underrepresented populations. Designing equity in research collaboration can also mitigate exploitation of participants: situations in which those who provide the data are least likely to benefit from the innovations that follow. Participatory research designs are an example of efforts to recognize participants as research partners.

59.3.3 Crossing Traditional Domains

Data science initiatives often involve moving or combining information from formerly distinct data activities. Confounding distinctions between clinical, research, and public health contexts, cross-sectoral efforts can generate uncertainty given how distinct norms and legal governance schemes have traditionally provided guidance based on these different purposes. Data scientists must attend to these considerations from the initiation of project design.

59.3.4 Ancillary Care Obligations

Resource-poor settings can also lead to data science operating in contexts where unmet health needs are prevalent. Global health ancillary care frameworks help teams reflect on the obligations generated by identification of previously unrecognized health burdens.

59.3.5 Privacy Challenges

Data science can also disrupt norms of data management and governance that have previously worked to provide protection from unwanted disclosure. Surveillance data have often been anonymized to protect patient privacy and facilitate destigmatization of public health data collection activities. However, advances in data science can lead to unintended revelations about both individuals and groups. For example, HIV phylogenetic analyses provide information about distinct strains of the virus, which can potentially reveal migratory pasts, incarceration history, and exposure of third parties [19]. Data science presents opportunities for innovation in developing community-engaged models of data sharing, interpretation, and dissemination that recognize these trade-offs.

59.3.6 Individual vs Aggregate Results

Data science responsibilities are tied up in public discourse around transparency of data use and dissemination of results [20]. Data science, especially far along the translational pathway, can produce results that have health implications for the individual. This can generate questions of when data scientists have a duty to disclose this information, even when discovered by chance. Secondary use of data sets can also generate questions about who bears responsibility for subsequent data use or dissemination of results.

59.4 Conclusion

Global health ethics frameworks are especially relevant to attending to justice and the future of scientific dividends. Intellectual property, scalability, and cost-effectiveness are central considerations to any intervention capable of impacting global health outcomes. Data science for global health will need to confront the tension between the development of big data as an industry driven by market dynamics and a vision of equitable health services delivery that is driven by population health needs. Data science ethical concerns in this arena include commercialization and resale of data [20].

Data science is not just innovating in how research, learning health systems, or population health insights can be gained. Increasingly, the big data revolution is changing what team science looks like, and who has a voice in knowledge production. Anticipatory shared governance schemes acknowledge that scientists' values alone should not determine knowledge production activities; communities should be included in the process [18]. Data scientists have an opportunity to integrate public voices throughout a project, through collaborations with social scientists, community engagement, and citizen science. In global health, this will entail recognizing diversity and pluralism in what communities value.

Understanding Data Science	
Terms	Definitions
Data science	Field of study that develops and uses scientific methods, processes, algorithms, and systems to extract meaningful knowledge and insights from big data
Big data	Large quantity of information, characterized by its volume, diversity, and speed of accumulation
Equitable data science	Collecting and interpreting data in such a way that access, decision-making, and implementation is equitable
Data sharing	Data sharing is the practice of making the same data available to other users or applications, including other investigators, consumers, corporations, and governments
Data privacy	Data privacy is the concept of protecting patient and/or customer data from unethical use and distribution
Data transparency	Data transparency describes the situation whereby those who collect and analyze data enable individuals to know why their data are needed, how their information is gathered, where it is stored, how it is protected, and how it will be used

References

1. Wyber R, Vaillancourt S, Perry W, Mannava P, Folaranmi T, Celi LA. Big data in global health: improving health in low- and middle-income countries. Bull World Health Organ. 2015;93(3):203–8. https://doi.org/10.2471/BLT.14.139022.
2. Qingpeng Z, Gao J, Wu JT, Cao Z, Zeng DD. Data science approaches to confronting the COVID-19 pandemic: a narrative review. Philos Trans A Math Phys Eng Sci. 2022;380:20210127. https://doi.org/10.1098/rsta.2021.0127.
3. Hao X, Cheng S, Wu D, Wu T, Lin X, Wang C. Reconstruction of the full transmission dynamics of COVID-19 in Wuhan. Nature. 2020;584(7821):420–4. https://doi.org/10.1038/s41586-020-2554-8.
4. Kleinman RA, Merkel C. Digital contact tracing for COVID-19. CMAJ. 2020;192(24):E653–6. https://doi.org/10.1503/cmaj.200922.
5. Ozturk T, Talo M, Yildirim EA, Baloglu UB, Yildirim O, Rajendra AU. Automated detection of COVID-19 cases using deep neural networks with x-ray images. Comput Biol Med. 2020;121:103792. https://doi.org/10.1016/j.compbiomed.2020.103792.
6. Ong E, Wong MU, Huffman A, He Y. COVID-19 coronavirus vaccine design using reverse vaccinology and machine learning. Front Immunol. 2020;11:1581Published 2020 Jul 3. https://doi.org/10.3389/fimmu.2020.01581.
7. Alrajhi AA, Alswailem OA, Wali G, et al. Data-driven prediction for COVID-19 severity in hospitalized patients. Int J Environ Res Public Health. 2022;19(5):2958. https://doi.org/10.3390/ijerph19052958.
8. Khan MT, Kaushik AC, Ji L, Malik SI, Ali S, Wei DQ. Artificial neural networks for prediction of tuberculosis disease. Front Microbiol. 2019;10:395. Published 2019 Mar 4. https://doi.org/10.3389/fmicb.2019.00395.
9. Nagpal MS, Barbaric A, Sherifali D, Morita PP, Cafazzo JA. Patient-generated data analytics of health behaviors of people living with type 2 diabetes: scoping

review. JMIR Diabetes. 2021;6(4):e29027. Published 2021 Dec 20. https://doi.org/10.2196/29027.

10. Achilonu OJ, Fabian J, Bebington B, Singh E, Eijkemans MJC, Musenge E. Predicting colorectal cancer recurrence and patient survival using supervised machine learning approach: a south african population-based study [Published correction appears in front public health]. Front Public Health. 2021;9:694306. https://doi.org/10.3389/fpubh.2021.694306.
11. Macaulay BO, Aribisala BS, Akande SA, Akinnuwesi BA, Olabanjo OA. Breast cancer risk prediction in African women using random Forest classifier. Cancer Treat Res Commun. 2021;28:100396. https://doi.org/10.1016/j.ctarc.2021.100396.
12. Li Y, Luo YH, Wampfler JA, et al. Efficient and accurate extracting of unstructured EHRs on cancer therapy responses for the development of RECIST natural language processing tools: part I, the corpus. JCO Clin Cancer Inform. 2020;4:383–91. https://doi.org/10.1200/CCI.19.00147.
13. Jamthikar AD, et al. Artificial intelligence framework for predictive cardiovascular and stroke risk assessment models: a narrative review of integrated approaches using carotid ultrasound. Comput Biol Med. 2020;126:104043.
14. Chowdhury AS, Lofgren ET, Moehring RW, Broschat SL. Identifying predictors of antimicrobial exposure in hospitalized patients using a machine learning approach. J Appl Microbiol. 2019;128:688–96. https://doi.org/10.1111/jam.14499.
15. Lara RAN, Aguilera-Mendoza L, Brizuela CA, Pena A, Rio G. Heterologous machine learning for the identification of antimicrobial activity in human-targeted drugs. Molecules. 2019;24:13. https://doi.org/10.3390/molecules24071258.
16. Valles S. A brief history of the social concept of health and its role in population health science. In: Philosophy of population health science: philosophy for a new public health era. London: Routledge; 2018. p. 31–56.
17. Yearby R. Structural racism and health disparities: reconfiguring the social determinants of health framework to include the root cause. J Law Med Ethics. 2020;48(3):518–26. https://doi.org/10.1177/1073110520958876.
18. COHRED: Research fairness initiative. 2018. https://rfi.cohred.org/. Accessed 22 Jun 2022.
19. Molldrem S, Smith AK. Reassessing the ethics of molecular HIV surveillance in the era of cluster detection and response: toward HIV data justice. Am J Bioeth. 2020;20(10):10–23.
20. Martin KE. Ethical issues in the big data industry. MIS Q Exec. 2015;14(2):67–85.

60 How Innovations Can Impact on people's Life: The Continuum of Research in Global Health

Christian Lienhardt and Frank Cobelens

Abstract

Knowledge is at the heart of health research, and production of relevant evidence along the overall spectrum of research—from basic science for discovery to the development of new tools or strategies, and their optimal uptake—is essential to improve health globally. The intention of this chapter is to present how thinking *along the research continuum* provides a solid basis to identify where and how interactions and synergies can take place profitably towards a common goal, and avoid dispersion of means, energies and funding. Mapping institutions, programmes and teams involved in research for a given health condition and matching these to research needs and priorities at national and international levels is fundamental to improve the relevance, quality and efficiency of research. Capitalizing on greater recognition of the value of research for health and society, an *end-to-end* vision is proposed, encompassing the full continuum of research to gain evidence from multiple sources, for ultimately linking research, policy and practice.

Keywords

Research for health · Implementation research · Health policy and systems research · Translational research · Basic research

60.1 Introduction

The COVID-19 pandemic that stroke the world in the early 2020's resulted in more than 6 million lives lost and overstress of health care systems capacities worldwide. The scientific community has been raising up and responding to this new pandemic in an unprecedented way, leading to the development and administration of safe and efficacious vaccines worldwide less than 2 years after disease emergence. This remarkably rapid development of vaccines has been possible, thanks to decades of investment in health technology development (especially for the messenger RNA platform), the fast conduct of pivotal trials and the use of accelerated regulatory pathways, leading to radical improvements in the way the pandemic was managed [1]. This response to the pandemic evolved through multiple phases as new information and tools became available,

C. Lienhardt (✉)
Epidemiology and Population Health, Department of Infectious Disease Epidemiology, London School of Hygiene and Tropical Medicine, London, UK

Unité Mixte Internationale TransVIHMI (UMI 233 and U1175 INSERM), Institut de Recherche pour le Développement (IRD), Montpellier, France
e-mail: christian.lienhardt@ird.fr

F. Cobelens
Amsterdam University Medical Centers, University of Amsterdam, Amsterdam, Netherlands

Amsterdam Institute for Global Health and Development (AIGHD), Amsterdam, Netherlands
e-mail: f.cobelens@aighd.org

M. C. B. Raviglione et al. (eds.), *Global Health Essentials*, Sustainable Development Goals Series,
https://doi.org/10.1007/978-3-031-33851-9_60

requiring development of novel policies and subsequent social and behavioural changes, based on rapidly accruing and evolving evidence. This shows how research undertaken along the continuum, feeding and learning from each other's experiences and mistakes, can rapidly bear fruits, while requiring constant adjustments as new evidence arises. Similarly, to achieve the WHO target of *1 billion more people getting access to universal health coverage by 2025* [2], we need to enhance research along the whole spectrum to ensure appropriate development, delivery and uptake of new biomedical products needed to combat main global health issues.

60.2 From Bench to Bed to Health Policies: The Continuum of Research

In its 2013 Report, the WHO defines Health Research as *the development of knowledge with the aim of understanding health challenges and mounting an improved response to them* [3]. Knowledge is at the heart of health research: beginning from what is already known, scientists ask questions, construct hypotheses, and develop experiments that in turn generate new knowledge, in an ongoing dynamic cycle, with the view to transforming human health. There are several types of research along the research continuum. We consider here those categorized in the WHO report 2013 (basic/fundamental research; applied research; operational/implementation research; translational research; and health policy and systems research—Box 60.1), presented below in an *operationally focused* order**.** This provides a comprehensive view of the spectrum of research involved to improving health globally—from basic science for discovery to the development of new tools or strategies and their optimal uptake in health systems. The intention is to provide a way of *thinking about the research process along the continuum* with the view to identifying where and how interactions and synergies can take place towards a common goal rather than conducting research in 'silos'—as has been demonstrated in the case of TB (Box 60.2).

Box 60.1 Research Definitions Used in the WHO Report 2013: Research for Universal Health Coverage*

Basic research or **fundamental research** is experimental or theoretical work undertaken primarily to acquire new knowledge about the underlying foundations of phenomena and observable facts, without any particular application or use in view.

Applied research is original investigation undertaken to acquire new knowledge, directed primarily towards a specific practical aim or objective.

Operational research or **implementation research** seeks knowledge on interventions, strategies or tools so as to enhance the quality or coverage of health systems and services. The design could be, for example, an observational study, a cross-sectional study, a case-control or cohort study, or a randomized controlled trial.

Translational research, which moves knowledge gained from basic research to its application in the clinic and community, is often characterized as 'bench-to-bedside' and 'bedside-to-community'. The translation is between any of several stages: moving basic discovery into a candidate health application; assessing the value of an application leading to the development of evidence-based guidelines; moving guidelines into health practice, through delivery, dissemination, and diffusion of research; or evaluating the health outcomes of public health practice. This has also been called **experimental development research**.

Health policy and systems research (HPSR) seeks to understand and improve how societies organize themselves in achieving their collective health goals, and how different actors interact in the policy and implementation processes to contribute to policy outcomes. HPSR is an interdisciplinary blend of economics, sociology, anthropology, political science, public health and epidemiology that together draw a comprehensive picture of how health systems respond and adapt to health policies, and how health policies can shape—and be shaped by—health systems and the broader determinants of health.

Research for health covers a broader range of investigations than **health research**, reflecting the fact that health also depends on actions taken outside the health sector—in agriculture, education, employment, fiscal policy, housing, social services, trade, transport, and so on. This wider view of research will become increasingly important in the transition from the United Nations Millennium Development Goals to a post-2015 sustainable development agenda [3].

Box 60.2 The International Roadmap for Tuberculosis Research[*]

Research for TB elimination requires an intensification of efforts across a continuum from fundamental research (for improved diagnostics, treatment and prevention) to operational and health systems research (for improved performance and introduction of new health care delivery strategies).[**]

To this end, the *International Roadmap for Tuberculosis Research* was developed with the view to stimulate outcome-oriented research to develop revolutionary new TB diagnostics, treatment, and prevention tools and approaches, optimize the use of existing technologies and strategies, and ensure the uptake of new TB interventions within the larger frame of system-wide health care.

More than a simple research agenda, the *International Roadmap for Tuberculosis Research* outlines critical and priority areas for future scientific investment, with the aim of increasing and harmonizing funding and multi-disciplinary work across the research spectrum. It provides an *architecture* on which transformational and outcome-oriented research areas can be constructed. It is intended to promote organization of cross-disciplinary teams and attract all research-related constituents to the field, especially those in BRICS countries, who have a vital role to play. It provides a common platform for donors, researchers, implementers, and advocates by identifying the most important research questions. Thus, investigators studying processes with the potential to inform product development would greatly benefit from a thorough understanding of the realities of tuberculosis patient care and all involved logistics and decision algorithms, as well as general practices and expectations for developing clinical candidates of diagnostics, drugs, and vaccines. Exposing basic research scientists to the realities of tuberculosis control in endemic settings would allow better understanding of the challenges and realities of tuberculosis patient care and would provide a valuable opportunity to create a deeper sense of where tuberculosis research needs to be applied and create connections between basic and clinical/operational disciplines [4, 5].

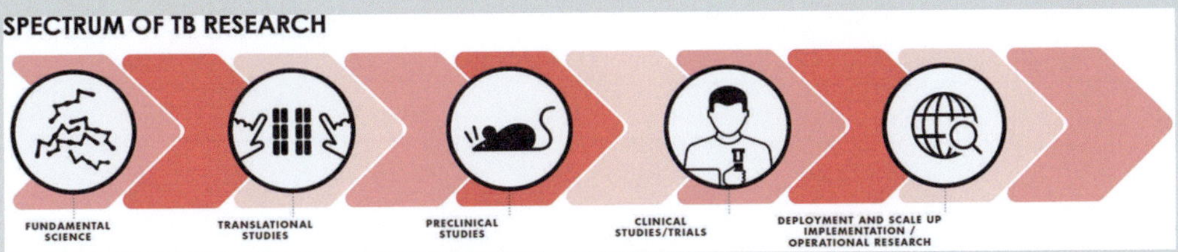

60.2.1 Basic and Fundamental Research

According to the UK Clinical Research Collaboration, basic research represents research *that underpins investigations into the cause, development, detection, treatment and management of diseases, conditions and ill health* [6]. Fundamental research is semantically broader than basic research, as it usually designates scientific studies that contribute to the understanding of a given ill-health condition, including its underlying biological or medical mechanisms, but also including its epidemiological and public health characteristics—such as the identification of determinants involved in the cause, risk or development of ill health conditions. Indeed, the difficulty in connecting basic scientific studies with tangible outcomes that would benefit patients, clinicians and programme managers has historically prevented interactions between the most basic and most applied disciplines of research. Thus, what comes out of basic science in terms of, for example, new drugs or vaccines, is often defined by technological opportunities rather than by well-established insights into what patients, health care workers, and policy-makers need. Such insights may arise from research looking at the expected health impact, acceptability and affordability of a given health product, in an 'end-to-end process' along the R&D chain, that transforms a rather limited 'single direction process' into a richer path with feedback loops from practice to (early) development. Thus, fundamental research spans several disciplines of science and can serve to connect these disciplines through cross-feeding, integrated projects. In this sense, fundamental research is crucial to the development of new tools and strategies for prevention, diagnosis and cure of ill-health conditions [7].

60.2.2 Translational Research

Translational research which moves knowledge gained from basic research to its application in the clinic, is often referred to as bench-to-bedside'. The translation is between any of several stages, for example, moving basic discovery on a candidate health product (a potential biomarker, a new chemical entity, a vaccine candidate) through pre-clinical experiments and assessing the clinical value and validity of this product leading to its potential use in the clinic. Thus, translational research includes all scientific experiments and studies that contribute directly to the development of new diagnostics, medicines or vaccines, leading to detection, prevention or treatment of disease and conditions.

A particular aspect of translational research is represented by clinical trials that are being used within the development pathway of new biological products [8], or to evaluate new public health interventions [9]. These trials comprise stepwise studies in human subjects to assess the efficacy, safety and validity of medical products after having been tested pre-clinically. Randomized controlled trials (RCTs) provide the strongest evidence of the efficacy and safety of a medical product to diagnose, treat or prevent ill health conditions. Clinical trials should be seen as a complete experimentation process, from the start (research question) until the end (proof of safety and/or efficacy of the tested product, procedure or intervention), ensuring validity and reproducibility of results.

60.2.3 Operational/Implementation Research

Down the line, it is critical to conduct research aimed at ensuring introduction and uptake of newest health products in policy and practice, as well as developing interventions that result in better health systems, or more efficient methods of service delivery. Operational/Implementation research (OR/IR) seeks to gather knowledge on interventions, strategies or tools to enhance the quality or coverage of health systems and services [10, 11]. According to WHO, OR is defined as '*the use of systematic research techniques for programme decision-making* to achieve a specific outcome. It provides policymakers and managers with evidence that they can use to improve programme operations' [12]. Thus, OR/IR can help evaluate the effectiveness of new tools or interventions and determine the conditions and requirements that maximize their effective use, but it can also assist identifying bottlenecks to implementation of existing policies and provide necessary evidence from the perspective of patients and health systems [13]. OR/IR studies are extremely useful at collecting information needed to guide policy-making and develop strategies on a global scale [14]. Methodological options range from observational studies (that may include qualitative components, for example, among small groups of patients or health care workers using direct observation of practice, focus group discussions or in-depth interviews) to randomized controlled trials evaluating strategies or interventions in which the primary outcomes would be determined by quantitative methods. In short, OR/IR can be understood as ranging from locally relevant research conducted to address locally defined problems to the evaluation of the potential impact of global policy recommendations.

60.2.4 Research in Global Health and Policy-Making

The importance of policy-making in building efficient health systems is increasingly recognized, drawing greater attention to research-informed policy-making eventually leading to essential health gains [15]. The use of research evidence is a complex, interdependent process that requires understanding of how research evidence is being produced and subsequently assessed and used by decision-makers—see Chap. 61. Research on health policy and systems covers all types of research investigating the organization and delivery of health services; health and welfare economics; health policy, ethics and research governance. This requires the production of robust research findings for bridging the evidence-to-policy gap [16]. Factors potentially enhancing recourse to this type of research often arise from priority setting exercises and the focus on issues arising at the interface between research and policy-making, including consideration of the 'end-users' needs. In this, research in global health can be defined as being *transnational* (focus on transnational health issues, determinants and solutions), *interdisciplinary* (involving many disciplines within and beyond the health sciences) and *integrated* (synthesis of population-based prevention with individual-level clinical care) [17].

60.3 The Importance of the *End-to-End Vision* to Structure Interdisciplinary Research and Collaboration

Effectively translating research into improved patient care and maximizing access to products requires optimal coordination among partners, so as to facilitate the seamless integration of new tools into current programmes—as exemplified by the search for new malaria vaccines (Box 60.3). Mapping institutions, programmes and teams involved in research for a given health condition and matching these to research needs and priorities at national and international levels is fundamental to improve the relevance, quality and efficiency of research. For this, fundamental researchers must learn how to give their studies the most impact on clinical needs and disease burden. In exchange, clinicians and public health specialists need to identify areas in which fundamental research can provide answers. This requires fresh thinking on how to fund and manage interdisciplinary science.[1] Considering the limitations in research funding, one suggested approach is to structure large, cross-cutting research initiatives, combining basic, clinical, health system, and social sciences. Such interdisciplinary, multicentre research projects, constructed around key thematic areas, could leverage support from a variety of funding organizations and allow synergy between different disciplines and sectors.

[1] In TB research, for instance, a network of longitudinal studies of patients and households are being used to identify biomarkers that characterize the various clinically relevant stages of TB, together with studies on how to prevent transmission and disease development.

Box 60.3 The Quest for a Malaria Vaccine: An 'End to End' Approach to Research and Development for Global Health

An estimated 1.7 billion cases of malaria and 10.6 million deaths have been averted over the past 20 years as a result of the scaling up of malaria control interventions worldwide [18]. Major reductions in malaria morbidity and mortality occurred between 2000 and 2015, thanks to the widespread use of insecticides for vector control and medicines for treatment and prevention that have become the standards of malaria control globally. However, all these products are unfortunately susceptible to emergence of biological resistances. An efficient and safe vaccine focusing on reducing malaria hospitalization and preventing severe disease and death, especially in young children who are most affected by the disease, would greatly help overcoming these barriers.

The first antiparasitic RTS,S/AS01 (RTS,S) malaria vaccine, recommended by WHO in 2021 to be given to children living in regions with moderate-to-high transmission of *Plasmodium falciparum* malaria, is a huge step forward in the fight against malaria [19]. The development of this vaccine took, however, more than 30 years, and, looking back, an *end to end* view of research and development with global health in mind could have shortened this development timeline. A series of Phase 3 trials of the RTS,S/AS01 vaccine showed partial efficacy against clinical and severe malaria in areas with moderate to high malaria transmission [20]. The pivotal phase 3 trial evaluated the efficacy of 3 or 4 doses of RTS,S/AS01 against various malaria endpoints in 8922 children aged 5–17 months and 6537 children aged 6–12 weeks at the time of the first dose. Efficacy varied according to the number of doses given and decreased from 51% (95% CI 47–55) to 39% (95% CI 34–43) against clinical and complicated malaria and from 45% (95% CI 22–60) to 29% (95% CI 6–46) against severe malaria as time since vaccination increased from 12 to 46 months [21]. Among a subset of children followed for a total of 7 years, vaccine efficacy against clinical malaria was 24% (95% CI 16–31, p <0.0001) for the 3-dose group and 19% (95% CI 11–27; p <0.0001) for the 4-dose group. Three safety signals were identified—i.e. an excess of meningitis, cerebral malaria and deaths among girls who had received RTS,S/AS01—that were thought to be chance findings.

Based on these results, RTS,S/AS01 vaccine received a *positive scientific opinion from the European Medicines Agency* in July 2015 [22]. However, WHO's Strategic Advisory Group of Experts (SAGE) on Immunization recommended further evaluation to address several gaps in knowledge (including on safety aspects) before considering wider country-level introduction. Subsequently, data on the effectiveness of RTS,S were generated through evaluation of a pilot phased introduction in Ghana, Kenya and Malawi. Pooled data across the three countries during the first 2 years of vaccine introduction showed that hospitalization with severe malaria among children eligible for at least three doses of vaccine was reduced by 29% (rate ratio 0.71 (95% CI 0.55–0.93)) and hospitalization was reduced by 21% (95% CI 7–32). The safety signals were not seen, supporting that those observed were chance findings. In total, RTS,S/AS01 vaccine was considered safe and well tolerated and, on 6 October 2021, *WHO recommended that this vaccine be used for the prevention of P. falciparum malaria in children living in regions with moderate to high transmission* [19]. Importantly, WHO recommended that the RTS,S/AS01 vaccine be provided as *part of a comprehensive malaria control strategy,* as highest impact in reducing malaria illness and death is achieved when multiple interventions are used concomitantly.

Several lessons can be learned from the various technical, regulatory, policy and investment planning hurdles that occurred along the way. The development of the vaccine took over 30 years, in part because malaria is a complex organism, and in part because malaria is a disease that affects low-income countries primarily. With a lack of a high-income market, a malaria vaccine was not prioritized, leading to potential loss of progress during the development pathway ('the first and second valleys of death'). The modest efficacy and safety signals seen in the phase 3 trial resulted in a recommendation for pilots, which further exasperated the situation because the manufacturer could not advance on plans to increase supply, resulting in another period of risk for bringing the vaccine forward. It has been suggested that *an end-to-end vision of vaccine development* would have helped avoiding pitfalls along the way, considering the true value-drivers, prospects for access and programmatic feasibility [23]. Such an *end-to-end vision* of research would arise from a wide, rigorous and objective review of the landscape of research along its continuum, from product development to potential health and societal impact, where late-stage research should reflect solid scientific justification, and a clear line of sight for access to the vaccine by the communities where research is undertaken. In this respect, the long road to development of the RTS,S vaccine opens doors for a new era of vaccine R&D that may be useful not only to a second malaria vaccine generation but also for the development of vaccines for infectious diseases affecting the poorest populations.

60.4 Conclusion

Recent decades have seen a greater recognition of the value of research for health and society. Guiding research and development of new health products or procedures can benefit greatly from an 'end-to-end' vision encompassing the full continuum of research, so as to develop highly suitable tools or interventions for effective health gains. This requires close collaboration between key stakeholders to guide development and implementation of new tools and create optimal synergy among researchers and research institutions, donors, programmes, health systems, patients and advocacy groups. In this way, efforts can be effectively carried out worldwide for enhanced, properly funded and sustainable research for better health. This requires considering the diversity of problems for which research can offer solutions, the benefits of gaining evidence from multiple sources, the relationship between study design and strength of inference, and the challenge of applying research findings from one setting to another, for ultimately linking research, policy and practice.

Acknowledgement The authors would like to thank Dr. Mary Hamel, from WHO, for her kind review of the malaria vaccine section.

References

1. Collins FS. COVID-19 lessons for research. Science. 2021;371(6534):1081. https://doi.org/10.1126/Science.abh3996.
2. WHO. Universal health coverage (UHC). 2022. https://www.who.int/news-room/fact-sheets/detail/universal-health-coverage-(Uhc).
3. World Health Organization: The world health report 2013: research for universal health coverage. WHO, Geneva, 2013. https://www.who.int/whr/2013/report/en/.
4. World Health Organization and Stop TB Partnership. An International Roadmap for Tuberculosis Research. Geneva, World Health Organization, 2011.
5. World Health Organization. A global action framework for TB research in support of the third pillar of WHO's end TB strategy. Geneva, 2015. WHO/HTM/TB/2015.26.
6. Medical Research Council on behalf of the UK Clinical Research Collaboration (UKCRC). UK clinical research collaboration health research classification system. 2018. http://hrcsonline.net/wp-content/uploads/2018/01/HRCS_Main_Handbook_v2_Feb2018.pdf
7. Lienhardt C. Fundamental research is the key to eliminating TB. Nature. 2014;507:401.
8. Pocock SJ. Clinical trials: a practical approach. London: Wiley; 1983.
9. Smith PG, Morrow RH, Ross DA. Field trials of health interventions–a toolbox. 3rd ed. Oxford (UK): Oxford University Press; 2015. ISBN-10: 0198732864ISBN-13: 9780198732860.
10. Zachariah R, Harries A, Ishikawa N, et al. Operational research in low-income countries: what, why, and how? Lancet Infect Dis. 2009;9:711–7.
11. Lobb R, Colditz GA. Implementation science and its application to population health. Ann Rev Public Health. 2013;34:235–51. https://doi.org/10.1146/annurev-publhealth-031912-114444. PMID:23297655.
12. World Health Organization. Operational research for malaria control: tutor's guide. WHO/HTM/RBM. Part II. Geneva, Switzerland: WHO; 2003. http://apps.who.int/malaria/docs/operational_research_tg.pdf.
13. Lienhardt C, Cobelens F. Operational research for TB control: the scope, the needs and the way forward. Int J Tuberc Lung Dis. 2011;15(1):6–13. PMID: 21276290.
14. Zachariah R, et al. Is operational research delivering the goods? the journey to success in low-income countries. Lancet Infect Dis. 2012;12:415–21. https://doi.org/10.1016/S1473-3099(11)70309-7. PMID:22326018.
15. Hanney S, Gonzalez-Block M, Buxton M, Kogan M. Health research policy and systems. The utilisation of health research in policy-making: concepts, examples and methods of assessment. Health Res Policy Sys. 2003;1:2.
16. Masood S, Kothari A, Regan S. The use of research in public health policy: a systematic review. Evidence Policy. 2020;16(1):7–43. https://bristoluniversitypressdigital.com/view/journals/evp/16/1/article-p7.xml
17. Koplan JP, Bond TC, Merson MH, et al. Towards a common definition of global health. Lancet. 2009;373:1993–5.
18. World Health Organization. World malaria report 2021. World Health Organization. 2021. https://apps.who.int/iris/handle/10665/350147. Licence: CC BY-NC-SA 3.0 IGO.
19. WHO. First-ever malaria vaccine recommendation now published in a position paper and in the WHO guidelines for malaria. 2022. https://www.who.int/news/item/04-03-2022-first-ever-malaria-vaccine-recommendation-now-published-in-a-position-paper-and-in-the-who-guidelines-for-malaria.
20. RTS,S Clinical Trials Partnership, Agnandji ST, Lell B, Soulanoudjingar SS, Fernandes JF, Abossolo BP, et al. First results of Phase 3 trial of RTS,S/AS01 malaria vaccine in African children. N Engl J

Med. 2011;365(20):1863–75. http://www.ncbi.nlm.nih.gov/pubmed/22007715; RTS,S Clinical Trials Partnership, Agnandji ST, Lell B, Fernandes JF, Abossolo BP, Methogo BGNO, et al. A phase 3 trial of RTS,S/AS01 malaria vaccine in African infants. N Engl J Med. 2012 Dec 13;367(24):2284.

21. RTS,S Clinical Trials Partnership. Efficacy and safety of RTS,S/AS01 malaria vaccine with or without a booster dose in infants and children in Africa: final results of a phase 3, individually randomised, controlled trial. Lancet. 2015;386(9988):31–45.
22. European Medicines Agency. First malaria vaccine receives positive scientific opinion from EMA [Internet]. Available from: www.ema.europa.eu.
23. Vekemans J, Schellenberg D, Benns S, et al. Meeting report: WHO consultation on malaria vaccine development, Geneva, 15–16 July 2019. Vaccine. 2021;39:2907–16.

61 Evaluation of Interventions in Global Health

Frank Cobelens and Christian Lienhardt

Abstract

Evaluations of health interventions aim to provide policy makers with evidence to decide about their scale-up. The key components of such evidence are the acceptability and feasibility of the intervention, its cost-effectiveness and affordability, and its effectiveness in terms of health outcomes. Acceptability can be evaluated throughout the intervention's development, mainly through qualitative research. Cost-effectiveness and affordability are generally assessed through modelling and may require collecting health system and patient costing data. Health outcomes should be carefully defined based on their relevance, validity and applicability. Health effectiveness can be evaluated through various study designs that have different applications during the evaluation process and produce different levels of confidence in the results. Key choices are experimental (randomized allocation of the intervention) versus quasi-experimental comparison, individual versus group-wise intervention allocation, and the desired level of pragmatism and the generalizability of the results beyond the setting in which the evaluation was done.

Keywords

Intervention evaluations · Cost-effectiveness · Affordability · Quasi-experimental studies · Experimental studies

61.1 Introduction

Health interventions are key to improving global health. They can be diagnostic, therapeutic or preventive, cover any health field, and be carried out by a broad range of providers across the full spectrum of health systems. Examples of interventions in global health are new drug combinations for treating malaria, vaccination against SARS-CoV-2, m-health to improve adherence to antiretroviral therapy, kangaroo care for preterm infants and subsidized private health insurance.

Public health or health service interventions are often complex as they involve several interconnected components and different stakeholders and can impact at various levels. Since the components of a complex health intervention

F. Cobelens (✉)
Amsterdam University Medical Centers, University of Amsterdam, Amsterdam, Netherlands

Amsterdam Institute for Global Health and Development (AIGHD), Amsterdam, Netherlands
e-mail: f.cobelens@aighd.org

C. Lienhardt
Epidemiology and Population Health, Department of Infectious Disease Epidemiology, London School of Hygiene and Tropical Medicine, London, UK

Unité Mixte Internationale TransVIHMI (UMI 233 and U1175 INSERM), Institut de Recherche pour le Développement (IRD), Montpellier, France
e-mail: christian.lienhardt@ird.fr

M. C. B. Raviglione et al. (eds.), *Global Health Essentials*, Sustainable Development Goals Series,
https://doi.org/10.1007/978-3-031-33851-9_61

can each affect its outcome and health impact, it is important that such interventions are carefully designed, taking into account biomedical (e.g. the efficacy of a vaccine), socio-behavioural (e.g. its acceptance by the target population) and resource allocation (e.g. staffing needs) aspects. In this chapter, we will focus on such complex public health or health service interventions.

61.2 Background

For the development and evaluation of complex interventions, different phases have been proposed to mirror those of clinical development of drugs or vaccines [1]. In this analogy, in the "preclinical" phase the intervention is conceived based on theory. Phase 1 includes formative research to describe the target population for the intervention, how to reach them and how to influence their behaviour. Phase 2 is exploratory and develops the optimum intervention focusing on acceptability to target groups and providers, and feasibility of the delivery. Phase 3 is the formal evaluation where the intervention's health effects are established. Finally phase 4 evaluates health and other impacts once it has been implemented. In this chapter, we will refer to these phases to clarify the suitability of various evaluation approaches along the intervention development pathway.

For interventions to reach health impact, they need to be widely accessible. The "ambition or process of expanding the coverage of health interventions" [2] is known as *scaling up*, which includes making available the financial, human, logistic and capital resources needed. Scaling up an intervention requires policy decisions by those responsible for its implementation, such as national or local governments or health care delivery organizations. These decisions will be based on various considerations that include effectiveness and expected health impact, feasibility and acceptability, cost-effectiveness and affordability. The ultimate aim for evaluations of health interventions is therefore to provide policy makers with evidence about these key considerations for scaling up.

61.3 Aim

This chapter aims to outline the key components of policy-relevant evidence and approaches to evaluating effectiveness in global health and to provide recommendations for choices in study design.

61.4 Policy-Relevant Evidence

Several frameworks exist for evaluating evidence about health interventions, generally based on systematic reviews of scientific literature. Most important for global health is the GRADE framework (Chap. 83), the standard for developing policy recommendations by the World Health Organization and several other international organizations. It weighs the strength of the recommendation for or against use of an intervention and the quality of the evidence for that recommendation separately, explicitly and in a transparent manner. The evidence includes health outcomes in terms of benefits and harms, and the importance of these outcomes to those affected, as well as the intervention's acceptability, feasibility, and resource and equity implications. Evaluations of health care interventions therefore need to address each of these elements, either separately in various phases of development, or collectively in a single study.

61.4.1 Health Outcomes

An important consideration in the design of any evaluation is the health outcomes that the study should look at and that the intervention is meant to improve. These can be *process indicators* (e.g. treatment adherence, utilization of services) or *impact indicators* (e.g. morbidity, quality of life, survival), depending on the type of intervention and its development phase. A study can have several health outcomes but generally one is defined as the primary. Careful selection of the primary outcome is important because that defines the data analysis, and the key message in reporting the results and the study's sample size that should be sufficient to detect a statistically significant change in the primary outcome (Table 61.1).

61.4.2 Acceptability and Feasibility

The acceptability of a health intervention reflects the extent to which people delivering or receiving that intervention find it appropriate. It is a multifaceted construct for which several theoretical frameworks exist. Often applied is the one by Sekhon et al. [3] that distinguishes seven components: how an individual feels about the intervention, the perceived effort required to participate in the intervention, the fit of the intervention with the participant's values, the extent to which the participant understands the intervention and how it works, the extent to which benefits, profits or values must be given up to engage in the intervention, the extent to which the intervention is perceived as likely to achieve its purpose, and the participant's confidence that they can perform the behaviour(s) required to participate. This theoretical framework considers these components prior to participating, while participating, and after participating in the intervention. Although acceptability is the prime focus of phase 2, it can be studied in each development phase using qualitative as well as quantitative methods.

The feasibility of an intervention primarily reflects its health system requirements, such as trained staff, clinical or laboratory infrastructure, surveillance systems and other conditions to make the intervention work (think of air-conditioned facilities or internet connection). It is important to list and quantify the critical feasibility conditions for the intervention, as that will determine its scalability.

61.4.3 Cost-Effectiveness and Affordability

The cost-effectiveness of a health intervention is the additional cost per unit improvement in the

Table 61.1 Considerations in defining the primary outcome for the evaluation of health effects

Consideration	Related question(s)	Example
Relevance	Is the outcome relevant to participants and the health care system? Will it change or influence clinical or public health policy?	For the evaluation of introducing a new diagnostic for malaria, sensitivity and specificity of the test compared to a reference standard are relevant, but ultimately important to policy makers is the extent to which it will lead to better health outcomes for malaria patients such as timely cure
Validity	Can the outcome be feasibly ascertained in all study participants with limited misclassification?	In a randomized trial of a vaccine against tuberculosis, a disease that is difficult to diagnose with certainty, if only microbiologically confirmed cases are counted in the outcome, some cases will be missed (false-negative outcomes) and a larger sample size is required. If also non-confirmed cases are counted, the outcome will include patients who do not have tuberculosis (false-positive outcomes), and the trial will underestimate the true protective efficacy
Applicability	Is the outcome likely affected by the intervention at reasonable scale? Can the expected difference in primary outcome due to the intervention be determined as statistically significant within a reasonable sample size?	The more directly the outcome is affected by the intervention, the larger the effectiveness that can be expected and hence the smaller the required sample size. A m-health intervention to improve treatment adherence for antiretroviral therapy would be expected to have a large effect on sustained HIV viral suppression, but a small effect on survival since that is affected by many other factors. While mortality may be a more relevant outcome from a public health perspective, it requires a much larger sample size than viral suppression, potentially making the study much more resource intensive

health outcome achieved by the intervention. It is generally quantified in cost-effectiveness analyses (CEA) as the incremental cost-effectiveness ratio (ICER), defined as the increment in cost divided by the increment in health outcome improvement. To make decisions about allocation of resources, policy makers need to be able to compare the cost-effectiveness of different interventions (Box 61.1).

Box 61.1 Health Outcome and Cost Components for Cost-Effectiveness Evaluations (CEA)

The health outcome or *effectiveness component* is often expressed as life years gained by the intervention after adjustment for the quality of life (quality-adjusted life years, QALYs) or the extent of disability (disability-adjusted life years, DALYs) that remains after the intervention. DALYs or QALYs are generally inferred from a health outcome measured in the evaluation such as a disease incidence or cure rate, and DALY estimates from the literature. DALYs are being estimated for a large variety of health conditions and populations using standard methodology developed by the Institute of Health Metrics and Evaluation as part of the Global Burden of Disease project [4]. DALYs or QALYs allow comparisons of cost-effectiveness of different interventions to achieve different health outcomes. CEAs can also base their effectiveness component directly on the health outcomes measured in the evaluation. Examples are cost per case of malaria diagnosed, or cost per patient that has well-controlled hypertension. These types of effectiveness measures allow comparisons of cost-effectiveness of different interventions to achieve the same health outcome. The *cost component* of a cost-effectiveness analysis requires collection of cost data as part of phase 2 and/or 3 of the evaluation. It can be restricted to cost borne by the health system (*health system perspective*) or also include cost borne by the health system users (*societal perspective*). The health system costs of an intervention can be estimated in two ways: top-down and bottom-up. Top-down costing takes into account the total expenditures for services, whereas bottom-up costing calculates the exact cost input for each element in those services on a per-participant basis, also taking into account overhead costs such as building space. The latter is more reflective of the true cost of the intervention but requires more detailed data collection and disregards inefficiencies such as underutilization of services. Cost data are sometimes sourced from literature. While that avoids direct cost data collection, it may result in biased CEA estimates since the health effectiveness of the intervention may be related to the effort put into it and thereby to its total cost.

Cost-effectiveness is generally determined through CEA models in which a hypothetical cohort of individuals with certain demographic and health characteristics is followed up for the health outcome [5]. It then compares introduction of the intervention with no intervention (the *base case*) for health outcome and total cost related to the intervention, with parameter values for the effectiveness of cost components derived from the evaluation study. CEAs allow choices about resource allocation by comparing the ICER of the intervention with a predefined threshold that defines an intervention as being cost-effective, or with the ICERs of other interventions for the same or different conditions. However, that an intervention is deemed cost-effective does not mean that it is also affordable given a country's or organization's budget. Therefore, a budget impact analysis may be needed in which the intervention's cost and effectiveness data from the evaluation are applied, usually through modelling studies, into the future to the population in which it is to be scaled-up [6].

61.5 Approaches to Evaluating Effectiveness

The level of confidence that policy makers have in the evidence of effectiveness of an intervention depends on the design of the evaluation: experimental or quasi-experimental. In experimental designs or *trials,* the allocation of the intervention to units of observation (e.g. people, clinics, villages) is *randomized,* i.e., based on chance; in quasi-experimental designs the allocation is purposeful. Randomization avoids that the intervention is preferentially given to those considered to benefit most (or least), which would produce biased results. Provided the sample size is large enough it also avoids confounding by underlying determinants of the health outcome. Therefore, experimental studies are considered to provide strong evidence of effectiveness. Quasi-experimental studies provide moderate evidence but have the advantage that they generally have smaller numbers of group units, lower cost and fewer logistical challenges.

61.5.1 Experimental Study Designs

Trial designs are defined by the unit of randomization (individuals or groups) and how the intervention is allocated over time. In *individually randomized trials,* individual participants are randomized to either (the intervention arm) or not (the control arm) receive the intervention. In *cluster-randomized trials* groups are randomized into intervention and control arms. The intervention can be introduced for all units concurrently (parallel designs) or stepwise over time. In *stepped wedge* or *phased implementation trials* the sequence by which the intervention is introduced is randomized across the groups. In *cross-over designs,* the intervention is started in one arm and after a predefined period switched to the other. In *factorial designs,* combinations of interventions are compared.

While individually randomized trials can be relevant in the evaluation of certain global health interventions such as preventive treatment or vaccines, group-randomized trial are used most often, especially in phase 3 (Table 61.2). Group-randomized trials pose specific challenges. Individual observations within clusters are not statistically independent, which means that the sample size required for the trial needs to be larger than if it were individually randomized. The adjustment factor (the *design effect*) depends on assumptions about how alike individuals are within and between clusters with regard to the primary outcome [7]. The overall sample size is a trade-off between the number of clusters and the number of individuals in each cluster. The larger the number of clusters the smaller the design effect and the overall sample size needed, the smaller the number of clusters the easier the logistics. Note that trials with small numbers of clusters (less than 2 × 15) are prone to bias and confounding. In those cases, it is advised to match the randomized intervention-control pairs based on relevant baseline characteristics including the primary outcome.

Table 61.2 Reasons for preferring group (cluster) randomization in intervention trials

Reason	Examples
Intervention provided at cluster level	Mosquito breeding site reduction in a village New system of quality improvement in health care facilities
Cluster-specific factors likely determine effectiveness	Success of the intervention for individual patients depends on attitude of the physician or quality of the laboratory
Complex intervention in which various components are decisive for its success	Introduction of a health insurance system
To take account of indirect effects	Insecticide-impregnated bed nets can provide direct protection against malaria to those sleeping under the bed nets but also indirect protection to others in the same dwelling or village because of reduced transmission
Logistic or acceptability reasons	If it is easier or more acceptable to the users if all in a clinic or village receive the intervention than if it is provided to only some randomly selected individuals

Stepped wedge trials are increasingly used in global health. They allow evaluation of the health effectiveness of an intervention while it is being rolled out. This may have advantages if the policy decision about scale-up of the intervention has already been taken or if withholding the intervention to the control arm is regarded undesirable or unethical. Therefore stepped wedge trials are typically conducted in phase 4. Since comparisons are made over time within clusters as well as concurrently between clusters the sample size determination and statistical analysis are complex [8].

61.5.2 Quasi-Experimental Study Designs

Quasi-experimental study designs used in global health compare the level of the health outcome before with that after the introduction of the intervention at the individual or group level. The simplest version is the *uncontrolled before-after comparison*, in which all individuals or groups receive the intervention. Its key limitation is that changes in health outcome may occur over time through other causes than the intervention, leading to over- or underestimation of its true effect. One way of dealing with this bias is the *controlled before-after comparison* in which a control group (individuals, villages, clinics), that is selected to be similar to the intervention group, does not receive the intervention. The *difference-in-difference* approach refines this design by estimating the intervention's effect on the health outcome through multivariable adjustment for changes over time in other characteristics. These designs are often used in phase 2 of the intervention development pathway. An approach often used in phase 4 is the *interrupted time series analysis* that plots the trend in level of health outcome over time and looks for sudden changes in that trend from the moment the intervention was introduced. An example is changes in medication use before versus after introduction of health insurance. It can also include a control group, for example, a geographic unit where the intervention has not (yet) been introduced.

61.6 Generalizability and Pragmatism: Recommendations

Evidence about an intervention should reflect what can be expected when the intervention is scaled-up. The extent to which the results of an intervention trial can be generalized to real-world implementation is known as its level of pragmatism. For example, eligibility criteria for study participants can be highly restricted, such as only participants with no comorbidities who are likely to adhere to the intervention. At the other end of the spectrum is allowing everyone into the study regardless of these conditions. With highly restricted eligibility criteria the intervention's effectiveness measured by the study will not be affected by comorbidities nor diluted by poor adherence. The trial thereby provides an estimate of effectiveness under optimal conditions, also known as efficacy (*explanatory trial*). Conversely, a trial with highly relaxed eligibility criteria will provide an estimate of effectiveness for the entire population that accesses the intervention when it is implemented in routine practice (*pragmatic trial*). There are several other components of a trial that determine its position on the continuum from explanatory to pragmatic, such trial setting, primary outcome, approach to follow-up and flexibility in delivering the intervention. The Pragmatic–Explanatory Continuum Indicator Summary (PRECIS-2) tool can help making decisions about the level of pragmatism when designing the evaluation [9].

Explanatory trials are generally required for regulatory approval of drugs or vaccines. For complex health interventions, they can be useful to answer the question whether the intervention *can work in principle*. To provide evidence for policy decisions, trials need to have a high level of pragmatism to answer the question whether the intervention *will work in practice*. One should note:

- There is a trade-off between the internal validity of the trial (the extent to which it yields unbiased results) and the generalizability of the study results. Highly pragmatic trials may have elements that introduce bias (e.g. high rates of loss to follow-up). Careful consideration of such elements is important to achieve meaningful results.

- Pragmatism may be conflated with weak health systems. There is no point in studying an intervention within a health system that is not capable of implementing that intervention effectively. Before the study is undertaken, one should make sure the health system conditions such as training, staffing or laboratory are at the level that is required for that setting or country. The quality of implementation of an intervention is known as its *fidelity*, and should be measured as part of the evaluation [10].
- Even with highly pragmatic trials, the generalizability of the results for complex health interventions will often be limited to similar settings and populations. To enable broader policy decisions the evaluation should be done across settings and populations. At the minimum, the health system setting in which the evaluation is done should be adequately described so that policy makers can make judgements about the generalizability of its results beyond that setting.

References

1. Campbell NC, Murray E, Darbyshire J, et al. Designing and evaluating complex interventions to improve health care. BMJ. 2007;334:455–9.
2. Mangham LJ, Hanson K. Scaling up in international health: what are the key issues? Health Policy Plan. 2010;25:85–96.
3. Sekhon M, Cartwright M, Francis JJ. Acceptability of healthcare interventions: an overview of reviews and development of a theoretical framework. BMC Health Serv Res. 2017;17:88.
4. GBD 2019 Diseases and Injuries Collaborators. Global burden of 369 diseases and injuries in 204 countries and territories, 1990–2019: a systematic analysis for the Global Burden of Disease Study 2019. Lancet. 2020;396:1204–22.
5. Sanders GD, Neumann PJ, Basu A, et al. Recommendations for conduct, methodological practices, and reporting of cost-effectiveness analyses: second panel on cost-effectiveness in health and medicine. JAMA. 2016;316:1093–103.
6. Mauskopf JA, Sullivan SD, Annemans L, et al. Principles of good practice for budget impact analysis: report of the ISPOR task force on good research practices–budget impact analysis. Value Health. 2007;10:336–47.
7. Hayes RJ, Bennett S. Simple sample size calculation for cluster-randomized trials. Int J Epidemiol. 1999;28:319–26.
8. Hemming K, Haines TP, Chilton PJ, Girling AJ, Lilford RJ. The stepped wedge cluster randomised trial: rationale, design, analysis, and reporting. BMJ. 2015;350:h391.
9. Loudon K, Treweek S, Sullivan F, Donnan P, Thorpe KE, Zwarenstein M. The PRECIS-2 tool: designing trials that are fit for purpose. BMJ. 2015;350:h2147.
10. Rychetnik L, Frommer M, Hawe P, Shiell A. Criteria for evaluating evidence on public health interventions. J Epidemiol Community Health. 2002;56:119–27.

Part IX

Governance of Global Health

62 Global Governance in Health

Eduardo Missoni

Abstract

Complex transnational inter-organizational networks, actors, and processes interact in different dimension of health-related global governance. The role and authority of the World Health Organization has been eroded over the past decades by the emerging of new public and private global actors, and increasingly hybrid multistakeholder initiatives and organizations with a powerful impact on health and related policies at all levels. Global health diplomacy, extended beyond intergovernmental relations is a constitutive part of the system of global health governance. The promotion of a heavily market-led, multistakeholder and financial mechanisms is a striking trend. There is an urgent need for wider and more equitable representation of people and their real needs. A new regulatory and ethical framework of reference is needed, together with the "decolonization" of global health policies led by few powerful transnational actors and framed on autoreferential Western concepts.

Keywords

Global governance · Intergovernmental stakeholders · Governmental agencies · Non-state actors · Global health philantrophy

62.1 Introduction

With the acceleration of the globalization process and the emerging role of transnational non-state actors (NSA), traditional policy-making processes and the international coordination and steering mechanisms faced new challenges. Governance processes progressively involved a much broader range of public and private actors pushing for a *multistakeholder* approach.

The term governance has been used to refer to multiple concepts. In the area of global health, we are mainly concerned with complex transnational inter-organizational networks and international regimes, as well as actors and processes around which very diverse expectations and interests interact leading to global policies with an impact on health determinants and health systems worldwide.

E. Missoni (✉)
SDA Bocconi School of Management, Bocconi University, Milan, Italy
e-mail: eduardo.missoni@unibocconi.it

M. C. B. Raviglione et al. (eds.), *Global Health Essentials*, Sustainable Development Goals Series,
https://doi.org/10.1007/978-3-031-33851-9_62

62.2 From International to Global Governance in Health

Historically, national, and subnational level authorities have assumed primary responsibility for the health of the population. At the origins of International Health Governance, there was the expansion of trade beyond national borders. Nation-States felt the need to establish common international rules to prevent the spread of disease, including for example the adoption of quarantine practices. Institutional structures, rules, and mechanisms were established during the nineteenth century to protect and promote human health across national borders, including the creation of the International Sanitary Conference in 1851, the International Sanitary Bureau (later the Pan American Sanitary Bureau) in 1902, the *Office International d'Hygiene Publique* (OIHP) created in Paris in 1907, and the Health Organization of the League of Nations, established in 1920.

The post-World War II governance system was rooted in the United Nations (UN) as a center for harmonizing the actions of nations in the attainment of their common ends and was based on international law.

The establishment of the World Health Organization (WHO) in 1948 as the UN specialized agency for health, with its pledge to universality, although strongly defined by the sovereignty of its member states, opened a new period in international health governance, and represented the first step toward a more complex system of interactions beyond *international* relations, i.e., intergovernmental relations [1]. The WHO Constitution allowed for official relations with non-governmental organizations (NGOs) and professional groups beyond national governments.

Over time, the number of intergovernmental organizations active in the field of health has grown dramatically. The elaboration of international public health norms and policies is the result of the contribution of a growing number of multilateral organizations. In particular, in the UN system, beyond the WHO, several funds and programs (e.g., UNICEF, UNFPA, WFP), and other entities of the UN, such as UNAIDS, other specialized agencies (e.g., ILO, FAO, the World Bank), and UN-related organizations (such as IOM, IAEA, or the WTO) have been increasingly involved.

Starting in the 1980s, neoliberal ideas became dominant and with the fall of the Berlin wall market economy became hegemonic "colonizing" also global health. Capital and market mechanisms progressively prevailed over state authority, creating governance gaps that have encouraged actors from business and civil society sectors to assume roles previously considered an exclusive prerogative of the State [2].

The role of old and new Non-State Actors (NSAs) with very diverse interests and influence (NGOs, global philanthropy, transnational companies, and investors) grew considerably, including with the creation of transnational hybrid multistakeholder entities such as coalitions, alliances, and all sorts of variously structured public-private partnerships, undermining WHO's role and authority, with a powerful impact on health and related policies at all levels (see Table 62.1).

The primacy given to the state was challenged and the concept of Global Health Governance (GHG) emerged [1] concerned with the multiple and diverse health-related actors, regimes, interactions, and policy-making processes that govern issues of transnational and global relevance in health systems and public health services [3].

The increased awareness of the importance of the social, economic, political, and environmental determinants of health and the influence of decisions made in global policy-making arenas outside the "health sector" (such as those governing international security, trade, environment, migration, and others) led to emphasize health in global governance. Thus, some authors highlighted the importance of the health outcomes of those policies and suggested the need of a "global governance *for* health" to foster health worldwide [4, 5].

Some authors added the notion of governance for global health referring to the actors and processes that act at national and regional level to contribute to global health governance and/or to governance for global health [6].

Table 62.1 Actors in Global health governance and financing

Actors	At the origins of the "development era" 1950s–1970s	Increasing importance 1980s–1990s	New and emerging 2000s–today
Intergovernmental (multilateral and multistakeholder)	WHO, UNICEF, UNFPA	World Bank, UNAIDS, European Union	Global public-private partnerships – GAVI Alliance – Global Fund to fight HIV/aids, tuberculosis, and malaria Multistakeholder and super-multistakeholder initiatives (e.g., Covax)
Governmental agencies and their groupings	OECD-DAC countries	G7/G8	BRICS countries (China, India, Russia, Brazil, South Africa) Other emerging economies G20
Non-state actors	Philanthropic Family foundations (e.g., Rockefeller, Ford, Wellcome Trust	Transnational Corporations Civil Society Organizations (e.g., Oxfam, MSF, Save the Children)	Global philanthropy/ Philanthrocapitalism – Bill and Melinda Gates Foundation Global financial mechanisms Civil Society Networks (e.g., People Health's Movement)

Both global health governance and global governance *for* health are basically based on two approaches: the legislation-based approach typical of international binding agreements (the so-called hard law)—typical of trade agreement—involving sanctions for those who do not respect the rules; and the moral norms derived from internationally recognized human rights (the so-called soft law) characterized by the absence rules binding partners to their commitments, as in the case of international declarations and resolutions, whose implementation relies more on domestic civil society pressure than international censure and rules [7].

62.3 Negotiation and Power Relations

Although the idea of global governance is presented as a collaborative process among involved actors, power relations continue to play the main role in the definition of the political agenda.

The geopolitical weight of leading states and, indirectly, of the national and global forces that influence their positions, still determines the dynamics and the limits of international governance, as well as the development and execution of policies in areas sensitive to their interests. Few "Western" countries or blocks (i.e., the European Union) still play a predominant role, which is however challenged by emerging economies and powers, such as China and the other countries in the BRICS group (Brazil, Russia, India, China, and South Africa) and others mostly in the G20 group in general.

Global health has been recognized as a "pressing foreign policy issue of our time" [8]. States' foreign policy priorities and practices define global health policies in multilateral negotiations and policy-making and the relationship between foreign policy and global health is often described as Global Health Diplomacy (GHD) acting in intersectional fields such as security, governance, development, human rights, trade, and the global public good for health [9].

GHD, a constitutive part of the system of global health governance, may play a positive role in global governance *for* health, but may also become an instrument the *Realpolitik* strategy in pursuing states' interests using health as a means to enhance other foreign policy goals (e.g., to expand their geopolitical influence through health aid) [6, 9]. "Vaccine diplomacy" has been a remarkable example of this approach, during the Covid-19 pandemic [10].

The concept of GHD has been extended to capture "multistakeholder diplomacy" with the involvement of NSAs in the multi-level and multi-actor negotiation processes that shape the global policy environment for health [6] as part of the wider complex system of influences, interests, and power balances that define health-related global governance [3].

The gravitational center of GHG, once restricted to the WHO, the World Bank, and the USA, arguably the single most influential governmental actor [1], became especially crowded over the last two decades.

The WHO is mandate of coordinating and directing authority has been progressively eroded. For decades, WHO has been suffering from the dependance on both public and private donors' heavily earmarked voluntary contributions, exposing the Organization to heavy external influences (Box 62.1).

Box 62.1 WHO Opening to the Private Sector

Can we still rely on the World Health Organization? It has not openly opposed the greed of the major global pharmaceutical companies and its director-general, Gro Harlem Brundtland, has deferred to them [...] Dr. David Nabarro, executive director at Dr. Brundtland's office, justifies the director-general's chosen course of action:

> We certainly need private financing. For the past decade governments' financial contributions have dwindled. The main sources of funding are the private sector and the financial markets. And since the American economy is the world's richest, we must make the WHO attractive to the United States and the financial markets.—(Jean-Loup Motchane, Health For All or Riches for Some: WHO's Responsible? *Le Monde diplomatique*, July 2002).

Member States themselves, especially the largest donors, contributed to undermine WHO's credibility and sustainability showing inconsistency between their global health discourse and their policies. On the one side, they proclaimed aid effectiveness principles requiring the reduction of existing aid fragmentation, on the other side they generated and/or supported a plethora of new players [3]. Against the priorities expressed in WHO's own governing forums, Member States' funding may reflect a different set of priorities [11].

New private and hybrid multistakeholder players entrusted with unprecedented amounts of funding are actively shaping global health policies, eroding the centrality of international institutions [12].

Powerful "philanthrocapitalists" [13] (led by the Bill and Melinda Gates Foundation), private investors, and corporate actors act well beyond open transactions to pursue their own interests and shape the global agenda. Information and mass-media control, lobbying, financing and control of institutions, programs, research, "revolving doors,"[1] are just a few of the mechanisms of "capture of the regulator"[2] used to directly or indirectly influence international policy-making. The push toward *multistakeholder* governance represents an additional mechanism of influence and capture of the policy-maker (Fig. 62.1).

[1] "Revolving doors" describes a situation in which personnel moves between roles as legislators and regulators, on the one hand, and representatives of the industries affected by the legislation and regulation, on the other.

[2] "Capture of the regulator" refers to a phenomenon that occurs when a regulatory agency that is created to act in the public interest, instead acts in ways that benefit incumbent actors it is supposed to be regulating.

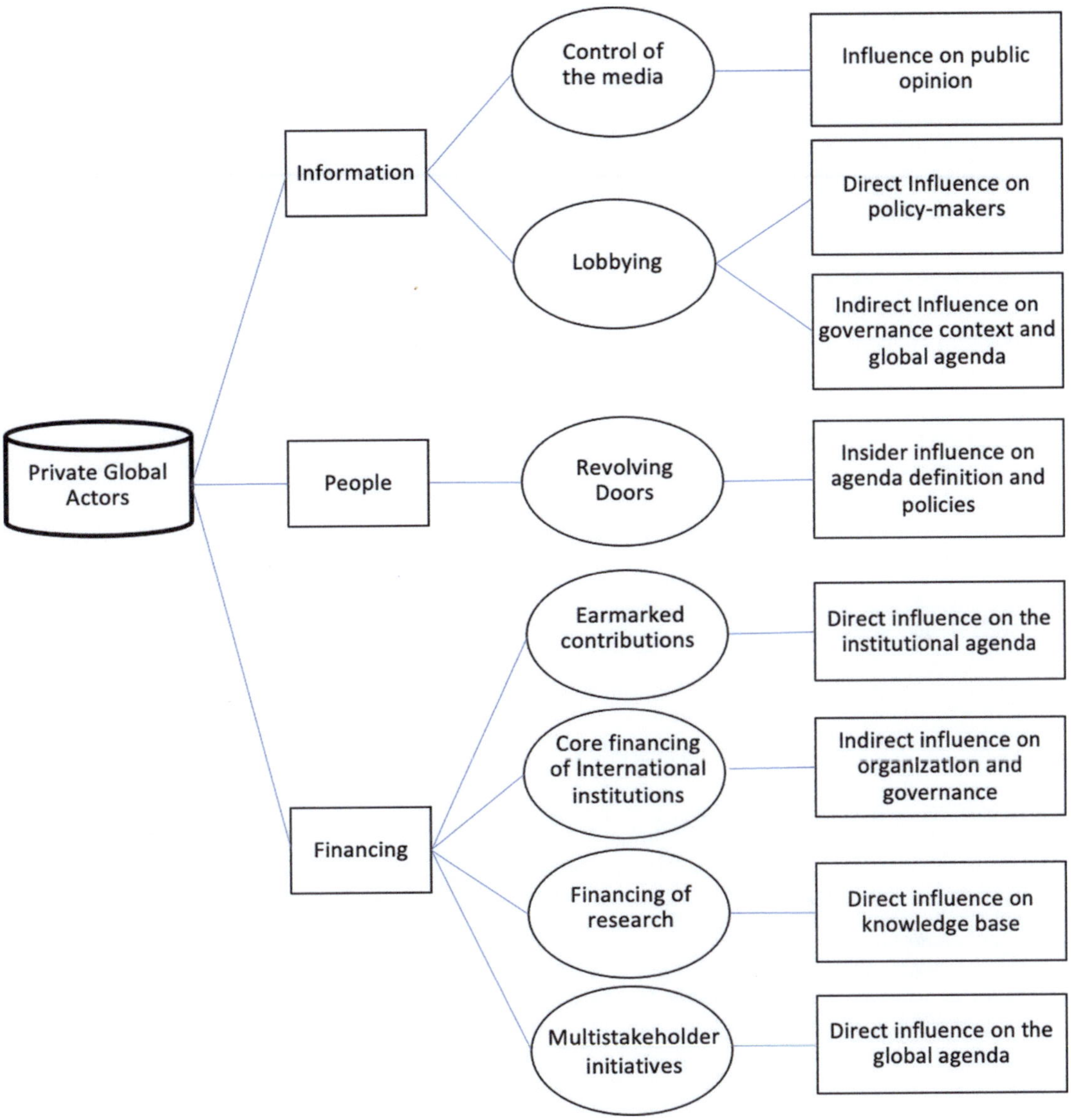

Fig. 62.1 Global Private Actors' mechanisms of capture of the policy-maker and influence on global governance. Source: Matteucci and Missoni, 2022. Modified

62.4 The Quest for a New Ethical Framework

The proliferation and increased power of very diverse transnational agents and the promotion of a heavily market-led, multistakeholder, and financial mechanisms[3]—which find an emerging gravitational center in the World Economic Forum, the private initiative of a single individual and his "Great Reset" project to impose "multistakeholder capitalism"—is a striking trend, which led to the current complexity of global governance, characterized for being multilayered, with interactions at multiple levels, from global to sub-state; multisector and multi-actor. The "polycentric" [14] or rather "chaotic nature" [10] of the current governance architecture represents a serious obstacle to transparent, democratic, fair, and effective collective action.

[3] Such as the International Financial Facility for Immunizations (IFFIm), the Advance Market Commitment (AMC) or Unitaid.

A rethinking of the traditional bureaucratic model of postwar intergovernmental organizations is still lacking. In an increasingly unequal and unfair globalized world, the need for wider and more equitable representation of people and their real needs is striking and requires a new regulatory and ethical framework of reference, together with the "decolonization" of global health policies remarkably led by few powerful transnational actors and framed on autoreferential Western concepts [15].

References

1. Dodgson R, Lee K, Drager N. Global health governance. A conceptual review. Discussion Paper no. 1, Centre on Global Change & Health. London and Geneva: London School of Hygiene & Tropical Medicine—Department of Health & Development, World Health Organization. 2002.
2. Jang J, McSparren J, Rashchupkina Y. Global governance: present and future. Palgrave Commun. 2016;2:15045.
3. Missoni E, Pacileo G, Tediosi F. Global Health Governance and Policy: an introduction. Abingdon: Routledge; 2019.
4. Frenk J, Moon S. Governance Challenges in Global Health. N Engl Theatr J. 2013;368(10):936–42.
5. Lee K, Kamradt-Scott A. The multiple meanings of global health governance: a call for conceptual clarity. Glob Health. 2014;10:28. https://doi.org/10.1186/1744-8603-10-28.
6. Labonté R. Health in all (foreign) policy: challenges in achieving coherence. Health Promot Int. 2014;29(Suppl. 1):i48–58.
7. Oslo Ministerial Declaration. Global health: a pressing foreign policy issue of our time. Ministers of Foreign Affairs of Brazil, France, Indonesia, Norway, Senegal, South Africa, and Thailand. Lancet. 2007;369(9570):1373–8.
8. McInnes C, Lee K. Global health and international relations. Cambridge: Polity Press; 2013.
9. Missoni E. Expectations on the health silk road after the pandemic. In: Amighini A, editor. China after Covid-19: economic revival and challenges to the world; 2021. p. 88–107.
10. Kickbusch I, Nikogosian H, Kazatchkine M, Kökény M. A guide to global health diplomacy. Better health—improved global solidarity—more equity. Geneva: Graduate Institute of International and Development Studies; 2021.
11. Lidén J. The World Health Organization and Global Health governance: Post-1990. Public Health. 2014;128(2):141–7. https://doi.org/10.1016/j.puhe.2013.08.008.
12. Helble M, Zulfiqar A, Lego J. A comparison of global governance across sectors: Global Health, trade, and multilateral development finance. ADBI Working Paper Series, Asian Development Bank Institute. 2018.
13. Dentico N, Seitz K. Philanthrocapitalism in global health and nutrition: analysis and implications. Spotlight on sustainable development. 2019. https://www.2030spotlight.org/sites/default/files/spot2019/Spotlight_Innenteil_2019_web_sdg3.pdf. Accessed 21 May 2022.
14. Tosun J. Polycentrism in global health governance scholarship. Comment on "our challenges that global health networks face". Int J Health Policy Manag. 2017;7(1):78–80.
15. Affun-Adegbulu C, Adegbulu O. Decolonising global (public) health: from Western universalism to global pluriversalities. BMJ Glob Health. 2020;5:e002947. https://doi.org/10.1136/bmjgh-2020-002947.

The World Health Organization

63

Marcos Cueto

Abstract

Since the mid-nineteenth century physicians, diplomats, commerce leaders, and politicians have been discussing and implementing an international-health global system that ranges from epidemiological-surveillance agreements of transnational epidemics to institutions promoting social and medical reforms of the living conditions of the poor. Of all these efforts the work of the World Health Organization, WHO (created in 1948) has been the boldest attempt to reach an international understanding among nations of the need of articulation of their action in matters of disease control. However, the WHO has been the house of two different perspectives to control health that can be summarized as a biomedical and technical approach and a socio-medical perspective. During the past few years, old and new historical actors, like officers of the WHO, health activists, and bilateral agencies, have been part of these perspectives and discussed if health is, or not, a global public good.

Keywords

World Health Organization · Global health governance · Global health players · Global health policy · Global health diplomacy

M. Cueto (✉)
Casa de Oswaldo Cruz, Fiocruz,
Rio de Janeiro, Brazil

63.1 Introduction

Since the origins of nations in the Middle Ages, there were official municipal, regional, and state regulations to control transnational diseases. The first and diverse quarantines were established then—although suffering from discontinuity—and their regulation were implemented with little or great political force. However, it was only in the nineteenth century when agreements, alliances between countries and the seeds of the first stable epidemiological institutions emerged. They emerge with the development of a notion dear to medical officers and diplomats: "international health." Primarily, it was associated to responses to control or mitigate pandemic threats usually perceived to be coming to Western Europe from "the East." Thanks to new steamship and railroad technology, increased and rapid world commerce, immigrants and travel allowed cholera, and later yellow fever and bubonic plague, to leave their traditional endemic sites in colonies and poor areas of India, the Caribbean and China and reach the recently industrialized nations of "the West." Physicians, business leaders, and politicians converged on the need to protect their patients, economic enterprises, and territories from epidemic outbreaks by standardizing quarantine and other border health controls and since 1851 signed a series of agreements to articulate some kind of epidemiological-surveillance and disease-control methods. Only

M. C. B. Raviglione et al. (eds.), *Global Health Essentials*, Sustainable Development Goals Series,
https://doi.org/10.1007/978-3-031-33851-9_63

in the late nineteenth century, a series of international sanitary rules were subscribed to among governments and during the interwar period (1919–1939) a fledgling health agency of the League of Nations promoted the development of "international health." A new official narrative tried to emerge in a world that was still crossed by populism and nationalism arguing that public health was good for global commerce, peace, and the solidarity among nations.

However, the League of Nations Health Organization had limited power and its attempts to incorporate national health boards was usually unsuccessful. It was only with the creation of the United Nations at the end of the Second World War that a more powerful health agency emerged. With headquarters in Geneva, the WHO was formally launched in 1948 when its Constitution was approved, thanks to the backing of the United States and the Soviet Union; the two superpowers that emerged after the War.

This chapter describes the role of WHO in global health, how it changed over time and some of the challenges it has been facing.

63.2 The First Years of the WHO: 1948–1988

During its early years, the new organization made an effort to establish its independence and to set its own agenda for international health despite inevitable political entanglements and budgetary constraints. The WHO attempted this by emphasizing its "technical" role as a clearinghouse for epidemiological information, an organizer of emergency relief in international health crises, and as a constructor of a network of medical experts around the globe.

The WHO was created when the influence of European social medicine, at its peak in the 1930s, was still strong. The state of the world, especially the worldwide economic depression and the social and political disruptions that followed from it, was of major significance for social medicine. These trends allowed the health officers of the League to follow interests in social medicine. Diseases that had been approached largely from technical perspectives were mainly considered in the broader context of income, working hours, diet, and living conditions. This broad vision was incorporated into the Preamble to the 1948 WHO Constitution that basically stated that health was not only the absence of disease but good living conditions but was downplayed in the eradication initiatives of the 1950s and 1960s that reflected the rise to dominance of the biomedical view, which glorified technical interventions as the answer to all health problems.

By the turn of the late twentieth century, the WHO had contributed to positive world medical trends such as significant advances in life expectancy, reductions in infant mortality, the control of malaria, the eradication of smallpox, and the spread of immunization campaigns. In addition, the WHO helped to control neglected tropical diseases, limited the consumption of tobacco, supported the right to health of colonial and developing nations, and promoted links between human rights and health.

63.3 The Coexistence of Two Socio-Medical Approaches to Protect Health

For all its achievements, the WHO has not been free of a major internal tension. Two socio-medical approaches coexisted during much of the lifespan of the WHO. One was biomedically and technically focused, illustrated by the malaria eradication campaign launched by the World Health Organization in the 1950s. The other was the approach, known as Primary Health Care, embodied in the Alma-Ata Declaration of 1978 supported by WHO and UNICEF, which prioritized holistic prevention programs, coordination with other governmental sectors like education and finances, community participation, and conceived health as a tool of social reform to reduce poverty. The WHO's twists and turns were in part the result of internal gyrations along a path marked by the changing fortunes of the two perspectives, neither of which achieved complete dominance. The

Alma-Ata perspective presumes that large changes in health require large social transformations and views health as an essential right of citizenship and one of the fundamental duties of nation states. The other perspective emphasizes technologically driven health interventions and programs organized around disease control and, in the rare case, eradication. In this perspective, public health is validated as a tool for economic productivity and national security, in contrast to the Alma-Ata perspective, which links public health to the goals of solidarity and equity. A few WHO programs, such as smallpox eradication and the Global Program on AIDS in the 1970s, successfully blended the two perspectives, but the WHO's major programs have tended to reflect one agenda or the other.

Two experiences that followed a similar path were, first: in the 1980s the Global AIDS Program asserted a close link between public health, social reform, and human rights. In the second place, during the early twenty-first century, the WHO-appointed but independent Commission on Social Determinants of Health advocated interventions to end unjust unfair relations and political realities that lead to poor health and massive health disparities between and withing countries.

The technically focused perspective was hegemonic in the disease-control and eradication campaigns of the 1950s and 1960s, the population control and family-planning programs of the 1970s, and the Selective Primary Health Care interventions of the 1980s such as immunization and diarrheal control. More recently, the advocated of a technical intervention on health have promoted a restricted version of Universal Health Care—with a package of limited interventions—that is not synonymous with the construction of solid health systems. Supporters of this perspective portray disease and poverty as "natural" conditions that new technologies, good administration, charitable funding, and intelligently cost-effective programs can control. Advocates of this perspective criticize advocates of the other for being too idealistic and for asking public health workers to solve problems beyond their reach, such as poverty and seemingly unbridgeable gaps between the rich and the poor.

63.4 The Struggle of Adapting to Recent Global Geo-Political Changes and to the Proliferation of Global Health Players

The WHO's ambivalent and shifting embrace of the social-medical and technocratic perspectives has shaped the organization internally but has also influenced its ability to deal with dramatically changing external realities. In the late twentieth century, the agency had difficulty adapting to global geo-political changes, like the emergence of the leading role in health of the World Bank, the Bill and Melinda Gates Foundations and several Public Private partnerships and began to lose control of its budget. It simultaneously lost authority in the international arena and was trapped by the growing weight of bureaucratic procedures and even accusations of corruptions. It also had to contend with the new reality of "economic globalization" with links to neoliberal politics. This new political-economic context was dramatically different from what prevailed during the early years when WHO operated with nation states confident in UN agencies. Another important external change that came in the wake of the AIDS epidemic was a dramatic increase in health activism. As it was built to deal with governments, the WHO lacked the flexibility to deal with civil society organizations. Then with the turn of the twenty-first century, the proliferation of non-state actors, the relative disempowerment of nation states, and the growing hegemony of global caretaker organizations like the World Bank, the International Monetary Fund, the World Trade Organization, and new transnational philanthropies (like the Gates Foundation) have compromised the UN system as a whole. The World Trade Organization has supported the intellectual property of big pharma in all nations making drugs and treatments private goods instead of public good as advocated by activists. To make matters few supranational decisions could be taken by an agency conceived to work by consensus and its existence was made more difficult with authoritarian populist and anti-globalization governments that are dangerously challenging multilateralism and global health governance.

63.5 Conclusion

As the main forum for discussions of health issues of global concern and the boldest attempt to coordinate and lead the work of governments during the second half of the twentieth and early twentieth first centuries, the WHO can play a crucial role in reinventing Global Health and in equitable and swift responses to transnational health emergencies (like the ongoing discussion on a novel health treaty on pandemics). The future viability of the WHO is a question that must be responded to by analyzing its complex past which indicates the pertinence of recovering the beliefs that any individual and country in the world has the right to physical and mental health, that health cannot be reduced to a responsibility of medical doctors and has to count with the participation of social scientists, activists, and patients, and that free and open multilateral cooperation between nations is imperative.

Further Reading

Babinski MA. For the good of humanity: Ludwik Rajchman, medical statesman. Budapest: Central European University Press; 1998.

Beigbeder Y. World Health Organization: achievements and failures. New York: Routledge; 2018.

Bhattacharya S. Expunging variola: the control and eradication of smallpox in India, 1947–1977. New Delhi: Orient Longman; 2006.

Clift C. The role of the World Health Organization in the international system. London: Chatham House; 2013.

Cueto M. The origins of primary health care and selective primary health care. Am J Public Health. 2004;94(11):1864–74.

Cueto M, Brown T, Fee E. The World Health Organization, a history. New York: Cambridge University Press; 2019.

Espinosa M. Epidemic invasions: yellow fever and the limits of Cuban Independence, 1878–1930. Chicago: University of Chicago Press; 2009.

Farley J. Brock Chisholm, the World Health Organization and the cold war. Vancouver: UBC Press; 2008.

Gorsky M, Sirrs C. Universal health coverage as a global public health goal: the work of the International Labour Organisation, c.1925-2018. História ciencia saúde-Manguinhos. 2020;27(Suppl. 1):71–93.

Lee K. Historical dictionary of the World Health Organization. Lanham: Scarecrow Press; 1998.

Lee K. World Health Organization (WHO). New York: Routledge; 2009.

Lindén J. The World Health Organization and Global Health Governance: post-1990. Public Health. 2014;128(2):141–7.

Litsios S. The third ten years of the World Health Organization, 1968–1977. Geneva: World Health Organization; 2008.

Packard R. History of global health: interventions into the lives of other peoples. Baltimore: Johns Hopkins University Press; 2016.

Sayward AL. The birth of development: how the World Bank, Food and Agriculture Organization, and World Health Organization changed the world, 1945–1965. Kent: Kent State University Press; 2006.

64 Global Health and International Politics During the COVID-19 Pandemic

Marta Dassù

Abstract

The chapter tracks the debate on global health in the international political agenda during the Covid-19 pandemic. It focuses on the role of multilateral institutions and global summitry, in particular the G20, in strengthening health systems across the world, including by championing a One Health approach and proposing innovative mechanisms to finance pandemic preparedness and response.

Keywords

Global health and international politics · Multilateral institutions · Global summitry · Finance for health preparedness · International development

64.1 Introduction

The outbreak of the Covid-19 crisis demonstrated that no country, alone, could cope with the spread of the virus. Since 2019, responses to the health emergency have been varied, with governments around the world adopting a diverse policy mix of social distancing, lockdown measures and travel bans, some of which are still in effect at the time of writing. Furthermore, despite some progress, vaccination rates across countries remain extremely uneven, due to both manufacturing and distribution issues, exposing a divide among the North and the Global South.

If the latest pandemic brought into light the shortcomings existing in the global health infrastructure, it has also recasted the role of multilateralism and international organizations. These can play a key role in fostering cross-country collaboration and support a more equitable distribution of resources among health systems which vary greatly in terms of funds and capabilities [1].

The European Union represents a paradigmatic example, albeit on a regional level, of the benefits of multilateralism. In front of the first uncoordinated responses to the COVID-19, the EU Commission took over the joint procurement of vaccines, with the consent of Member States, to prevent internal competition from undermining efforts to rein in the pandemic. There are lessons to be learned from the European experience as global institutions move forward to strengthen international public health [2].

M. Dassù (✉)
Aspen Institute Italia, Rome, Italy
e-mail: marta.dassu@aspeninstitute.it

M. C. B. Raviglione et al. (eds.), *Global Health Essentials*, Sustainable Development Goals Series,
https://doi.org/10.1007/978-3-031-33851-9_64

64.2 Multilateralism and Global Institutions

While not perfect, nor without missteps, the World Health Organization (WHO) played an important role in coordinating the response to the Covid-19 pandemic. In April 2020, thanks to the spear-heading of the WHO, The Access to COVID-19 Tools (ACT) accelerator was launched: a global collaboration scheme, bringing together international health organizations, national governments, scientists, businesses, and civil society to boost the development, production, and equitable access to COVID-19 tests, treatments, and, most importantly, vaccines—under the COVAX pillar [3, 4].

Most importantly, health played also a key role in global summitry: in the past years, both the BRICS and G7 made global health commitments, and so did the G20, which attempted to shape the global health agenda to tackle vaccine inequality and put forward comprehensive proposals to build health system preparedness and resilience [5].

Compared to the other groups, the G20 is more representatives, comprising more than 80% of the world's GDP, 75% of global trade and 60% of the planet's population; at the same time, it is by definition more flexible than the WHO, which helped in increasing its immediate impact [6].

64.3 The Italian G20 Presidency and the Rome Declaration

In 2021, as the vaccine rollout gained traction, the Italian G20 Presidency spear-headed the effort—on the basis of the path paved by the previous G20 Saudi Presidency—to foster the implementation of a multi-sectoral, evidence-based One Health approach to build preparedness and strengthen the resilience of health systems in front of future crisis.[1]

Among the most important milestones, was the issuing of the Rome Declaration, the concluding document of the Global Health Summit, co-hosted in May 2021 by Italy and the European Commission, and endorsed by the leaders of the G20, as they pledged to take a series of actions to accelerate the end of the coronavirus emergency and better prepare for future pandemics [7].

In the Rome Declaration, the G20 championed an approach based on the paradigm of One Health, striving for a set of integrated programs and policies across multiple domains, including food safety and the control of zoonotic diseases. The stress was put on the need to enhance the current multilateral health architecture built around the WHO. Principles 9 and 12 of the declaration, for instance, called for greater coordination in research, development, and innovation of both pharmaceutical and non-pharmaceutical tools, as well as developing assistance and response capacities to support low-income and crisis-affected countries, favoring the transfer of know-how through data sharing and licensing agreements. Principle 4, on the other hand, underscored the importance of an open and multilateral trading system as a guarantee for secure and reliable global supply chains for medical tools and equipment to avoid the heightened international tensions that followed in the wake of the great trade collapse of 2020.

The stated goal of the Rome Declaration was that of establishing a multi-stakeholder health governance system, promoting meaningful and inclusive dialogue between international institutions, national governments, local communities, and private actors. With various countries still divided between those that rely on hospital-centered healthcare models and those that favor a more decentralized bottom-up approach, fostering a transparent and trustworthy system of international cooperation can bring about not only better health, but also an acceleration of development and advancement in social inclu-

[1] According to the One Health High Level Expert Panel, convened by the FAO, UNEP, WHO, and WOAH, "One Health is an integrated, unifying approach that aims to sustainably balance and optimize the health of people, animals and ecosystems. It recognizes the health of humans, domestic and wild animals, plants, and the wider environment (including ecosystems) are closely linked and inter-dependent [...]" [10].

sion, in line with the Sustainable Development Goal Agenda.

Not all the principles of the Rome Declaration, however, were immediately operationalized, indicating a chasm between words and action: the Declaration of the G20 Health Ministers which followed their meeting at the beginning of September 2021, contained more detailed yet limited provision, such as: (1) the commitment by the G20 Health Ministers to support a joint work plan on One Health, developed by the WHO, OIE, FAO, and UNEP; (2) the commitment to contribute to the action plan of the jointly managed ILO, OECD, and WHO Working for Health Programme, to bolster the recruitment and improve the training of the health workforce, and lastly (3) the support for the establishment of the COVAX Humanitarian Buffer, to intervene in instances of state failure and conflict, covering the basic health needs of people in areas controlled by non-state armed groups that are inaccessible to governments [8].

64.4 International Politics and Finance for Health Preparedness

One of the critical issues that has taken center stage in the debate within international institutions pertains to the financing needed to support global pandemic prevention, preparedness, and response (PPR). The Rome Declaration explicitly recognized the need for enhanced, streamlined, and sustainable mechanisms to finance the preparedness of health systems and rapidly mobilize resources in a coordinated manner to support surge capacity, stressing the importance to leverage on blended finance, including public and private funds, as well as philanthropic and international financial institutions funds.

Earlier in 2021, the G20 had also established a High-Level Independent Panel on Financing the Global Commons for Pandemic Preparedness and Response, which, in parallel, suggested the creation of a Global Health Threats Fund to distribute $15 billion annually for pandemic PPR. As a response, the G20 Finance and Health Ministers, which met in late October that year, decided for the establishment of Joint Finance-Health Task Force, with the aim of developing coordination arrangements between Finance and Health Ministries and encourage effective stewardship of resources to address the existing financing gaps in PPR [6].

This represented the signature move of the Italian G20 2021 Presidency, establishing a legacy that is set to be taken up by the G20 2022 Indonesian Presidency, as the Joint Finance-Health Task Force is co-chaired by the two. At the end of June 2022, the G20 Health and Finance ministers met to discuss the establishment of a Financial Intermediary Fund (FIF) for PPR, under the trusteeship of the World Bank.

64.5 Conclusions

While global summitry is making important headways towards building a cohesive global health infrastructure, shortcomings will need to be addressed: the G20 still lacks a serious commitment towards health policy harmonization and a more homogenous pandemic preparedness tool. The absence of the Heads of State of both China and Russia from the Rome summits, moreover, underscores how growing international tensions risks undermining sound global governance on health matters. This is a problem that affects also the G7 and the BRICS forum, overly focused on geopolitical great-power rivalry.

Another important matter, going forward, will be that of deciding a common taxonomy to keep track of investments on health system strengthening. While it is more cost-effective to build health system resilience than it is to cope with the costs of mitigating a pandemic, it is necessary—as argued by Hatice Kücük and Alan Donnely, Executive Director and Chairman of the G20 Health Development partnership—to define a common global framework to demonstrate that finance towards One Health is producing consistent and measurable results [9].

References

1. Dunn-Georgiou Elisha. Four pillars part 2: multilateral support. 2022. https://globalhealth.org/four-pillars-2-multilateral/. Accessed 20 Jun 2022.
2. Bongardt A, Torres F. Europe's vaccine paradox: from supply to demand issues. Interconomics. 2021;56:130–1. https://doi.org/10.1007/s10272-021-0966-9.
3. Adhanom Ghebreyesus Tedros. Building a better global health framework. 2022. https://www.project-syndicate.org/commentary/four-priorities-for-improving-global-health-security-by-tedros-adhanom-ghebreyesus-2021-11. Accessed 24 Jun 2022.
4. WHO. What is the ACT-accelerator. 2020. https://www.who.int/initiatives/act-accelerator/about. Accessed 6 Nov 2022.
5. McBride B, Hawkes S, Buse K. Soft power and global health: the sustainable development goals (SDGs) era health agendas of the G7, G20 and BRICS. BMC Public Health. 2019;19:815. https://doi.org/10.1186/s12889-019-7114-5.
6. Fidler David P. The G20 Disappoints on Global Health, but that's OK with the United States. 2021. https://www.thinkglobalhealth.org/article/g20-disappoints-global-health-thats-ok-united-states. Accessed 24 Jun 2022.
7. Rome Declaration. Governo italiano. 2021. https://www.governo.it/sites/governo.it/files/documenti/documenti/Approfondimenti/GlobalHealthSummit/GlobalHealthSummit_RomeDeclaration.pdf. Accessed 23 Jun 2022.
8. Declaration of the G20 Health Ministers. 2021. G20 Italia 2021. https://www.salute.gov.it/imgs/C_17_pagineAree_5459_8_file.pdf. Accessed 24 Jun 2022.
9. Kücük, Hatice; Donnely, Alan. Financing new global health emergency framework is within reach. 2022. https://www.politico.eu/sponsored-content/financing-new-global-health-emergency-framework-is-within-reach/. Accessed 24 Jun 2022.
10. WHO. Tripartite and UNEP support OHHLEP's definition of "One Health". 2021. https://www.who.int/news/item/01-12-2021-tripartite-and-unep-support-ohhlep-s-definition-of-one-health. Accessed 6 Nov 2022.

65 Essentials of Global Health Diplomacy

Michaela Told

Abstract

This chapter addresses the rapidly evolving field of global health diplomacy. It briefly traces the historical roots of global health diplomacy in the nineteenth century and links it to the practice of today. As the intersection of health and foreign policy is at heart of global health diplomacy, this chapter highlights the political dimensions of global health negotiations and decision-making processes. In doing so, it refers to global health diplomacy as an instrument of governance and a tool of managing interdependence. Global health diplomacy today goes beyond the multilateral diplomacy and involves different actors across different sectors. The framing of the global health issues is essential to be effective in the different venues, and it allows to contextualize global health diplomacy within the larger ecosystem. The chapter concludes by outlining the different forms of diplomacy and briefly outlines the roadmap ahead.

Keywords

Diplomacy · Global health · Foreign policy · International relations · Global health diplomacy

65.1 Introduction

In the past two decades, global health diplomacy has emerged as a distinct field of study and the COVID-19 pandemic has prominently illustrated its magnitude, complexity, and its changing nature. Diplomacy in its traditional meaning of managing international relations between states and governments has evolved into a practice that addresses global challenges in a rapidly changing interdependent world. Health has fundamentally contributed to this development and is today an integral part of international relations and diplomacy. This chapter outlines the key concepts involved in global health diplomacy, its growing scope, as well as the challenges and issues at stake.

65.2 Historical Roots

Already back in ancient times, health diplomacy was practiced when medical doctors have traded herbal medicines, offered services of healing to neighboring countries and acted as ambassadors

M. Told (✉)
Global Studies Institute, University of Geneva, Geneva, Switzerland

HI5 Governance, Geneva, Switzerland
e-mail: michaela@hi5governance.ch

M. C. B. Raviglione et al. (eds.), *Global Health Essentials*, Sustainable Development Goals Series,
https://doi.org/10.1007/978-3-031-33851-9_65

to build relations [1]. In the literature, however, the starting point of global health diplomacy is mostly traced back to the first International Sanitary Conference in 1851 because states came together to standardize international quarantine regulations to hinder the spread of infectious diseases, namely cholera, plague, and yellow fever, across Europe as it negatively impacted the trade and shipping industry [2]. This gathering featured already some characteristics that apply to global health diplomacy still today: states set up a governance mechanism with its rules, norms, and processes in order to negotiate a collective solution and make decisions on a common challenge that crossed geographical and sector boundaries and impacted all states involved. Even though the first sanitary conferences were not successful, they did pave the way for new international health institutions to be created in the following years and decades that served multilateral negotiation and decision-making processes. Box 65.1 provides an account of WHO as actor in global health diplomacy and some of the intergovernmental processes as of August 2022.

Box 65.1 WHO as Actor in Global Health Diplomacy

The World Health Organization, established in 1948 as a specialized agency within the UN system and with its mandate to "to act as the directing and coordinating authority on international health work" (WHO Constitution, article 2(a)), is the main venue for global health diplomacy.

The main decision-making body within the WHO is the World Health Assembly (WHA) where all member states come together in May each year to make decisions on a wide range of health issues. The Executive Board (EB) is a second governing body which gives effect to the decisions and policies of the WHA and consists of 34 regionally selected member states.

These two governing bodies can mandate intergovernmental processes to take place. These processes are usually open to all member states but can have varying tasks that will determine also whether or not final decision-making would be referred back into the governing bodies. There are currently four processes ongoing which are:

1. The Member State Mechanism on substandard and falsified medical products: functioning since 2012 as a platform for collaboration, policy formulation, and capacity building.
2. The Agile Member State Task Group: established in 2022 to strengthen WHO's budgetary programmatic and financing governance and to analyze challenges in governance for transparency, efficiency, accountability, and compliance, and to devise recommendations.
3. The Intergovernmental Negotiating Body (INB) to draft and negotiate a WHO convention, agreement or other international instrument on pandemic prevention, preparedness, and response: set up in the response of the COVID-19 pandemic after the Special Session of the WHA in December 2021 with a specific mandate to negotiate a legally-binding instrument.
4. The Working Group on Amendments of the International Health Regulation (IHR) (2005): running in parallel to the INB to amend the IHR, building on the lessons learned from the various review panels that examined the functioning of the IHR and the global health security architecture during the COVID-19 pandemic.

WHO coordinates first and foremost member states, but it also participates as actor in different health and non-health fora to promote health and wellbeing. The increasing complexity of health issues and its role in health emergencies manifested its technical, convening, and normative power in health.

Source: who.int.

65.3 Global Health and Foreign Policy

At the heart of global health, diplomacy is the intersection of health with foreign policy. This requires reconciling two policy communities serving different interests: protecting and promoting national interests as foreign policy objectives with the objectives to improve population health and to achieve health equity [3]. The Ministers of Foreign Affairs of Brazil, France, Indonesia, Norway, Senegal, South Africa, and Thailand have acknowledged in 2007 this intersection and declared that "global health is one of the most pressing foreign policy issues of our time" [4]. Since then, the UN General Assembly has passed not only every year a resolution on "Global Health and Foreign Policy" but also has seen a number of health issues being discussed (Fig. 65.1).

The integration of health into political fora, such as the UN General Assembly (Fig. 65.1), the UN Security Council (Fig. 65.2) or the meetings of the G7 and G20, is critical not only to align interests and create impact but it also raises the awareness of the centrality of health issues. States' foreign policy priorities and engagement in global health are defined by their political value system and therefore can greatly vary across states but safeguarding national security and developing relationships and partnerships remain always in focus. COVID-19 has well illustrated the importance of health on all domains of life, the entanglement of health issues in state-to-state political relationships, as well as the need for cross-border cooperation that goes beyond the narrowly defined security concepts. Navigating the complexity of global health issues entails an understanding of the power dynamics and power asymmetries between the actors involved [7]. The use of soft power, i.e., the art to influence or persuade others, is therefore essential to both global health and foreign policy. The prerequisite for successful global health diplomacy is not only to speak a common language and adapt it to the stakeholders across different policy domains but also to recognize that it is an essentially political process [8].

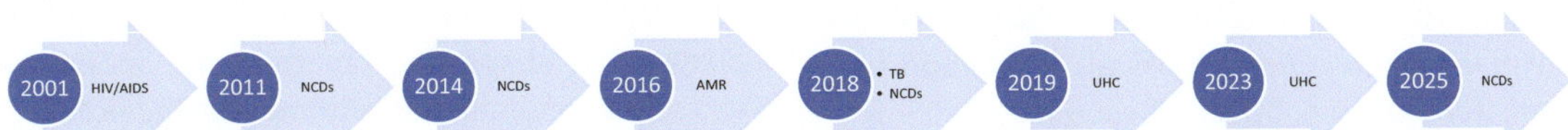
2001
HIV/AIDS
2011
NCDs
2014
NCDs
2016
AMR
2018
• TB
• NCDs
2019
UHC
2023
UHC
2025
NCDs

Fig. 65.1 High-level meetings on health at the UN GENERAL ASSEMBLY (Source: adapted from Rodi et al. [5])

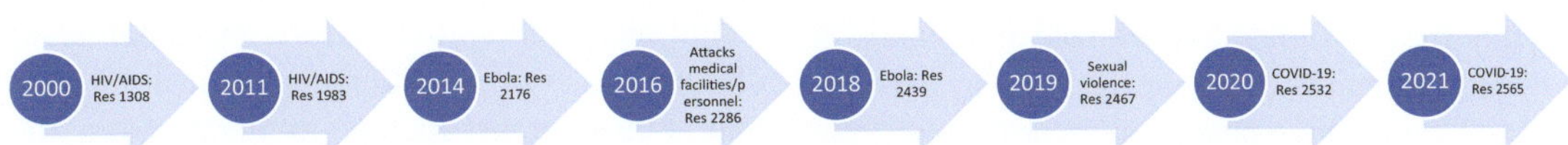

Fig. 65.2 Resolutions on health at the UN Security Council (Source: adapted from Sekalala et al. [6])

65.4 Multifaceted Complexity

Global Health Diplomacy aims at finding policy solutions that improve health for all. It basically means to apply a health lens to global challenges and involves processes of negotiations and decision-making at national, regional, and global level. It becomes an instrument of governance and a tool to manage interdependence, necessitating an understanding on where and how decisions are reached, in which ways negotiations are organized, who is involved, and what instruments are at hand [9]. At the global and regional level, the decision-making processes remain largely among states within the multilateral system of the UN, international organizations, regional alliances, and other political fora, even though the larger ecosystem has changed dramatically: a wide range of non-state actors, including NGOs, the private sector, academia, philanthropic organizations and foundations, participate and influence the negotiation processes and digital diplomacy, i.e., the use of the internet and social media, has changed the diplomatic practice. These changes also concern, among others, the need and the possibility today to include the voices of affected or marginalized communities, to empower patient groups and practitioners at local level, and to recognize and listen to the experts in countries of the Global South. This brings along a new complexity of negotiations that vertically involves more actors across all levels and horizontally connects different sectors.

Global health has expanded its scope of negotiations and decision-making from health to other areas, such as trade, development, humanitarian affairs, human rights, and climate mitigation. It entails to examine the role health can play in building and maintaining peace and security, especially also in times of uncertainty. Successful global health diplomacy involves an awareness of the interconnectedness of global health negotiations and of the different processes that may take place in various venues at the same time, potentially influencing one another. For example, in the context of the COVID-19 pandemic, equitable and affordable access to vaccines was discussed, among others, at WHO, the World Trade Organization, the Human Rights Council, IOM, UNICEF, and most of the other international organizations. In addition, it was also on the agenda of G7 and G20 meetings, and triggered new procurement mechanisms to be established, such as the COVAX Facility and the African Vaccine Acquisition Trust (AVAT), and other financing mechanisms, such as the Pandemic Fund.

The ability to address the same issue across different sectors requires tailoring the issue to the respective audience and framing it accordingly in order to secure attention and often also resources. Many global health issues can be framed in more than one way. Anti-Microbial Resistance (AMR) is frequently framed as medical issue, as political issue, as security issue, as development issue, and as economic issue. The framing not only shapes the level of priority, but it also provides different entry points for the negotiation and decision-making processes, both at global and national level. It pre-defines the context of the negotiation and can therefore be used as a conscious and strategic choice in global health diplomacy to influence the decision-making process [10].

The contextualization within the governance sphere depends largely on the health issues at stake within society and the broader public debates that shape this environment, including the socio-economic, the cultural, and the political context. The strive for human dignity for all, health equity, social justice, and human rights, including the important call to decolonize global health must underpin all efforts in global health diplomacy, even if different political interests may influence or attempt to derail from this broader vision. The principles of solidarity, transparency, accountability, inclusiveness, and multilateralism have to be re-enforced and strengthened to be able to act not only in health emergencies

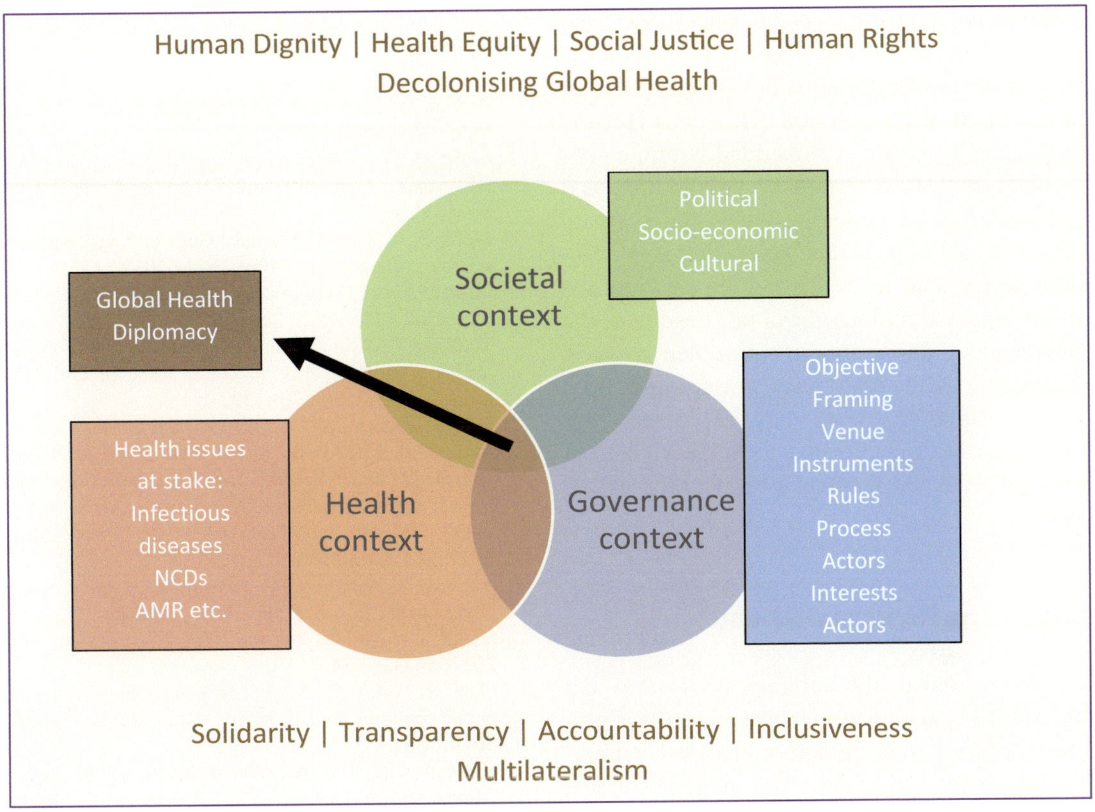

Fig. 65.3 The ecosystem of global health diplomacy

but also to effectively address issues at stake (Fig. 65.3) [11].

65.5 "For Health" Diplomacy

The multitude of health issues that are addressed through global health diplomacy manifests itself in issue diplomacy, such as NCD diplomacy, AMR diplomacy, vaccine diplomacy, or One Health diplomacy [9]. They all highlight the health problem that needs a collective solution, involving different actors, sectors, and countries and are intertwined with foreign policy, involving negotiations, relationship building, cooperation, and securitization. Health security has become a cross-cutting framing theme penetrating most topics and is mostly linked to the perception of threat and national security concerns. At the same time, the more people-centered approach of human security is central to global health diplomacy as it brings empowerment, human development, and human rights back in focus [12].

The interconnectedness of issues and the complexity of global health has led to the emergence and proliferation of "For Health" diplomacy that wants to create a positive impact on health and wellbeing through diplomacy on non-health issues in non-health fora: disaster diplomacy for health, migration diplomacy for health, science diplomacy for health and climate diplomacy for health are just a few of these examples. The emergence of these forms of diplomacy are mostly linked to uncertainty, crisis situations, the related urgency to act and the realization that health must be considered as an integral part of the solution. This "For Health" diplomacy, however, is embedded within a geopolitical context of increased polarization and fragmentation of powerful states and political alliances, as well as increased extremist tensions at national level. This often restricts the ability to act at national level and results in the emergence of new actors to claim their space in diplomacy: public diplomacy, grassroots or civil society diplomacy, and city diplomacy are involving those actors that leverage change at national level and feeding it up it to the global level.

65.6 The Roadmap Ahead

The navigation of the complex ecosystem and the effective participation in global health diplomacy requires from all actors involved a mindset and skills that allow to engage amidst competing interests and to negotiate for better health at home and abroad. Amidst rising nationalism with its spillover effects on health, solidarity remains a critical value to find collective solutions. Building trust and fostering a social contract between those involved is essential that allows to build relationships and partnerships, achieve cooperation, and conduct negotiations which are at the core of diplomacy and more than ever need to be nurtured in and for global health.

References

1. Badeau JS. Diplomacy and medicine. Bull N Y Acad Med. 1970;46(5):303–12.
2. Fidler D. The globalization of public health: the first 100 years of international health diplomacy. Bull World Health Organ. 2001;79(9):842–9.
3. McInnes C, Lee K. Global health and international relations. Cambridge: Polity Press; 2012.
4. Ministers of Foreign Affairs of Brazil, France, Indonesia, Norway, Senegal, South Africa, and Thailand. Oslo Ministerial Declaration—global health: a pressing foreign policy issue of our time. Lancet. 2007;369(9570):1373–8.
5. Rodi P, Obermeyer W, Pablos-Mendez A, Gori A, Raviglione MC. Political rationale, aims, and outcomes of health-related high-level meetings and special sessions at the UN General Assembly: a policy research observational study. PLoS Med. 2022;19(1):e1003873.
6. Sekalala S, Williams CR, Mason MB. Global health governance through the UN Security Council: health security vs. human rights? Aust J Int Aff. 2022;76(1):27–34.
7. Gore R, Parker R. Analysing power and politics in health policies and systems. Glob Public Health. 2019;14(4):481–8.
8. Kickbusch I, Liu A. Global health diplomacy—reconstructing power and governance. Lancet. 2022;399:2156–66.
9. Kickbusch I, Nikogosian H, Kazatchkine M, Kökeny M. A guide to Global Health Diplomacy. Geneva: The Graduate Institute; 2021.
10. Shiffman J, Shawar YR. Framing and the formation of global health priorities. Lancet. 2022;399:1977–90.
11. The Lancet COVID-19 Commission Global Health Diplomacy and Cooperation Task Force. Global diplomacy and cooperation in pandemic times: lessons and recommendations from COVID-19. London: The Lancet Commission; 2021.
12. Malik SM, Barlow A, Johnson B. Reconceptualizing health security in a post-COVID-19 world. BMJ Glob Health. 2021;6:e006520.

Financing Global Common Goods for Health

66

Gavin Yamey

Abstract

Global public health is under threat from challenges that transcend the boundaries of individual nation states, including pandemics and antimicrobial resistance. Activities that can curb these transnational threats are called global common goods for health (CGH). These goods cannot be fully funded through the private market because providing them is subject to market failures—either because they are global public goods or because of the large health externalities they generate. Central to the case for investing in global CGH are (1) the very large health and economic returns of such investment and (2) the high health and economic costs of inaction. In the years leading up to the COVID-19 pandemic, about $5–7 billion was spent annually on global CGH. A conservative estimate of the cost of funding a range of high priority CGH is about $50 billion annually. Mechanisms to close the financing gap include resource mobilization, pooling, and strategic purchasing.

G. Yamey (✉)
Center for Policy Impact in Global Health, Duke Global Health Institute, Duke University, Durham, NC, USA
e-mail: gavin.yamey@duke.edu

Keywords

Global common goods for health · Global public health · Global health financing · Public goods · Global health investments

66.1 Introduction

Global public health is under threat from several challenges that transcend the boundaries of individual nation states. These challenges include pandemics, antimicrobial resistance (AMR), and the cross-border spread of risk factors for non-communicable diseases (NCDs), such as tobacco and alcohol. Activities that can curb these transnational threats are called global common goods for health (CGH). This chapter examines the types of global CGH, how much funding CGH have received, the "price tag" for adequately funding a range of high priority CGH, and potential mechanisms for mobilizing additional funding.

66.2 Types of Global Common Goods for Health

In its 2021 report, *Financing Common Goods for Health*, the World Health Organization defined CGH as "the core population-based functions or interventions that are essential to the health and well-being of entire societies"

M. C. B. Raviglione et al. (eds.), *Global Health Essentials*, Sustainable Development Goals Series,
https://doi.org/10.1007/978-3-031-33851-9_66

Table 66.1 Categorizing global common goods for health

Category of CGH	Examples
Supporting global public goods	• Development of new medicines, vaccines, and diagnostics for neglected diseases • Setting of international norms, standards, and guidelines • Intellectual property sharing • Knowledge generation and sharing • Global surveillance of biological, chemical, and physical pathogens/threats • Market shaping • Population, policy, and implementation research
Managing cross-border and global externalities	• Control of cross-border disease movement • Curbing the cross-border marketing of addictive and other unhealthy goods • Pandemic preparedness and response • Curbing antimicrobial resistance
Fostering leadership and stewardship	• Global advocacy for marginalized populations (e.g., refugees, men who have sex with men, transgender people) • Convening for consensus building on policies and priorities • Health and cross-sectoral advocacy (e.g., education, trade, environment)

[1]. Yazbeck and Soucat note that CGH have two key characteristics. First, they cannot be fully funded through the private market because providing such goods is subject to market failures. The market fails either because CGH are public goods (they are non-rival and non-excludable, i.e., multiple people can use them and nobody can be excluded) or because of the large health externalities they generate [2]. Second, investing in such goods has enormous health and economic benefits.

At national level, examples of CGH include regulating the safety of medicines, health taxes (e.g., tobacco taxes), and vector control. CGH can also be global in nature—the global market fails because they are global public goods (GPGs) or the externalities they generate are transnational. Global CGH are the focus of this chapter.

Building on a taxonomy developed by the *Lancet* Commission on Investing in Health (CIH) [3], Yamey and colleagues propose that global CGH be classified into three types (Table 66.1) [4]:

- *Providing GPGs*, for example, generating and sharing health knowledge, developing new health technologies to tackle neglected diseases.
- *Managing negative regional and global cross-border externalities*, for example, tackling AMR, pandemic preparedness and response (PPR).
- *Fostering global health leadership and stewardship*, for example, global cross-sectoral advocacy for health, convening for negotiation.

66.3 The Case for Investing in Global CGH

Central to the case for investing in global CGH is the very large health and economic returns. For example, from 2011 to 2020, the return on investment for one dollar invested in global vaccination against 10 pathogens in 94 low- and middle-income countries was $US 19.8 [5]. Market shaping—in which governments, donors, and procurers use their purchasing power, financing, influence, and technical expertise to "address the root causes of market shortcomings and influence markets for improved health outcomes" [3]—has helped expand global access to vaccines. For example, in 2001, only one manufacturer was supplying the pentavalent DTP-HBV-Hib vaccine at the Gavi, the Vaccine Alliance (Gavi) price of $US 3.50 per dose. Gavi's market shaping efforts meant that by 2017, there were five suppliers and the lowest price offered was $US 0.68 per dose [6].

The high cost of inaction is another rationale for funding global CGH. Under-funding PPR, for example, can have catastrophic health, social, and economic consequences, as seen with the COVID-19 pandemic. At the time of writing this, 6.5 million people have been killed by the illness; the economic losses caused by COVID-19 are predicted to be $US 13.8 trillion from 2020 to 2024 [7].

66.4 Trends in Financing Global CGH

Given the global market failures and large externalities described above, global CGH should be collectively funded mostly by public financing, complemented by private and philanthropic support. To date, most funding for global CGH has come from official development assistance (ODA). The CIH notes that ODA for global CGH (or "global functions"), which brings transnational benefits, is distinct from ODA for "country-specific functions," i.e., aid that is given to an individual country for national disease control that benefits that country alone (e.g., support to reduce national maternal mortality) [3].

How much ODA is invested in global CGH versus country-specific support? Schäferhoff et al. [8], estimated that in 2013, out of a total of $22 billion in external assistance for health, only one fifth (21%, $4.6 billion) was directed at global CGH (14% of ODA went to providing GPGs, 4% to managing cross-border externalities, and 3% to fostering leadership). In a follow-up study, the authors found that the proportion of ODA directed at global CGH rose to 29% in 2015, in the wake of the west Africa Ebola epidemic, then fell again to 24% in 2017 (Fig. 66.1) [9]. These findings, say the authors, provide "empirical evidence that international funders are prone to 'cycles of panic and neglect'." In other words, funding for global CGH has tended to be reactive rather than proactive—funding rises during crises ("panic") and then falls once the crisis recedes ("neglect"). Breaking these cycles will be crucial to ensuring sustained financing for global CGH.

The reactive nature of funding for global CGH is also in the most recent ODA data, available for 2020, the year when COVID-19 was declared a pandemic [10]. In 2020, ODA for health rose to US$29.1 billion, up from $22.2 billion in 2019, a 31% increase; almost two-thirds of the increase resulted from donor funding for global COVID-19 control.

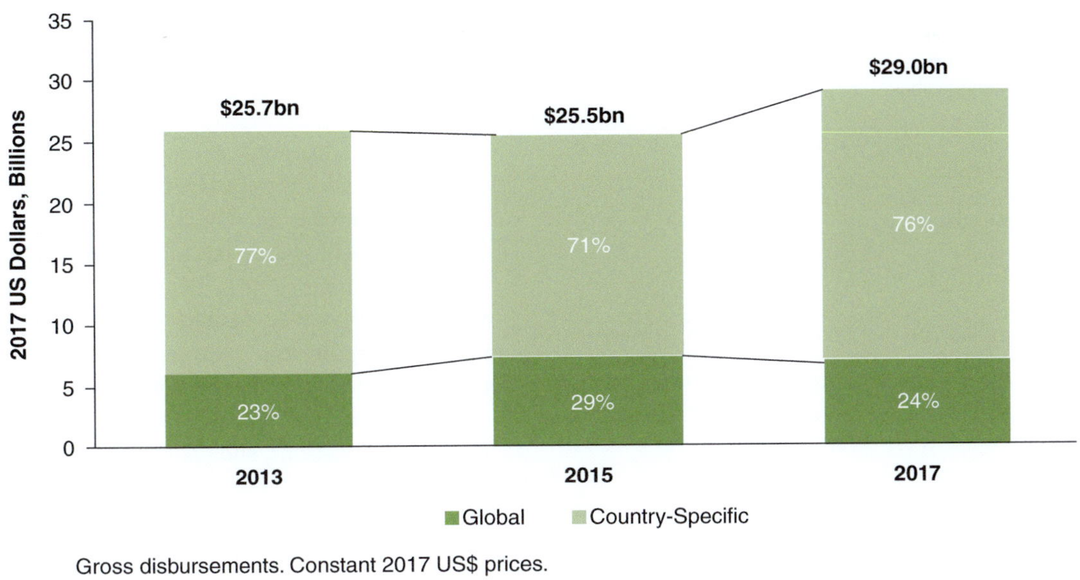

Fig. 66.1 Donor funding for global common goods for health ("global") versus country-specific support in 2013, 2015, and 2017. Figure from Ref. [9] (distributed under the terms of the Creative Commons Attribution 3.0 IGO License (https://creativecommons.org/licenses/by/3.0/igo/))

66.5 The Financing Gap for High Priority CGH

As noted, in the years leading up to the COVID-19 pandemic, about $5–7 billion was spent annually on global CGH. This amount fell short of what was needed to fund a set of high priority international collective action activities.

A conservative estimate of the cost of funding a range of high priority CGH is about $50 billion annually (Table 66.2). This is a sum of the estimated annual costs to fund: product development for neglected diseases [11]; polio eradication activities [12]; a pooled procurement mechanism for non-communicable diseases [6]; knowledge generation and distribution activities [6]; malaria eradication [13]; and a fit-for-purpose PPR system [14].

Table 66.2 The estimated annual "price tag" for a range of high priority global common goods for health

Activity	Annual estimated cost ($US, billions)	Source of estimate
Product development for neglected diseases	3.0	Reference [11]
Polio eradication	1.0	Reference [12]
WHO's core activities	0.24	Reference [4]
Pooled procurement mechanism for non-communicable diseases	1.2	Reference [6]
Knowledge generation and distribution activities, including population, policy, and implementation research	0.6	Reference [6]
Malaria eradication	2.0	Reference [13]
PPR	41.6 (31.1 at the national level and 10.5 billion at the international level)	Reference [6]
Total	**49.64**	

66.6 Mechanisms to Close the Financing Gap

Based on a WHO framework that conceptualizes ways to finance health [15], mechanisms to close the financing gap for CGH can be organized into resource mobilization, pooling, and strategic purchasing (Fig. 66.2):

- Resource mobilization mechanisms include global taxation, voluntary earmarking, and reallocation of ODA. An existing global tax mechanism is the airline tax that UNITAID uses to raise revenue. There is a strong case for global carbon and financial transaction taxes, both of which could help support CGH. Voluntary earmarked mechanisms for CGH include the Coalition for Epidemic Preparedness Innovations (CEPI) and the Financial Intermediary Fund for Pandemic Preparedness (FIF). As middle-income countries graduate from ODA, there will be opportunities to "reallocate ODA to areas where governments have natural incentives to underinvest," [6] including CGH.
- Pooled mechanisms include pooled R&D funds, R&D coordination platforms (e.g., the new Global Antimicrobial Resistance Research and Development Hub), and multilateral agency support for CGH (e.g., the World Bank has a new funding window for GPGs).
- As Yamey et al. note, several global health agencies have "progressively developed a 'strategic purchasing' function through the development of prioritization models to allocate their funding" [4]. Examples of CGH funded in this way include (1) the Global Fund's support for "Strategic Initiatives" (investments that cannot be delivered through country grants, and that include CGH, such as malaria elimination), and (2) IDA's funding of the East Africa Public Health Laboratory Network.

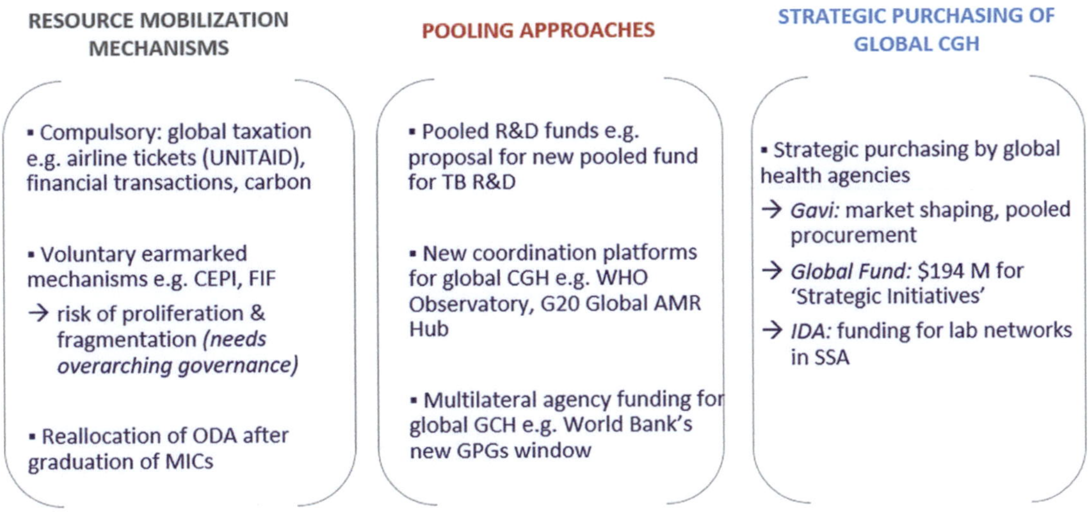

Fig. 66.2 Mechanisms to close the CGH financing gap

References

1. WHO. Financing common goods for health. Geneva: World Health Organization; 2021. https://www.who.int/health-topics/common-goods-for-health#tab=tab_1
2. Yazbeck AS, Soucat A. When both markets and governments fail health. Health Syst Reform. 2019;5(4):268–79.
3. Jamison DT, Summers LH, Alleyne G, et al. Global health 2035: a world converging within a generation. Lancet. 2015;382:1898–955.
4. Yamey G, Jamison DT, Hanssen O, Soucat A. Financing global common goods for health: when the world is a country. Health Syst Reform. 2019;5(4):334–49.
5. Sim SY, Watts E, Constenla G, et al. Return on investment from immunization against 10 pathogens in 94 low- and middle-income countries, 2011–2030. Health Aff (Milwood). 2020;39(8):1343–53.
6. Watkins DA, Yamey G, Schäferhoff M, et al. Alma-Ata at 40 years: reflections from the Lancet commission on investing in health. Lancet. 2018;392:1434–60.
7. Gopinath G. A disrupted global recovery. IMG Blog. 2022. https://blogs.imf.org/2022/01/25/a-disrupted-global-recovery/.
8. Schäferhoff M, Fewer S, Kraus J, et al. How much donor financing for health is channelled to global versus country-specific aid functions? Lancet. 2015;86(10011):2436–41.
9. Schäferhoff M, Chodavadia P, Martinez S, et al. International funding for global common goods for health: an analysis using the creditor reporting system and G-FINDER databases. Health Syst Reform. 2019;5(4):350–65.
10. OECD Statistics. Creditor reporting system. 2022. https://stats.oecd.org/Index.aspx?DataSetCode=CRS1.
11. Young R, Bekele T, Gunn A, et al. Developing new health technologies for neglected diseases: a pipeline portfolio review and cost model. Gates Open Res. 2018;2:23.
12. Global Polio Eradication Initiative. Financial resource requirements: GPEI budget 2018. Geneva (Switzerland): GPEI; 2018. http://polioeradication.org/financing/financial-needs/financial-resource-requirements-frr/gpei-budget-2018/
13. Feachem RGA, Chen I, Akbari O, et al. Lancet commission on malaria eradication: malaria eradication within a generation: ambitious, achievable and necessary. Lancet. 2019;394(10203):1056–112.
14. World Bank and WHO. Analysis of Pandemic Preparedness and Response (PPR) architecture, financing needs, gaps and mechanisms. 2022. https://thedocs.worldbank.org/en/doc/5760109c4db174ff90a8dfa7d025644a-0290032022/original/G20-Gaps-in-PPR-Financing-Mechanisms-W0HO-and-WB-pdf.pdf.
15. Kutzin J. A descriptive framework for country-level analysis of health care financing arrangements. Health Pol. 2001;6(3):171–204.

Performance-Based Funding for Health

67

Daniel Low-Beer and Ronald Tran Ba Huy

Abstract

Performance and results-based financing, at their simplest, aim to focus health financing and negotiations between funders and implementers on results (Fritsche GB, Soeters R, Meessen B, Performance based financing toolkit. World Bank, 2014). They require both a measurement component where results are collected, shared transparently and verified, and a management component which defines decisions based on results (Low-Beer D, Afkhami H, Komatsu R, PLOS Medicine 4:e219, 2007).

There are benefits and weaknesses to this focus on results. The economic argument is that it allows to finance results directly and to reduce transaction costs by aligning the incentives of different partners on measurable results and outcomes (Khanna M, Loevinsohn B, Pardhan E, BMC Medicine 18:224, 2021).

The weaknesses are that it requires verified measurable results, can distort overall incentives in the country, and is more difficult to apply to less measurable but equally important areas like prevention (Meessen B, Soucat A, Sekabaraga C, Bull WHO 89:153–6, 2011).

This section follows the emergence of performance-based funding, its strengths and weaknesses, and how it was consolidated into the routine business of health financing mechanisms. It highlights the challenge of the Sustainable Development Goals (SDGs) to raise the focus of performance-based funding to the ambitious goals of impact which are set for 2030.

Keywords

Results-based financing · Performance · Development effectiveness · Incentives · Public private partnership · SDGS · Health impact · Evaluation · Health diplomacy of data

67.1 Introduction

At the start of this century, there was an eruption of new partners in global health governance, Bill Gates programming global health rather than software, non-governmental organisations and people living with HIV formally governing a US$20 billion Global Fund to fight AIDS, TB and Malaria, GAVI and financial markets launching bonds to support vaccines, the US announcing a US$15 billion global programme on AIDS, the musician Bono selling RED products alongside his music [1].

D. Low-Beer (✉)
World Health Organization, Geneva, Switzerland

R. T. B. Huy
World Food Programme, Rome, Italy

M. C. B. Raviglione et al. (eds.), *Global Health Essentials*, Sustainable Development Goals Series,
https://doi.org/10.1007/978-3-031-33851-9_67

Central to the effort to get such diverse partners to work together, was the implementation of a results agenda, and building performance-based funding into the funding mechanisms and development principles that emerged [2]. As much as a technical agenda, the partners required a common language, a diplomacy of data to negotiate health, align and consolidate their efforts. As Richard Manning comments "International cooperation for better health outcomes has developed through a number of periods of creativity usually followed by periods of consolidation" [3].

This section follows the emergence of performance-based funding, its strengths and weaknesses, and how it was consolidated into the routine business of health financing mechanisms. It highlights the challenge of the SDGs to raise the focus of performance-based funding to the ambitious goals of impact for 2030.

67.2 Measuring and Managing for Results

The results agenda has a long history in education and then health [2, 4]. Two agendas "measuring" and "managing" programmes for results came together at the start of the twenty-first century.

From the 1980s UNICEF had used a results focus to guide health interventions in vaccination and oral rehydration therapy [2]. Furthermore, the collaboration of WHO and the World Bank led to the comprehensive measurement of the Global Burden of disease, and their joint report "Investing in Health" in 1993 [5]. This marked the integration of health and development issues, health as a contributor and outcome of economic development [6].

As Sen noted "At all levels of development the three essential capabilities are for people to lead a long and healthy life, to be knowledgeable, and to have access to the resources needed for a decent standard of living" [6]. This was captured in the Human Development Index and reports.

The measurement initiatives were influential in putting health at the heart of the International Development Goals of 1996 and the MDGs in 2001 with their specific goals and targets.

The second theme is on the management side of "managing for results", largely outside mainstream development. This comes from innovations particularly in the public sector, first in education and then health, and from private foundations on returns on social investments [7].

Performance-based funding and rewards were introduced in the public sector in the United States starting in Tennessee and became widespread in the 1990s in education and health [2]. The World Bank increasingly built performance incentives into its programmes and helped convene the International Roundtables on Managing for Results in 2002 and 2004.

The measurement and management agendas came together as a focus of the new partners who set up public private health initiatives, and performance-based funding was built into their business and governance models.

67.3 Implementing Performance-Based Funding

Performance and results-based financing, at their simplest, aim to focus health financing and negotiations between funders and implementers on results. They require both a measurement component where results are collected, shared transparently and verified, and a management component which defines decisions based on results [8].

The OECD describe results-based funding as "a mechanism through which a funder is willing to make payments to an implementer who assumes responsibility for achieving predefined results. The rationale behind this approach is to link financing more directly with outputs and outcomes, rather than inputs and processes" [2, 9].

There are three important requirements to achieve the benefits of this approach.

1. **Ownership**—the targets and the means of implementation need to be owned by the country or implementer, for the benefits in terms of transaction costs and incentives to be achieved.
2. **Investment in measurement**—to support the focus on results 5–10% of the funding amount should be invested in strengthening country data systems including verification. There is an asymmetry of information in implementation so the focus should be on country data systems, getting countries to manage by results.
3. **Balance of outputs and impact**—the results should not just focus on outputs but also have separate ratings for outcomes and impact. Performance should be verified independently to both the implementer and grant management and published transparently.

There is a subtle difference between results and performance-based funding. Results-based financing provides the apparent simplicity of funding result directly, for example, paying 100 dollars per person on HIV treatment might allow support to 30 million people for less than 3 billion p.a. with limited grant transaction costs. Performance-based funding focuses on the difference between results and targets and uses this as a basis to finance improved performance at all levels of performance, including responding to the uncertainty, risks and discovery process of implementation.

A programme that is underperforming can be a good opportunity for additional financing, if investments to improve performance can be revealed, for example, in Ethiopia when zero bednets were delivered against a target of 2 million, the supply chain issues were diagnosed, allowing investments in an underperforming grant to accelerate results dramatically. As the Minister of Health mentioned "we were in the 'red zone' and we both saw the problem, performance-based funding allowed us to think through implementation" [1]. Performance-based funding should aim to improve results at all levels of performance, to stretch and accelerate a well performing grant, to invest in capacity in underperforming grants and to reprogramme the strategy in the poorest performers [2].

Six characteristics of performance-based funding have been identified [10]:

1. **General goals** reflecting the interests of main stakeholders.
3. **Targets** established for each indicator.
4. **Performance data** to measure achievement relative to targets and investment in country measurement systems.
5. **Funds allocated according to uniformly applied, easily understood mechanisms** and business rules relating funding to attainment of targets.
6. **Evaluation and adjustment** to respond to the changing goals of the performance-based funding system and to refine and correct operational problems in its application.

67.4 Strengths and Weaknesses of a Focus on Results

There are benefits and weaknesses to this focus on results. The economic argument is that it allows to finance results directly and to reduce transaction costs by aligning the incentives of different partners on measurable results and outcomes [11].

The weaknesses are that it requires verified measurable results, can distort overall incentives in the country if not owned, needs to define quality as well as quantity of deliverables, and is more difficult to apply to less measurable but equally important areas like prevention [12].

In practice, there is considerable overlap and complexity in the approaches, with different definitions illustrated in Table 67.1, adapted from [13]:

Table 67.1 Different approaches to results-based financing with definitions and examples (adapted from [13])

Mechanism	Definition	Example
Performance-based grants	Links grant recipient performance to access to and amount of funding disbursed to recipient based on clear ratings and business rules	The Global Fund to fight AIDS, TB and malaria
Cash on delivery	Funders pay aid recipients based on achievement of mutually agreed upon and verified progress towards a goal—Recipients can use funds as they decide	A donor pays a national government for registered births and provides additional payments for each registered child who survives to age five
Social or development impact bonds	A public private partnership that allows private investors to front capital for public projects that deliver social outcomes. If the project succeeds, investors are repaid by the government (social impact bonds) with interest	In 2017, USAID launched the first health development impact bond in Rajasthan, India to reduce maternal and new-born deaths by improving the quality of maternal care in health facilities
Incentive payments to facilities or individuals for results	Paying public or private health facilities or individuals monetary or nonmonetary incentives based on achievement of agreed upon performance indicators	The World Bank has supported implementation of large-scale PBF pilots in 30 countries. Programmes vary but each involves paying for improved quantity and quality of services with robust verification

67.5 The Diplomacy of Data

The MDGs saw performance-based funding built into the new financing mechanisms and the principles of aid effectiveness—"achieving development results—and openly accounting for them—must be at the heart of all we do" (Accra Action Agenda 2008) [2].

As much as a technical agenda, it supported the efforts of diverse partners to work together [14, 15], often with little else in common except a commitment to results, a partial lingua franca for health diplomacy. Results were built into the business models of a range of individual partners in different ways as shown in Table 67.2:

The SDGS have provided a focus on impact and on integrated results across health (with an integrated health area 3—ensure health lives and promote well-being at all ages, compared to MDGs 4–6 on separated parts of health).

Most importantly, data is not measured afterwards (the results against targets of the MDGs) but is an upfront part of how development is managed and implemented. Data is defined as one of the three systematic issues in the implementation of sustainable development in SDG 17, with targets to build country capacity for data disaggregated by income, gender, age, race, ethnicity, migration, disability and geographical location (SDG 17.18).

There is an additional target for countries to measure their own performance and progress (SDG 17.19). The challenge is for countries to manage their own programmes for results and use results to align diverse partners with the diplomacy of data [1]. At the same time, data is seen as the most valuable economic resource in wider management, and its ownership a key issue of societal debate [16].

The challenge of the SDGs will be the extent to which performance-based funding can be integrated into implementation with disaggregated data, the focus on impact, and basing performance on how countries themselves measure and manage for results.

Table 67.2 How partners have included results-based approaches showing the characteristics and challenges

	Selected results approaches	Key characteristics	Challenges
GAVI	Performance-based funding	Strong use of incentives and rewards for good performance. Use of partner estimates and country reporting with validation. Defined baselines for support	Unintended effects of incentives on reporting, data quality issues. Incentives to improve less-performing grants
Global Fund	Performance-based funding	Explicit performance rating for each disbursement. Actions defined for each level of performance. Transparent M&E frameworks with funding of M&E plans	Country data quality and transaction costs can be issues. Challenge to balance impact and quality with number of services delivered
PEPFAR	Target-based financing	Overall programme targets set and reported to Congress. Strong building of M&E capacity and support of independent impact surveys	Challenges in showing HIV prevention impact. Some issues of alignment with national reporting and consistency of performance-based disbursement rules
World Bank	Results-based financing and output-based aid	Performance incentives actively decentralised to local and health worker level. Results included in conditional loans	Evaluation showed need to explicitly measure goals of programmes during implementation. Results-based financing used only in selected projects

References

1. Low-Beer D. Innovative health partnerships–the diplomacy of diversity. Singapore: World Scientific; 2012.
2. Low-Beer D. Managing for results: a "common currency" to coordinate health development, in Low-Beer D (2012) innovative health partnerships. Singapore: World Scientific; 2012.
3. Manning R. Origins and diversity of health partnerships in Low-Beer D (2012) innovative health partnerships. Singapore: World Scientific; 2012.
4. Fritsche GB, Soeters R, Meessen B. Performance based financing toolkit. Washington: World Bank; 2014.
5. World Bank. Investing in health (World Development Report). New York: Oxford University Press; 1993.
6. Sen A. Development as freedom. New York: Oxford University Press; 1999.
7. Jongbloed B, Vossensteyn H. Keeping up performances: an international survey of performance-based funding in higher education. J High Educ Policy Manag. 2001;23(2):127–45.
8. Low-Beer D, Afkhami H, Komatsu R. Making performance-based funding work for health. PLoS Med. 2007;4(8):e219.
9. OECD. Technical workshop on results-based funding, workshop report. Paris: OECD; 2014.
10. Plowman B. How the big three AIDS donors define and use performance to inform funding decisions. Washington: Center for Global Development; 2008.
11. Khanna M, Loevinsohn B, Pardhan E, et al. Decentralized facility financing versus performance-based payments in primary health care: a large-scale randomized controlled trial in Nigeria. BMC Med. 2021;18:224.
12. Meessen B, Soucat A, Sekabaraga C. Performance-based financing: just a donor fad or a catalyst towards comprehensive health-care reform? Bull World Health Organ. 2011;89(2):153–6.
13. Management Sciences for Health. The AIDSTAR-two project. In: The PBF Handbook: Designing and Implementing Effective Performance-Based Financing Programs, vol. 1.0. Cambridge: Management Sciences for Health; 2011.
14. Basinga P, Gertler P, Binagwaho A, Soucat A, Sturdy J, Vermeersch C. Effect on maternal and child health services in Rwanda of payment to primary health care providers for performance: an impact evaluation. Lancet. 2011;377(9775):1421–8.
15. Shroff Z, Bigdeli M, Meessen B. From scheme to system: findings from ten countries on policy evolution of results based financing in health systems. Health System Reform. 2017;3(2):137–47.
16. Economist. The world's most valuable resource is no longer oil, but data, May 6th. 2017. Economist, London.

International Cooperation and Development

68

Francesco Castelli and Beatrice Formenti

"Yet there is still so much to be done."
António Guterres
United Nations Secretary-General
Remarks at the UN General Assembly, 2020

Abstract

The international community is currently facing global challenges that call for a global, multilateral and integrated response. This requires a profound rethinking of the modalities of international cooperation, with implications for both the aid architecture and overall development governance, overcoming the paralysis of economic growth, which is more means than end. Now more than ever, a cooperation for development designed with a multidimensional, multisectoral and participatory approach is needed.

Keywords

International cooperation · Adi effectiveness · Global health donors · Governance for health · Multilateral organizations

68.1 The State of the World

Peace, diplomacy and international cooperation are fundamental conditions for the world to progress toward the Sustainable Development Goals (SDGs) and beyond. We are at an unprecedented moment in the history of humankind and of our planet. For the second year running, the world is no longer making progress on the SDGs. COVID-19 pandemic has triggered the first increase of extreme poverty after more than two decades of decline. While economic output should rise to pre-COVID-19 levels aided by stimulus packages and access to vaccines, for many low-middle income countries (LMICs) long-term scarring will be more severe [1]. But COVID-19 was not just the primary threat, as it exacerbated pre-existing vulnerabilities. About 700 million people still live on less than US$1.90 per day and 1.3 billion are multidimensionally poor, where women and people with disabilities are overrepresented [2]. 274 million people are estimated to be in need of humanitarian assistance in 2022—a remarkable increase from 235 million people 1 year ago, which was already the highest figure in decades [1]. 2010–2019 was the hottest decade on record, with climate change and extreme weather-related disasters boosting risks and vulnerabilities, disrupting livelihoods and threatening lives, causing misery and hunger for millions of people. Over 2 billion people lack access to safe drinking water, with preventable diarrhoeal diseases still among the five top causes of death in low-income countries [1]. Half of the world's population cannot obtain essential health services and about 23 million children worldwide missed basic childhood vaccines in 2021. Globally, levels of hunger remain alarmingly

F. Castelli (✉) · B. Formenti
UNESCO Chair "Training and Empowering Human Resources for Health Development in Resource Limited Countries", University of Brescia, Brescia, Italy
e-mail: francesco.castelli@unibs.it; beatrice.formenti@unibs.it

M. C. B. Raviglione et al. (eds.), *Global Health Essentials*, Sustainable Development Goals Series, https://doi.org/10.1007/978-3-031-33851-9_68

high, with up to 811 million people undernourished and 193 million acutely food insecure and in need of urgent assistance, especially women and children under 5 years old [3]. The 70% of people in crisis in 2021 were in 10 food crisis countries: the DRC, Afghanistan, Ethiopia, Yemen, northern Nigeria, the Syrian Arab Republic, the Sudan, South Sudan, Pakistan and Haiti [3]. Prospects for serious global food insecurity in 2022 are projected to deteriorate further. In particular, the ongoing war in Ukraine threatens to exacerbate the already serious vulnerabilities, not only because of the impact of the war on global prices and supplies of food and energy, but for the millions of people displaced in protracted need of aid. Today, the number of people forcibly displaced worldwide because of conflict, violence, human rights violations and climate shocks has now reached for the first time the striking milestone of 100 million [4].

68.2 International Cooperation: How it Started and How it Continues

Over the last century, the landscape of international cooperation, from the first international public initiatives carried out during European colonialism and religious charity, has changed and evolved until today—still a time of great rethinking.

The structure and purpose of current international cooperation can be traced back to two major events following World War II: (1) the Marshall Plan, a US-sponsored package to recover European countries, and (2) the founding of international organizations, including today's United Nations, International Monetary Fund and the World Bank. In particular, in 1945 the UN Charter formulated the notion of international development as "to employ international machinery for the promotion of the economic and social advancement of all peoples". Following Europe's recovery—seen as a prototype of foreign aid's success–the Organisation for Economic Co-operation and Development (OECD) was constituted in 1961 to enhance recovery programmes and supervise foreign aid. "Development" has become a metaphor for economic growth with Official Development Assistance (ODA) as a western instrument for establishing the market economy promoted by the member countries of the Development Assistance Committee (DAC) of the OECD.

Despite aid, economic growth failed to alleviate poverty. The one-way North-South dialogue and dependency led the UN to adopt a resolution in 1974 "to involve the active and equal participation of the beneficiary countries in the formulation and application of all decisions". This new paradigm has led to rethinking cooperation as endogenous and in line with the needs of each society (basic needs approach).

In the 1990s—years of market liberalization and financial deregulation—a succession of wide-ranging international debates redefined the global development agenda by focusing on the fight against poverty, laying the groundwork for a deepening path that led to the Millennium Declaration in 2000. Although the several milestones achieved during the MDGs, one of the most commonly cited concerns is that these goals were defined by few stakeholders with little involvement of LMICs despite they had the primary responsibility for achieving these goals [5].

It was in 2015 that, overcoming the traditional North-South approach, the 2030 Agenda was adopted introducing 17 universal SDGs and bringing the concept of "development" finally to a global dimension [6].

The changeover is still ongoing, as in 2019 EU Commission President Ursula von der Leyen stated the need to move from a "donor-beneficiary relationship" to "equal opportunities partnerships" between the EU and other countries [7].

Nowadays, after more than 50 years of international development cooperation and despite 1 billion people having been lifted out of extreme poverty within a generation, the world is not on track to achieve many human development-related SDGs. Why? What has gone wrong? The effectiveness of development cooperation is heated debated, for which three major thinking-silos—somehow opposite—may be distinguished: (1) aid levels have been too low, and a specific and increased level of aid would reduce poverty (Sachs 2005) [8]; (2) foreign aid is not only ineffective but even harmful because it creates dependency and prevents countries from searching for their own solutions (Easterly 2014, Moyo 2010) [9, 10]; (3) evidence-based policymaking that leverages experimental and quasi-experimental approaches may help devise effective and specific aid programmes (Banerjee and Duflo 2011) [11].

The impact of international aid is complex and multi-channel, and it is added to other global and local interdependencies. The world today can no longer be divided into North-South, and the development concept and its strategies must reflect this multilevel dimension.

68.3 Rethink the Future of International Cooperation

Initially based on North-South relations, international cooperation is today confronted with substantial global transformations. The environmental impact of economic growth, the technological and digital revolution, globalized trade and growing inequalities have made traditional "aid" paradigms inadequate in many ways. This is compounded by greater complexity because of the emergence of new players in the global arena. The world has become multipolar, with transnational non-state actors, economic forces, global philanthropy and civil society actors exerting greater influence.

The general landscape of international development cooperation has changed due to changing economic and geopolitical balances. More recently, some emerging economies, such as the so-called BRICS (Brazil, Russia, India, China and South Africa), have assumed an increasing role in international cooperation, often widely differing from the OECD approach. Having been receptors of official assistance, many of the emerging donors may be bringing positive innovations to the cooperation landscape; on the other hand, it is also possible that those same donors do not treasure the mistakes of traditional ODA. This is why the shared alignment with the same principles is fundamental for the effectiveness of cooperation. Transnational corporations also exert increasing influence, directly or indirectly, on governments and multilateral processes: both the private sector in financing international programmes, philanthropic initiatives and global public-private partnerships, and the growing landscape of non-governmental organizations. Although the cooperation machinery needs new supporters, the threat of non-coordination and conflicts of interests between transnational actors is to further fragment the already crowded aid architecture, lacking a global vision and addressing singular challenges "vertically", weakening the UN system and multilateral management. The fragmentation and poor coordination of cooperation undermines the potential benefits for recipient countries, better evaluation of effectiveness and a comprehensive approach to cooperation. The global development agenda requires multidimensional coordinated cooperation that shifts from traditional bilateral relations to multinational, south-south, triangular and horizontal cooperation between local governments [12].

Although absolute poverty has decreased, poverty in a new geography is emerging, with growing inequalities between and within countries, making redistributive policies even more urgent. To fulfil the goals of the 2030 Agenda, re-conceptualizing development in order to "leave no one behind" is urgently needed. The globalization era's growing interdependence extends the concept of development to a planetary level, needing worldwide cooperation to create and implement policies that secure the conservation and access to global public goods, with an increasing focus on environmental and climate challenges [12].

Given the global scope and the indivisibility of the SDGs, the proposed solutions must maintain a planetary, integrated and determinant-oriented assessment. In an increasingly fast-paced and innovative world, despite the need to pursue digital cooperation, the risk could be to lose sight of the social and structural roots, such as the lack of access to basic services, chasing the technological and cutting-edge solution.

The 2030 Agenda, and even more the required paradigm shift, need a thorough examination of governing processes. While on the one hand it appears necessary to identify new structures capable of encompassing the variegated plurality of actors in the development cooperation system and linking their activities to the broader sustainable development agenda, it is crucial to clearly identify the shared approach and distinguish the responsibilities [13]. This is not completely new. Already in 2005, with the Paris Declaration, countries, multilateral institutions and civil societies signed the principles that the international community must adhere in order to make development cooperation more effective: *Ownership* of the receiving countries; *Alignment* and Donor *Harmonization*; *Managing* for verifiable results; and *Mutual accountability*. So the international community already has good shared tools [14].

This calls for a profound rethinking of the modalities of international cooperation, with implications for both the aid architecture and overall development governance. New analytical approaches are needed, as well as a revision of the indicators and the concept of development to overcome the paralysis of economic growth, which is more means than end. Cooperation strategies for development should be designed with a multidimensional, multisectoral and participatory approach and be based on tailor-made country diagnoses [13]. Development needs to be seen as a multifaceted process in addressing the structural challenges of a given country, rather than a one-size-fits-all approach based on income-grouping countries, as human development should be about "expanding human freedoms and opening more choices for people to chart their own development paths according to their diverse values" [15].

Disclaimer The authors are responsible for the choice and presentation of views contained in this article and for opinions expressed therein, which are not necessarily those of UNESCO and do not commit the Organizations.

References

1. United Nations Office for the Coordination of Humanitarian Affairs (OCHA). Global humanitarian overview. 2022.
2. UNDP (United Nations Development Programme). 2022 special report on human security. New York; 2022.
3. World Food Programme. Global report on food crises (GRFC 2022). Global Network against Food Crises. 2022. https://www.wfp.org/publications/global-report-food-crises-2022.
4. UNHCR. UNHCR: Ukraine, other conflicts push forcibly displaced total over 100 million for first time. 2022. https://www.unhcr.org/news/press/2022/5/628a389e4/unhcr-ukraine-other-conflicts-push-forcibly-displaced-total-100-million.html.
5. Fehling M, Nelson BD, Venkatapuram S. Limitations of the millennium development goals: a literature review. Glob Public Health. 2013;8(10):1109–22. https://doi.org/10.1080/17441692.2013.845676. Epub 2013 Nov 25. PMID: 24266508; PMCID: PMC3877943.
6. UN. Transforming our world: the 2030 agenda for sustainable development. New York: United Nations; 2015.
7. Riccardo Roba, ISPI (Italian Institute for International Political Studies). Toward a new paradigm for EU International Cooperation. 2021. https://www.ispionline.it/en/pubblicazione/toward-new-paradigm-eu-international-cooperation-28982.
8. Sachs J. The end of poverty: economic possibilities for our time. New York: Penguin Press; 2005.
9. Easterly W. The tyranny of experts: economists, dictators, and the forgotten rights of the poor. New York: Basic Books; 2014.
10. Moyo D. Dead aid: why aid makes things worse and how there is another way for Africa. London: Penguin Books; 2010.
11. Banerjee A, Duflo E. Poor economics: a radical rethinking of the way to fight global poverty. New York: Public Affairs; 2011.
12. Missoni E, Pacileo G, Tediosi F. Global Health governance and policy: an introduction. Abingdon: Routledge; 2019.
13. Economic Commission for Latin America and the Caribbean (ECLAC)/Organisation for Economic Cooperation and Development (OECD). Emerging challenges and shifting paradigms: new perspectives on international cooperation for development (LC/PUB.2018/16), Santiago. 2018.
14. OECD/DAC. Paris declaration on aid effectiveness, high level forum, Paris. 2005. February 28–March 2, 2005. https://www.oecd.org/dac/effectiveness/parisdeclarationandaccraagendaforaction.htm.
15. UNDP (United Nations Development Programme). Human development report 2020: the next frontier: human development and the Anthropocene. 2020. New York.

International Law and Global Health

69

Pedro A. Villarreal and Claudia Nannini

Abstract

This chapter provides a brief overview of some of the core international law instruments in the field of global health. Such overview includes legally binding rules developed both under the Constitution of the World Health Organization (WHO), as well as beyond its purview. Instruments created within the WHO and enshrining the protection of human health as the main object and purpose consist of Regulations dealing with Nomenclature and the cross-border spread of disease—namely, the International Health Regulations (IHR) of 2005—as well as the Framework Convention on Tobacco Control. Other international law regimes are correlated to human health, even though they might not foresee it as the central object and purpose. In particular, multilateral human rights frameworks such as the International Covenants on Civil and Political Rights, on the one hand, and on Economic, Social and Cultural Rights, on the other hand, are a necessary stepping-stone towards the fulfilment of the "highest attainable physical and mental well-being". Furthermore, the existing three international conventions on drug control regulate the use and abuse of substances for medical and other purposes. These instruments are by no means the only ones relevant for global health goals, as others may have important effects on the provision of healthcare products and services to populations around the world.

Keywords

International law · International Health Regulations (IHR) · Health regulations · World Health Organization · Framework Convention on Tobacco Control

69.1 Introduction

The core goals of global health require an effective coordination between different countries, i.e. states, in order to achieve "the highest attainable standard of physical and mental well-being" (Preamble, Constitution of the WHO). Such goals may lead to the creation of legal obligations for states, represented by governmental authorities. Public international law is needed, in so far as global health goals that go beyond a single state can only be achieved through concerted efforts.

P. A. Villarreal (✉)
German Institute for International and Security Affairs, Berlin, Germany

Max Planck Institute for Comparative Public Law and International Law, Heidelberg, Germany
e-mail: villarreal@mpil.de

C. Nannini
World Health Organization, Geneva, Switzerland
e-mail: nanninic@who.int

M. C. B. Raviglione et al. (eds.), *Global Health Essentials*, Sustainable Development Goals Series,
https://doi.org/10.1007/978-3-031-33851-9_69

Consequently, a series of international law instruments are currently in force, with human health as part and parcel of their object and purpose. Nevertheless, the intersection between international law and global health is not limited to those instruments. Instead, a fragmented set of different fields contribute to the improvement of human health. This includes human rights law, international drug control, and international intellectual property law, to mention a few.

This chapter provides an overview of different legal instruments directly correlated to global health and their main obligations for states. The aim is to emphasize how states, namely their governments, must fulfil a number of rules in the aegis of reaching the highest attainable standard of physical and mental well-being of their population.

69.2 The WHO's Legal Instruments

69.2.1 The Constitution of the WHO

The Constitution of the WHO is the founding treaty of the Organization. It was adopted on 22 July 1946 in the context of the International Health Conference held in New York and entered into force on 7 April 1948. It defines the WHO's objective as being "the attainment by all peoples of the highest possible level of health"[1] and identifies the functions to achieve such objective, which include to direct and coordinate international health work.[2] Furthermore, the Constitution establishes the general normative framework governing WHO's functioning. Importantly, the Constitution empowers the World Health Assembly (i.e. the main decision-making organ of the Organization) to adopt three types of normative instruments: conventions or agreements, regulations and recommendations.

Conventions or agreements are legally binding instruments that, under Article 19 of the Constitution of the WHO, may be adopted by the World Health Assembly with respect to any matter falling within the organization's competence. Like other international treaties, any convention or agreement adopted by the Assembly becomes binding only upon those Member States that have ratified it, or otherwise expressed their consent to be bound by it, in accordance with their constitutional processes. The Assembly has made limited use of its authority to adopt conventions or agreements on health matters as only one convention has been adopted so far: the WHO Framework Convention on Tobacco Control.

Regulations are also legally binding but, unlike conventions or agreements, may be adopted only with respect to five specific health-related areas.[3] Furthermore, regulations automatically come into force for all Member States after a given time period has passed from the notification of their adoption by the Assembly, except for those Member States that reject them or file reservations by a set deadline.[4]

Finally, recommendations may be adopted on any matter falling within WHO's competence but are not legally binding.[5] They carry different designations (e.g. codes, global strategies, plans of actions, roadmaps or frameworks) and are the legal tool most widely used by the World Health Assembly.

69.2.2 WHO Regulations

Since the creation of WHO, the World Health Assembly has adopted two regulations: the Nomenclature Regulations and the International Health Regulations.

[1] Article 1 of the WHO Constitution.

[2] Article 2(a) of the WHO Constitution.

[3] In accordance with Article 21 of the Constitution, these are: (a) sanitary and quarantine requirements and other procedures designed to prevent the international spread of disease; (b) nomenclatures with respect to diseases, causes of death and public health practices; (c) standards with respect to diagnostic procedures for international use; (d) standards with respect to the safety, purity and potency of biological, pharmaceutical and similar products moving in international commerce; (e) advertising and labelling of biological, pharmaceutical and similar products moving in international commerce.

[4] Article 22 of the WHO Constitution.

[5] Article 23 of the WHO Constitution.

The Nomenclature Regulations, first adopted in 1948, require WHO Members States to compile mortality and morbidity statistics in accordance with the revision of the International Statistical Classification of Diseases, Injuries and Causes of Death (ICD) in force at any given time. The ICD itself is an Assembly-adopted instrument but does not constitute a regulation per se.

The International Health Regulations, in their currently applicable version of 2005 ("IHR (2005)") are intended under its Article 2 "to prevent, protect against, control and provide a public health response to the international spread of disease in ways that are commensurate with and restricted to public health risks, and which avoid unnecessary interference with international traffic and trade". While their predecessors, the international Sanitary Regulations of 1951 and the IHR of 1969, applied to a pre-determined set of diseases, the IHR (2005) apply to any public health risk, regardless of its origin or nature. They represent the only internationally applicable normative framework for the prevention and detection of diseases, and the coordinated response against public health emergencies of international concern. Since their adoption, the IHR (2005) have been amended only twice with respect to narrowly defined aspects, particularly: in 2014 to provide for the validity of certificates affirming life-long duration of the protection from yellow fever vaccination; and in 2022, to shorten the time period required for the entry into force of, and for rejecting or filing reservations to, any future amendments to the instrument. The latter reform illustrates how the COVID-19 pandemic has rejuvenated discussions around, inter alia, the potential need to further amend the instrument.[6]

69.2.3 The Framework Convention on Tobacco Control

The WHO Framework Convention on Tobacco Control (FCTC) was adopted by the World Health Assembly on 21 May 2003 to combat the global tobacco epidemic and came into force on 27 February 2005.[7] It is almost universal in membership as it counts, at the time of writing, 182 States Parties. Under its Article 3, the FCTC establishes a general normative framework for the adoption of tobacco control measures at the national, regional and international level in order "to reduce continually and substantially the prevalence of tobacco use and exposure to tobacco smoke". It is complemented by a Protocol to Eliminate Illicit Trade in Tobacco Products, adopted in 2012 and entered into force in 2018.

69.3 Global Health and International Human Rights

Human rights enshrined at the international level are a key legal component for the improvement of the "physical and mental well-being" of all persons. These rights constitute obligations for states towards their own populations and, under certain circumstances, towards people beyond their territories. While a number of international human rights instruments exist, two thematic instruments stand out in terms of their multilateral reach: the International Covenant on Economic, Social and Cultural Rights[8]; and the International Covenant on Civil and Political Rights.[9] These two international treaties do not have universal validity, as there are notable absent countries in each of them. Nevertheless, they are in force across most of the planet, with both

[6] An intergovernmental process was established in 2022 to consider potential targeted amendments to the instrument, for consideration in May 2024 (decision WHA75 (9) (27 May 2022) 'Strengthening WHO preparedness for and response to health emergencies').

[7] WHO Framework Convention on Tobacco Control (adopted 21 May 2003, entered into force 27 February 2005) 2302 UNTS 166.

[8] Currently with 171 states parties. See https://indicators.ohchr.org

[9] Currently with 173 states parties. Ibid.

instruments combined encompassing the vast majority of the world population.

69.3.1 The International Covenant on Economic, Social and Cultural Rights

The clearest formulation on obligations towards the population of a country is found in Article 12 of the International Covenant on Economic, Social and Cultural Rights. The first paragraph of this provision affirms every person's right to "the enjoyment of the highest attainable standard of physical and mental health". The contents of this right are further fleshed out by the provision's second paragraph, which refers to the inclusion of policies to: reduce the rates of stillbirths and infant mortality as well as the healthy development of the child; improve environmental and industrial hygiene; prevent, control and treat epidemic and endemic (i.e. communicable), occupational and other diseases; and creating conditions ensuring access to medical services for treating "sickness".

The contents of the right to health were further interpreted by the United Nations Committee on Economic, Social and Cultural Rights, an authoritative body with the mandate to clarify what obligations entail for national authorities. Importantly, General Comment 14 formulated four criteria that healthcare services must comply with, namely: availability, accessibility, acceptability and quality. It is worth underscoring that these obligations apply to all healthcare providers, and not just those directly run by states.

69.3.2 The International Covenant on Civil and Political Rights

The International Covenant on Civil and Political Rights foresees a number of rights which can lead to fostering the improvement of people's health. The clearest example is the right to life, enshrined in its Article 6. The protection of human life necessarily requires upholding health. Thus, in its General Comment No. 36, the United Nations Human Rights Committee, tasked with interpreting the Covenant, included multiple aspects of access to medical services as an essential component of the right to life.

By contrast, several civil and political rights are linked to the protection of human health in a contingent manner, that is, depending on certain circumstances. For instance, protecting health during communicable disease pandemics may require restricting individual liberties related to free movement and assembly, particularly through the adoption of non-pharmaceutical interventions. To the extent these measures may be considered necessary to mitigate the spread of the disease, the public health justification will be key in determining whether restrictions are justified from a legal perspective.

69.4 International Drug Control

There are also international law rules applicable to the production, trade or traffic and use of substances which are both necessary for medical research and products, as well as harmful when they are misused. The need to regulate the international traffic of such substances led to the creation of three separate Conventions: the Single Convention on Narcotic Drugs of 1961—amended through a Protocol in 1972—the Convention on Psychotropic Substances of 1973 and the Convention Against Illicit Traffic in Narcotic Drugs and Psychotropic Substances of 1988. These conventions establish, under their Preambles, obligations to limit the production, traffic or trade and use of such substances throughout countries, to the amount strictly necessary for "medical and scientific use".

The three Conventions on drug control encompass substances considered to pose the highest risk of abuse at the time of their adoption, which are divided across schedules with varying degrees of stringent regulation. The provisions in force allow for flexibility in adding new substances not foreseen at the moment of the drafting of the text or, as in the case of cannabis, to be moved from one schedule to another one. The consequence of such reclassification can pave the way to laxer or more stringent policies for monitoring the use of these substances in a given country.

The Single Convention on Narcotic Drugs has multiple provisions on cannabis, coca leaf and opium, while including other derivates thereof. The Convention on Psychotropic Substances envisages very similar commitments with regard to a list of chemical precursors. Lastly, the United Nations Convention Against Illicit Traffic in Narcotic Drugs and Psychotropic Substances mandates states to impose harsher criminal law sanctions on illicit activities related to substances falling within the purview of all three Conventions.

The monitoring of the implementation of states' commitments in the Conventions is undertaken by the United Nations Office on Drugs and Crime. This body reports on both the volume in known traffic and overall trends in the abuse of substances. In 2016, legal obligations in these three Conventions were the subject of debates at the United Nations General Assembly on whether punitive approaches are well suited to control the use and abuse of these substances. So far, however, efforts at global reform have fallen short.

69.5 Conclusions

The legal instruments referred to in this chapter tackle the protection and improvement of human health as their object and purpose. Nevertheless, other health concerns may be found in other fields of law. An example is the norms on patent protection under the Paris Convention for the Protection of Industrial Property of 1883, within the framework of the World Intellectual Property Organization; and the World Trade Organization's Agreement on Trade-Related Aspects of Intellectual Property Rights (TRIPS). These two international law instruments, among other regional agreements, determine access to new medicines and other medical technologies, which may be protected under a patent granting its holder a monopoly over "making, using, offering for sale, selling, or importing" the product in question. Addressing these legal frameworks is inevitable in the calculation of how to expand access to healthcare products subjected to intellectual property rules.

As the COVID-19 pandemic has elicited legal reform processes at the WHO and beyond, questions on the role of international law in achieving better health outcomes have taken centre stage. In that endeavour, the ambitious definition of health in the Preamble of the Constitution of the WHO still resonates more than seven decades after its adoption. Meaningful ways forward must pay heed to how rights of, and obligations for states under international law can shift discourses and practices at the national level.

Further Reading

Beigbeder Y. L' Organisation mondiale de la santé. Paris: PUF; 1997.

Boister N, Jelsma M. Inter se modification of the UN drug control conventions. An exploration of its applicability to legitimize the legal regulation of cannabis markets. Int Comm Law Rev. 2018;20:456–92.

Burci GL, Toebes B, editors. Global Health Law, Elgar research handbook. Cheltenham: Elgar; 2018.

Burci GL, Vignes C-H. The World Health Organization. The Hague: Kluwer Law International; 2004.

Fidler DP. From International Sanitary Conventions to Global Health Security: The New International Health Regulations. Chin J Int Law. 2005;4:325–92.

Gostin L. Global Health Law. Cambridge: Harvard University Press; 2014.

Gostin L, Meier BM, editors. Foundations of Global Health & Human Rights. Oxford: Oxford University Press; 2020.

Solomon SA. Instruments of Global Health Governance at the World Health Organization. In: Kickbusch I, Lister G, Told M, Drager N, editors. Global Health Diplomacy. Concepts, Issues, Actors, Instruments, Fora and Cases. New York: Springer; 2013. p. 187–98.

United Nations. United Nations Commentary on the Single Convention on Narcotic Drugs, 1961; Commentary on the Convention on Psychotropic Substances, 1976; United Nations Convention against Illicit Traffic in Narcotic Drugs and Psychotropic Substances, 1988.

United Nations Committee on Economic, Social and Cultural Rights. General Comment No. 14: The Right to the Highest Attainable Standard of Health (Art. 12), adopted at the Twenty-second Session of the Committee on Economic, Social and Cultural Rights. 2000. (Contained in Document E/C.12/2000/4).

United Nations, Human Rights Committee. General Comment No. 36, Article 6: The Right to Life, Adopted by the Committee at its 124th session. 2018. (CCPR/C/GC/36).

Advocacy and Communication in Global Health

70

Bettina Borisch and Francesco Rio

Abstract

Advocacy has been recognized as one of the four most important enabler functions for the implementation of Public Health measures. Advocacy tools are well known but not always applied. Advocacy comes into action when a need for health improvement is recognized. On the basis of knowledge and evidence advocacy argues in favour of a cause or policy. This will frequently involve change. At the Global Health level, advocacy will interact with states, supra-national organizations, and corporates as well as civil society.

Keywords

Global health advocacy · Health communication · Health promotion · Social media · Health diplomacy

70.1 Introduction

Advocacy and communication are critical components of global health. They are essential for building awareness, understanding, and support for health-related issues and for promoting policies and programs that can improve health outcomes. In this chapter, we will explore the role of advocacy and communication in global health and discuss the key strategies and tactics that are used to effectively communicate and advocate for global health issues. Advocacy in global health refers to the process of raising awareness and building support for health-related issues and policies. It involves identifying key stakeholders, building coalitions and partnerships, and developing and communicating effective messages. Advocacy can be used to influence policies and programs at the local, national, and global levels, and it is a critical tool for promoting health equity and addressing the needs of marginalized populations. In the context of Global Health (GH), communication has the aim to promote and improve the health of individuals, communities, and the society as a whole. GH communication deals mostly with global health issues directly related to human behaviour, which is at the core of many public health challenges. But the global level also includes communication at supra-national levels as well as communication using the multilateral system—both the UN organization as well as NGOs and Global Foundations.

Recognition of the multiple level complexity of human behaviour modification and the challenges addressing it in global settings is it critical in addressing global health communication implementation. The levels of both individual

B. Borisch (✉)
Université de Genève, Geneva, Switzerland
e-mail: bettina.borisch@unige.ch

F. Rio
World Health Organization, Geneva, Switzerland

M. C. B. Raviglione et al. (eds.), *Global Health Essentials*, Sustainable Development Goals Series,
https://doi.org/10.1007/978-3-031-33851-9_70

and structural modifications are to be targeted. These basic requirements have been declared at the first International Conference on Health Promotion, "health promotion is the process of enabling people to increase control over, and to improve, their health. To reach a state of complete physical, mental, and social well-being, an individual or group must be able to identify and to realize aspirations, to satisfy needs, and to change or cope with the environment. Health is, therefore, seen as a resource for everyday life, not the objective of living. Health is a positive concept emphasizing social and personal resources, as well as physical capacities. Therefore, health promotion is not just the responsibility of the health sector, but goes beyond healthy life-styles to well-being" [1]. This means for global health communication that these different levels have to be tackled—communication on the institutional structural level will include advocacy.

Effective health communication is relevant to increase health risk perception at individual and collective level. The community level may be the workplace, the regional group or even the larger national group of concerned people. Following the then created awareness, health communication should then reinforce/encourage behaviours leading to better health; this is best done with the establishment of new social norms, creation of enabling structures and the overall usage of a health positive narrative. Health Communication can then help advocate for the availability of services and other forms of support. As pointed out in the Ottawa Charter, the empowerment of the individual and its group is key to change their health conditions.

70.2 Strategies and Tools Used in Advocacy and Communication in Global Health

There are several main strategies and tools that are used in advocacy and communication in global health. To build up a strategy, the prerequirements is to have the vision, the goal, and the evidence that supports it. Then, tools will be used according to the respective case. One important tool is to build coalitions and partnerships. This can involve working with other organizations and groups to raise awareness and build support for health-related issues. For example, organizations that work on issues related to maternal and child health may partner with organizations that work on issues related to women's rights and education to build a broader coalition of support.

Another tool is to use multiple channels to communicate and advocate for health-related issues. This can include using traditional media such as television and newspapers, as well as newer forms of media such as social media and mobile phone technology. It is important to use multiple channels because it can reach a wider audience and different audiences may prefer different type of communication channels. It needs to tackle the difficult to reach parts of population in particular.

For certain audiences, it is good to use evidence-based data and research to support advocacy and communication efforts. This can involve using data to demonstrate the impact of a particular health issue or to show the effectiveness of a particular policy or program in other places/countries. By using data, it can help to build support for a particular issue and also to make a stronger case for a policy change.

It is always important to engage with and empower communities. This can involve working with communities to identify and address health-related issues and to build support for policies and programs that can improve health outcomes. Community engagement can also help to build local capacity to address health-related issues, and it can help to ensure that policies and programs are responsive to the needs of local communities.

70.3 Areas of Global Health Communication

Research in five major areas of health communication inquiry have generated strong evidence demonstrating that strategic health communication can help reduce health risks, incidence, morbidity, and mortality and improve the quality of life. Large number of health determinants cross boarders globalization enhances the phenomenon, and therefore global health communication will eventually extend to health diplomacy. The latter can be defined both as a system of organization and as communication and negotiation processes that shape the global policy environment in the sphere of health and its determinants. Other areas include the (1) communication in the delivery of care—interpersonal and group communication, intercultural communication, verbal/nonverbal communication and organizational communication; (2) the communication in health promotion—mass communication, journalism, strategic communication, and health campaign communication; (3) health risk communication—environmental communication, public affairs, international communication, intercultural communication, journalism, strategic communication, and campaign communication; (4) e-health communication—computer-mediated communication, digital communication, information sciences, media studies, journalism, and strategic communication; (5) communication in managing health care systems—organizational communication, group communication, public relations, and strategic communication; (6) health diplomacy—ways to communicate and advocate for political action to negotiate long-term agreements for health and global collective action.

70.4 The Importance of Engaging Stakeholders: Major Players in Global Health Governance Advocacy

As defers from the complexity of GH communication, this task needs the collaboration of several stakeholders. Involvement of stakeholders, including governments, funding agencies, health services providers, and civil society is crucial to the success of any GH communication policy design and implementation. In the ever-changing GH governance, the "classical" part is located in the UN-system's multilateral organization. First and foremost, of all the World Health Organization (WHO) itself but in addition all the UN organizations that also pertain to health. Examples are the World Intellectual Property Organization (WIPO), the International Labor Office (ILO), and many others more including intergovernmental organizations outside the UN system. A lot of the agenda setting and consequently communication in GH is now in the hands of big funding agencies, some of which can be classified as charity capitalism. Due to their financial power, they dominate the discourse and the communication and governance particularly in some smaller countries with weak health care systems. The private sector (including some think tanks) and public–private partnerships have a crucial influence on global health but play a more hidden role in the global health governance. Academia and their institutions and journals are important knowledge providers for GH communication. On another level plays the civil society organizations (CSO) and their diverse non-governmental organization (NGOs). NGOs reach from pure humanitarian-aid to clear advocacy-oriented groups. The interactions between governments, UN agencies, and the CSO/NGOs world are yet to be clarified. Securing involvement of civil society and communities in the response and ensuring inclusive and accessible health care, especially for the most marginalized and vulnerable populations, can never be emphasized enough. It remains a challenging task to really include the populations most concerned into the multi-stakeholder activities. In places with strong health care systems, the service providers themselves are an important voice and can both be partners to promote or hinder global health. In privately managed health care, they may be a decisive factor in the lobby work with governments and supra-national institutions. Lastly, the role of the rule of law, the influence of lawmakers and legal experts is underestimated when it comes to GH communication. All these groups are major players in GH advocacy—where a last global actor is the broad world of media. These are the classical medias as well as the social media and further forms of communication. The newly identified "infodemic" that parallels the COVID-pandemic is a demonstration of their power in GH communication.

70.4.1 Media Representation: Social Media

With the growth of social networking in health care and the rising influence of social media on individual health care, social media is attracting the attention of researchers, clinicians, health care organizations, and policymakers intrigued by its affordability, influence, and virtually universal reach.

Social media hold a great potential in disseminating health-related information as they provide the public, patients, and health professionals with a platform to exchange on different health matters potentially affecting population health outcome and so be used in GH communication. Prerequisite is that their usage does not increase inequity among groups or discriminates parts of populations.

In conclusion, advocacy and communication are critical components of global health. They are essential for building awareness, understanding, and support for health-related issues and for promoting policies and programs that can improve health outcomes. To be effective, advocacy and communication strategies must be tailored to the specific audience and use evidence-based data, multiple channels and engage with communities. The role of advocacy and communication in global health is crucial for creating a more equitable, efficient, and effective health system.

References

1. The Ottawa Charter for Health Promotion, https://www.who.int/teams/health-promotion/enhanced-wellbeing/firstglobal-conference (accessed 02708/2023).

Further Reading

Abdalla SM, Solomon H, Trinquart L, et al. What is considered as global health scholarship? A meta-knowledge analysis of global health journals and definitions. BMJ Glob Health. 2020;5:e002884.

Centers for Disease Control and Prevention. Gateway to Health Communication: Health Communication Basics. n.d. https://www.cdc.gov/healthcommunication/healthbasics/index.html.

Charalambous A. Social media and health policy. Asia Pac J Oncol Nurs. 2019;6(1):24–7. https://doi.org/10.4103/apjon.apjon_60_18. PMID: 30599012; PMCID: PMC6287377

Conrad PA, Meek LA, Dumit J. Operationalizing a one health approach to global health challenges. Comp Immunol Microbiol Infect Dis. 2013;36(3):211–6, ISSN 0147-9571,. https://doi.org/10.1016/j.cimid.2013.03.006.

Kickbusch I, Kökeny M. Bull World Health Organ. 2013;91:159–159A. https://doi.org/10.2471/BLT.13.118596.

Kreps GL. The value of health communication scholarship: new directions for health communication inquiry. Int J Nurs Sci. 2020;7(Suppl 1):S4–7. Published 2020 May 30

Nutbeam D, Kickbusch I. Health promotion glossary. Health Promot Int. 1998;13(4):349–64.

WHO. Communicating for health. WHO strategic Framework for effective communications. n.d. https://www.who.int/about/communications.

Yale News Ten Principles to Strengthen Global Health. n.d. https://news.yale.edu/2010/12/22/ten-principles-strengthen-global-health.

Part X

New Visions in the Era of Sustainable Development

From MDGs to SDGs

71

Emanuela Parotto and Ariel Pablos-Méndez

Abstract

The United Nations (UN) Millennium Development Goals (MDGs) set out eight goals by the target date of 2015 aimed at reducing poverty, improving health of women and children and promoting education, gender equality, environmental sustainability and global partnerships. Although the MDGs achieved positive results mobilizing attention to important and neglected global issues, they have been criticized for their "one-size-fits all" approach for all countries. As the MDGs era came to a close in 2015, a new UN Agenda established 17 Sustainable Development Goals (SDGs) by 2030. The SDGs formulation engaged many stakeholders and provides a broader approach to sustainability, considering the three development pillars (economic, social and environmental) for people, planet, prosperity, peace and partnership. Despite the well-documented negative impact of the COVID-19 pandemic on their achievement, the post-pandemic strategies could offer new opportunities to strengthen the SDGs path and to satisfy the 2030 Agenda.

E. Parotto (✉)
Departmental Unit in Anesthesia and Intensive Care in Complex Surgery and Transplant Surgery, Azienda Ospedale Università, Padua, Italy

A. Pablos-Méndez
Division of General Medicine, Columbia University Medical Centre, New York, NY, USA

Keywords

Human development · Sustainability · Millennium development goals · Sustainable development goals · COVID-19 pandemic impact

71.1 Aim of the Chapter

The aim of this chapter is to explore the transition from Millennium Development Goals (MDGs) to Sustainable Development Goals (SDGs). The first section covers the MDGs, the context in which they were developed and their achievements and limitations. In the second section the chapter describes the SDGs, and the third section discusses the transition from MDGs to SDGs and the impact of COVID-19.

71.2 Millennium Development Goals (MDGs)

The formulation of Millennium Development Goals (MDGs) originated during the 1990s, when the world agenda for economic and social development was redefined following the end of the cold war [1]. There was an increasing need to redefine the meaning, goals and measurements for development. The concept of "human development" was adopted to underline the basic

M. C. B. Raviglione et al. (eds.), *Global Health Essentials*, Sustainable Development Goals Series,
https://doi.org/10.1007/978-3-031-33851-9_71

objective "to create an enabling environment for people to enjoy long, healthy and creative lives" [2].

The Millennium Summit was a meeting of 191 world leaders, from 6 to 8 September 2000, held at the United Nations (UN) headquarters in New York City to ratify the Millennium Declaration and the MDGs for 2015. The declaration aimed at reaffirming a human-based development approach to overcome the narrow paradigm of growth and to focus on human, sustainable and fair welfare [1]. The MDGs set out 8 goals (Fig. 71.1) with different targets (18 total targets) by 2015 and specific indicators (48 total indicators) to monitor progress from 1990 levels. The MDGs mobilized attention to important but neglected global issues and achieved much progress. Globally, the number of people living in extreme poverty and undernourished declined by more than half in 2015. The under-five mortality rate declined from 90 to 43 deaths per 1000 live births between 1990 and 2015 and maternal mortality dropped by 45 per cent worldwide. The primary school net enrolment rate reached 91 per cent in 2015. Most significantly, the MDGs made huge progresses in fighting HIV/AIDS, malaria and tuberculosis and reducing mortality by nearly half [3]. As a result, the median life expectancy in the world surpassed 70 years. The MDGs also recognized the importance of a global partnership with high-income nations reforming their domestic and international policies related to agriculture, trade and sustainable development; enhancing the effectiveness of their aid programs and helping poor countries reduce their debt burdens [4].

The MDGs agenda has been criticized on various points. With respect to the process of formulation and implementation, the MDGs were formulated by a small group of experts without wide consultation or stakeholders engagement. The resulting agenda excluded important dimensions of development such as governance, climate change and human right. The goals took a "one-size-fits all" approach for all countries despite hugely divergent starting points, financial resources and capacities, and followed an aid-centric approach focused on low-income countries. Further, MDGs represent the apex of an extremely "vertical" approach to health interventions neglecting health systems and ignoring the non-linearity of progress [5]. Finally, it was hard to assess the health MDGs because the most basic life indicators, such as births and deaths, are not directly registered in the poorest countries [5].

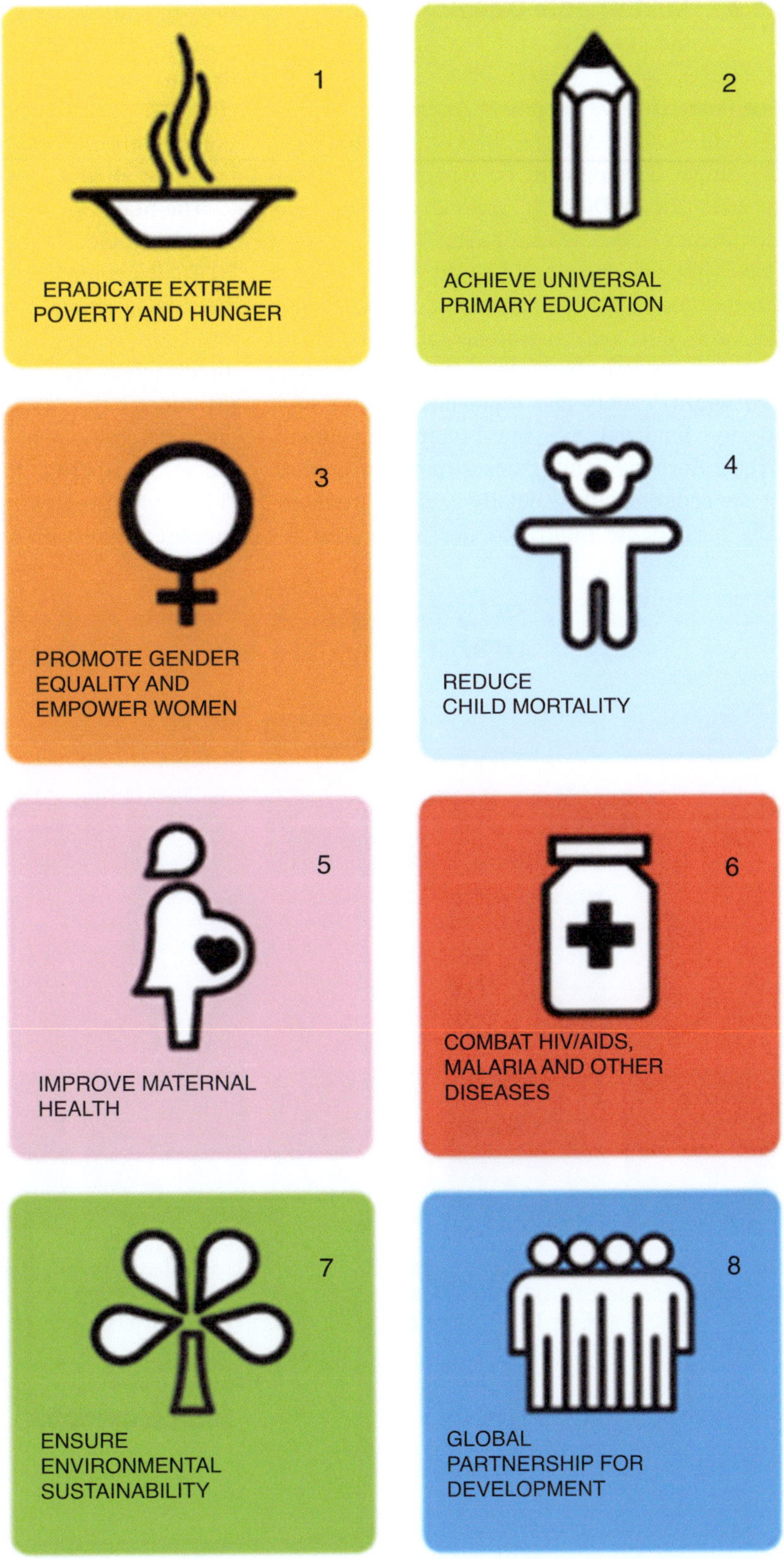

Fig. 71.1 The United Nations (UN) Millennium Development Goals (MDGs) [3] (this figure is published with the permission of the United Nations Development Programs, UNDP)

71.3 Sustainable Development Goals (SDGs)

The Post-2015 Development Agenda was a process led by the UN from 2012 to 2015 to define the global development framework that would succeed the MDGs. It started with the UN Conference on Sustainable Development (UNCSD), also known as Rio 2012, Rio + 20 or Earth Summit 2012, and it aimed at reconciling the economic and environmental goals of the global community. By the end of the Conference, 193 world leaders and representatives of civil society finalized the non-binding document, "The Future We Want", "ensuring the promotion of an economically, socially and environmentally sustainable future for our planet and for present and future generations" [6]. The conference ignited an intergovernmental process which led to the 17 SDGs and their 169 targets (Fig. 71.2); this time health got only one direct goal to "ensure healthy lives and promote well-being for all at all ages".

The SDGs are a universal call to action to end poverty, protect the planet, and ensure that by 2030 all people enjoy peace and prosperity [7]. The SDGs are strongly linked to the "Triple bottom Line" concept of balancing interests in three dimensions: economy, social and environment [8]. Indeed, the SDGs embrace all dimensions of human development and sustainability: People, Planet, Prosperity, Peace and Partnership (the "Five Ps"); progress on one P must balance and support progress on others [9].

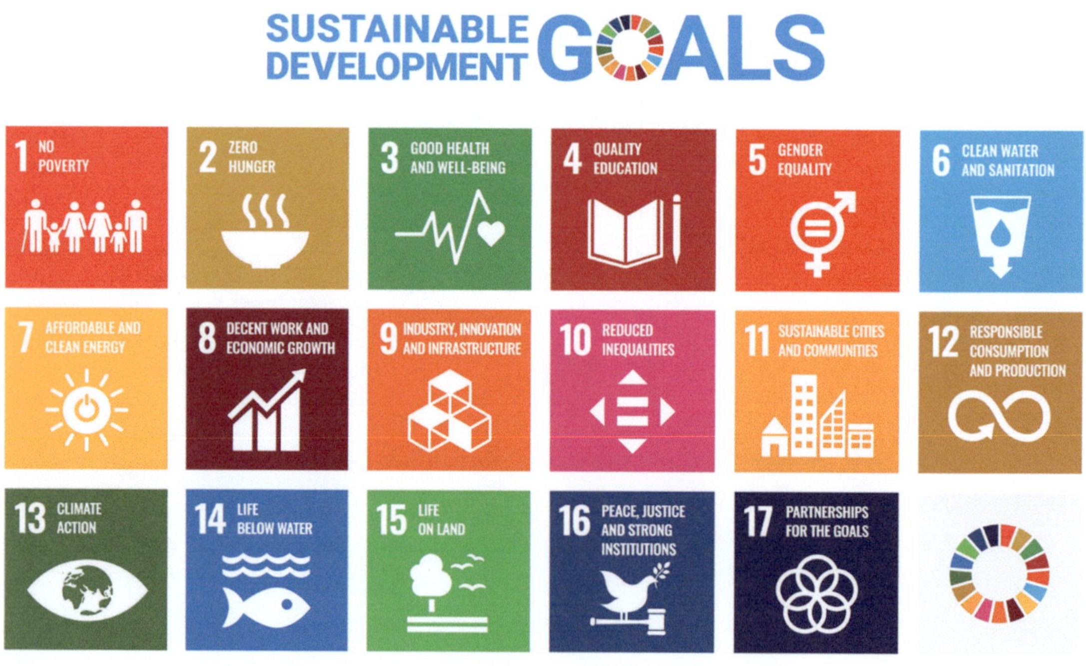

Fig. 71.2 The United Nations (UN) Sustainable Development Goals (SDGs) [11] (this figure is published with the permission of the UN. The content of this book chapter has not been approved by the United Nations and does not reflect the views of the United Nations or its officials or Member States)

71.4 Transition from MDGs to SDGs and the Impact of COVID-19

The formulation of the MDGs was largely development-oriented, led by development champions and motivated to increase international aid. In general, they achieved positive results in poverty reduction, gender disparity, school education, health-related goals, access to drinking water and mobilization of financial resources of global partnership. On the other hand, MDGs have not succeeded in decreasing the malnourished population, sanitation or environmental sustainability, and the "one-size-fits-all" approach prevented implementing plans from global to national and local levels, leading to a significant achievements' variability among different countries. The SDGs were built on the development success of the MDGs taking a broader stakeholder engagement and the blessing of governments at the planning stage and addressing the economic, social and ecologic domains of sustainable development. They set universal goals for both developing and developed countries, including issues such as climate change, human rights, human security targets to be tailored at regional, national or local levels [8]. Domestic resource mobilization and country ownership will be a hallmark of the SDGs.

Given measurement delays and lag time to results, the first SDGs reports to the UN were still early when the COVID-19 pandemic arrived and the evolving global crisis will exert a deep impact on the ability to deliver in the intended timescales, creating large uncertainties about their achievement at planetary level [10]. COVID-19 has not only stopped work towards some of these goals but has largely shifted the immediate focus of governments and international agencies involved to dealing with the imminent havoc of the pandemic. The global recession caused by COVID-19 was accompanied by a retrocession in the SDGs achievements, with some disarray in functioning of political systems (SDG 16) and partnerships (SDG 17) [10].

The UN SDGs Report 2021 gave a sobering assessment of the 2030 Agenda: the global poverty rate is projected to be 7%, missing the SDG1 target of eradicating poverty; world hunger and child malnutrition are worsening, with an additional 70–161 million people experiencing hunger. The pandemic has shortened life expectancy, stalling or reversing progresses obtained in maternal health, child health and reproductive health; deaths from tuberculosis are increasing after decades declining [11]. The implications concerning school and education are catastrophic, with 101 million children falling below the minimum reading proficiency threshold. Women have faced increased domestic violence, child marriage is projected to rise again, and job losses and underpaid work are increasing. The pandemic is exacerbating existing inequalities within and among countries. Notwithstanding the global economic slowdown, concentrations of major greenhouse gases continue to increase.

Although the COVID-19 pandemic threatened the SDG's achievement, the challenges could lead to an open transformation. After an MDGs era propelled by globalization, a new era will see greater political demand for social protection by governments [12]. Post-pandemic strategies should create synergies across several SDGs simultaneously, strengthening social protection systems and public services (including health systems, education, water and sanitation and other basic services); increasing investments in science, technology and innovation (including improvement of data and information systems) and investing in clean energy and industry [10]. In the context of COVID-19 pandemic crisis, sustaining Universal Health Coverage (UHC) emerges as a critical step to build resilient health systems and to promote more inclusive and fairer societies [13].

71.5 Conclusions

In 2015, the MDGs came to a close and the success of the UN formula energized a more ambitious post-2015 agenda with 17 goals and scores of targets. The SDGs formulation engaged many stakeholders and provides a broader approach to sustainability, considering the three development pillars (economic, social and environmental) for people, planet, prosperity, peace and partnership.

The SDGs achievement is threatened by the aftermath of COVID-19; despite the well-documented negative impact of the pandemic, the SDGs framework offers the best path to satisfy the 2030 agenda and the post-pandemic strategies could offer new opportunities to strengthen the system interactions of the SDGs and achieve the world we want.

References

1. Missoni E, Pacileo G, Tediosi F. Global Health Governance and Policy: an introduction. 1st ed. England: Routledge; 2019. p. 11–20.
2. United Nations. Human development report 1990. Published for the United Nations (New York) Development Programme. New York: Oxford University Press; 1990. p. 10.
3. United Nations. The Millennium Development Goals Report 2015. New York: United Nations Development Programme. UNDP; 2022. https://www.undp.org/publications/millennium-development-goals-report-2015.
4. Wilkinson R, Hulme D, editors. The millennium development goals and beyond: global development after 2015. London: Routledge; 2012. p. 288.
5. Vandemoortele J. The MDG Story: Intention Denied. In: Development and change, vol. 42; 2011. p. 1–21.
6. Environment UN. Rio+20 outcome document the future we want. UNEP-UN Environment Programme. 2017. http://www.unep.org/resources/report/rio20-outcome-document-future-we-want.
7. Dpi campaigns. Take action for the sustainable development goals [Internet]. United Nations Sustainable Development. 2022. https://www.un.org/sustainabledevelopment/sustainable-development-goals/.
8. WHO. Health in 2015: from MDGs to SDGs [Internet]. 2022. https://www.who.int/publications-detail-redirect/9789241565110.
9. Elkington J. Partnerships from cannibals with forks: the triple bottom line of 21st-century business. Environ Qual Manag. 1998;8(1):37–51.
10. Fenner R, Cernev T. The implications of the Covid-19 pandemic for delivering the sustainable development goals. Futures. 2021 Apr;128:102726.
11. UN. SDG Indicators [Internet]. 2022. https://unstats.un.org/sdgs/report/2021/.
12. Pablos-Méndez A, Raviglione MC. A New World health era. Glob Health Sci Pract. 2018;6(1):8–16.
13. Pablos-Mendez A, Cavanaugh K, Ly C. The new era of health goals: universal health coverage as a pathway to the sustainable development goals. Health Syst Reform. 2016;2(1):15–7.

Globalization, Socio-Economic Development, and Health

72

Eduardo Missoni

Abstract

Globalization is described as the growing interconnection between human societies beyond geographical boundaries, at increasing speed and impact on ideas, culture, and behaviours. Global health policies have been associated to development strategies, and the idea itself of "development" has been "colonized" becoming a metaphor of economic growth. The neoliberal ideas and policies increased inequalities worldwide concentrating wealth in the hands of small sectors. Those ideas also affected the definition, consistency and sustainability of the development agenda 2030. Counter-hegemonic processes are needed in defence of the sovereignty of local communities with human and ecosystem's health as the new indicator of "development".

Keywords

Globalization · Global health policy · Health determinants · International politics · Health and development

E. Missoni (✉)
SDA Bocconi Management School, Bocconi University, Milan, Italy
e-mail: Eduardo.missoni@unibocconi.it

72.1 Introduction

In its essential meaning, Global Health (GH) is inherently linked to the "effects of globalization on health" and the interactions of global determinants (including political, economic, social, cultural, and ecosystemic) with national and local systems [1].

Globalization can be understood as the growing interconnection between human societies beyond geographical and political boundaries, whereby the acceleration of those processes, mainly mediated by technological progress on the one side and the expansion of capitalism and market economy, have been the characterizing features since the second half of the twentieth century [1]. Development instinctively associated with human progress and a positive social and economic transformation to eradicate historical injustices, has instead become a metaphor of economic growth. Economics prevailed over all other aspects of life and well-being influencing the international "development" agenda and the establishment of an unsustainable growth society with severe impact on ecosystems and human health.

In this chapter, an overview is presented of the links between globalization, development, and health.

M. C. B. Raviglione et al. (eds.), *Global Health Essentials*, Sustainable Development Goals Series,
https://doi.org/10.1007/978-3-031-33851-9_72

72.2 Three Interconnected Dimensions of Globalization

As a result of globalization, social relations have undergone transformations in three essential dimensions: space, temporal, and cognitive [2].

The transformation of the **spatial dimension** refers to changes in the way people interact in physical and territorial space. Information and communication technology allowed for the creation of virtual communities and social networks no matter an individual's location. The concept of geographical boundaries becomes increasingly blurred. In a licit or illicit way, people, money, technology, goods, information, ideas, pollution, but also vectors and etiologic agents of diseases easily cross these boundaries.

Alongside the traditional international community of Nation States, powerful non-state transnational actors, both private entities (businesses, foundations, non-governmental organizations, social movements) and hybrids (multi-stakeholder alliances, initiatives, and public-private partnership organizations), contribute to modifying the world's power and governance structures (see Chap. 62). They all play a role in influencing policies and decision-making processes, previously an exclusive prerogative of international, i.e. intergovernmental institutions [1].

In its **temporal dimension**, globalization affected the use and value of time [2]. Our lives are moving at speeds we have never experienced before and so does our consumption and waste production. Pollution and climate change reflect the acceleration of global transformation processes. Equally, the spread of communicable diseases across national boundaries is achieved with unprecedented speed, thanks to population mobility and the speed of transport.

Finally, the **cognitive dimension** concerns change in the production and exchange of knowledge, ideas, laws, beliefs, values, cultural identities, and other mental processes that define our ability to interpret reality [2].

Financed, dominated, and often literally colonized by the market and the few hegemonic interconnected global forces behind it, too often mass media, educational institutions, expert committees, scientists, consulting companies, and communication experts all serve this transformation [2]. Globalized behaviours are part of the daily life of the vast majority of world population. Global brands became an integral part of daily life [3]. Global health policies are not exempt of these influences, and there is an increasing quest for their "decolonization". Indeed, they have been associated to development strategies, and the idea itself of "development" equally needs to be decolonized [4].

72.3 Development

In the aftermath of World War II, "development" emerged as a new discourse serving the emerging power of the USA to justify the dismantling of colonial empires and gain access to new markets [5]. "A bold new program" for the "improvement and growth of underdeveloped areas" would contribute to the expansion of US commerce [6].

Development became the universal ideal that should guide the progress of the "underdeveloped" world, i.e. "economically backward regions". The term "development" became a metaphor of economic growth measured through the increase of the gross domestic product (GDP), and economics towered over all other aspects of life and well-being. Conceived in technocratic and quantitative terms, "development" soon became "the password for imposing a new kind of dependency, for enriching the already rich world and for shaping other societies to meet its commercial and political needs" [7].

The evidence of the quantitative restraints of the ecosystem and the "limits to growth" were authoritatively pointed out since the early 1970s by a Club of Rome commissioned report. Despite the call for "a fundamental revision of human behavior and, by implication, of the entire fabric of present-day society" to avoid "the tragic consequences of an overshoot" [8], growth has been considered the most desirable effect of "development" and has been converted into a "global faith" [5].

Neoliberal ideas, championed in the 1980s by the Reagan Administration in the USA and the Thatcher Government in Great Britain and fostered by the International Monetary Fund (IMF) and the World Bank (WB) further emphasized the dominion of the market, promoted the reduced role of the State and the removal of every barrier blocking any market penetration. Neoliberal structural adjustment policies (SAPs) initially imposed to developing countries were later globalized, especially after the fall of the Berlin wall and following economic crises. They came with large-scale privatizations, reduced taxation for the benefit of higher incomes, cuts in public spending and the dismantling of education, health and social systems, the financial deregulation and the free movement of capital, the uncontrolled exploitation of environmental resources and lastly, the export-oriented industrial production. Inequalities grew and wealth concentrated in the hands of small sectors that emerged from the expansion of the economy [1].

In 1987, the Our Common Future Report, led by Dr. Brundtland who would later become WHO's DG, introduced the concept of "sustainable development" defined as: "development that meets the needs of the present without compromising the ability of future generations to meet their own needs" [9]. The report recognized the limits of the biosphere to absorb the effects of human activities, however insisted on technology as the way toward *a new era of economic growth* [9]. Sustainable development was just another masking operation to prevent the radical questioning of the effects of economic growth [5].

New approaches to development were proposed in the 1990s. The seminal work of the Nobel laureate Amartya Sen, inspired UNDP's first annual flagship report in1990 where the concept of "human development" was adopted, questioning economic growth and GDP as efficient indicators of progress. The report stated that "the basic objective of development is to create an enabling environment for people to enjoy long, healthy and creative lives" [10].

In 2000, The Millennium Declaration, signed by all Heads of State and Government proclaimed the "fundamental values" of equality, freedom, solidarity, tolerance, respect for nature and shared responsibility [11]. However, the eight Millennium Development Goals (MDGs) to be reached by 2015, lacked a systemic vision and were focused only on low-income countries.

The development agenda was redefined again in 2015 with the launch of the "Agenda 2030" and its "universal" and "indivisible" 17 Sustainable Development Goals (SDG) [12] (see Chap. 71).

These goals aim to put an end to poverty by 2030, combat inequalities, ensure lasting protection of the planet and its resources, and create the conditions for "shared prosperity", and "sustainable, inclusive and sustained" growth [12]. However, the latter is evidently an oxymoron: sustained growth is not sustainable.

The fundamental contradiction between sustainability and indiscriminate, sustained economic growth led to a vision of "de-growth". An alternative post-growth societal project based on voluntary equitable downscaling of production and consumption that increases human well-being and enhances ecological conditions at the local and global level, counteracting the omnipresence of market-based relations in society [13].

Box 72.1 Degrowth as an Opportunity

"The construction of an alternative society requires the end of the infernal cycle of unlimited growth of needs and products—and of the endless frustration it breeds; it also requires to restrain selfishness, i.e. individualism resulting from massive uniformity. The first objective can be achieved by self-limitation leading to frugal affluence; the second, by the rehabilitation of the spirit of giving and the promotion of conviviality".

"Degrowth is an opportunity, an invitation to find another possible world. It is also an invitation to live in it, here and now, and not just in some hypothetical future which we will probably never know, no matter how attractive it seems. This other world is already part of ours. It is also in us".

(Serge Latouche, Degrowth and the paradoxes of happiness

Annals of the Fondazione Luigi Einaudi. Volume LIV, June 2020: 133–152).

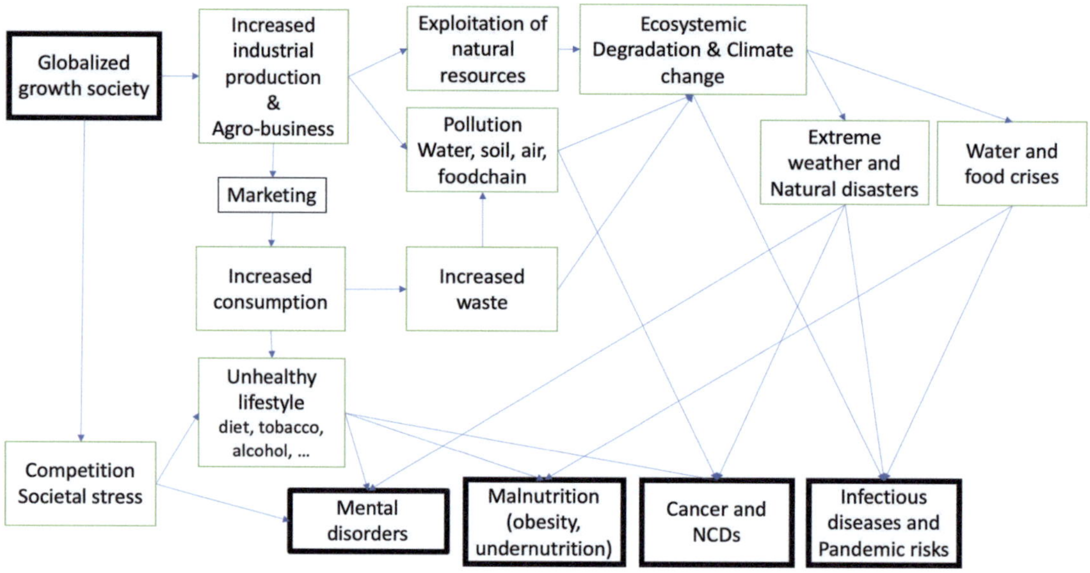

Fig. 72.1 Disease pathways of globalized growth society

That "growth has become humanity's cancer" [4] is not just a metaphor. A direct relation exists between economic growth and the incidence rate of cancer, which increases linearly with per capita income, even after controlling for population ageing, improvement in cancer detection, and omitted spatially correlated variables [14]. Disease pathways of the globalized growth society can be synthetically represented (see Fig. 72.1).

Box 72.2 A Humanity of Humility

We must grow essential needs products, quality products, hygienic products, and degrow the unhealthy products of industrial agriculture, artificial products, and products that are only propelled by advertising but have no intrinsic value. We should account for what must grow and what must degrow […].

As for globalization, we should favour everything that fosters cooperation and culture and, at the same time, be able to partially unglobalize so to save territories, natural environments, and cultures that are under the threat of desertification. We should think the world over […].

Today, one of humanity's big problems is that we are sorcerer's apprentices who created machines that are becoming more powerful than we are and dominate us. We created forces that can annihilate us.

We have become too proud, and we must fall back to a humanity of humility […].

Today we see more and more, especially as part of transhumanism, the pride of human beings who set out to conquer nature at the same time when, because of this pride, they are destroying it.

(Edgar Morin. Uniting the best of Africa and the West. *New African*—17/01/2022)

There is an urgent need to "decolonize our imaginaries" dominated by growth, as a starting point for a paradigmatic shift in the inspiring values of human society [4].

Universal attainment of health, defined as a "complete physical, mental and social wellbeing", goes well beyond healthcare and disease control. It concerns the common "planetary destiny" that all living beings share [15]. Emphasis on "one health" (see Chap. 76) and "planetary health" (see Chap. 77) contribute to reaffirm the health determinants and human rights approach which inspire GH. Nevertheless, global health studies and policymaking must abandon the top-down, colonial, market-based development perspective. Aware of global interconnectedness and power dynamics, "g-local" counter-hegemonic processes are needed in defence of the sovereignty of local communities with human and ecosystem's health as the new indicator of "development".

References

1. Missoni E, Pacileo G, Tediosi F. Global Health Governance and Policy: an introduction. Abingdon: Routledge; 2019.
2. Lee K. Global dimensions of health. In: Parsons L, Lister G, editors. Global Health: a local issue. London: The Nuffield Trust; 2000.
3. Klein N. No logo: taking aim at the brand bullies. Toronto: Knopf Canada; 2000.
4. Latouche S. Farewell to growth. Cambridge: Polity Press; 2010.
5. Rist G. Lo sviluppo. Storia di una credenza occidentale, Torino: Bollati Boringhieri; 1997. (Original title in French: Rist G. Le Dévelopment. Histoire d'une croyance occidental, Paris: Presses de la Fondation Nationale de Sciences Politiques; 1996
6. Truman H. Truman's inaugural address. Washington: Library & Museum; 1949. https://www.trumanlibrary.org/whistlestop/50yr_archive/inagural20jan1949.htm
7. George S. How the other half dies. The real reasons for world hunger. Harmondsworth: Penguin Books; 1976. p. xvii.
8. Meadows DH, et al. The limits to growth: a report for the Club of Rome's project on the predicament of mankind. New York: Universe Books; 1972. p. 185–96.
9. WCED. Our common future. World commission on environment and development. Oxford: Oxford University Press; 1987.
10. UNDP. Human Development Report 1990. Concept and measurement of human development. New York: United Nations Development Program; 1990.
11. UN. United Nations Millennium Declaration, UN document: Resolution A/RES/55/2, 18 September 2000.
12. UN. Transforming our world: the 2030 agenda for sustainable development. New York: United Nations; 2015. https://sustainabledevelopment.un.org/post2015/transformingourworld
13. Demaria F, et al. What is degrowth? From an activist slogan to a social movement. Environ Values. 2013;22(2):191–215.
14. Luzzati T, Parenti A, Rughi T. Economic growth and cancer incidence. Ecol Econ. 2018;146:381–96.
15. Morin E. La Voie. Pour l'avenir de l'humanité. Paris: Librairie Arthème Fayard; 2011.

73 Aiming for Better Health in Cities

Meelan Thondoo and Mark Nieuwenhuijsen

Abstract

Cities are important hubs for economic growth and social advancement but are also hotspots for disease and deaths. Two-thirds of the world's population will live in cities by 2050; therefore, models and strategies to decrease the impacts of urbanization on health are urgently needed. The chapter uses salient urban health pathways to guide reflection on a potential strategic and integrated approach to health in cities. It is relevant to city decision-makers and implementers who are acting on health through different sectors and pathways. Urban populations are at higher risk of falling sick due to existing chronic diseases, lack of physical activity, unhealthy food behaviours, and unequal exposure to socio-economic inequity. The chapter refers to four current models addressing these risks by reducing speed in cities, increasing active travel, green spaces, considering inequity and building strong governance can make cities more healthy, inclusive, and sustainable. Further research is needed on how best to develop new urban models that are relevant to cities of Africa and Asia where urbanization rates are the highest; only then will it be possible for cities to fully achieve their potential in safeguarding health of people and planet.

Keywords

Urbanization · Urban health · Inequity · Climate change · Urban models

73.1 Introduction

The impacts of global urbanization on health are complex. Health challenges in cities are closely interlinked and crosscut many sectors. One action on a particular health problem in a sector can affect others and often in unpredictable ways (see some sectors in Box 73.1). The COVID-19 pandemic has shown how cities responses to health can be fragmented rather than strategic and integrated. Knowledge exchange, collaboration, and communication between health and non-health actors in cities remain scarce. As a result, health is rarely on the urban agenda and non-health actors remain unaware of the health impacts of their decisions and actions. This chapter uses salient urban health pathways to guide reflection on a potential strategic and integrated approach to health in cities. We consider urban health as the field of enquiry examining the linkages between the urban context and the distribution of death and disease within resident populations. This chapter can be helpful to city actors who

M. Thondoo (✉) · M. Nieuwenhuijsen
IS Global Barcelona Institute for Global Health, Barcelona, Spain
e-mail: mark.nieuwenhuijsen@isglobal.org

M. C. B. Raviglione et al. (eds.), *Global Health Essentials*, Sustainable Development Goals Series,
https://doi.org/10.1007/978-3-031-33851-9_73

have reflected on lessons learnt during the recent COVID-19 pandemic, where urban populations were at higher risk of falling sick due to existing chronic diseases, lack of physical activity, unhealthy food behaviours, and unequal exposure to socio-economic inequity.

Box 73.1 Some Sectors of Relevance to Health

Housing	Commercial	Biomass
Food	determinants	burning
systems	Citizen engagement	Energy supply
Violence	Corruption	Waste
Crime	Digitalization	Safe water
Mobility	E-commerce	Sanitation
Care	Migration	Sewage
systems	City/health	Infections
Education	governance,	COVID-19
Drugs	Informal	Public and
Smoking	settlements	private spaces
	Noise	

73.2 Background

Cities are important hubs for economic growth and social advancement but are also hotspots for disease and deaths. Cities cover 3% of the planet, yet emit 78% of all global greenhouse gas emissions, absorb 80% of final global energy, and consume 60% of domestic water [1]. Cities also concentrate on people with higher degrees of vulnerability. These trends will continue as the proportion of urban dwellers will increase to two-thirds of the world's population by 2050 [2]. Evidence shows that unless cities are properly designed to achieve equitable, sustainable, and environmental goals, people will continue to suffer avoidable disease and death. Urban risk factors currently drive a triple health threat in cities: communicable diseases, including infectious diseases like COVID-19, tuberculosis, dengue, and diarrhoea; noncommunicable diseases, including heart disease, stroke, asthma, cancer, diabetes, and depression; and finally, violence and road traffic injuries.

Health risks in cities will remain as 40% of urban populations still do not access adequate sanitation and as an estimated 91% of people in urban areas breathe polluted air. Air pollution kills around 4–9 million people each year, while 3.2 million people die of lack of physical activity and 1.2 million perish in traffic accidents [3]. Poorly designed urban transport systems affect health as private motorization limits access to green spaces and increases barriers to safe physical activity. Finally, cities everywhere face growing risks due to climate disasters that are predicted to increase in severity, frequency, intensity and impact, threatening health through food and water insecurity, water- and vector-borne diseases, malnutrition, decrease in natural resources, and threat to biodiversity.

73.3 Urbanization and Health

Urbanization in cities can affect physical and mental health through a wide range of factors such as polluted water runoff, destruction of green space, non-regulation of motor vehicle use, an increase in accident rates, and intensification of urban heat. Here, we provide a brief review of the different pathways through which urban environments affect health.

Air pollution (AP) increases steadily with urbanization and is one of the greatest environmental risk factors for diseases including pneumonia, asthma, chronic respiratory diseases, stroke, and cardiovascular diseases, across all age groups [4]. AP sources include mass motorization, industry activity, and use of coal for power and heat in homes. Currently, 90% of all deaths in the world occur in poorer countries [2] with an increase in average of deaths across African and Asian regions [5]. An important consideration of air pollution flow is that populations bearing the consequences of exposure can be located far from the original source of emission. For instance, evidence shows that 41–53% of premature mortality in the United States due to air pollution was due to emissions generated in another state [6].

Climate change affects urban health through an increase in temperatures, rise in CO_2 emissions, and extreme weather events. Floods, droughts, and mudslides are affecting people, livelihoods, and access to city services across the globe. The increase in temperatures is also affecting people across the world with 37% of heat-related deaths that is estimated to be attributed to anthropogenic climate change [7]. By 2030, approximately US$4 trillion of assets will be at risk from climate events [8]. Urban areas are particularly vulnerable as they can be more than 5 °F warmer than surrounding areas creating urban heat island effects and causing hospitalization, heat exhaustion, exacerbation of existing health disorder and deaths every year. The need to use cooling technologies and appliances also strains the environment through an increase in pollution and energy use.

The lack of green space and biodiversity has been associated with lower likelihood of physical activity, decreased functional status, higher cardiovascular disease risk, and less longevity among older populations. It is estimated that 60% of the world's population do not have access to green spaces despite evidence of health benefits and potential to save 43,000 lives per year in cities [9]. Currently, only a quarter of all trips in cities are done by car but infrastructure for motorization takes up to 60% of public space. If transport systems are reviewed, this public space can be freed for green areas which would benefit all age groups by providing safe, healthy, sustainable green spaces for transit, work, and play.

Inequity in cities is characterized by informal structures, gentrification, economic disparities, spatial segregation, and post-colonization. These factors highly influence the health of urban populations as they drive unequal levels of exposures and vulnerability to air, noise, and water pollution, toxic substances, sedentary lifestyles, and access to socio-economic opportunities. With bad distribution of income and resources, poverty exacerbates inequity as it is closely correlated with inadequate housing, limited access to health care and decreased social capital. The issue of inequity is particularly relevant for developing countries where between 60 and 94% of urban dwellers live in slums characterized by overcrowded housing, unsafe working conditions, lack of access to clean water and decent sanitation, and social exclusion.

Effective governance is a critical lever for cities to gather autonomy and resources to engage into evidence-based and inclusive policy-making and informed citizenry [10]. Effective governance means that local authorities and national governments can promote sustainable investments, design accessible services, and scale up energy efficiency to the benefit of the people. Equity-driven governance places socially vulnerable groups at the centre of decisions to ensure no-one is left behind. To increase governance, city actors can tap into innovative city networks that are advancing climate action and promoting health through sustainable urban development. Examples include the International Society of Urban Health (ISUH), C40 Climate Leadership Group, WHO Healthy Cities, Local Governments for Sustainability (ICLEI), and United Cities and Local Governments (UCLG). These networks provide tools and resources, best practices, campaigns and technical support for monitoring indicators, evaluating progress and designing policies.

73.4 Approach to Solutions

Multi-sectoral and systemic approaches are needed to address change in cities. We need healthier environments and more resilient populations; therefore, new urban models should be explored (see examples in Table 73.1). Overall, these models show that reducing speed in cities, increasing active travel, green spaces, considering inequity, and building strong governance can make our cities more healthy, inclusive, and sustainable. A crucial step forward is to explore new urban models that are adapted to cities of Africa and Asia where 90% of 2.5 billion urbanites will live by 2050 [11].

Table 73.1 New urban models

New urban model	City of focus	Description
The 15-min city model	Paris	All destinations should be within 15-min walk from residence with access to all services, opportunities, and commodities.
The low-traffic neighbourhoods	London	Places characterized by residential streets, bordered by main or "distributor" roads where "through" motor vehicle traffic is discouraged or removed.
The superblock model	Barcelona	A 400 x 400 m unit aiming to recover space for the community, improve biodiversity, move towards sustainable mobility, and encourage social cohesion.
The car-free neighbourhood	Freiburg	Based on a five-prong transport strategy to extend public transport networks, promote cycling, restrain and channel motor traffic, and manage parking space.

73.5 Main Conclusions

City-level action is a key and strategic opportunity to improve global health and well-being of people and planet. Cities are the main implementers of health-relevant policies across different sectors and can react quickly to social needs. The scale and complexity of urban health challenges means that approaches across sectors and pathways must draw on solid evidence and collaborative strategies. Challenges remain on how best to develop new urban models that are relevant to cities of Africa and Asia where urbanization rates are the highest. Decision-making and actions must focus effective governance to reduce inequities while anticipating future needs. Only then will cities fully achieve their potential to restore and safeguard human health while contributing their share to sustainable development and the long-term conservation of the planet.

References

1. Landrigan PJ, Fuller R, Acosta NJR, et al. The lancet commission on pollution and health. Lancet. 2017;391(10119):462–512.
2. United Nations. World urbanization prospects: the 2014 revision, highlights. Department of Economic and Social Affairs. Population Division, United Nations Published online. 2014.
3. Nieuwenhuijsen MJ, Khreis H, Mueller N, Rojas-Rueda D. Health impact assessment of transport planning and policy. In: Advances in Transportation and Health. Amsterdam: Elsevier; 2020. p. 309–28.
4. Goshua A, Akdis CA, Nadeau KC. World Health Organization global air quality guideline recommendations: executive summary. Allergy. 2022;77(7):1955–60.
5. Southerland VA, Brauer M, Mohegh A, et al. Global urban temporal trends in fine particulate matter (PM2·5) and attributable health burdens: estimates from global datasets. Lancet Planet Health. 2022;6(2):e139–46.
6. Dedoussi IC, Eastham SD, Monier E, Barrett SRH. Premature mortality related to United States cross-state air pollution. Nature. 2020;578(7794):261–5.
7. Vicedo-Cabrera AM, Scovronick N, Sera F, et al. The burden of heat-related mortality attributable to recent human-induced climate change. Nat Clim Chang. 2021;11(6):492–500.
8. Bai X, Dawson RJ, Ürge-Vorsatz D, et al. Six research priorities for cities and climate change. Nature. 2018;555:23.
9. Barboza EP, Cirach M, Khomenko S, et al. Green space and mortality in European cities: a health impact assessment study. Lancet Planet Health. 2021;5(10):e718–30.
10. Tonne C, Adair L, Adlakha D, et al. Defining pathways to healthy sustainable urban development. Environ Int. 2021;146:106236.
11. Thondoo M, de Vries DH, Rojas-Rueda D, et al. Framework for participatory quantitative health impact assessment in low-and middle-income countries. Int J Environ Res Public Health. 2020;17(20):7688. https://doi.org/10.3390/ijerph17207688.

74 Climate Change and Human Health

Tara Neville, Diarmid Campbell-Lendrum, Marina Maiero, Arthur Wyns, and Maria Neira

Abstract

Climate change has profound and wide-ranging effects on human health and health systems, and the impacts of climate change undermine public health advancements. The health sector is mobilizing to protect population health and build climate resilient and sustainable health systems. However, sector-wide cuts in global greenhouse gas emissions are urgently required to preserve our ecological and human systems. The health community plays a critical role in ensuring future population and planetary health through advocacy, policy development, evidence strengthening and health response.

Keywords

Health · Climate change · Health impacts · Health co-benefits · Resilient health systems · Sustainable health systems

74.1 Introduction

Climate change is one of the most urgent global health challenges facing the world. Scientific evidence demonstrates that the earth is warming at an unprecedented rate [1]. In 2021, the global mean temperature was 1.11 °C higher than pre-industrial levels with each of the past four decades warmer than the preceding decade [1, 2]. Emissions of greenhouse gases caused by human activities are the main driver of this change in the global climate [1].

Climate change is increasing the intensity and frequency of extreme weather events such as storms, floods, droughts, heatwaves and wildfires. We have now reached a point where these weather and climate extremes have caused irreversible damage to natural and human systems, affecting every aspect of our society including people's health and well-being [3]. Over 3 billion people are estimated to live in situations that are considered highly vulnerable to the impacts of climate change [3]. Adaptation can strengthen the resilience, reduce the vulnerability, and enhance the adaptive capacity of populations to climate change, but there are limits to these efforts.

Low and lower-middle income countries and small island developing states suffer the greatest health consequences of climate shocks and stresses, despite contributing the least to historical global emissions. Within countries there can

T. Neville (✉) · D. Campbell-Lendrum · M. Maiero · A. Wyns · M. Neira
World Health Organization, Geneva, Switzerland
e-mail: nevillet@who.int; campbelllendrumd@who.int; maierom@who.int; neiram@who.int

M. C. B. Raviglione et al. (eds.), *Global Health Essentials*, Sustainable Development Goals Series,
https://doi.org/10.1007/978-3-031-33851-9_74

also be large disparities in those most vulnerable to the impacts of climate change. Populations living in poverty, the elderly, women, children, Indigenous Peoples, outdoor workers, the socially isolated and individuals with pre-existing medical conditions provide examples of groups at highest risk [3, 4].

The global response to climate change is currently insufficient to avert widespread and severe consequences. The 2022 report of the Intergovernmental Panel on Climate Change emphasized that 'Climate change is a threat to human well-being and planetary health. Any further delay in concerted anticipatory global action on adaptation and mitigation will miss a brief, rapidly closing window to secure a liveable and sustainable future for all' [3].

74.2 Climate-Sensitive Health Risks

The 2023 World Health Statistics report summarizes the main health risks associated with climate change and key objectives for a comprehensive health response [4]. In line with this report, Fig. 74.1 illustrates examples of major health risks associated with climate change and the exposure pathways by which climate hazards, vulnerability factors and health system resilience can affect health outcomes. Several factors, including the natural environment, socio-economic conditions, demographic factors, health system functioning and individual health status, play a significant role in mediating the health risks of climate change [5].

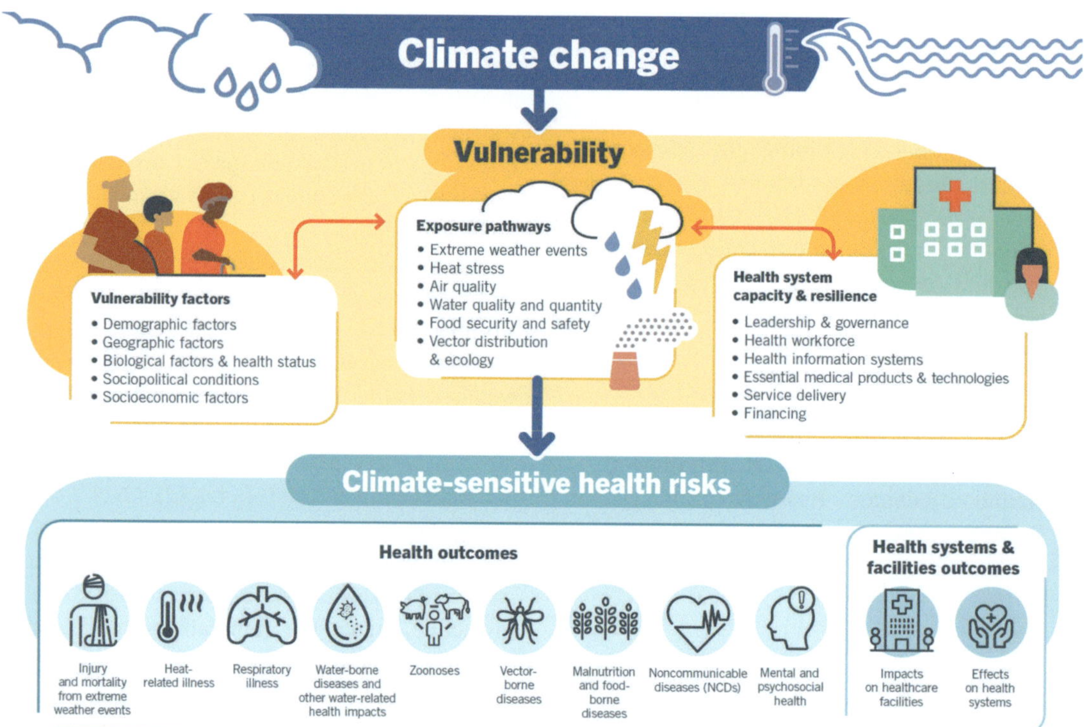

Fig. 74.1 Major health risks associated with climate change [6]

74.2.1 Direct Health Impacts

Extreme weather events such as storms, floods, droughts, heatwaves and wildfires have a direct impact on health by causing injuries, illnesses and deaths. All regions are experiencing climate extremes but vulnerability to these hazards differ. Evidence has shown that between 2010 and 2020, regions with high vulnerability to climate change experienced 15 times higher mortality from extreme weather events than regions with very low vulnerability [3]. An increase in the likelihood of concurrent or cascading extreme events is also being observed [1], making disaster preparedness and response even more challenging.

74.2.2 Indirect Health Impacts

The indirect health impacts of climate change may pose the largest long-term threat to public health and health systems.

Some of the world's most virulent infections are highly sensitive to weather and climate conditions. Each year over 700,000 people die from vector-borne diseases, many being children under 5 years of age [7]. Conditions for the transmission of mosquito-borne, tick-borne and rodent-borne diseases are increasing in many regions and spreading to new areas. This raises the risk of infection and outbreaks, particularly if adequate prevention measures are not in place [8].

Climate change degrades the foundations of human health: air, water, soil, food, shelter and security, leading to higher risk of water-borne diseases, food-borne diseases and malnutrition [3]. In 2020, about 770 million people in the world faced hunger, primarily in Africa and Asia. Women and children were at high risk with 22% of children under five affected by stunting [9]. Globally, there are about 600 million cases of foodborne illnesses each year [10] and approximately 2 billion people lack access to safe drinking water [11]. These health risks are expected to worsen with climate change. Additionally, acute and cumulative mental health stresses are higher when confronted with climate-related traumatic events, displacement, loss and future insecurity [12].

Damaged health care facilities and critical infrastructure from storms, flooding and rising sea levels can also limit access to and delivery of health services [13].

Climate change is often considered a threat multiplier because it amplifies global health and development challenges. Inequity, urbanization, biodiversity loss, ecosystem destruction, water and food insecurity and conflict will be more difficult to address under intensifying climate pressures. In this context, climate change threatens the achievement of the Sustainable Development Goals (SDGs) and undermines past public health gains [4].

74.3 Health Co-benefits of Climate Change Mitigation

Many policies and individual actions have the potential to both reduce greenhouse gas emissions and produce major health benefits. Several of the sectors driving greenhouse gas emissions—including energy, transport, industry, agriculture and waste—are also sources of harmful air pollutants. Each year, air pollution causes approximately 6.7 million deaths primarily due to cardiovascular diseases, respiratory illnesses and cancer [14]. Transitioning from polluting forms of energy, such as fossil fuels, towards renewable energy sources can bring air quality improvements and lower the incidence of illness and premature deaths from air pollution [15].

Promoting safe walking and cycling as part of sustainable urban planning, can reduce carbon emissions and bring multiple health benefits through increased physical activity, reduced air pollution and lower noise levels [4, 5].

While climate change is a driver of food insecurity, the global food system also contributes between 21 and 37% of global greenhouse gas emissions [16]. In high income countries, a transition towards plant-based diets, lower red meat consumption and less food waste offers an opportunity to mitigate climate change while lowering the health burden of diet-related non-communicable diseases. Sustainable agriculture and food production in low- and middle-income countries can protect local environments, lower emissions and promote food and nutrition security [4].

Research has shown that global climate action aimed at limiting warming to below 2 °C, could save millions of lives due to improvements in air quality, diet and physical activity [17]. Health benefits from climate change mitigation also provide cost-savings for health systems and improved productivity from a healthier workforce. These economic gains can offset the costs of mitigation and provide a strong motivation for climate action.

74.4 Actions for a Healthy Population and Planet

74.4.1 Build Climate Resilient and Sustainable Health Systems

Building climate resilient and sustainable health systems involves a systematic and comprehensive approach to strengthening all core functions of a health system so it can respond and adapt to the health risks of climate change, (see Fig. 74.2) [18]. To do this, accurate vulnerability and adaptation assessments of the health system are required [19]. Governments are scaling up action in this area to better inform their health policies and programmes [20, 21]. Multisectoral collaboration with other health-determining sectors is also needed to ensure resilience across all aspects of health service provision and the protection of public health.

The health sector is responsible for approximately 4–5% of global greenhouse gas emissions [16, 22]. Health systems can decarbonize through measures such as sustainable procurement prac-

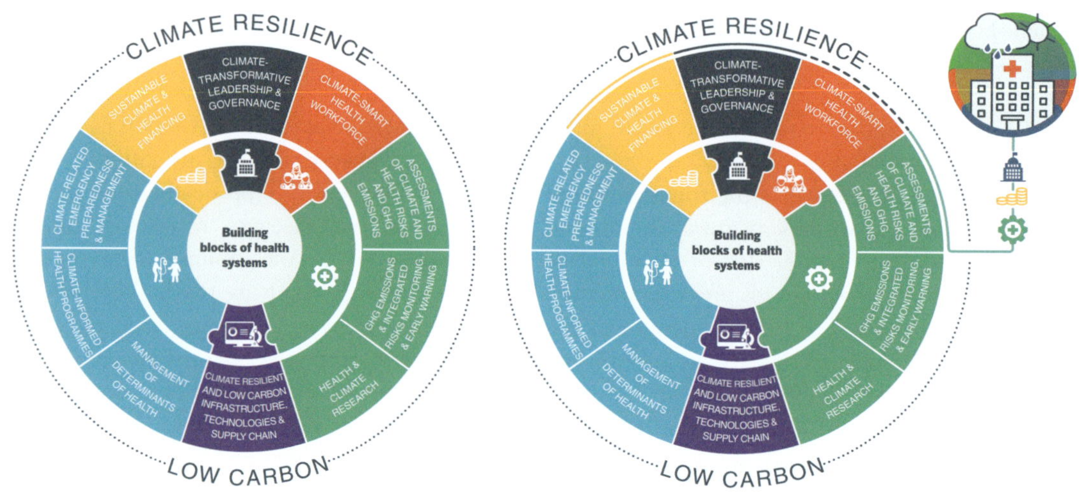

Fig. 74.2 Adapted from conceptual and operational framework for climate-resilient and low-carbon health systems. The health system response to climate change should build on the core 'building blocks' of health systems: leadership, workforce, information systems, infrastructure and technologies, service delivery and finance (inner ring); adding additional functionality and capacity specifically to build resilience to climate shocks and stresses, while minimizing carbon emissions (outer ring)

tices, more efficient or renewable energy sources, waste reduction and optimizing the use of resources. Implementing these measures can bring multiple health system benefits by contributing to a higher quality of care, greater accessibility, more reliable services, reduced occupational hazards from air pollution and waste, and reduced costs [13, 22].

74.4.2 Achieve Global Health and Climate Change Goals

Given the interconnectedness of natural, economic, social and human systems, action in the health sector alone is not enough to protect human health. Coherence in health and climate policies and their effective implementation is necessary [23]. In 2015, two international agreements were implemented that provide overarching goals for climate change and health. The United Nations Framework Convention on Climate Change (UNFCCC) Paris Agreement and the 2030 Agenda for Sustainable Development.

The Paris Agreement sets out clear targets to limit global temperature rise to well below 2 °C above pre-industrial levels. The agreement recognizes the intrinsic link between the natural environment and human well-being, specifying that climate change action should respect and promote 'the right to health' [24].

Under the UNFCCC, countries set out their mitigation commitments and adaptation priorities through their Nationally Determined Contributions (NDCs) and National Adaptation Plans (NAPs). By reflecting health priorities in NDCs and NAPs, governments can ensure that health considerations are an integral part of national and international climate policies and processes while maximising synergies with health goals. As such, health can be a powerful argument to galvanize political and financial support for accelerated climate action [23].

74.4.3 Mobilize the Strength of the Health Community

Effectively tackling climate change and maximizing benefits for health requires broad public support. Health professionals are often a trusted voice in society. They have direct contact with patients and communities and witness the health impacts of climate change first-hand. Health professionals and health organizations have become increasingly engaged in raising awareness and taking action to address the health risks of climate change. As climate change intensifies the health community will play a critical role in advocacy, evidence generation, policy development and building health system resilience and sustainability [23].

References

1. IPCC. Summary for Policymakers. In: Masson-Delmotte V, Zhai P, Pirani A, Connors SL, Péan C, Berger S, Caud N, Chen Y, Goldfarb L, Gomis MI, Huang M, Leitzell K, Lonnoy E, Matthews JBR, Maycock TK, Waterfield T, Yelekçi O, Yu R, Zhou B, editors. Climate change 2021: the physical science basis. contribution of working group I to the sixth assessment report of the intergovernmental panel on climate change. Cambridge: Cambridge University Press; 2021. p. 3–32. https://doi.org/10.1017/9781009157896.001.
2. State of the Global Climate 2021. WMO-No.1290. Geneva: World Health Meteorological Organization. 2022. https://public.wmo.int/en/our-mandate/climate/wmo-statement-state-of-global-climate.
3. IPCC. Summary for policymakers. In: Pörtner H-O, Roberts DC, Poloczanska ES, Mintenbeck K, Tignor M, Alegría A, Craig M, Langsdorf S, Löschke S, Möller V, Okem A, editors. Climate change 2022: impacts, adaptation, and vulnerability. Contribution of Working Group II to the sixth assessment report of the Intergovernmental Panel on Climate Change. Cambridge: Cambridge University Press; 2022. https://doi.org/10.1017/9781009325844.001.
4. World Health Organization. World health statistics 2023: monitoring health for the SDGs, sustainable development goals. https://apps.who.int/iris/handle/10665/367912.
5. WHO. COP24 special report: health and climate change. Geneva: World Health Organization;

2018. https://www.who.int/publications/i/item/9789241514972.
6. WHO. Quality Criteria for Health National Adaptation Plans. Geneva: World Health Organization; 2021. https://www.who.int/publications/i/item/9789240018983.
7. World Health Organization. Vector-borne diseases. 2020. https://www.who.int/news-room/fact-sheets/detail/vector-borne-diseases. Accessed 20 Jun 2022.
8. WHO. Protecting health from climate change. Geneva: World Health Organization; 2009. https://www.who.int/publications/i/item/9789241598880.
9. FAO, IFAD, UNICEF, WFP and WHO. The state of food security and nutrition in the world 2021. Transforming food systems for food security, improved nutrition and affordable healthy diets for all. Rome: FAO; 2021. https://doi.org/10.4060/cb4474en.
10. World Health Organization. Estimating the burden of foodborne diseases. https://www.who.int/activities/estimating-the-burdenof-foodborne-diseases.
11. WHO, UNICEF & World Bank. State of the world's drinking water: an urgent call to action to accelerate progress on ensuring safe drinking water for all. 2022. https://www.apps.who.int/iris/handle/10665/363704.
12. WHO. Mental health and climate change policy brief. Geneva: World Health Organization; 2022. https://www.who.int/publications/i/item/9789240045125.
13. WHO. WHO guidance for climate-resilient and environmentally sustainable health care facilities. Geneva: World Health Organization; 2020. https://www.who.int/publications/i/item/9789240012226.
14. Global Health Observatory. Air pollution data portal. 2022. https://www.who.int/data/gho/data/themes/air-pollution?lang=en. Accessed 20 Jun 2022.
15. WHO. Preventing disease through healthy environments. A global assessment of the burden of disease from environmental risks. Geneva: World Health Organization; 2016. https://www.who.int/publications/i/item/9789241565196
16. Romanello M, McGushin A, Napoli C, Drummond P, Hughes N, et al. The 2021 report of the lancet countdown on health and climate change: code red for a healthy future. Lancet. 2021;398:1619–62. Published Online October 20, 2021. https://doi.org/10.1016/S0140-6736(21)01787-6.
17. Hamilton I, et al. The public health implications of the Paris Agreement: a modelling study. Lancet Planet Health. 2021;5(2):e74–83. https://doi.org/10.1016/S2542-5196(20)30249-7.
18. World Health Organization. Conceptual and Operational Framework for Building Climate Resilient and Low Carbon Health Systems (in press).
19. WHO. Climate change and health: vulnerability and adaptation assessment. Geneva: World Health Organization; 2021. https://www.who.int/publications/i/item/9789240036383
20. WHO. WHO health and climate change global survey report. Geneva: World Health Organization; 2021. https://www.who.int/publications/i/item/9789240038509
21. WHO COP26 health programme. World Health Organization. https://www.who.int/initiatives/cop26-health-programme. Accessed 20 Jun 2022.
22. Health Care Climate Action. Global road map for health care decarbonization: a navigational tool for achieving zero emissions with climate resilience and health equity. [Website]. Health care without harm. https://healthcareclimateaction.org/roadmap. Accessed 20 Jun 2022.
23. WHO. COP26 special report on climate change and health: the health argument for climate action. Geneva: World Health Organization; 2021. https://apps.who.int/iris/bitstream/handle/10665/346168/9789240036727-eng.pdf?sequence=1&isAllowed=y.
24. Paris Agreement. Bonn: United Nations framework convention on climate change. 2015. https://unfccc.int/files/meetings/paris_nov_2015/application/pdf/paris_agreement_english_.pdf. Accessed 20 Jun 2022.

The Ecology of Agri-Food System

75

Stefano Bocchi

Abstract

The model of industrial agriculture, modeled on the criteria by the green revolution of the last century, after having allowed a significant increase in the production of some crops, has demonstrated increasing critical points over decades. The substantial negative impacts on natural resources (i.e., land, water, air, and biodiversity), the unsustainable dependence on fossil fuels, the spread of malnutrition, and the unequal distribution of wealth push to find an alternative model. Agroecology proposes a systemic approach to redesign and manage agri-food systems that can also face the current challenges: facing climate change, regenerating ecosystems, and spreading food security within a vision based on the emerging concept of global health and on the vision proposed by Agenda 2030. A renewed cultural and ethical framework, where thanks to peaceful and democratic institutions, the interests of safeguarding the commons and general well-being prevail, will also make it possible to identify the best technological innovations. The contribution of agroecology to the realization of the 2030 Agenda for Sustainable Development appears crucial.

Keywords

Agroecology · Double helix · Sustainable multifunctional agriculture · Nutrition-sensitive agriculture for global health

75.1 Historical Background of the "Green Revolution"

The "Green Revolution" was a powerful strategy of innovation of the agricultural model designed in the 40s in the United States and spread throughout the world since the end of the Second World War. The promoters of this model focused the innovation on some important crops and their yield improvement, through genetic techniques. The so-called extension service would have disseminated the new technological package including the high-yielding variety, and other products such as fertilizers (containing nitrogen, phosphorus, and potassium), new irrigation systems, mechanization, and pesticides. The cost of fossil energy required in production processes and "incorporated" into the products was relatively low. The new production model of modern agriculture was designed on industrial schemes, concentrating either on the production in selected areas and the control of the value chain. The farm was no longer designed and managed as a dynamic, complex, biological, and evolving system, part of the territory, but as an industry.

S. Bocchi (✉)
Department of Environmental Science and Policy, University of Milan, Milan, Italy
e-mail: stefano.bocchi@unimi.it

M. C. B. Raviglione et al. (eds.), *Global Health Essentials*, Sustainable Development Goals Series,
https://doi.org/10.1007/978-3-031-33851-9_75

The "Green Revolution" achieved the goal of increasing the yields of some important crops. The global food production increased by 150–200%, and the new agri-food system was defined as one of humanity's most significant achievements, potentially able to face the challenges of hunger on the planet [1].

The dark side of industrial agriculture would have appeared clearly in the last decades of the twentieth century when it was possible to globally analyze, with more scientific instruments, new diseases of biotopes (erosion, soil fertility, decrease of nutrient, salinity, water table pollution) of biocenosis[1] (natural enemies' loss, new dangerous pest appearance, genetic resistance, reduction of natural feedback mechanisms), and of Landscape Unit [2].

The negative consequences of the green revolution were numerous: biodiversity reduction (75% of the agrobiodiversity), soil degradation, desertification (50% of the cultivated area), landscapes trivialization, weakening of farms in the supply of ecosystem services, greenhouse gas (GHG) emissions (19–29% of global emissions), reduction in diets variability, heavy reliance on fossil fuels, water, air, and soil pollution, unequal wealth distribution. The agri-food system is showing its weaknesses concerning other aspects such as unsustainable use of resources, food insecurity, uncertainty due to climate change, global loss of productivity of cultivated soil by 0.2% per year, unhealthy diet models [3].

75.2 The Impact of Food on Human and Planetary Health

The "Green Revolution" brought the availability of nutrient-rich and calorie-dense foods, often heavily processed, and changes in dietary behaviors. This, coupled with hastily urbanization and increase of countries' income, created favorable conditions for malnutrition and diseases.

Malnutrition, disproportionally affecting a growing part of the world's population and arising from unsustainable diets and lifestyles, is a wide-spectrum term covering deficiencies, excesses, and imbalances in energy and nutrient intake. Therefore, it has three different expressions: (1) overweight and obesity, (2) undernutrition, and (3) micronutrient-related malnutrition (diets poor in vitamins and minerals, the "hidden hunger").

75.2.1 Non-communicable Diseases

Globally, among the top 10 most common diseases, 6 are non-communicable diseases (NCDs) caused by unhealthy lifestyles (e.g., low physical activity, fat-rich diets, tobacco smoking) [4]. Most commonly, overweight and obesity are the leading causes of NCDs, except for chronic undernutrition resulting in stunting.[2] As the income of countries increases, disease patterns are rapidly shifting from infectious diseases to NCDs in a phenomenon known as "epidemiological transition" (Chaps. 2, 4, and 5). Contrary to what is expected, however, lower-middle-income countries (LICs/LMICs) are experiencing high burden of overweight and obesity, and consequently of NDCs, especially in populations aged under 70 years (i.e., the double burden of NCDs and communicable diseases).

75.2.2 Communicable Diseases

Most of the communicable, maternal, neonatal, and nutritional diseases (CMNNDs), globally, are associated to poverty and undernutrition. Therefore, there is a clear epidemiological pattern in LICs and LMICs where CMNNDs have the highest burden of diseases.

[1] Biocenosis: a biological association of different organisms forming an integrated and self-regulating community living in a given environment

[2] Stunting is defined by WHO as the impaired growth and development experienced by children because of poor nutrition, recurrent infections, and insufficient psychosocial stimulation.

Table 75.1 The main environmental pollutants

Pollutants	Main sources or vectors	Notes
Heavy metals (HMs)	Pesticides and fertilizers can contain traces of heavy metals	HMs can be adsorbed and accumulated in plants contaminating food chains
Endocrine-disrupting chemicals (EDCs)	Compounds and products used in pesticides, food packaging, and food contact materials	EDCs can alter the (human) endocrine function of exposed subjects (especially for chronic exposures)
GHG, PM (indoor air pollutants)	Low-resource settings food cooking, heating, and lighting based on household fuel combustion	Women and children are threatened by indoor air pollution in many LICs
GHG, PM (outdoor air pollutants)	The agri-food system produces GHG (e.g., methane and carbon dioxide (CO_2))	The level of GHG emissions is highly dependent on diet composition
Antimicrobials	In agriculture and husbandry of livestock, the use of antibiotics is widespread	Emergence of anti-microbial resistance
Plastic and microplastic	Widespread use of plastics in different sectors and human activities	
Others: Pharmaceutical and per- and poly-fluoroalkyl substances (PFASs)	Several thousands of PFASs are used in a wide range of applications	

Globally each year there are 600 million people affected by foodborne diseases, a subset of CMNNDs, 420,000 of which die, especially children under-5 years of age (30% of foodborne diseases). The vast majority of foodborne diseases are diarrhea and Campylobacter gastroenteritis (96 million) [5]. Pathogens causing foodborne diseases in humans have frequently developed resistance to antimicrobials because of their extensive use in agriculture and livestock husbandry, and to other non-antimicrobial compounds (e.g., heavy metals, HMs).

75.2.3 Environmental Pollutants in Food

In the past years, evidence has accrued regarding the importance and the impact of environmental pollution and chemical contamination in human food chain. An overview of the most frequent pollutants is reported in Table 75.1.

75.3 Approach to Solutions

Springmann et al. [6] observed that "the agri-food system is the major driver of climate change, changes in land use, depletion of freshwater resources, and pollution of aquatic and terrestrial ecosystems through excessive nitrogen and phosphorus inputs.". If both food patterns will not move from meat-based animal proteins to plant-based protein intake, and industrial agriculture will not adopt nutrition-sensitive multifunctional forms, natural resources that underpin the quality of life (i.e., air, water, soil, biodiversity, and natural biome) will be further degraded [7].

The Food and Agriculture Organization (FAO) [8] recently underlined the importance of the contribution of agri-food system to the realization of the 2030 Agenda for Sustainable Development [9], ending poverty (SDG 1), hunger and malnutrition (SDG 2), and responding to climate change (SDG 13) while achieving inclusive growth (SDGs 5, 8, 10), building resilient communities (SDG 11) and sustainably managing natural resources (SDGs 6, 7, 14, 15); all goals clearly connected each other.

75.3.1 The Double Helix of Agroecology

Within the agri-food systems, sustainability can be originated by a double helix: (1) balanced sustainable healthy diets, whose main features are indicated by the World Health Organization (WHO) [5] from one side; and, on the other side, (2) the ecosystem-services supply from agroecosystems. Modern agroecology offers the principles and practices for the connection of the two helixes. Such crucial change can be described in terms of a transition from market-based agriculture to sustainable nutrition-sensitive agriculture [10]. Nutrition-sensitive agriculture (NSA) is an approach that seeks to maximize agriculture's contribution to nutrition, linking agriculture to sectors that address the several causes of malnutrition, including education, food policy, health, and social protection [11].

Many are the connections between NSA and multifunctional agriculture (MFA) because NSA instead of focusing on cash crops to be sold on the global market invites communities of farmers to improve agrobiodiversity by using the land to cultivate many crops including fruits, vegetables, and breeding small livestock (multifunctional farming systems).

Finally, an environmentally sustainable diet, in addition to being healthy, should be acceptable from a social, economic, and ethical point of view with respect, among other, to food needs and food security issues, culinary tradition, farming system resilience (e.g., risks due to yield or price variability), employment, and farmers working conditions.

References

1. Bocchi S, Villa S, Orlando F, Grimoldi L, Raviglione M. Agrofood system and human health. In: Environmental alteration leads to human diseases. A planetary approach, vol. 2021. New York: Springer; 2022. p. 131–65.
2. Ingegnoli V. Planetary health: human impacts on the environment. In: Environmental alteration leads to human diseases. A planetary approach, vol. 2022. New York: Springer; 2022. p. 95–130.
3. Clark M, Hill J, Tilman D. The diet, health, and environment trilemma. Annu Rev Environ Resour. 2018;43:109–34.
4. WHO. The Global health observatory. 2020. https://www.who.int/data/gho/data/indicators. Accessed 29 Jun 2020.
5. WHO. Connecting global priorities: biodiversity and human health: a state of knowledge review. World Health Organization and Secretariat of the Convention on Biological Diversity. 2015.
6. Springmann M, Clark M, Mason-D'Croz D, et al. Options for keeping the food system within environmental limits. Nature. 2018;562:519–25.
7. FAO. Polluting our soils is polluting our future. 2020. http://www.fao.org/fao-stories/article/en/c/1126974/. Accessed 15 Jul 2020.
8. FAO. Background notes on sustainable, productive and resilient agro-food system. 2019. https://www.fao.org/3/ca5385en/ca5385en.pdf.
9. United Nations. Transforming our world: the 2030 Agenda for Sustainable Development. A/RES/70/1. New York. 2015.
10. Gliessmann S. Agroecology: the ecology of sustainable food systems. 3rd ed. Boca Raton: CRC Press; 2016. p. 405.
11. FAO Nutrion-sensitive agriculture and global soil partnership. 2017 https://www.fao.org/global-soil-partnership/areas-of-work/soil-fertility/nutrition-sensitive-agriculture/en/. Accessed 19 June 2022.

One Health

76

Eric Cardinale and Ilaria Bernotti

Abstract

As its name suggestes, Global Health aims to approach health issues broadly and comprehensively both from a geographical and a conceptual point of view. In this demand, the human–animal–ecosystem interface cannot be left behind: the One Health approach, an improved integration among disciplines that enhances cross-sectoral collaboration between stakeholders at different levels, is paramount.

It increases public health efficiency and effectiveness through a better understanding of diseases and risk factors through shared efforts that will benefit human, animal, and ecosystem health. Successful results were already achived in key Global Health issues, such as zoonotic diseases, antimicrobial resistance, and food safety but a lot remains to be done.

The integration that led to these promising outcomes was not spontaneously achieved, but it was structured through methodological principles, guidelines, and related transaction costs. However, the procedural shift is a highly rewording effort that have multiple but still unattempt field of application.

Keywords

One Health · Health collaboration · Multisectoral approach · Preventive medicine · Zoonoses · Pandemic prevention · Food safety · Antimicrobial resistance

76.1 Introduction: Historical Basis and Definitions

"An integrated, unifying approach that aims to sustainably balance and optimise the health of people, animals and ecosystems": this is the One Health's (OH) definition proposed by the One Health High-Level Expert panel (OHHLEP) in December 2021 [1] (Fig. 76.1). Even with a clear definition in mind, understanding how it is practically applied and which added value it provides to the Global Health landscape might be more challenging.

To clarify these crucial concepts, it is wise to start from the beginning. The recognition of interlinkages between humans, animals (domestic and wild), and the wider environment's health by the OHHLEP is not a new assumption. From early philosophers (e.g., Xenophon) on, many

E. Cardinale
ASTRE, University of Montpellier (I-MUSE), CIRAD, INRAe, Montpellier, France
e-mail: eric.cardinale@cirad.fr

I. Bernotti (✉)
Department of Veterinary Preventive Medicine, The Ohio State University, Columbus, OH, USA
e-mail: bernotti.1@osu.edu

M. C. B. Raviglione et al. (eds.), *Global Health Essentials*, Sustainable Development Goals Series,
https://doi.org/10.1007/978-3-031-33851-9_76

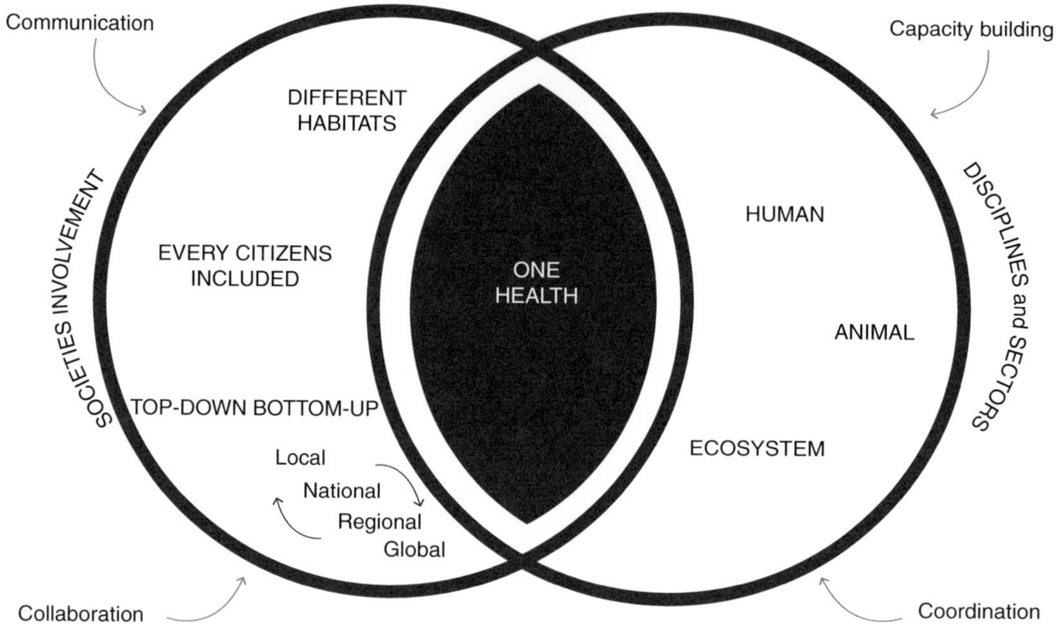

Fig. 76.1 The One Health approach (Based on "Tripartite and UNEP support OHHLEP's definition of 'One Health'," WHO 2021)

integrative thinkers highlighted biological similarities and coexistence's mutual benefits between humans and animals. Indeed, countless improvements in socio-economic conditions and breakthroughs in health and scientific research were allowed by the close interface between humans, animals and their shared environment. This proximity, however, is not bereft of risks, and the current era of emerging and re-emerging pandemics is highlighting it.

In fact, after centuries in which it was casted aside, in the second half of the twentieth century One Health regained strength just as a broader conceptual term, fuelled by pandemic threats and conservation issues. It evolved from "One Medicine" (interaction between human and animal health) in the 1960s to the "One World, One Health" of the Manhattan Principles on zoonoses in 2004 [2]. And today, a new Quadripartite agreement – among the World Health Organization (WHO), World Organisation for Animal Health (WOAH, former OIE), United Nations Environment Programme (UNEP), and Food and Agriculture Organization (FAO) – has been signed to provide a legal and formal framework for the four organizations to tackle the challenges at the human, animal, plant, and ecosystem interface using this integrated and coordinated One Health approach [3].

Since this awareness gained new global consensus, parallel but slightly different health approaches have arisen. EcoHealth and Planetary Health, for example, are frequently handled as One Health synonymous: they indeed share core focus and values but do differ in contributing sciences. Planetary Health approaches animals and ecosystems as enhancers of human wellbeing, while EcoHealth encompasses a broad range of disciplines (scientific, humanistic, and social sciences) at the same level [4, 5].

76.2 Methods and Approaches

One Health acts upon health systems that work collaboratively, with multisectorality, and transdisciplinarity at the local, regional, national, and global levels toward the highest level of effectiveness and efficiency. It applies a system thinking perspective to solve complex problems; it covers the policies, processes, practices and people, the roles each play and how they interact to function effectively to solve public health threats [6] (Fig. 76.2).

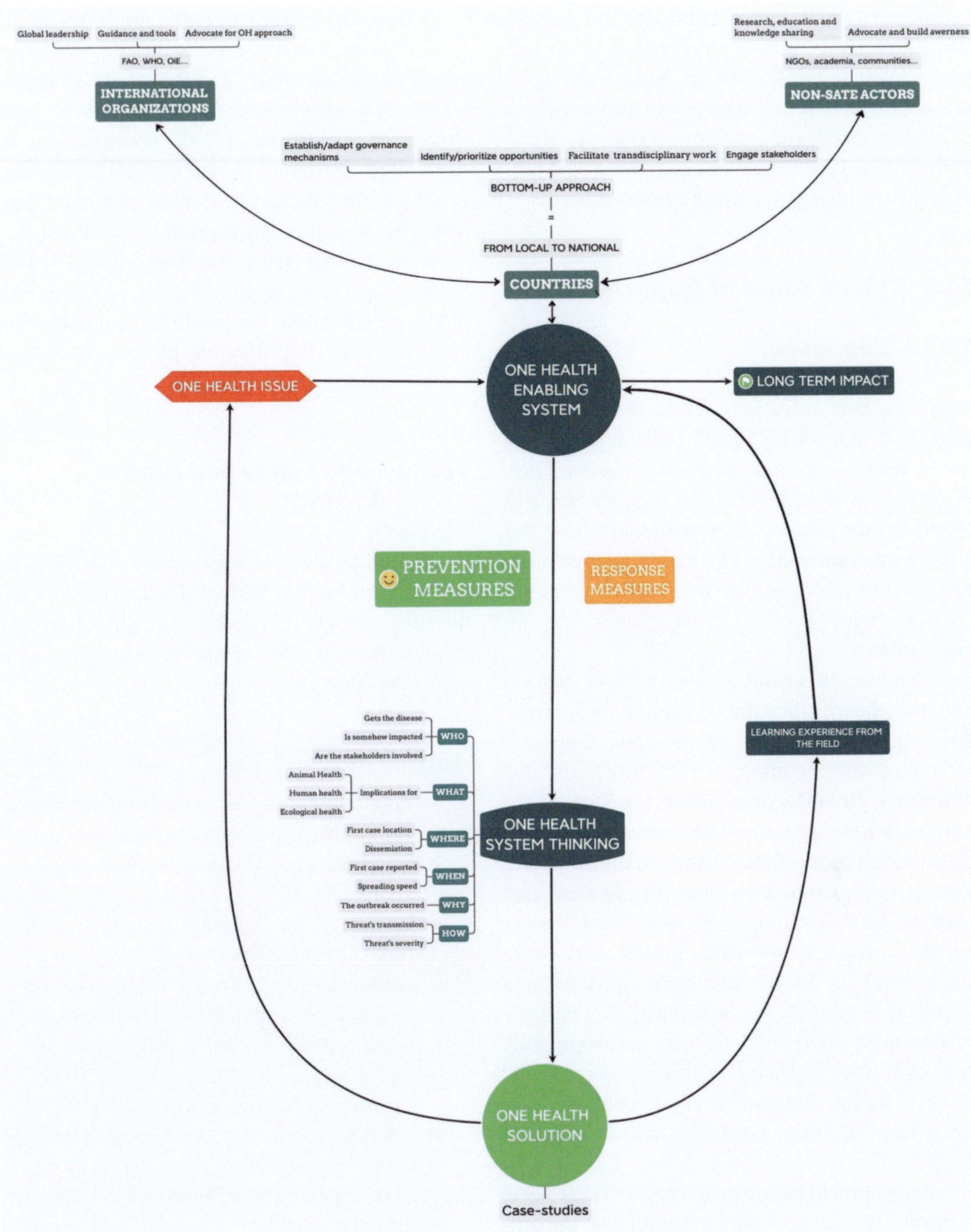

Fig. 76.2 The system thinking in One Health approach: A One Health enabling system (i.e., the interdisciplinary, international, and intersectoral collaboration between countries, international organizations, and non-state agents) works toward prevention measures to avoid health crisis rather than dealing with the response phase. In both cases, however, solutions are found following the One Health system thinking approach. It's a bottom-up approach where outcomes and feedback from the field are the most valuable gained knowledge to enhance the enabling system. If a long-term impact is aimed, especially in a Sustainable Development Goals' prospective, greater involvement of hotspots' populations is needed

These structures have to be planned and settled preventively before any emergence to happen. COVID-19's devastating burden proved it: prevention and preparedness are less costly in each dimension (i.e., health, economy, socio-political), and they enhance ecosystems and populations' resilience against multiple scenarios.

76.3 Major Areas of Application

76.3.1 Zoonoses

Zoonoses are infectious diseases caused by pathogens that could "jump" (technically "spill-over") from non-human to human species. These diseases may have a bacterial, viral, or parasitic origin or may involve unconventional agents that allow human spreading. The main routes of transmission are direct animal contacts and indirect contacts with vectors, food, water, or the environment.

Zoonotic infectious diseases have been a human concern since the beginning of animals' domestication. 10,000 years later, they still remain a significant cause of mortality and morbidity globally, accounting for 75% of the current emerging infectious diseases (EIDs). Since 1980, more than 87 new zoonotic and/or vector-borne EIDs have been discovered and, over the last 15 years, 15 of them were deadly zoonotic or vector-borne global outbreaks (both viral as Ebola and coronaviruses and bacterial as plague and anthrax) [7]. The phenomenon is sharpened by our anthropogenic way of living: intensive farming, international trades, social inequality, and conflicts are examples of this burden's avoidable risk factors.

Sheep' brucellosis, for example, is an issue for both the (human) public health and the animal industry's sectors. Livestock's vaccination campaigns are a win-win solution: livestock breeders save losses in animals' treatments and lack of productions while the health sector indirectly registers less cases in humans (as it originates essentially from livestock and livestock products) [8].

A vaccination campaign that improves human health through interventions in the veterinary sector is the case study on rabies in N'Djamena, Chad. The cost-effectiveness of human post-exposure prophylaxis (PEP) accompanied by mass dogs' vaccination was proved to be more profitable than human PEP alone just in 5 years' time after a single campaign of vaccination.

Several other risky interfaces could benefit from a systemic approach and, despite each pathogen and context's peculiarity, standardized practices could be effective prevention tools at the community and personal levels.

76.3.2 Food Safety and Food Security

In the food safety field, appropriate guidelines for animal care help to reduce foodborne zoonotic diseases' (FBD) outbreaks, that spread through meat, eggs, dairy, or even some vegetables' consumption (Box 76.1).

Box 76.1 Foodborne diseases

- Foodborne diseases arise from the consumption of food or associated products contaminated with pathogens or chemicals.
- Cases can be sporadic or outbreaks (if linked by a common source).
- Outbreaks are generally acute yet relatively short and with regional impacts (e.g., *Salmonella spp., Campylobacter, Escherichia coli, Staphylococci, Listeria,* or Norovirus).
- Incidents can be prolonged due to lengthier incubation periods or long-term exposure (e.g., bovine spongiform encephalopathy, melamine-contaminated milk products).
- Increased internationalization of food production chains and its economic importance calls for measures to identify, prevent, and manage risks of contamination before they occur.

As an instance, *Salmonella enterica ssp. enterica* is the leading cause of bacterial food-borne disease outbreaks in developed countries as long as a public health concern in developing countries especially from poultry meat and eggs' consumption [9]. Senegal provides a successful OH example because of the numerous works that performed situational analysis to mitigate risks found at each unit of production. Differences between farms (between laying hens and broiler chickens), slaughter infrastructures, regional or international consumption sector, and the cold chain (frozen products as opposed to fresh products) were all identified as potential points of outbreak's risk. On this evidence, professionals and consumers were taught specific training and sensitization sessions that made them aware of correct preventive measures.

76.3.3 Antimicrobial Resistance

Antimicrobial resistance (AMR) is the issue that epitomizes One Health principles [10]. Misusage of antimicrobials in animals leads to residues in animals' tissues and their excreta: their consumption poses some risks for human health while excreta challenges waters and soils' safety. Moreover, excessive antimicrobial use (AMU) in crops themselves constantly exposes who is fed with them (regardless if human or animal) to subtherapeutic doses. Some types of bacteria that cause serious infections in humans have already developed resistances to most or to all the available treatments.

Professionals (e.g., veterinarians, physicians, ecologists, and agricultural professionals) must work collaboratively to ensure that antimicrobial products are used judiciously and to preserve antimicrobial efficacy, especially for the human compound.

According to WHO, some countries are using a total amount of antibiotics in animals that is 4 times larger than the one used for humans [11]. A shift toward a more conscientious AMU in agricultural and livestock systems showed to be a good policy practice to mitigate the threat. Both World Organisation for Animal Health (WOAH) and WHO had indeed recommended an overall usage reduction in food-producing animals to help preserve their effectiveness for human medicine. In Europe, regulations have forbidden AMU as growth promoters while in the United States, consumer preferences have driven companies to reduce AMU in animals. Even without antimicrobilas, animals are able to remain healthy and complete their production cycles: farms' management and biosafety measures are the key resources. Sweden is a successful model in the field: its strong underpinning policy framework is integrated into all relevant governmental systems, and is supported by adequate human, infrastructural, and operational resources in all sectors of the One Health triad, driven actively both by practitioners on the ground as well as local role models and champions [12].

76.4 Main Conclusions

As previously explained, the One Health approach enables an effective and efficient usage of limited resources to catalyze better public health outcomes. Results may be simply measured as reduced morbidity and mortality, or by cost-benefit analyses using economic data. Advantages are not limited to improved public health outcomes, strengthened management systems and coordination across health sectors but also linked to increased return of investments. Costs are indeed reduced by avoiding duplication of activities and performances may further benefit by improving synergies (e.g., shared laboratory facilities). Reduced risks from zoonotic diseases are reflected in reduced indirect societal losses: impacts on small producers' livelihood, poorer nutrition, trade, and tourism's restriction are all elements that brought the global costs of some recent zoonotic outbreaks to tens of billions of dollars. The added value in each of the sectors can justify the investments as an advocacy tool, helping policy-makers to understand how to share "one-healthily" costs and benefits across sectors is a winning decision.

COVID-19 pandemic gave an unprecedented momentum to One Health research and its integration in policy making as a diplomacy tool. We have to act in this direction, since all these synergies between animal health, public health, and environmental specialists applied at the local, national, and global levels undoubtedly contribute to the continuous and simultaneous improvement of public health and animal health worldwide.

References

1. One Health High-Level Expert Panel (OHHLEP), Adisasmito WB, Almuhairi S, Behravesh CB, Bilivogui P, Bukachi SA, et al. One Health: a new definition for a sustainable and healthy future. PLoS Pathog. 2022;18(6):e1010537.
2. Evans BR, Leighton FA. A history of One Health. Rev Sci Tech OIE. 2014. [cited 2022 Jun 21];33(2):413–20. https://doi.org/10.20506/rst.33.2.2298.
3. WHO. Quadripartite Memorandum Of Understanding (MoU) Signed For A New Era Of One Health Collaboration. https://www.who.int/. 2022 [cited 2022 Jul 7]. https://www.who.int/news/item/29-04-2022-quadripartite-memorandum-of-understanding-(mou)-signed-for-a-new-era-of-one-health-collaboration.
4. Lerner H, Berg C. A comparison of three holistic approaches to health: One health, ecohealth, and planetary health. Frontiers. 2017;4:163. [cited 2022 Jun 21]. https://doi.org/10.3389/fvets.2017.00163/full.
5. Morand S, Guégan J-F, Laurans Y. From One Health to EcoHealth, mapping the incomplete integration of human, animal and environmental health. Iddri Issue Brief. 2020 ;(4):784. [cited 2022 Jul 7]. https://www.iddri.org/en/publications-and-events/issue-brief/one-health-ecohealth-mapping-incomplete-integration-human.
6. Yasobant S, Bruchhausen W, Saxena D. Applications of systems thinking for health system research: a one health perspective. SAGE Publications Limited; 2020. [Cited 2022 Jun 21]. https://doi.org/10.4135/9781529730739.
7. Bhattacharya S, Singh A. Fixing accountabilities and finding solutions to tackle acute (communicable) diseases viewed as collateral damage due to errors of omission and commission in primary care. J Family Med Prim Care. 2019. [cited 2022 Jun 21];8(3):784. https://doi.org/10.4103/jfmpc.jfmpc_45_19.
8. Gomo C. Brucellosis at the wildlife/livestock/human interface; 2015. [Cited 2022 Jun 21. https://doi.org/10.5772/61212.
9. Cardinale E, Perrier Gros-Claude JD, Rivoal K, Rose V, Tall F, Mead GC, et al. Epidemiological analysis of salmonella enterica ssp. enterica serovars Hadar, Brancaster and Enteritidis from humans and broiler chickens in Senegal using pulsed-field gel electrophoresis and antibiotic susceptibility. J Appl Microbiol [Internet]. 2005. [cited 2022 Jun 21];99(4):968–77. https://doi.org/10.1111/j.1365-2672.2005.02618.x.
10. Robinson TP, Bu DP, Carrique-Mas J, Fèvre EM, Gilbert M, Grace D, et al. Antibiotic resistance is the quintessential One Health issue. Trans R Soc Trop Med Hyg. 2016. [cited 2022 Jun 21];110(7):377–80. https://doi.org/10.1093/trstmh/trw048.
11. Stop using Antibiotics in healthy animals to preserve their effectiveness. WHO 2017; [cited 2022 Jun 21]. https://www.who.int/news/item/07-11-2017-stop-using-antibiotics-in-healthy-animals-to-prevent-the-spread-of-antibiotic-resistance.
12. Eriksen J, Björkman I, Röing M, Essack SY, Stålsby LC. Exploring the One Health perspective in Sweden's policies for containing antibiotic resistance. Antibiotics. 2021. [cited 2022 Jun 21];10(5):526. https://doi.org/10.3390/antibiotics10050526.

77 Planetary Health: From Concept to Action

Josep M. Antó and Cathryn Tonne

Abstract

Today we live in the Anthropocene, a new epoch characterized by the profound disturbances that industrial societies have caused in the Earth's natural systems, resulting in an unprecedented existential threat to humans and most species. Planetary Health has emerged as a new interdisciplinary and transdisciplinary approach focused on understanding and addressing the impacts of human activities on natural systems and their consequences for human health and that of other species. Planetary Health adopts approaches from the sciences of complex systems to analyze the multiple interactions between social systems and natural systems and propose solutions to preserve the health of humans and other species within the sustainable limits of the Earth. Ethics is central to Planetary Health as it involves a strong focus on identifying the winners and losers from global environmental change and the need to protect the most vulnerable and future generations. Likewise, consistent with the timescale of the current transgression of planetary boundaries, there is a unique sense of urgency in Planetary Health to implement transformative mitigation and adaptation strategies.

Keywords

Planetary Health · Earth systems · Sustainability · Planetary boundaries · Global Health

J. M. Antó (✉)
ISGlobal, Barcelona Institute for Global Health, Barcelona, Spain

Universitat Pompeu Fabra (UPF), Barcelona, Spain

CIBER Epidemiología y Salud Pública (CIBERESP), Barcelona, Spain
e-mail: josepm.anto@isglobal.org

C. Tonne
ISGlobal, Barcelona Institute for Global Health, Barcelona, Spain

Universitat Pompeu Fabra (UPF), Barcelona, Spain

CIBER Epidemiología y Salud Pública (CIBERESP), Barcelona, Spain
e-mail: cathryn.tonne@isglobal.org

77.1 Introduction

During the last decades, scientific evidence has unequivocally shown that human activity has profoundly altered the Earth's climate system and biodiversity resulting in an unprecedented existential threat for humans and other species [1]. The understanding of the scale of human impacts on Earth systems has led to the formulation of the Anthropocene [2], a new geological epoch characterized by negative impacts on natural systems due to human activities and which replaces the Holocene, a 10,000 year-long period characterized by a stable climate. Planetary boundaries

M. C. B. Raviglione et al. (eds.), *Global Health Essentials*, Sustainable Development Goals Series,
https://doi.org/10.1007/978-3-031-33851-9_77

have been defined to delineate the safe operating space for humanity with respect to the Earth system. Recent assessments indicate that four of nine proposed planetary boundaries have been exceeded due to human activities [3]. Many of the Earth's subsystems react in non-linear, often abrupt ways, and are particularly sensitive around tipping points of certain key variables.

Current rates of degradation of natural systems are leading to ecosystem disruption, increasing the risk of cascading effects which could massively affect human societies, particularly the living conditions of future generations and today's most vulnerable populations [4]. In response to the Anthropocene, a group of experts convened as the Rockefeller-Lancet Commission on Planetary Health proposed to shift the prevailing human health paradigm by adopting the concept of Planetary Health [5]. In this chapter, we describe the concept of Planetary Health, highlighting its added value to Global Health.

77.2 What Is Planetary Health?

Earlier concepts of human health did not consider the fact that improvements in health may be directly and indirectly associated with the degradation of natural systems and resources which are a necessary requirement for human health. Planetary Health makes these links explicit. The Rockefeller-Lancet Commission [5] defined Planetary Health as "the highest possible standard of health, well-being, and equity worldwide through the judicious attention to the human systems that shape the future of humanity and the Earth's natural systems that define the safe environmental limits within which humanity can flourish." Since then, Planetary Health has evolved as a solutions-oriented transdisciplinary field and social movement focused on analyzing and addressing the impacts of human disruptions to natural systems on human health and all life on Earth (i.e., the Planetary Health Alliance). Since its initial formulation, the Planetary Health approach is increasingly capturing imaginations across society, growing rapidly to including the launch of new scientific journals including the Lancet Planetary Health, several textbooks [6, 7], and being readily taken up in education and the arts [8, 9].

77.3 Key Components of Planetary Health

Defining elements of a Planetary Health approach include the focus on upstream drivers of human health, in particular, the relationship between humans and nature [6]. Drawing heavily from ecology, it leverages systems thinking and approaches to understand the complex systems shaping human health and the potential for unintended consequences. It involves a strong focus on identifying the winners and losers of global environmental change, protecting the most vulnerable, and quantifying externalities to more accurately evaluate the social and environmental costs of human activities [6]. Ethics, norms, and values are central to Planetary Health, for example, in understanding how human health came to be seen apart from that of other species and how to tip the scales in public health to better balance the needs of all species and between current and future generations. Finally, there is a unique urgency in Planetary Health to shift the steep trends of the past six decades in greenhouse gas emissions, resource use, environmental degradation, and ecosystem disruption to ensure human health can continue to improve. These defining features are embedded in the Helsinki Declaration, a call for action to support Planetary Health [10] (see Box 77.1).

Box 77.1: The Helsinki Declaration on Planetary Health

H: Human health depends on our ability to sustain Planetary Health. Awareness of the strong interlinkage between human and Planetary Health must be raised.

E: Equity is the guiding principle to ensure societal balance, which is a prerequisite for any successful action. Nature conservation and restoration do not succeed without social justice.

L: Long-term goals are to take priority over short-term political victories or economic gains.

S: Short-term actions, like reducing air pollution, chemical contamination, and ending smoking, have fast and radical impacts on health and should be actively promoted, as they also sustain Planetary Health.

I: Interventions among and planned with communities and citizens produce relevant results for political decisions and models for societal learning.

N: Nature is us, we are nature. Nature is both inside and outside of us, and well-functioning, sustainable, and biodiverse natural systems are essential for human health and survival.

K: Knowledge emerges from scientific insights and innovations proceed to action only when co-created by scientists, citizens, and policy makers.

I: Impact-oriented actions for Planetary Health must be continuously evaluated and adjusted accordingly.

Reproduced with permission from: https://thl.fi/en/web/thlfi-en/-/the-time-to-act-is-now-helsinki-declaration-on-planetary-health-calls-for-commitment-from-the-eu

See also references

77.4 What Is the Value Added to Global Health?

Planetary Health involves a paradigm shift compared to Global Health. First, Planetary Health broadens the scope beyond the health of all people worldwide by integrating human health with the health of other species and Earth's natural systems. Whereas global health has incorporated a social sciences approach in dealing with health inequalities and equity, Planetary Health focus on the intersection between social systems and ecosystems. Second, a Planetary Health perspective reveals that delivering the goals of Global Health (i.e., improving health and health equity for all people worldwide) requires protecting and restoring the natural systems on which human health depends. This implies a significantly broader view of the ethical considerations and values underpinning health to explicitly account for the value of non-human species. Third, Planetary Health is the natural evolution of Global Health which further extends the emphasis on transnational health issues, determinants, and solutions by focusing on the consequences for human health of global-scale changes in the biosphere. Like Eco-Health and One Health (see Chap. 76), Planetary Health further expands the interdisciplinary links seen in Global Health to include integration of disciplines such as ecology and Earth sciences [11].

77.5 Challenges and Responses Toward Securing Planetary Health

The Rockefeller-Lancet Commission presented a taxonomy of challenges in Planetary Health including those related to imagination, knowledge, and implementation. This taxonomy serves to guide identifying solutions and pathways for transformation.

77.5.1 Imagination Challenges

Challenges of the imagination have to do with ethical values and our concept of health [6]. The dominant paradigm that separates human health from that of natural systems is relatively recent. Planetary Health has a particular emphasis on concepts of health and values in indigenous cultures, which define themselves according to the inextricable links to the lands and natural resources where they live or from which they have been displaced. Many of today's pressing public health issues arise from ways of thinking that do not value the lives of other species, or nature either due to its inherent value or due to the services it provides to humans (i.e., ecosys-

Table 77.1 Examples of Planetary Health actions

Planetary Health actions	Example(s)	Levers for change
Meet food needs within environmental limits	Sustainably increase food from the Sea to meet future demand by improving management of wild fisheries, policy reform of mariculture, advancing feed technology for mariculture, shifting demand [15]	• Governance (e.g., policy reform) • Finance (e.g., price controls, subsidies) • Technology (e.g., intellectual property rights for new innovations) • Individual and collective action (e.g., demand for seafood)
Maximize health co-benefits from climate change mitigation	Place health at the center of climate and other policies to maximize benefits and minimize harms. [17]	• Governance (e.g., account for health implications of policy decisions) • Technology (e.g., air pollution emission controls) • Individual and collective action (e.g., shift toward plant-based diets and active travel)
Manage chemicals within safe planetary boundaries	• Prioritize pollution prevention and health protection nationally and internationally; • Mobilize, increase, and focus funding and international technical support for pollution control • Establish systems to monitor and control pollution • Build multisectoral partnerships for pollution control [19]	• Governance (e.g., government policy to remove lead from gasoline) • Finance (e.g., adopt polluter pays principle) • Technology (e.g., emissions control)

tem services). Similarly, many of today's pressing environmental and equity issues arise from focusing on short-term gains, without consideration of the longer-term consequences of human activities and their impacts on the well-being of future generations.

77.5.2 Knowledge Challenges

Knowledge challenges result from inadequate understanding of the interactions between social and natural systems and the impact of these interactions on human health. Addressing these challenges requires new models and methods capable of dealing with complexity as well as inter- and transdisciplinary approaches [12]. In responding to the inherent complexity of the Anthropocene's challenges, Planetary Health adopts a holistic approach to knowledge aimed at capturing the multiplicity of links and interactions, across different systems. This type of approach requires the development and application of new methods suited to modeling complex systems, scenario-based modeling, as well as developing the necessary cross-disciplinary alliances [13].

77.5.3 Implementation Challenges

The most consequential, however, are implementation challenges. These relate to how we apply existing knowledge to put in place solutions to protect health and natural systems. Levers for transformative change which have been identified in the context of achieving the Sustainable Development Goals are equally relevant for identifying Planetary Health solutions. These include governance (local, national, and global scale), economy and finance, individual and collective action, and science and technology [14]. Key areas in which planetary health action is being proposed [10] include (Table 77.1): strategies to cover food needs within environmental limits including issues like sustainable aquaculture [15] and the promotion of low-environmental impact diets [16], mitigation of climate change to achieve the goals of the Paris agreement [17], sound management of chemicals within the planetary boundaries [18, 19], climate neutral and sustainable cities and metropolitan conurbations [20] and decarbonized and sustainable health systems [21].

77.6 Concluding Remarks

Planetary health is a relatively recent concept that redefines public health goals by framing them within the safe environmental boundaries within which humanity can flourish. As a field, it is fostering the development of transdisciplinary alliances, new theoretical and methodological approaches suited to complex systems, and is informing new solutions that simultaneously promote human health, sustainability goals, and equity. Planetary Health brings urgency and a call to action to reverse the negative impacts of human activities on natural systems that underpin human health and well-being. As a social movement, Planetary Health goes far beyond the scientific community, forging a broad alliance including engaged citizens, educators, health practitioners, civil society, and funders to ensure a healthier planet for current and future generations.

References

1. https://report.ipcc.ch/ar6/wg1/IPCC_AR6_WGI_FullReport.pdf.
2. Waters CN, Zalasiewicz J, Summerhayes C, Barnosky AD, Poirier C, Gałuszka A, et al. The Anthropocene is functionally and stratigraphically distinct from the Holocene. Science. 2016;351(6269):aad2622.
3. Steffen W, Richardson K, Rockström J, Cornell SE, Fetzer I, Bennett EM, et al. Planetary boundaries: guiding human development on a changing planet. Science. 2015;347(6223):1259855.
4. Bergstrom DM, Wienecke BC, van den Hoff J, Hughes L, Lindenmayer DB, Ainsworth TD, et al. Combating ecosystem collapse from the tropics to the Antarctic. Glob Chang Biol. 2021;27(9):1692–703.
5. Whitmee S, Haines A, Beyrer C, Boltz F, Capon AG, de Souza Dias BF, et al. Safeguarding human health in the Anthropocene epoch: report of The Rockefeller Foundation–Lancet Commission on planetary health. Lancet. 2015;386(10007):1973–2028.
6. Myers SS, Frumkin H. Planetary health - protecting nature to protect ourselves. Island Press; 2020. [cited 2022 Feb 24]. https://islandpress.org/books/planetary-health.
7. Haines A, Frumkin H. Planetary health: safeguarding human health and the environment in the Anthropocene|Fifteen Eighty Four|Cambridge University Press. 2021 [cited 2022 Jun 21]. http://www.cambridgeblog.org/2021/07/planetary-health-safeguarding-human-health-and-the-environment-in-the-anthropocene/.
8. Antó JM, Martí JL, Casals J, Bou-Habib P, Casal P, Fleurbaey M, et al. The planetary wellbeing initiative: pursuing the sustainable development goals in higher education. Sustainability. 2021;13(6):3372.
9. Visions and voices of a healthy planet: A healing arts event for world health day 2022. [cited 2022 Jun 28]. https://www.who.int/news-room/events/detail/2022/04/05/default-calendar/visions-and-voices-of-a-healthy-planet-a-healing-arts-event-for-world-health-day-2022.
10. Halonen JI, Erhola M, Furman E, Haahtela T, Jousilahti P, Barouki R, et al. The Helsinki Declaration 2020: Europe that protects. Lancet Planet Health. 2020;4(11):e503–5.
11. Buse CG, Oestreicher JS, Ellis NR, Patrick R, Brisbois B, Jenkins AP, et al. Public health guide to field developments linking ecosystems, environments and health in the Anthropocene. J Epidemiol Community Health. 2018;72(5):420–5.
12. Steffen W, Richardson K, Rockström J, Schellnhuber HJ, Dube OP, Dutreuil S, et al. The emergence and evolution of earth system science. Nat Rev Earth Environ. 2020;1(1):54–63.
13. Cerdá M, Keyes KM. Systems modeling to advance the promise of data science in epidemiology. Am J Epidemiol. 2019;188(5):862–5.
14. Independent group of scientist. Global sustainable development report 2019: The future is now – science for achieving sustainable development. 2019. https://sdgs.un.org/es/node/24576.
15. Costello C, Cao L, Gelcich S, Cisneros-Mata MÁ, Free CM, Froehlich HE, et al. The future of food from the sea. Nature. 2020;588(7836):95–100.
16. Springmann M, Wiebe K, Mason-D'Croz D, Sulser TB, Rayner M, Scarborough P. Health and nutritional aspects of sustainable diet strategies and their association with environmental impacts: a global modelling analysis with country-level detail. Lancet Planet Health. 2018;2(10):e451–61.
17. Hamilton I, Kennard H, McGushin A, Höglund-Isaksson L, Kiesewetter G, Lott M, et al. The public health implications of the Paris agreement: a modelling study. Lancet Planet Health. 2021;5(2):e74–83.
18. Landrigan PJ, Fuller R, Acosta NJR, Adeyi O, Arnold R, Basu NN, et al. The Lancet commission on pollution and health. Lancet. 2018;391(10119):462–512.
19. Fuller R, Landrigan PJ, Balakrishnan K, Bathan G, Bose-O'Reilly S, Brauer M, et al. Pollution and health: a progress update. Lancet Planet Health. 2022;6(6):e535–47.
20. Tonne C, Adair L, Adlakha D, Anguelovski I, Belesova K, Berger M, et al. Defining pathways to healthy sustainable urban development. Environ Int. 2021;146:106236.
21. Salas RN, Maibach E, Pencheon D, Watts N, Frumkin H. A pathway to net zero emissions for healthcare. BMJ. 2020;1(371):m3785.

Equity, Inclusivity, and Diversity as Drivers of Global Health—Recommendations for Global Health Research, Education, and Practice

78

Astrid Berner-Rodoreda, Núria Casamitjana, Guenter Froeschl, Catherine Kyobutungi, J. Jaime Miranda, Kabir Sheikh, and Jolene Skordis

Abstract

Global Health recognizes the interconnectedness of communities across the world in terms of health problems and solutions; yet, despite being foundationally different from international and tropical health, the term maintains a focus on low- and middle-income countries. The practice of global health is not a one-way street and, in order to follow a truly global and equitable approach, inclusiveness and diversity need to be ingrained and structural issues, such as inequity in accessing medical products and diagnostics, gender and income inequalities, among others, tackled. We contend that Global Health research, education, and practice require a truly participatory system in order to make fundamental changes to the present Northern-dominated Global Health agenda.

Keywords

Equity · Inclusivity · Diversity · Global health education · Global health research

A. Berner-Rodoreda
University of Heidelberg, Heidelberg, Germany
e-mail: astrid.berner-rodoreda@uni-heidelberg.de

N. Casamitjana (✉)
Barcelona Institute for Global Health—University of Barcelona, Barcelona, Spain
e-mail: nuria.casamitjana@isglobal.org

G. Froeschl
University Hospital, LMU Munich, Munich, Germany
e-mail: Guenter.Froeschl@med.uni-muenchen.de

C. Kyobutungi
African Population and Health Research Center (APHRC), Nairobi, Kenya
e-mail: CKyobutungi@aphrc.org

J. J. Miranda
Universidad Peruana Cayetano Heredia, Lima, Peru
e-mail: jaime.miranda@upch.pe

K. Sheikh
Alliance for Health Policy and Systems Research, World Health Organization, Geneva, Switzerland
e-mail: ksheikh@who.int

J. Skordis
University College London, London, UK
e-mail: j.skordis@ucl.ac.uk

M. C. B. Raviglione et al. (eds.), *Global Health Essentials*, Sustainable Development Goals Series,
https://doi.org/10.1007/978-3-031-33851-9_78

78.1 Introduction to the Issue

All humans are considered equal [1]; yet, means to lead a healthy life are not equally accessible. Social and economic barriers are common, not only between richer and poorer nations but also within countries and communities. Discrimination and structural inequities can be based on gender, sexual orientation, ethnicity, age, profession, education, disability, religion, and practically any characteristics of individuals or a community. These inequities bear upon the possibilities to meaningfully participate across different aspects of society, shaping job and research opportunities, representation at leadership level of institutions and organizations, policy formulation or, more operational aspects such as the procurement of consumables—all of which are relevant motors of global health policy.

Equity and inclusiveness are core concepts in the Sustainable Development Goals [2]. To achieve more inclusiveness and diversity in Global Health, the multi-dimensionality and intersectionality of disadvantages overlapping across gender, World Bank categorization of country of origin, stage of researcher's career, and other factors, need to be further appreciated and addressed [3]. Fruitful collaboration in terms of research and publication necessitates an equitable approach drawing on inclusivity and diversity [4]. Despite its intentions to convey a 'health for all', and thus a truly global approach to overcome health inequities, Global Health has failed to do so even (or also) in terms of Global Health research and practice [5] as well as Global Health education [6].

78.2 Background

Global Health addresses the globalization of health and recognizes the interconnectedness between communities in terms of health problems and health solutions. Unlike previous terms such as tropical medicine or international health, Global Health applies to all countries irrespective of regional or income characteristics, yet its emergence from those previous concepts and the usage of the term predominantly by scholars in the Global North have led to it being viewed as also linked to colonialism and 'othering' in describing health situations in low- and middle-income countries (LMICs) [7].

A global response to infectious diseases such as HIV, Ebola, and COVID-19, to name a few, has revealed structural injustices that amplify their negative impacts on society, and the global response to these have shown inequity in accessing life-saving diagnostics, therapeutics, and vaccines, due to differing levels of country income and a tendency of the Global North to impose solutions on the Global South without making the learning reciprocal. Similar examples can be also be made from the worldwide rise of non-communicable diseases, including obesity. Additional drivers of inequities in health are gender issues, socio-economic disparities, and exclusion of affected and often marginalized groups in decision-making.

78.3 Aims of the Chapter

In order to achieve equitable health in the domains of research, practice, and education, we should consider an equity approach which takes diversity and inclusiveness into account at all levels-community, researchers, students, educators. To this end, the current shortcomings in the areas of global health research, practice, and education, will be shown (description of issues), and truly participatory and equitable global health approaches will be suggested (approach to solutions).

78.4 Description of the Issues

Equity is fundamental when working in global health, it should be present in any partnership or collaboration, especially in transboundary and intercultural contexts, regardless of the country's level of income. Inequities arise from lack of joint agreement and planning; uneven distribution of tasks, responsibilities and resources; absence of mutuality in learning, data sharing and a reciprocal transfer of skills; as well as an inequitable distribution of profits and rewards, amongst others [8].

In the case of research collaborations, these shortcomings have been acknowledged, yet power differentials and unequal access to resources continue to exist between Northern and Southern researchers, expressing themselves in a number of ways, e.g., the attendance to Global Health conferences is lower for researchers from the Global South due to travel costs, visa challenges, and fewer accepted research presentations [9]. In the academic publishing environment, only a third of editors are female and a third are based in LMICs, thus showing a persistent male and Northern dominance [4].

To address inequity issues in global health education, action is required with special attention to the pervasive use of a competency-based education frameworks and curricular content that ignores the above-mentioned origins of Global Health [10]. Also, learning experiences still seem to be mainly provided for Northern scholars to those in the Global South, when it should be obvious that Global Health is not a one-way street [6, 11]. While efforts are being made to increasingly confront power asymmetries and colonialism in Global Health education in high-income countries, a bolder approach is needed to ensure that scholars from the Global South equally share their expertise with those from the Global North.

Prevailing imbalances in Global Health are also noticeable with regard to governance representation in organizations. The annual review of the equality- and gender-related policies and practices of 200 global organizations showed that out of 2024 board seats across 146 global health organizations, up to 75% of governing bodies and 82% of funding bodies were held by nationals of high-income countries. In terms of gender, 1% of seats in the non-profit sector were held by female nationals of low-income countries, and none on for-profit boards. [12].

Further, inequalities persist between global health practitioners and the communities they are intended to partner with [13]. This constitutes another inequity that is often ignored and will have to be addressed in order to achieve an inclusive approach to global health.

78.5 Approach to Solutions and Options

Equity, diversity, and inclusion should be core principles of agenda setting, planning, and financing of Global Health delivery, teaching, and research; and, therefore, close monitoring of these indicators is essential to ensure adequate accountability. Structural barriers that drive entrenched inequities and exclusion need to be identified and, correspondingly, adequate mechanisms for representation and meaningful involvement of actors at all levels, e.g., service deliverers and (marginalized) communities, institutions from North and South, international and national actors in Global Health endeavours need to be pursued, including but not limited to a diverse representation of actors from different countries, backgrounds, and gender. Positive and negative lessons for Global Health research, practice, and education, more so given the recent learnings from the COVID-19 pandemic, can support in identifying barriers and shortcomings, but can also act as catalysts towards change.

The Swiss Academy of Sciences (2018) has proposed key principles for research partnerships including joint agenda setting, clarifying responsibilities, sharing data and networks, pooling profits and rewards for Global Health research, which meaningfully encompass the meaning of Global Health research. We propose that such principles should also be adapted to Global Health education and practice to ensure meaningful inclusion of diverse groups (Fig. 78.1).

Box 78.1: Recommendations to Achieve Equity, Inclusiveness, and Diversity in Global Health

- Power asymmetries between nations, populations, and differing social standings have to be recognized and addressed in all Global Health settings.
- The Global Health agenda with regard to research, education, and practice has to be set under recognition of local expertise and concerns.
- Empowerment as another form of paternalistic approach should be replaced by a guiding principle of equal opportunities, where decision making powers can evolve.
- The intersectionality of gender, income-levels, age, and experience has to be addressed to achieve diversity and inclusivity.
- Marginalization of populations has many faces, and focussing on characteristics like gender or ethnicity will not suffice. Reasoning by decision makers should be based on the fundamental human rights approach to health.

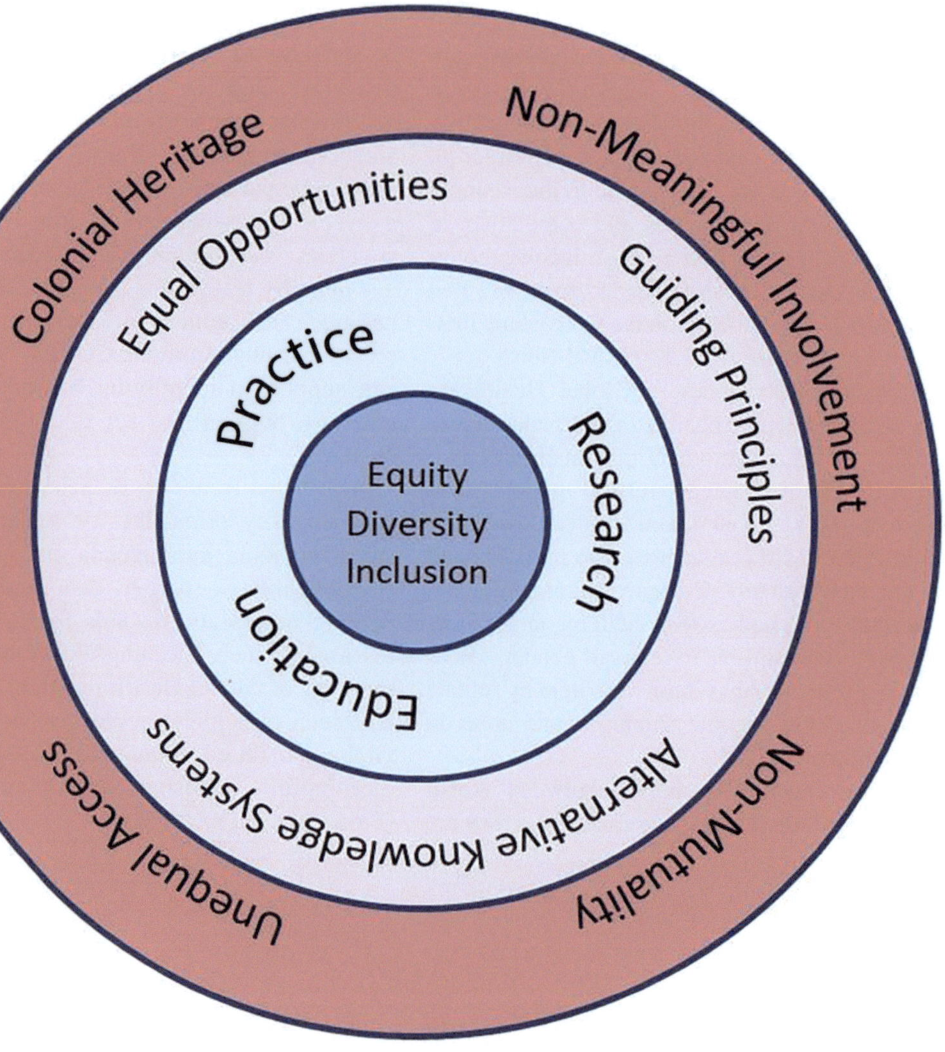

Fig. 78.1 Issues, domains, approaches, and principles in Equity, Diversity and Inclusion

78.6 Conclusions

Inequities are a key barrier to achieve universal health for all, they are entrenched through history, self-sustaining power asymmetries, economic interests, conceptions, and stigmatization of marginalized groups. Tackling inequities will amplify the goals of diversity and inclusion, and this calls for a fundamental transformation and cannot be reduced to making a few cosmetic changes. A truly participatory system of equitable agenda setting, ranging from research funding to the making of health policy, securing diversity and meaningful representation of actors and institutions across Global Health research, practice, and education areas would make fundamental changes to the present Global North-dominated agenda and modus operandi.

References

1. United Nations General Assembly. Universal declaration of human rights. Geneva: United Nations; 1948. https://www.un.org/en/about-us/universal-declaration-of-human-rights.
2. United Nations General Assembly. Transforming our world: the 2030 agenda for sustainable development. New York: United Nations General Assembly; 2015.
3. Sheikh K, Bennett SC, El Jardali F, Gotsadze G. Privilege and inclusivity in shaping Global Health agendas. Health Policy Plan. 2017;32(3):303–4. https://doi.org/10.1093/heapol/czw146.
4. Nafade V, Sen P, Pai M. Global Health journals need to address equity, diversity and inclusion. BMJ Glob Health. 2019;4(5):e002018. https://doi.org/10.1136/bmjgh-2019-002018.
5. Berner-Rodoreda A, Rehfuess EA, Klipstein-Grobusch K, Cobelens F, Raviglione M, Flahaut A, Casamitjana N, et al. Where is the 'global' in the European Union's Health Research and innovation agenda? BMJ Glob Health. 2019;4(5):e001559. https://doi.org/10.1136/bmjgh-2019-001559.
6. Eichbaum QG, Adams LV, Evert J, Ho M-J, Semali IA, van Schalkwyk SC. Decolonizing Global Health education: rethinking institutional partnerships and approaches. Acad Med. 2021;96(3):329–35. https://doi.org/10.1097/ACM.0000000000003473.
7. Bain LE, Nanyonjo A, Blake V, Tembo J, Nkongho F, Bates M. How do we 'decolonize global health'? J Prev Diagn Treat Strat Med. 2022;1(1):4.
8. Swiss Academy of Sciences. A guide for transboundary research partnerships. 2018, 3rd edition. https://kfpe.scnat.ch/en/about_kfpe/uuid/i/13beb0f7-4780-5967-a257-bd6cc3d5e424-A_Guide_for_Transboundary_Research_Partnerships_3rd_edition_-_2018.
9. Velin L, Lartigue J-W, Johnson SA, Zorigtbaatar A, Kanmounye US, Truche P, Joseph MN. Conference equity in Global Health: a systematic review of factors impacting LMIC representation at Global Health conferences. BMJ Glob Health. 2021;6(1):e003455. https://doi.org/10.1136/bmjgh-2020-003455.
10. Sayegh H, Harden C, Khan H, et al. Global health education in high-income countries: confronting coloniality and power asymmetry. BMJ Glob Health. 2022;7:e008501. https://doi.org/10.1136/bmjgh-2022-008501.
11. Miranda JJ, Garcia PJ, Lescano AG, Gotuzzo E, Garcia HH. Global health training – one way street? Am J Trop Med Hyg. 2011;84(3):506.; author reply 507. PMID: 21363994; PMCID: PMC3042832. https://doi.org/10.4269/ajtmh.2011.10-0694a.
12. Global Health 50/50 report. Boards for all? A review of power, policy and people on the boards of organisations active in Global Health. London, UK; 2022.
13. Urmitapa D. Decolonizing "community" in community psychology. Am J Community Psychol. 2018;62(3–4):272–82. https://doi.org/10.1002/ajcp.12281.

79 Rethinking Knowledge in Global Health

Emilie Koum Besson and Madhukar Pai

Abstract

In global (public) health, the way we define knowledge and knowers is not neutral and directly affects the outcome of health interventions. The COVID-19 pandemic highlighted both the limitations of the current knowledge ecosystem in global health and the positive impact of nationally and locally informed public health interventions. From this perspective, this chapter aims to increase readers' understanding of these limitations and guide them in efforts to improve interactions between and within diverse knowledge systems.

This chapter is divided into three main sections. Firstly, we briefly illuminate the roots of decolonial science in global health and the importance of social sciences in public health practice. Secondly, we describe common biases that act as barriers to change in the global health knowledge ecosystem and introduce a change management approach to rethink the way different forms of knowledge are currently generated, understood, used, disseminated, and legitimized. Thirdly, we define the concept of Emancipatory Health Interventions (EHIs), the role of global actors in their design, and present a case study to guide actors in efforts to identify existing EHIs and normalize practices in the future.

Keywords

Global health · Decoloniality · Decolonizing global health · Global health equity · Knowledge cultivation

79.1 Colonial History in Global Health Knowledge Ecosystem

79.1.1 Introduction to Decolonial Science

Throughout history, those seeking to expand colonial missions used public health as a façade of benevolence to disguise their true motivations [1]. "I now firmly believe in the tropical colonisation by the white race…" were the words of Patrick Manson in 1900. As the father of tropical medicine, Manson arguably founded global health education.

Global health architecture still mimics its colonial origins [2]. Gender (men) and ancestry

E. Koum Besson
The Global Fund to Fight AIDS, Tuberculosis and Malaria, Geneva, Switzerland

M. Pai (✉)
School of Population and Global Health, McGill University, Montreal, Canada
e-mail: madhukar.pai@mcgill.ca

M. C. B. Raviglione et al. (eds.), *Global Health Essentials*, Sustainable Development Goals Series,
https://doi.org/10.1007/978-3-031-33851-9_79

(white European) dominates and dictates funding streams, authorship of publications, leadership of agencies, composition of boards, editorial board positions, awards, and even participants at "international" conferences. In institutions, systems of privilege are sustained by processes and practices rooted in saviourism instead of agency [3]. In practice, the COVID-19 pandemic response underscored how systems of power, hidden behind calls for "generosity" over equity, ensured a prolonged pandemic and limited the expected impact of vaccination in LMICs [4].

Global health is not neutral, reciprocal, diverse or equitable. Global health is not global.

Disrupting the current global health architecture does not aim to introduce a new definition but to move beyond the binaries that oppose Euro North-American regions (i.e. Global North) considered as the norm from other regions (i.e. Global South) by creating space for different ways of doing and being to co-exist and flourish [5, 6].

In The Black Pacific: Anti-Colonial Struggles and Oceanic Connections (2015), postcolonial researcher Robbie Shilliam defines decolonial science as the *cultivation* rather than the *production* of knowledge. He argues that knowledge production is an imperialist endeavour that aims to prolong and accumulate knowledge so that (post)colonized people can only consume or extend someone else's knowledge of themselves while *knowledge cultivation* is a creative process that requires actors to reflect on the past and centre themselves in the matter of their inquiry. Fostering *knowledge cultivation* offers a pathway towards acknowledging the past wrongdoings, unlearning entrenched negative practices, and embracing a future rooted in self-reliance that matches the historic aspirations of decolonization movements.

79.1.2 Brief History of Global Health Education Colonial Origins

Global health education's history is indissociable from theories around the supremacy of the white race that underpin racism and served to justify colonialism and its legacies. It continues to bear (harmful) assumptions so engrained that they have long been mistaken for facts [7, 8]. While decolonial studies, critical development studies, critical race theory, and whiteness studies offer a lot to global health, many students have never been introduced to these fields.

Global health originates from colonial and tropical medicine, created during colonialism as an effort to protect the health of white colonists and keep indigenous population used as labour force alive. Following political decolonization (i.e., independence movements), it was renamed international health with a novel emphasis placed on the notion that formally colonized actors were incapable of addressing their health issues without the "development or technical assistance" or "aid" of former colonizers.

It was Frantz Fanon who first defined global health as a system where public health is used as a colonial tool to westernize the world.

The doctor always appears as a link in the colonialist network, as a spokesman for the occupying power.

His work provides a framework to facilitate our understanding of the current asymmetries of power and privilege in health as well as the origins of the resistance emanating from Global South actors, indigenous communities in the Global North, and people with Global South ancestries living in the Global North [9].

The COVID-19 pandemic underscored the importance of Fanon's work to gain insight into the limitations of global health responses in the absence of active mechanisms to transcend global health origins and make it actively anti-supremacist, anti-oppressionist, and anti-racist [10]. At the global, national, and interpersonal level reaching health equity worldwide will only be achieved by actively working towards applying a decolonial lens to health globally [11]. This, in turn, will require us to address how knowledge is legitimized.

79.1.3 How Can we Foster Knowledge Cultivation?

Rather than defining national boundaries or a specific category of actors, this chapter aims to guide public health actors over the world, passionate about achieving health equity to answer the question: how do we rethink the way we interact with different forms of knowledge? This approach is guided by the words of Paul Farmer:

> *Global health is not a discipline or a field but rather a collection of problems*

The way we generate, understand, use, disseminate, and legitimize knowledge is intertwined with our culture and geographies. The current knowledge hierarchy—inherited from colonial administrations—that assumes the superiority of "Western scientific knowledge" (i.e., Euro-North-American) and Global North experts over ancestral and Indigenous ways of knowing and experts in and from the Global South hinders innovation and progress in addressing health inequities [12]. To inform the design of fit-for-purpose interventions and policies that meet the specific needs of diverse communities, public health actors must break these hierarchies and learn how to foster knowledge plurality—a system that learns from and equally values every form of knowledge derived from all regions.

In this chapter, our decolonial approach to rethinking knowledge in global health aims to normalize the design of health interventions liberated from colonial hierarchies of knowledge and knowers and which reflect the collective power and agency of people to determine their own destiny. We called them Emancipatory Health Interventions (EHIs).

An in-depth discussion of colonial legacies and the debates around global solidarity/cooperation is beyond the scope of this chapter. However, additional reading is referenced [13].

79.2 Critical Steps to Understand and Change the Current Knowledge Ecosystem

79.2.1 Common Barriers to Knowledge Ecosystem Change

Change is not a moment, a task, or a checklist. It is a process. Before diving into our three-steps change management approach to addressing asymmetries in the current global health knowledge ecosystem, we identify some common barriers to change.

- *Problem blindness*—Just because some practices are common does not make them acceptable. Actors' inability to properly name issues is a barrier to change. Problematizing the normal means naming and stigmatizing issues to allow collective solutions to emerge. For example, the Black Lives Matter and Decolonising Global Health movements did not introduce new issues but rather—through social media—increased access to terminologies (for example, intersectionality, epistemic injustice) from social sciences scholars working at the intersection of colonialism, racism, and health.
- *Framing bias*—Public health issues can be linked to behaviour and/or environment which means that framing should never be limited to the notion that a group should mimic another that is seemingly "performing better". Doing so effectively negates the role of culture, socio-economic, gender, sexual orientation, and potential differential access. The way we frame issues inform the approaches chosen. For example, talking about *hard-to-reach groups* versus *hard-to-reach services* often activates different public health responses. The former places the onus on communities and the latter on the public health system. The more distant one is from an issue/community, the more likely they are to misdiagnose or misrepresent them due to lower contextual, cultural, and practical understanding of the constraints of communities at risk. It manifests when actors in the Global North promote policies or conceptualize issues in a way that is disconnected from the realities of communities in the Global South (i.e., "Debates" around remunerating Community Health Workers).
- *Ignoring positionality*—Actors' understanding of health issues is informed by their proximity to the environment of communities at risk. The academic literature is only the collection of what has been written by those who

have been historically granted access to publications in academic journals (e.g., mostly Euro-North American scholars) rather than the sum of all knowledge on a specific context. Here, bi- and multi-cultural actors—including diasporic communities—who work at the intersection of the Global North and the Global South (also known as double agents or brokers) can play in important role in reducing the gaps between national/local versus international understanding to address framing biases [14].

- *Analysing problems and not successes*: There is a tendency in the Euro-North American scholarship to approach changes in terms of *what is not working and need to be fixed* rather than *what is working and how can it be reproduced*. Successes are not best practices but instead reflects the way an intervention functions at its best. Analysing and sharing successes are a way to show communities at risk that things can be done differently and give them a sense of what changes would mean for them in practice. Additionally, by placing their environment rather than theories at the centre of the change through learnings from other communities closest to them, positive outcomes become more relatable which ultimately increases sense of ownership. Here, the objective is to normalize pre-defined outcomes rather than scale up.

In summary, the current knowledge ecosystem is contaminated with conscious and unconscious biases. Thus, moving towards embracing all forms of knowledge cannot be achieved without critically thinking about what is currently taught, how it is taught, and the positionality of the teachers.

79.2.2 From Saviourism to Unleashing Agency of Communities

To the question "why did you chose the field of global health?" students often answer, "I want to help". While compassion and altruism are central in efforts to reach health equity globally, global health should no longer be a "safe space" to enact saviour fetish of "helping", inherited from colonialism [15].

Global health education is not neutral. In 1970, in the Pedagogy of the Oppressed, Paulo Freire described how a teacher, by simple virtue of having power over the curriculum, the dispensation of knowledge and what is allowed to be taught can influence how students think with respect to values, attitudes, and beliefs. When students and communities are expected to be passive recipients of "knowledge" and interventions with no say in design or content, agency is removed, and the "help" becomes a tool to oppress voices in societies [16].

In this section, we define saviourism as all practices, policies, and attitudes that reinforces privilege and power by placing the perspective of the "saviour" above the agency of communities. The saviour or charity model implies that the right to health is given by others (e.g., licenced or donated) rather than taken by communities to make sense of their world in their own terms (e.g., emancipatory) [17, 18]. An excellent contemporary example is vaccine donations as the way to achieve COVID-19 vaccine equity rather than a TRIPS intellectual property waiver and technology transfer that would allow countries to make their own products and be self-reliant.

Saviourism is displayed when actors:

1. Do not question the origins and legitimacy of current asymmetries of power.
2. Do not challenge the parameters sets by those who are not affected by the issues (e.g., global health priorities, intellectual property laws).
3. Prioritize quick fixes that create an endless cycle of reactions rather than allowing structures and systems to learn and adapt by focusing solely on what is achieved rather than how it is achieved.
4. See global health as charity, aid or philanthropy, rather than equity, justice, reparations, and solidarity.

Reaching health equity requires a paradigm shift that removes the control over the content and type of knowledge from the hand of the "teacher" and instead promotes agency to enable students/communities to construct their own meaning through experience within their sociocultural contexts.

Unleashing the agency or self-determination of communities at risk means moving towards self-regulation of the learning [16]. These communities should no longer be used as a mean to implement interventions and policies largely already designed by people who are far removed from their environment. To move beyond this subject/object relationship, public health actors globally should invoke the ability of communities at risk to understand their problems better than anyone else, actively engage with resources, accept responsibility, take control of, make mistakes in learning, and see how those choices impact their lives [17].

79.2.3 From Hierarchies of Knowing to Global Public Health

The idea of global health as an academic discipline and a field reinforces hierarchies of knowledge and knowers and disconnects health interventions from their regional/national/local public health systems. The distance between those who define and have the power to shape the agenda and those whose lives are impacted by these issues continues to maintain avoidable, unfair, and structural inequalities between actors.

Can a field be "global" when it is primarily taught in the Global North and therefore, the expertise relies on geographies and ability to afford costs of attendance (e.g., tuition fees, cost of living, visa)? What differentiates global health actors from national public health actors in countries which are the targets or intended recipients of global health interventions? [19].

Rather than attempting to answer these questions, we are introducing the concept of *global public health*. It is neither a new name for global health nor a novel discipline. It is the acknowledgement that health is indissociable from the social, cultural, economic, historic, and geographic specificities of a country. While current global health practices and policies places others before communities, applying a *global public health* lens demands that the design of health interventions be always informed by those impacted by the issues and led by those whose lived experience and positionality is closest to the realities of the communities being served. It breaks hierarchies of knowledge and knowers by centring the voices of national public health actors and defining global health actors as enablers or allies whose role is to facilitate knowledge sharing and global cooperation.

79.2.4 From the Foreign Gaze to Reconnecting Knowledge to its Context

The foreign gaze is a concept coined by Seye Abimbola to describe entrenched power asymmetries in global health partnerships between the actors who fund and set the agenda and the settings where the research and interventions are conducted. It reflects a disconnect between knowledge and their social, cultural, economic, and geographic context that seems to shift the responsibility to address health issues on "others". When the value of data and knowledge is based on parameters set by others rather than the impact on communities, it weakens communities' ownership of these issues and its consequences.

Who we imagine we write and work for (i.e., gaze), and the position or standpoint from which we write, and work (i.e., pose) informs the success of global health interventions [20]. Recentring public health work towards the local/regional gaze is key to addressing health inequities globally.

79.3 Freeing Public Health Interventions from Colonial Legacies

79.3.1 A Framework to Reimagine Global Health Knowledge Ecosystem

The design of health interventions freed from colonial legacies starts with delinking entrenched assumptions that development, progress, and modernity are synonyms with the westernization of the world [21]. It is about fostering the natural evolution of local ways of doing in a way that contextualize the idea of health as a fundamental and inalienable human right [8, 22, 23]. In Table 79.1, we presented some of the ways in which coloniality currently manifests in the global health knowledge ecosystem and proposed solutions to improve interactions between knowledge systems in the future.

79.3.2 Defining Emancipatory Health Interventions and Example in Practice

We define emancipatory health interventions as projects where the:

1. Data are collected with the primary aim to increase and expand the knowledge of people on the frontline and the communities at risk as opposed to addressing "gaps in the literature".
2. Design of the interventions is driven by people with lived experience, in the communities at risk or those closest to them as opposed to foreign actors.
3. Communities at risk and those closest to them are encouraged to develop products and tools specific to their environment first rather than attempting to answer to "global needs".
4. Demand for the interventions, and assessment of their successes and failures is articulated by the communities at risk or those closest to them as opposed to international donors' agendas.
5. Monitoring of projects is primarily designed to support communities at risk learning and advocacy efforts in the long term rather than for compliance to donors' reporting requirements.

Table 79.1 Reimagining global health knowledge ecosystem interactions

Current global health knowledge ecosystem		Re-imagined global health knowledge ecosystem	
Coloniality of power	Institutions and actors in the Global North control financial resources, health research and health policy agenda, as well as knowledge prioritization decision-making	Capacity strengthening and sharing with local, national, and regional health actors with onus placed on local, national, and regional health organizations to set health agenda. (e.g. reinforcing the role and voice of national public health experts, agencies, and regional entities like Africa CDC over "international" organizations)	Unleashing the agency of community
Coloniality of knowledge	Perceived inherent superiority of euro-north American ways of doing and knowing over "others"	Foreign knowledge should be complementary to national knowledge systems rather than seek to assert its dominance and/or try to erase them (e.g. integrating traditional healers in health interventions, designing contextualized community mental health interventions, acknowledging the origins of health interventions like mindfulness beyond the foreign gaze, recognizing the contribution of "othered" knowledge systems to euro-north American model)	Reconnecting knowledge to its context
Coloniality of being	Legitimized superiority of euro-north American knowers mirrored by the legitimized inferiority of non-euro-north American knowers. Binary of modern/rational/civilized versus traditional/irrational/uncivilized	Knowledge systems should be equally valued, studied, and respected. (e.g. diversify teaching and learning to include global south led interventions like the friendship bench in Zimbabwe (see case study below), COVID-19 vaccines manufactured in low and middle-income countries, Ife medical school of primary health care in Nigeria, Indian & Chinese Indigenous medical systems, etc.)	Fostering global public health

Public health interventions should enable people with lived experience, communities at risk and those closest to them to speak for themselves and advance their own struggle. Recentring public health interventions towards the local/regional gaze is key to addressing health inequities globally.

A practical example of what we recognize as an Emancipatory Health intervention is the Friendship Bench intervention [24]. Zimbabwean psychiatrist, Dixon Chibanda built from his knowledge of its context and community, collaborated with national and international actors, and used foreign knowledge systems and resources to develop a fit-for-purpose and contextualized intervention that meet the needs of the communities the intervention aimed to serve. Beyond the internationally recognised success of this intervention, current attempts to normalize its unique approach to mental health support in both Global South and Global North settings underscore the importance of community ownership in the success of public health interventions.

79.4 Conclusion

Rethinking knowledge in global health is a process of unlearning and challenging harmful conscious and unconscious practices and processes in the current knowledge ecosystem to create space for diverse knowledge systems to flourish. This change cannot be summarized into tasks and is better understood as an intentional and continuous process to critically engage with the dominant teaching and learning environment until currently other(ed) knowledge systems can co-exist, develop, and freely generate the knowledge necessary to address the issues of the communities they represent.

We believe that this novel global public health environment, centred around the cultivation of knowledge, shared learning across countries, between and within communities, will enable the design of the Emancipatory Health interventions needed to address health inequities and make sustainable changes worldwide.

Any public health actors can contribute to the emancipatory project, but foreign/distant/Global North actors cannot be the drivers of emancipation. They need to start with confronting their past, reflecting on their gaze and humbly working towards building trustworthiness and allyship rather than relying on saviour tropes that demand blind trust, unchallenged obedience and reinforce power and privilege by removing communities' agency.

Disclaimer The views expressed in this article do not necessarily represent the views of the organizations the authors work at.

References

1. Gregg A. Colonizing Fertility: Modern and historic case studies of the powerful exploiting the fertility of the powerless in Africa from the era of colonization forward. 2020 [cited 2022 Feb 3]. https://storymaps.arcgis.com/stories/8b5186f12e754dd8868bc6775 43d9666.
2. Pai M. Global health still mimics colonial ways: here's how to break the pattern. [cited 2021 Jul 30]. https://theconversation.com/global-health-still-mimics-colonial-ways-heres-how-to-break-the-pattern-121951.
3. Odjidja EN. What is wrong with global health? So-called glorified data collectors in low-income regions. Lancet Glob Health. 2021;9(10):e1365. [cited 2021 Sep 15]. http://www.thelancet.com/article/S2214109X21003715/fulltext
4. Watson OJ, Barnsley G, Toor J, Hogan AB, Winskill P, Ghani AC. Global impact of the first year of COVID-19 vaccination: a mathematical modelling study. Lancet Infect Dis. 2022;0(0):1–10. [cited 2022 Jun 27]. http://www.thelancet.com/article/S1473309922003206/fulltext
5. Khan T, Abimbola S, Kyobutungi C, Pai M. How we classify countries and people—and why it matters. BMJ Glob Health. 2022;7(6):e009704. [cited 2022 Aug 29]. https://gh.bmj.com/content/7/6/e009704
6. Koum Besson ES. Confronting whiteness and decolonising global health institutions. The Lancet. 2021;397(10292):2328–9. [cited 2021 Jul 29]. http://www.thelancet.com/article/S0140673621013210/fulltext
7. How eugenics shaped statistics—Nautilus|Science Connected. [cited 2022 May 16]. https://nautil.us/how-eugenics-shaped-statistics-9365/.
8. Naidu T, Abimbola S. How medical education holds back health equity. Lancet. 2022;400(10352):556–7. [cited 2022 Aug 29]. http://www.thelancet.com/article/S0140673622014234/fulltext

9. Ali SH, Rose JR. The post-colonialist condition, suspicion, and social resistance during the West African Ebola epidemic: The importance of Frantz Fanon for global health. Soc Sci Med. 2022;305:115066. [cited 2022 Jun 17]. https://doi.org/10.1016/j.socscimed.2022.115066.
10. Abimbola S, Pai M. Will global health survive its decolonisation? Lancet. 2020;396:1627–8.
11. Horton R. Offline: COVID-19 is not a pandemic. Lancet. 2020;396:874. [cited 2020 Nov 21]. www.thelancet.com.
12. Nordling L. How COVID-19 changed African R&D—Harvard public health magazine. Harvard Public Health 2022 [cited 2022 Jun 20]. https://harvardpublichealth.org/how-covid-19-changed-african-rd/.
13. Koum Besson ES, Rose Clarke A, Aleka Kebede M, Ismail Z, Pensa S. Introduction to Decoloniality & Anti-racism in global health Student toolkit. [cited 2022 Jun 27]. https://researchonline.lshtm.ac.uk/id/eprint/4664957.
14. Pai M. Double Agents in global health. Forbes. 2022 [cited 2022 Feb 6]. https://www.forbes.com/sites/madhukarpai/2022/02/06/double-agents-in-global-health/?sh=188df3cc1a2e.
15. Warren RC, Forrow L, Hodge DA, Truog RD. Trustworthiness before Trust — Covid-19 Vaccine Trials and the Black Community. N Engl J Med. 2020. [cited 2021 Nov 18];383(22):e121. https://doi.org/10.1056/NEJMp2030033.
16. The Pedagogy of Learner Agency—Unleashing the Power of Learner Agency. [cited 2022 Jun 27]. https://edtechbooks.org/up/peda.
17. Manji F. NGOs and Social Justice in Africa: The missionary position: NGOs and development in Africa. 2014. [cited 2022 Feb 4]. http://thinkingafricangos.blogspot.com/2014/08/the-missionary-position-ngos-and.html.
18. Kwete X, Tang K, Chen L, Ren R, Chen Q, Wu Z, et al. Decolonizing global health: what should be the target of this movement and where does it lead us? Glob Health Res Policy. 2022. [cited 2022 Mar 3];7(1):1–6. https://doi.org/10.1186/s41256-022-00237-3.
19. King NB, Koski A. Defining global health as public health somewhere else. BMJ Glob Health. 2020;5(1):e002172. [cited 2022 Aug 29]. https://gh.bmj.com/content/5/1/e002172
20. Bhakuni H, Abimbola S. Epistemic injustice in academic global health. Lancet Glob Health. 2021. [cited 2021 Aug 31];9:e1465. https://doi.org/10.1016/S2214-109X.
21. Koum Besson ES. How to identify epistemic injustice in global health research funding practices: a decolonial guide. BMJ Glob Health. 2022;7(4):e008950. [cited 2022 Jun 27]. https://gh.bmj.com/content/7/4/e008950
22. Boum Y, Kwedi-Nolna S, Haberer JE, Leke RRG. Traditional healers to improve access to quality health care in Africa. Lancet Glob Health. 2021;9(11):e1487–8. [cited 2022 Aug 29]. http://www.thelancet.com/article/S2214109X21004381/fulltext.
23. Ranchod K, Guimarães DS. Transcending global health dogma: an indigenous perspective. Lancet Glob Health. 2021;9(10):e1357–8. [cited 2021 Sep 15]. http://www.thelancet.com/article/S2214109X21003429/fulltext.
24. Chibanda D, Weiss HA, Verhey R, Simms V, Munjoma R, Rusakaniko S, et al. Effect of a primary care-based psychological intervention on symptoms of common mental disorders in Zimbabwe: a randomized clinical trial. JAMA. 2016;316(24):2618–26.

80 Strengthening Global Health and Health Diplomacy Capacity in the Global South

Elil Renganathan and Precious Matsoso

Abstract

Global health and health diplomacy are closely linked and have emerged as critical to the global discourse on Public Health. The increasing borderless nature of health and the influence of determinants that go beyond health require a special skill set and capacity. Furthermore, the changing Global Health environment, with the increasing prominence of health in the global development agenda and the increasing number of fora and health actors engaged in health policy-making, has posed challenges for the Global South to engage actively and effectively in an inclusive manner. This needs to be addressed urgently through strengthening capacity in Global Health and health diplomacy.

Keywords

Global Health · Health diplomacy · World Health Organization · Global South

E. Renganathan (✉) · P. Matsoso
Sunway University, Bandar Sunway, Malaysia

Health Regulatory Science Platform, Division of Wits Health Consortium, Department of Pharmacy and Pharmacology, University of Witwatersrand, Johannesburg, South Africa
e-mail: elil@sunway.edu.my; pmatsoso@HRSP.co.za

Global Health has been defined in different ways over the years [1–4]. Raviglione (Chap. 1, Global Health Essentials) proposes the following updated definition: *Global Health relates to issues that transcend national boundaries, are important to many countries at the same time and require global cooperation. Global Health, in seeking equitable access to healthcare for people in all countries, pursues universal health coverage (UHC), and furthermore, it is multi-disciplinary and extends beyond the health sciences.*

More recently, health diplomacy has emerged as a critical area closely linked to Global Health, and contributing to discourse on issues such as health governance, global public health goods, health security, trade and intellectual property. It has been defined as the multi-level processes that shape and manage the global policy environment for health [5, 6].

Developments over the past two decades also raise a number of important issues:

- *How global is global health?* One key issue is the voice given to the Global South in Global Health and its influence on setting the Global Health agenda to reduce health inequities. The discussion over the pertinence of who designs interventions and who receives them has been ongoing for the past two decades. Disparities in the level of engagement by the Global South in Global Health agenda both because

M. C. B. Raviglione et al. (eds.), *Global Health Essentials*, Sustainable Development Goals Series,
https://doi.org/10.1007/978-3-031-33851-9_80

of the lack of capacity and the lack of opportunities are well documented, and some of the reasons for this are addressed by Pai and Besson (Chap. 79, Global Health Essentials).

- The *increasing borderless nature of health* requires a better understanding and appreciation of critical influences and determinants that go beyond health, such as trade, intellectual property, One Health and Planetary Health. While countries have cooperated to fight health threats in the past, globalization, international trade and travel have contributed to an increasingly borderless world. As Global Health moves beyond the medical field and becomes an integrated part of foreign, security and trade policies, there has been increased influence of determinants of health that transcend national borders, thus requiring intersectoral and multi-stakeholder diplomacy and collaborative action to find global solutions.
- Historically the World Health Organization (WHO), and to a lesser extent the United Nations (UN) and its component agencies provided the critical platforms for governments (Global North and Global South) to discuss health-related matters in an inclusive and participatory manner. *Multiple fora have since emerged that address health-related issues* but do not necessarily engage the Global South in a more broadly inclusive and participatory manner, e.g. G7 and G20 health meetings; World Health Summit (Berlin); and World Economic Forum. The Global Health agenda is also shaped by agreements adopted by world leaders such as the UN Millennium Declaration (2000) and the 2030 Agenda for Sustainable Development, and far-reaching political commitments have been made in several UN global conferences, such as the UN International Conference on Population and development (1994). Health also features prominently in many international agreements, including the World Trade Organization (WTO) Declaration on the TRIPS Agreement and Public Health (2001); International Conferences on Financing for Development (2002, 2008 and 2015) and the World Summit on Sustainable Development (2002). (see also Box 80.1).

Box 80.1: Some Historical Context

- The UN role in promoting and protecting health was originally delegated to specialized agencies with WHO taking the leading role as directing and coordinating authority on international health.
- Over time, specific health topics have found their way back to UN agendas, especially in the context of global health.
- HIV became the first health issue to receive attention in the UN General Assembly in 2001, viewed as a health threat and a security issue that caught the attention of heads of state and multisectoral leaders and became a "whole of government" policy.
- The UN millennium development goals included health issues in a development agenda.
- UN has also included noncommunicable diseases (2011), antimicrobial resistance (2016), tuberculosis (2018) and universal health coverage (2019) on their agenda.
- Globalization triggered health debates beyond the health sector, with different diplomatic, political and economic perspectives.
- Health issues have evolved over the past 70 years and it is recognized that health governance at the global level must be relevant to the local context, taking community perspectives into account and embracing community engagement.
- Social media platforms have brought global health topics into households and community fora and this has subsequently fed into local and global discussions.
- Discussions at UN special sessions and high-level meetings on health issues are spearheaded by foreign affairs and international relations sectors. However, the same issues are also discussed in the

World Health Assembly, led by the health sector, with potential for diplomatic dilemmas and policy incoherence in global health.

- Kickbusch [7] questioned the ongoing referral of health matters to the UN, but the complexities of the global health environment (emerging diseases, climate change, geopolitics) are such that there are no clear-cut answers.
- Different fora have approached this situation by linking global health with foreign policy. A significant development in this regard was the UN General Assembly resolution on Global Health and Foreign Policy [8].
- Despite the existence of literature on the relationship between health and foreign policy, e.g. Feldbaum [9], Kickbusch et al. [5, 6] view foreign policy and health issues as a skills gap problem.

- The *dramatic increase in the number of health actors and international partnerships in health*, which are highly diverse in nature, scope and size, offers the potential to combine the strengths of public and private institutions, together with civil society, in tackling health problems. However, it also raises challenges such as duplication of efforts between initiatives, high transaction costs to governments and donors, unclear accountability especially when the non-State sector is involved, and lack of alignment with country priorities and needs.
- Not all countries of the Global South are equipped in terms of capacity, skills set, and resourcing to participate equitably and inclusively in Global Health negotiations that ultimately also shape their own health policies and outcomes. In some instances, negotiators from the Global South resort to guidance and advice from non-State actors, who do not necessarily provide objective viewpoints.

Faced with this reality, it is critical to redouble efforts to *strengthen capacity in both Global Health and in health diplomacy in the Global South*. This could be in the form of taught courses or other innovative means.

Traditionally, most postgraduate courses in Global Health have either been stand-alone courses (Master of Global Health or Certificate courses) or were included as elective subjects/modules in Master of Public Health (MPH) courses. These courses were mainly offered in institutions in the Global North. MPH courses in the Global South increasingly offer Global Health as a module but there is a need to expand this. One proposal is for universities in the Global South to consistently include a Global Health module with any MPH programme offered. Given the global and borderless nature of health, there is also a case to encourage undergraduate medical courses to consider including at least an elective module on Global Health in their programmes.

Health diplomacy is mainly taught as a certificate course by institutions in the North. Given the interdisciplinary dimension of health diplomacy, and that actors in this area also include officials from ministries of foreign affairs, other ministries such as trade and environment, and other government bodies, it is prudent to offer any taught courses to a broader target audience. For example, academic institutions in the South with capacity and expertise in health diplomacy could work with their health and foreign affairs ministries to provide appropriately designed courses. Courses across regions would also enhance capacity and promote collaboration in Global Health and health diplomacy. One such course is currently planned through a collaboration between universities in Malaysia, South Africa, and Italy.[1]

In order to enhance capacity, countries have devised innovative approaches to address shortfalls and create new avenues for learning. One approach is for countries to include younger and early-career officials in their delegations, allowing them to present interventions and engage in discussions on less contentious matters during Global Health governance meetings—an excel-

[1] Sunway University, Malaysia, University of Witwatersrand, South Africa, and University of Milan, Italy.

lent on-the-job-training opportunity. Another avenue for collaboration and learning is the presentation of regional interventions in global meetings with responsibility for intervention and leading on agenda items distributed among the countries of the region. This has led to good cooperation and effective representation of regional viewpoints in governance meetings.

In conclusion, the changing Global Health environment, with the increasing prominence of health in the global development agenda and the increasing number of fora and players engaged in health policy-making, has posed challenges for the Global South to engage much more actively and effectively in an inclusive manner. This needs to be addressed urgently through strengthening capacity in Global Health and health diplomacy.

References

1. Kickbusch I. The need for a European strategy on global health. Scand J Public Health. 2006;34:5615.
2. Koplan JP, Bond TC, Merson MH, Reddy KS, Rodriguez MH, Sewankambo NK, et al. Towards a common definition of global health. Lancet. 2009;373(9679):1993–5.
3. Beaglehole R, Bonita R. What is global health. Glob Health Action. 2010;3:5142.
4. Frenk J, Moon S. Governance challenges in global health. N Engl J Med. 2013;368(10):936–42.
5. Kickbusch I, Silberschmidt G, Buss P. Global health diplomacy: the need for new perspectives, strategic approaches and skills in global health. Bull World Health Organ. 2007a;85(3):230–2.
6. Kickbusch I, Novotny TE, Drager N, Silberschmidt G, Alcazar S. Global health diplomacy: training across disciplines. Bull World Health Organ. 2007b;85:971–3.
7. Kickbusch I. Global health diplomacy: how foreign policy can influence health. BMJ. 2011;342:d3154.
8. Foreign Ministers of Brazil, France, Indonesia, Norway, Senegal, South Africa & Thailand (Oslo). Oslo ministerial declaration-global health: a pressing foreign policy issue of our time. Lancet. 2007;369(9570):1373–8.
9. Feldbaum H. Building US diplomatic capacity for Global Health. Washington DC: Center for Strategic and International Studies; 2010.

Part XI

Methods in Global Health

Quantitative Methods: Basics of Epidemiology and Biostatistics

81

Giovanni Sotgiu and Maria Cristina Monti

Abstract

The chapter will describe epidemiological indicators adopted to evaluate the burden of disease, to estimate a risk related to an exposure, and to assess health status changes. Moreover, a few elements of epidemiological reasoning (bias, confounding, study designs) and a pragmatic framework of statistical reasoning will be presented. It will be described the role played by an appropriate methodology driven by a specific research question, the role of the study designs to address knowledge gaps and confounders.

Keywords

Epidemiology · Statistical analyses · Epidemiological indicators · Study design · Research study

G. Sotgiu
Clinical Epidemiology and Medical Statistics Unit, Department of Medicine, Surgery and Pharmacy, University of Sassari, Sassari, Italy
e-mail: gsotgiu@uniss.it

M. C. Monti (✉)
Biostatistics and Clinical Epidemiology Unit, Department of Public Health Experimental and Forensic Medicine, University of Pavia, Pavia, Italy
e-mail: cristina.monti@unipv.it

81.1 Epidemiological Indicators

Epidemiology is aimed at evaluating health status of a statistical population, describing natural history of diseases, and detecting causal or protective factors involved in their pathogenesis, with the final goal of adopting appropriate responses for disease control and prevention.

Epidemiological indicators are measures summarizing a specific health characteristic (or attribute) in a population, or sample, mainly to evaluate the burden of an event (or a disease) and the strength of association between (an) exposure(s) and an outcome. Based on this definition, health indicators are dynamic and depend on social, geographical, and temporal settings and their choice should be in agreement with objectives and design of a research study.

The absolute frequency is the count of events/attributes, or subjects with an event/attribute. However, it shows the limitation for spatial and temporal comparisons.

Relative measures can be expressed by ratios, proportions, and rates. A *ratio* indicates how many times one quantity is larger or smaller when compared to another; a *proportion* relates a part to a whole, therefore, in this case, the numerator is included in the denominator; whereas, a *rate* includes time as an additional dimension. All these indicators can be referred to the general population or to subgroups, and can be defined as:

M. C. B. Raviglione et al. (eds.), *Global Health Essentials*, Sustainable Development Goals Series,
https://doi.org/10.1007/978-3-031-33851-9_81

- "Crude" when the number of events are divided by the total population;
- "Stratum-specific" in case they are computed in subgroups of interest; and
- "Adjusted" when the resulting population indicator has been computed with methods to correct the potential effect of (a) certain variable(s) (i.e., confounding factors).

81.1.1 Measure of Occurrence

The health status of a population is usually described using *morbidity* and *mortality*, which describe the number of diseases and deaths, respectively, occurring in a population during an interval of time.

The main indicators describing morbidity in a population are prevalence and incidence. Incidence evaluates the occurrence of new events, triggering hypotheses on potential risks, whereas prevalence describes number of existing events in a population at a given time and it is useful to plan health services. The two measures are associated with one another as prevalence is directly proportional to incidence and duration of disease.

Prevalence is defined as the proportion of cases of events in a population at a given time (point prevalence) or in a time interval (period prevalence), and it is mainly adopted in cross-sectional studies (see Box 81.1).

Box 81.1 Study Design Classification Algorithm

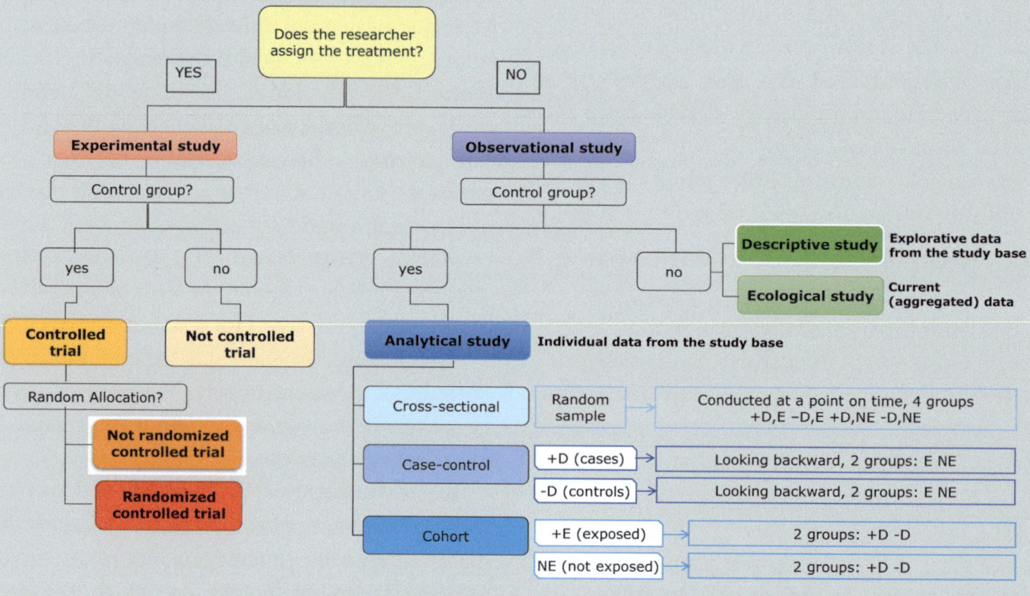

Descriptive

- Distribution of existing variables, outcome frequency, and history
- Important for the generation of broad hypotheses
- Used to relate groups morbidity or mortality differences of to their local environment (or setting)

Ecological

- Like descriptive studies except that the relationship between exposure and outcome is reported at the group-level
- Usually based on existing data, with no comparison group
- Risk to incur into the "ecological fallacy" when group-level results are inferred to individual level

Cross-sectional

- Conducted at a specific point in time and defined by the geographical context, with usually a random sample
- Outcome measure of occurrence: prevalence
- Exposure measure of effect: prevalence rate or relative risk
- Useful for acute effects, although the temporal exposure-outcome sequence cannot be assessed

Case-control

- Comparison groups based on the presence or absence of the outcome of interest
- Exposure histories collected «backward» from cases and controls; *population-based* or *hospital-based* or *nested within a cohort*
- Outcome measure of occurrence: none as it will be biased
- Exposure measure of effect: odds ratio
- Causality between exposure and outcome cannot be assessed

Cohort

- Comparison groups based on the presence or absence of the exposure of interest
- Follow-up of outcome happens prospectively unless the design is *retrospective/historical* (from a past point in time onward to mimic the follow-up)
- Outcome's measure of occurrence: incidence
- Exposure's measure of effect: relative risk
- *Longitudinal study/panel study*: health status or biological markers measured at several points in time

Non-controlled trial

- Subjects exposed to one intervention administered by the investigators
- Aimed at determine intervention's efficacy and safety

Controlled trial

- Subjects exposed to different interventions
- Subjects in the control group either receive the standard of care or a *placebo* intervention, if there is no current effective intervention
- *Randomized control trial*: groups are managed with a randomized allocation scheme where the intervention(s) is/are allocated to groups by chance
- *Blindness/masking*: participants and/or investigators and/or statisticians are unaware of the group allocation of the intervention(s) provided
- Based on the recruited statistical units: *clinical trials* (study participants); *field trials* (community members, free of disease); *community intervention trials* (whole communities)

$$\text{Prevalence} = \frac{\text{No.of cases of disease at a given moment (or time interval)}}{\text{Total population at the same moment (or time interval)}}$$

Incidence is defined as the proportion of new events occurring in a population at risk[1] (cumulative incidence) or the rate between the number of new events occurring in a population at risk in a period by the total person-time at risk.[2]

$$\text{Cumulative incidence} = \frac{\text{No.of new cases of disease}}{\text{Population at risk at baseline}}$$

$$\text{Incidence rate} = \frac{\text{No.of new cases of disease within a time interval}}{\text{Total person} - \text{time at risk}}$$

Incidence, therefore, measures the probability that an individual (at risk) could develop a disease during a specific time period. Furthermore, incidence rates describe how quickly an event occurs in a population, providing essential information for the comparison of different epidemiological scenarios.

Incidence is used in cohort studies, where participants are recruited and followed-up during a time period, with the aim of estimating the occurrence of an outcome.

Mortality rate (MR) represents the frequency of deaths in a defined population during a specified time interval. It is actually a ratio, having numerator and denominator with the same unit of measure. Considering the high variability in death by age, sex, socio-economic status, and other variables, a variety of mortality rates can be reported by specific groups or as adjusted rate.

Case fatality rate (CFR) is defined as the proportion of individuals who die from a specific disease among all individuals diagnosed with the same disease, over a specific time period. CFR measures the severity of disease and can range from 0 to 1, where values closer to 1 indicate a higher severity of the disease.

Mortality can be reported as *proportionate mortality* which describes the proportion of deaths, in a target population, attributable to different causes: the denominator includes all causes of deaths and it is useful to compare deaths in a precise context with mortality in the general population.

Infant mortality is an indicator of the health level, providing a measure of socio-economic status and healthcare delivery quality. It is calculated by dividing the number of deaths in children during the first year of life with the number of births during the same year. Similarly, *neonatal* and *post-neonatal mortality* describe the level of healthcare assistance in relation to the first 28 days and 1 year after birth, respectively.

Conversely, *survival rate* describes the number of patients alive among those diagnosed with a disease during a specific period.

Measures of disease/event frequency describe the burden. However, to assess the role of potential risk factors, comparison of two or more groups (exposed or not exposed) is needed.

81.1.2 Measures of Effect

The measures of effect quantify the strength of the relationship between exposure and outcome in analytical epidemiological research. They include ratio measures such as relative risk (RR) and odds ratio (OR), and difference measures such as the attributable risk (AR).

Relative risk compares the risk of an event occurrence between exposed and unexposed groups.

Odds ratio represents the measure of choice in case-control studies, where it is computed as the

[1]A population at risk includes only those subjects that do not have the condition of interest. Therefore, all subjects having the condition under investigation at the beginning of the study should be excluded, when possible.

[2]The total person-time at risk is the total time that participants are disease-free, thus at risk to acquire it.

ratio between the odds of an outcome in the exposed group and the odds of an outcome in the unexposed group.

		Outcome	
		Present	Absent
Exposure	Expose	*a*	*c*
	Non-exposed	*b*	*d*

where

a = number of persons exposed with the outcome
b = number of persons unexposed with the outcome
c = number of persons exposed without the outcome
d = number of persons unexposed without the outcome

$$\text{OR} = \frac{\text{odds of an event in exposed group}}{\text{odds of an event in unexposed group}}$$

$$\text{OR} - \frac{a}{c} \times \frac{d}{b} - ad / cb$$

Both OR and RR values range from 0 to ∞. A value equal to 1 means that both groups have the same risk of developing the outcome, values above 1 indicate that there is a positive association between exposure and outcomes, whereas below 1 implies that there is a negative association between exposure and outcomes. Because the incidence of disease in case-control studies is unknown, the OR only estimates the RR and it is useful for rare diseases.

Attributable risk, defined as the difference between the incidence of an outcome in exposed individuals and the incidence of an outcome in non-exposed individuals, is used in epidemiological cohort studies. AR describes the expected reduction of disease cases if the exposure is removed. Therefore, the AR represents the proportion of the outcome attributable only to a single risk factor and, consequently, it is not applicable to the study of multifactorial diseases.

None of the measures of effect, neither those measuring the strength of an association (i.e., OR and RR) imply a cause-effect relationship between exposure and disease. A causal relationship between exposure and outcome can be suggested by following the Bradford-Hill criteria (e.g., specificity of the causative role, temporal sequence, biological gradient, biological plausibility, coherence).

81.2 Epidemiological Reasoning and Study Design

Epidemiological reasoning is based on three major elements [1].

(a) Statistical association between an exposure and the outcome of interest is assessed in the study base (or study population).
(b) Inference on the outcome mechanism is hypothesized.
(c) Subsequent observation of the outcome frequency provides the potential refutation of the association.

Epidemiological reasoning is an iterative process of hypothesis generation and it must be carried out using the right study base and study design. The investigator should identify the most suitable *study base* to explore a specific research question; this means that both the distribution of exposures and outcome have to be comparable to the target population [2].

When systematic errors of the study design favor an inaccurate estimation of the role of an exposure on the outcome, health consequences can occur (epidemiological bias): the findings are spurious and the final conclusion diverges from the reality. The most frequently biases are selection (e.g., allocation, sampling) and information (e.g., interviewer, recall).

Some factors can also confound the relationship between exposure and outcome, increasing or decreasing the strength of their association. A *confounder* must show a significant association with the outcome and also with the exposure, and it should not be in the exposure-outcome pathway.

To evaluate the achievement of study-related standards for quality of evidence [3], it is key to assess the *study design* (Box 81.1). A study hypothesis usually derives from *observational studies* that describe the occurrence of an event (namely *descriptive/ecological* studies), then, an association between an outcome and an exposure is further confirmed through *analytical observational studies*.

The final step is to assess this association by intentionally administering the exposure to some individuals in *experimental studies*. They are performed when the role of an exposure could potentially improve health outcomes. As this might raise ethical issues, the performance of such studies should be supporting by the existence of an equipoise.[3]

When clinical trials cannot really represent the entire population, excluding individuals with vulnerable characteristics, for example, or there is an interest for obtaining evidence on the relative benefits and harms of interventions in real settings (without randomization), *real-world studies* could be considered. These studies often can be obtained with observational data capturing routine care (as electronic health records, billing databases, product and disease registries) to assess the safety and effectiveness of drugs and devices [4].

[3]As far as the researchers know, at the time of the study design there is not one "better" intervention/exposure.

81.3 Statistical Reasoning

The statistical reasoning for an epidemiological study starts with the planning phase, when ideally all details of conduction and analyses must be summarized in the *study protocol* [5, 6]; specifically, the *statistical plan* should be included to facilitate answering the research questions (Box 81.2). After data collection, the *statistical analyses* will really start. Different data mean different statistical methods and, hence, for being able to choose among plenty of summary statistics and statistical tests, the theoretical statistical framework should be clear to the research team [1, 7, 8]. Depending on the study design and the sample size [9], statistical analyses may include different descriptive and inferential phases (Box 81.2).

Box 81.2

Milestones of the Research protocol

- Define a *coherent measurerable* and *testable* research hypothesis
- Define the population of interest and study base
- Choose the best **study design** (Box1)
- Select key variables (outcomes, exposures and potential confounders)
- Compute the sample size
- **Prepare the Statistical plan before to start the data collection:**

•Sample size for being confident enough to accept or reject the null hypothesis (considering the primary endpoint of the study)
•Variables (with coding scheme or scale)
•Data repository structure and number of time points
•Descriptive statistics (to check the data and to describe the variables collected)
•Statistical models to capture the relationship between exposures and outcomes and control for confounders

Data collection →

Based on the statistical plan you can now detail the statistical analysis phases:

- **Data mining and data cleaning**: inspect the data to find internal inconsistencies, implausible or missing or outliers data using graphical representations and summary statistics
- **Descriptive statistics:** present and discuss the structure of the data. Quantitative and qualitative variables will need different summary statistics
- **Estimates of population parameters of interest** (like the mean or median or the proportion or morbidity and mortality indicators) **and their empirical measures of dispersion and confidence intervals**
- **Inference about the research hypotheses in the analytical studies:** comparison of the distribution of the estimated parameters in different population groups, time-periods or places by use of statistical tests
- **Multivariable statistical models:** multiple independent variables to assess, eventually, independent relationships with the outcome while adjusting for potential confounders
- **Goodness of fit and post-estimation diagnostics**: how well the statistical models fit the data and model assumptions evaluation

References

1. Arhens W, Pigeot I. Handbook of epidemiology. 2nd ed. New York, NY: Springer; 2014.
2. Hernberg S. Introduction to occupational epidemiology. Chelsea: Lewis Publishers; 1992.
3. Guyatt GH, GRADE Working Group. What is "quality of evidence" and why is it important to clinicians? BMJ. 2008;336:995–8.
4. Sherman RE, et al. Real-world evidence - what is it and what can it tell us? N Engl J Med. 2016;375(23):2293–7.
5. Schulz KF, et al. CONSORT 2010 statement: updated guidelines for reporting parallel group randomised trials. BMC Med. 2010;8:18.
6. Von Elm E, et al. The strengthening the reporting of observational studies in epidemiology (STROBE) statement: guidelines for reporting observational studies. Lancet. 2007;370(9596):1453–7.
7. Pagano M, Gauvreau K. Principles of biostatistics. New York: Chapman and Hall/CRC; 2018.
8. Cross C, Daniel WW. Biostatistics: a Foundation for Analysis in the health sciences. 11th ed. John Wiley & Sons; 2018.
9. Verma JP, Verma P. Determining sample size and power in research studies. A manual for researchers. Singapore: Springer; 2020.

82 Methods in Global Health: Disease Modelling

Melissa A. Penny and Pablo M. De Salazar

Abstract

Disease modelling utilizes statistical and mathematical models to address questions in biomedical sciences, ecology, epidemiology, and public health, for infectious and non-communicable diseases. When applied to Global Health, modelling improves our understanding of diseases affecting humans globally and supports decision making for improving health at the individual and population levels. While a range of topics can be examined, modelling does not necessarily aim to predict the future, but to analyze hypothetical scenarios to estimate the impact and economics of interventions, and to select between them to improve health outcomes. In this chapter, we outline basic concepts for understanding the use of models to improve disease knowledge; to design or evaluate interventions to reduce the disease burden; and to support Global Health decision-making. We provide several examples of applications and critical questions in disease modelling for Global Health.

M. A. Penny (✉) · P. M. De Salazar
Swiss Tropical and Public Health Institute, Allschwil, Switzerland

University of Basel, Basel, Switzerland
e-mail: melissa.penny@swisstph.ch; pablo.martinezdesalazar@swisstph.ch

Keywords

Disease modelling · Disease dynamic · Cost-effectiveness · Model performance · Disease burden

82.1 Introduction

Disease modelling is an intersectional discipline based on mathematical and/or statistical methods with a long history of development and use. Disease modelling aims to address biomedical sciences, ecology, epidemiology, and public health questions, ranging across types of disease (i.e., infectious vs. non-communicable diseases), biological levels (i.e., within host vs population levels), the type of data available (i.e., genomic vs. clinical data), or how uncertainty is addressed (i.e., deterministic vs. stochastic models). When applied to Global Health, generally, its goals include improving our understanding of diseases affecting humans globally and to support making informed decisions for policymakers, clinicians, and public health practitioners for improving health with interventions at the individual and population levels [1]. Many different types of models are helpful, including mechanistic models that capture, for example, dynamics of disease transmission or more causal models that attempt to capture the determinants leading to increased

M. C. B. Raviglione et al. (eds.), *Global Health Essentials*, Sustainable Development Goals Series,
https://doi.org/10.1007/978-3-031-33851-9_82

disease prevalence in a population or increased risk of disease development in an individual.

Models are generally simplified representations of real-life phenomena informed by existing evidence. They are particularly beneficial when observational evidence is sparse or experimental approaches to estimate the impact of disease interventions are limited or not feasible, too costly, or not ethical. Moreover, disease modelling can also support the evidence obtained from experimental and observational approaches.

However, the theoretical nature of disease modelling usually requires recognizing the limitations arising from the reduction, simplification, and potential lack of sufficient evidence in the assumptions intrinsic to formulating models. Thus, disease modelling is unavoidably entangled with more empirical sources of evidence: data is crucial to formulate the questions the model can answer, shaping its goals, validity, and usefulness.

82.2 Background

Models based on mathematical methods, including statistical and simulation models, are used in many areas, ranging from infectious diseases to physical systems, economics, and even in fields such as political science or music. A mathematical model uses mathematical or statistical equations to describe a real-life system or process, such as disease transmission dynamics. Models can be relatively simple systems of one or more equations, all the way through to complex algorithms that consider a large number of biological, epidemiological, or behavioral relationships. A model distils knowledge and can help explain and study a system and quantify the effects of the different assumptions or components described in it. By using simple models or simulating more complex ones, we can also make predictions about the behaviors of a system.

Disease models can be used to investigate disease features such as the distribution, transmission, or progression of a particular disease within an individual or population under different scenarios. Through simulation, they can be utilized to explore future disease trends and help to determine how to intervene to prevent disease, prevent transmission, or even cure or delay disease progression within an individual. However, simulation results from models are not necessarily predictions of the future. In contrast to models used for forecasts, for example, weather prediction models, mechanistic models of disease dynamics will not tell us exactly what the future will be—rather they add value to our current knowledge of today, as they give us a way to explore what could be under a range of different assumptions.

82.3 Aim of the Chapter

In this chapter, we describe basic concepts for understanding the use of models to improve disease knowledge; to design or evaluate interventions to reduce the disease burden; and to support Global Health decision-making.

82.4 Description of the Issue

Disease modelling is beneficial to compensate for lack of knowledge or when the questions posed cannot be addressed experimentally (i.e., in the real world) because of feasibility, cost or ethical barriers, or for extrapolating from limited evidence. Disease modelling and simulation can have different specific objectives, from understanding disease dynamics or disease progression at the clinical or the epidemiological level to informing decisions for preventing, curing, or reducing the burden of a particular disease.

A crucial aspect of disease modelling is understanding what models can and cannot do, namely, understanding a model's limitations. The limitations will differ depending on the nature of the model, its purpose, the time-frame of analysis, and the context to which the model will be applied. Moreover, limitations include the assumptions of disease biology, epidemiology, and disease progression used to formulate the model, how model output uncertainty is communicated, and the availability of empirical data to train the model or validate its outcomes. All these limitations will determine a model's usefulness and appropriateness. The question being posed drives how one will proceed with the modelling. What insight is needed, and what questions need answering is generally driven by the users as well as by the modellers themselves. Thus, it is essential that those who formulate the model engage in an iterative dialogue and communication with users of the modelling outcomes.

82.5 Approach to Solutions

Modelling can be useful at all stages and levels of a Global Health problem, including understanding its pathogenesis, estimating its trends, burden or dynamics over time or space, or guiding policy decisions about therapies or interventions (Table 82.1).

Mathematical models of diseases provide a formal approach to explore what could happen under a range of different hypothetical situations or scenarios. Models allow us to answer a range of these "*What if…?*" questions via simulation. The value of the models is not to predict the future but rather to compare what could happen if a particular intervention was implemented or not implemented. Or to compare "*What could happen?*" if intervention A was implemented rather than intervention B. This type of scenario analysis is a powerful approach to providing quantitative evidence for decision-making.

A root goal of disease modelling is concerned with evaluating, validating, and appraising the models that have been formulated. The goal here might also be to identify further data needed to answer different questions and to determine whether the models you developed were correct by comparing the model predictions against real data and future events. This goal remains relevant with further use of the models and commonly reflects features crucial for evaluating the model's outputs, such as accuracy, reliability, robustness, generalizability, and transportability (Box 82.1).

Table 82.1 Applications of modelling in Global Health as disease knowledge increases

Applications	Example of questions	Example model type
To understand disease pathogenesis and disease progression	*"What are the disease dynamics that lead to illness and mortality? What disease progression states or patient risk factors lead to adverse disease outcomes?"*	Within-host models of pathogen dynamics or of disease progression states (e.g., [9]). Causal analysis or covariate analysis to identify risk factors (e.g., [10])
To understand disease burden, transmission, and/or distribution	*"What is the disease burden and expected progression? What are the drivers or associated factors to its distribution?"*	Geospatial models to estimate the global burden of a disease [11]
To evaluate the impact of different interventions on disease burden or dynamics	*"How can we intervene?" "How and by how much a specific intervention might impact the disease burden, progression, or distribution?"*	With-host or epidemiological models quantifying the effect of interventions in reducing disease metrics (within-host or at population level)
To predict scenarios for supporting policy decisions	*"How much a certain decision costs?" "which combination of interventions maximizes public health impact under a limited budget?"*	Cost-effectiveness models
To identify what data is needed to answer different questions. To determine whether the models developed are sufficiently robust, and whether the model outputs are translatable to other settings or populations	*"How reliable are the model predictions?" "how much can we extrapolate the model's output across other settings or populations?"*	Machine-learning based models for parameterization and/or fitting

Box 82.1 Important Features for Evaluating Model Performance in Global Health

Characteristic	Definition
Accuracy	How close a final model output is to the targeted value accepted as correct?
Robustness	How correct remains a model output under invalid inputs?
Reliability	How close repeated model outputs are to each other?
Internal validity	How close is the model output to the value accepted as correct for a given population, setting, or event?
External validity	How generalizable is the model output to other populations, settings, or events? External validity in epidemiological and clinical models includes *generalizability*, which is concerned with making inferences from a possibly biased sample of a target population back to the whole population, as well as *transportability*, which is concerned with making inferences for a target population when the study sample and the target population are partially or entirely non-overlapping [12]

An application of modelling can be to understand the pathogenesis, burden, progression, and/or distribution of a particular disease. For example, in an outbreak of an emerging infectious disease, relatively little is known about the pathogen and therefore modelling is usually critical to elucidate the key factors that allow and support transmission, which in turn allows us to interpret how likely the disease is to invade a population that has never seen it before, and how quickly it will transmit in that population [2]. As an alternative example for non-communicable diseases, geospatial models can be used to evaluate the relationship between the distribution of specific environmental factors and their potential influence in increasing or decreasing the risk of a particular disease, such as cancer, depression, or hypertension [3].

A second use of disease models can aim to answer the question, *"How can we intervene?"* To this end, one might better understand the disease, and therefore, developing more specific models to explore diseases beyond their initial dynamics. However, it is worth noting that these questions might also be answered when there is still little information, such as the early stages of an emerging disease outbreak or to estimate potential impact of antimicrobial or drug resistance [4]. Nevertheless, one might aim to compare the impact of different interventions by creating *"what if"* scenario analyses or by further applying threshold concepts of mathematical epidemiology. The modelling of *"What if scenarios?"* allows you to quantify the impact on disease dynamics within a host or at a population level for a single intervention or mix of interventions.

A third use of modelling might aim to move beyond the relative comparisons of the impacts of interventions towards predictions for policy decisions. For example, within policy-relevant modelling, the expected cost of implementing different intervention scenarios is commonly calculated [5, 6]. Thus, one can aim to answer the question, *"How much a certain decision will cost?"* In this type of *"What if resources are limited in a setting?"* question, modelling helps predict how many disease cases could be averted under a given strategy with a limited number of interventions available or given a limited budget.

So while disease modelling can be helpful at all stages, levels and types of Global Health problems, modelling questions, and models themselves must be updated as more knowledge on the disease or epidemiology becomes available.

Finally, it is worth highlighting the role of engaging with Global Health stakeholders and equity in all aspects of modelling. When modelling is utilized to support public health decisions, the dialogue and communication required between modellers and decision-makers are iterative: as you analyze and incorporate different sources of data, develop new models, or undertake modelling and simulation, and as you communicate initial results, you may discover that your question needs refining or reframing altogether. This iterative process can be challenging. Therefore, communication between the modellers, the decision-makers, and partners is crucial to ensure diseases modelling addresses appropriate and relevant questions that yield model evidence to support decisions. Lastly, disease modelling can support understanding the equity implications of implementing public interventions and policies by simulating the distributional impacts on different population groups. Thus the development and use of models should proactively consider advancing health equity and the representation of populations experiencing the burden [7, 8].

82.6 Conclusions and Recommendations

Disease modelling helps improving our understanding of diseases at individual, population, or meta population levels, and to generate evidence when one cannot apply empirical methods due to feasibility, cost, or ethical limitations or for extrapolating from limited evidence. Modelling can be useful at all stages, levels, and types of Global Health problems: from estimating burden metrics in emerging disease outbreaks to evaluating the cost-effectiveness of prevention intervention deployed locally, nationally or globally to reduce burden, improve health outcomes, or eliminate a disease.

Yet, it is important to understand the limitations of disease models for interpreting their outcomes and their usefulness and appropriateness. The limitations of models will differ depending on factors such as the nature of the model, its purpose, time-frame, and the context to which is aimed to be applied. Lastly, disease modelling supporting policy-making requires an iterative dialogue between modellers and decision-makers that must commence from the beginning of the modelling process.

References

1. Heesterbeek H, Anderson RM, Andreasen V, Bansal S, De Angelis D, Dye C, et al. Modeling infectious disease dynamics in the complex landscape of global health. Science. 2015;347(6227):aaa4339.
2. Wu JT, Leung K, Bushman M, Kishore N, Niehus R, de Salazar PM, et al. Estimating clinical severity of COVID-19 from the transmission dynamics in Wuhan. China Nat Med. 2020;26(4):506–10.
3. Wang Y, Wang J. Modelling and prediction of global non-communicable diseases. BMC Public Health. 2020;20(1):1–13.
4. Fitzpatrick MC, Bauch CT, Townsend JP, Galvani AP. Modelling microbial infection to address global health challenges. Nat Microbiol. 2019;4(10):1612–9.
5. Penny MA, Verity R, Bever CA, Sauboin C, Galactionova K, Flasche S, et al. Public health impact and cost-effectiveness of the RTS,S/AS01 malaria vaccine: a systematic comparison of predictions from four mathematical models. Lancet. 2016;387(10016):367–75.
6. Divajeva D, Marsh T, Logstrup S, Kestens M, Vemer P, Kriaucioniene V, et al. Economics of chronic diseases protocol: cost-effectiveness modelling and the future burden of non-communicable disease in Europe. BMC Public Health. 2014;14(1):1–5.
7. Rajkomar A, Hardt M, Howell MD, Corrado G, Chin MH. Ensuring fairness in machine learning to advance health equity. Ann Intern Med. 2018;169(12):866–72.
8. Unwin HJT, Mwandigha L, Winskill P, Ghani AC, Hogan AB. Analysis of the potential for a malaria vaccine to reduce gaps in malaria intervention coverage. Malar J. 2021;20(1):1–11.
9. Camponovo F, Lee TE, Russell JR, Burgert L, Gerardin J, Penny MA. Mechanistic within-host models of the asexual plasmodium falciparum infection: a review and analytical assessment. Malar J. 2021;20(1):1–22.
10. Leopold SJ, Watson JA, Jeeyapant A, Simpson JA, Phu NH, Hien TT, et al. Investigating causal pathways in severe falciparum malaria: a pooled retrospective analysis of clinical studies. PLoS Med. 2019;16(8):e1002858.
11. Weiss DJ, Lucas TC, Nguyen M, Nandi AK, Bisanzio D, Battle KE, et al. Mapping the global prevalence, incidence, and mortality of plasmodium falciparum, 2000–17: a spatial and temporal modelling study. Lancet. 2019;394(10195):322–31.
12. Lesko CR, Buchanan AL, Westreich D, Edwards JK, Hudgens MG, Cole SR. Generalizing study results: a potential outcomes perspective. Epidemiology. 2017;28(4):553.

83 Qualitative Methods for Global Health in Operational, Implementation and Health Systems Research

Bogomil Kohlbrenner and Beat Stoll

Abstract

Qualitative methods in health research are key to understand and integrate the implication of social determinants as they are lived and impact health issues from concerned persons and communities' perspectives. Specifically, in applied global and public health research, three interconnected stratus can be distinguished: *operational research* focused on the district and hospital level and its actors; *implementation research* focused on bringing evidence-based practice to the field and give recommendations at the program level; *health systems research* which will focus on health systems and policy questions and recommendations that aren't disease specific. Here we focus giving an overview on qualitative research as it applies to these three levels in global health research. Specifically, we distinguish the classical and more contemporary research methods, the need to integrate a systemic and interdisciplinary perspective, and we propose the realist evaluation method as a key interdisciplinary approach well adapted to research in this setting.

B. Kohlbrenner (✉) · B. Stoll
University of Geneva, Geneva, Switzerland
e-mail: bogomil.kohlbrenner@unige.ch; beat.stoll@unige.ch

Keywords

Qualitative methods · Applied global health research · Operational research · Implementation research · Health systems research · Participant observation · In-depth interviews · Focus groups · Realist evaluation

83.1 Introduction to the Issue

Human health, health systems and services are complex touching on human frailty and integrated into larger social, economic, infrastructural, and environmental systems and their determinants of health. Strengthening health systems requires taking a systemic interdisciplinary approach that integrates concerned actors such as service providers or beneficiaries. Applied research to improve health should integrate impacted communities, beneficiaries, health care providers, managers, and policy makers depending on its focus and whom will directly benefit from the findings. There are today three overlapping domains in Global Health that focus on strengthening health systems as defined by Remme et al. They are "*operational research* predominantly, but not exclusively, of use to health care providers; *implementation research* predominantly of use to managers of programmes scaling up an intervention; and *research on the*

M. C. B. Raviglione et al. (eds.), *Global Health Essentials*, Sustainable Development Goals Series,
https://doi.org/10.1007/978-3-031-33851-9_83

health system as a whole (or one of its building blocks) of most use to those who manage or need to make policy for the health system" [1].

Qualitative research embraces social and systemic complexity by inductively researching from the concerned actors' perspectives: integrating their discourse, behaviours, beliefs and role in a larger social context; giving insight into why and how people do what they do; offering granularity and narrative to the lived experiences, and collected and researched data; giving insight into feasibility and acceptability from the actor's perspectives; and ideally integrating itself into an interdisciplinary approach to strengthen health systems that may also need to integrate other key research elements such as cost-effectiveness.

83.2 Background

The recognition of the need to integrate research focusing on strengthening health systems anchoring itself on how, why and what people do in the systems at different levels in order to ensure appropriate incorporation and adoption of interventions, has grown in the global health sector over the years; both with activists pushing for more local research and implementation decision capacity [2] and with donors recognizing this need. Interdisciplinary health research that integrates qualitative research has grown as a key approach responding to this [3]. Biomedical solutions are only a partial solution; to ensure interventions effectiveness within a given context, they must account for the socio-behavioural factors, such as power relations, cultural norms, beliefs, identities, gender norms, stigma, and socioeconomic status [4].

83.3 Aims of the Chapter

This chapter aims to offer a brief overview of three overlapping main fields of research that focus on health systems strengthening in global health (i.e., operational, implementation and health systems research) with a focus on qualitative methods used in health research and their current future developments. We will also propose the systems thinking approach as a framework and realist evaluation approach as a concrete example of a systemic methodology to address health issues that is especially well adapted to integrating qualitative methods.

83.4 The Issue

Applied research that aims to strengthen healthcare systems has historically and generally been categorized with overlap and a certain confusion in terminology between the three main paradigms. Taking Remme et al.'s [1] proposal to clarify these domains allows us to refine both the objects of study of each as well as the users of the research results. A World Health Organization (WHO)-led consortium of bilateral organizations defined the framework for operational and implementation research in 2008 giving momentum to this action-oriented research field [5].

83.4.1 Operational Research

Operational research in global health is the investigation of strategies, interventions, instruments or knowledge that can enhance the quality, coverage, and effectiveness of health systems or improve its performance or the health services, or disease control programs; by showing what works, and what does not in various contexts. Operational research can provide evidence to help healthcare workers and policymakers to adapt health interventions and services for maximum public health benefit. Its main focus is on the district level, hospital or local healthcare provision level. Its recommendations will be taken up mostly at that level. Results generalizability will be more focused on comparison and process than on specific local results.

83.4.2 Implementation Research

Implementation research focuses on bringing evidence-based medicine and practices to the field. Implementation science focuses on the uptake of evidence-based practices (EBP), and it is defined as "the scientific study of methods to promote the systematic uptake of research findings and other EBPs into routine practice, and, hence, to improve the quality and effectiveness of health services" [6]. As such, its recommendations will be considered primarily at the program manager level to inform how they orient health care provision. Results will aim to be taken up beyond the local context whilst considering the stakeholders and processes to be considered through the research. As with other fields of research standardization in scientific processes and common understandings of theories remain [7].

83.4.3 Health Systems Research

Health systems research generally focuses on research that is not disease-specific but concerns health system and policy questions that affect the performance of the health system as a whole [1]. It can focus on any of the 6 WHO building blocks of health systems: service delivery, information and evidence, medical products and technologies, health workforce, health financing, leadership and governance [8]. It often has a strong use of qualitative research and economics focused research methods to engage and understand stakeholder issues as part of multidisciplinary and international research teams. Approaches that integrate systems thinking and analysis can bring key insight as they allow the mapping and integration of the different stakeholders and institutions at all levels in the analysis [9].

83.5 Systems Thinking to Grasp Systemic Complexity

Systems thinking begins its analysis from the anti-reductionist perspective that posits that the system is more than the sum of its parts [10]. As such, the different systems exhibit properties that interact build their own dynamics creating relational ontologies [9]. Researching through this lens allows to put different agents on the same playing field for analysis be they representations, institutions or healthcare providers [11]. Integrating this approach allows the researcher to have a better grasp and capacity to analyse the complex realities that interact around health issues and health systems. Wernli et al. propose six global health dimensions through systemic lenses that should be considered for Global Health research and that integrates well into the framing of this type of research: considering the complexity of the situation with the health problem, its transnational dimension, the cross disciplinarily and trans-sectoral aspects of interventions, the dimension of sustainability, the affordability of innovations for such interventions and finally as well the respect of human rights and dignity for the population [12].

83.6 Qualitative Methods a Brief Overview

Qualitative methods in Global Health focus on giving voice to people's complex lived experiences of health, how they understand their world and specific issues, and how they behave and communicate in a social context. This "thick" data allows to gain insight into how and if a health system strengthening intervention can and should be led. Research can be done before an intervention to understand the context, but ideally will also accompany an intervention and/or its impact to adjust the recommendations and the intervention itself.

The limitations of qualitative research are generally that they capture a specific context in a specific timeframe with a comparatively small sample size. Another difficulty is that qualitative research requires time and building relationships with informants especially with participant observation. Mitigation strategies include a strong focus on reflexivity of the researcher's implication in the research and clarifying it in the research results to reduce bias; integrating different researchers both from the discipline and across disciplines to compare and discuss; and adapt the research and its analysis and presentation. As qualitative research will be more hypothesis building, integrating it in a research process with quantitative methods that will be hypothesis testing in a mixed method approach can lead to a stronger recognition.

Examples of qualitative methods to respond to these challenges are:

Participant observation means entering the context of study and building rapport with people to become a participant observer, someone who is in place and part of the social context. This requires time and relationship building. This will allow the researcher to observe and discuss directly with the concerned actors in situ, test his questions and observations and refine the research iteratively in the given social context.

In-depth interviews can be part of participant observation, but also be lead independently. In contrast to more quantitatively and closed questions focused questionnaires, in-depth interviews will develop more open-ended questions and the interviewee will be encouraged to develop his thoughts through a non-directive approach. This approach allows to deepen the understanding through the narrative of the concerned actors' perspectives and when comparing interviews both between interviewees and with the same interviewee over time, strengthening the global perspective.

Focus groups allow the researchers to confront perspectives and engage them in conversation over a given subject. The researcher must here take the role of moderator and facilitator to ensure the different participants take part and are able to constructively exchange and give their perspectives. The group dynamics are used to gain insights that may not be gained through inter-individual exchanges with the researchers. The main limitation to be accounted for in this approach is the issue of power dynamics and inhibition and this may lead to in participants that will depend on who is part of the group.

Mixed methods and new real-time data collection (for example, through social-network data analysis, or patient forums/chats) integrates the qualitative and quantitative approaches through interdisciplinary collaboration. This will enrich research results, but researchers must clarify terms, paradigms and understandings together in order to avoid misunderstandings in the way they analyse and speak of the data and of the different forms of data. This has been called the fourth research paradigm in health research services by Rapport and Braithwaite and holds its own limitations due to complexity, but also promises on improving research strength and validity [3].

This being a very limited overview we recommend Taylors et al. [13], as well as Mack's [4] books on qualitative research.

These approaches allow to grasp the lived realities of the actors in the health system and benefiting communities and inform on key data, limitations and possible paths for implementation in research that aims to strengthen health systems, accounting for the social realities and dynamics that will influence an intervention. But, to ensure larger validity and adoption by the different stakeholders these approaches should also integrate other health strengthening implementers and approaches, in the optic of pragmatically strengthening the health system with the stakeholders.

83.6.1 Realist Evaluation

Based on the importance of context and the social components underlined in the qualitative approach, we propose the realist evaluation [14] as a specific methodology well adapted to applied global health research in its different levels. The realistic evaluation (RE) starts with the basic assumption that the context of a given program is central and effects are not just guaranteed by the action.

The RE seeks not only to understand if a program works (cause and effect relationship) but above all what works, for whom and under what circumstances. The basic premise is that what works in a certain context does not necessarily work in a different, self-adapting environment. Classical scientific experimental studies demonstrate null-hypothesis falsification tests, and the RE demonstrates by multi-side and interdisciplinary case studies. In RE, the context is seen as central and confounding factors, which are an integral part of the context, that cannot be controlled and even contribute to the final effect. RE thus highlights the essential elements to activate in order to achieve a given result in a given context.

A realistic-inspired evaluation of a given project therefore does not amount to asking only whether the program works or not as in a classical experimental approach using the concept of linear relationships for the factors influencing the effect and where confounding factors are either eliminated or randomly controlled. For RE, confounding factors are part of the context, which means this cannot be controlled and which contributes to the effect of the program.

The RE uses complexity of systems with nonlinear relationships and feedbacks. The objectives of this mapped complexity system will be to define which is ultimately of lesser use and to know why and how and for whom such a program works. The RE aims to understand which intervention produces which effect in which context and what are the mechanisms by which an intervention produces a given effect. And then these results will thus help to determine if a given program could be implemented elsewhere and what conditions are necessary to trigger these mechanisms in which context and how to improve and sustain them.

83.7 Main Conclusions and Recommendations

It is important when doing applied Global Health research to be clear at which level your focus is and to whom the recommendations will most matter, on what or at what level it is lead. Qualitative research allows to integrate the concerned actors' perspectives and their realities to ensure a better understanding of implementation implications and issues. Accounting for its limitations as well as the perspectives of the concerned actors concerns in terms of data and application interdisciplinary approaches can strengthen results and validity for healthcare strengthening. Acknowledging complexity, building a relational understanding of the issues allows for a better understanding of what can be done at what level to strengthen the health system.

References

1. Remme JH, Adam T, Becerra-Posada F, D'Arcangues C, Devlin M, Gardner C, et al. Defining research to improve health systems. PLoS Med. 2010;7(11):e1001000.
2. Abimbola S, Negin J, Jan S, Martiniuk A. Towards people-centred health systems: a multi-level framework for analysing primary health care governance in low- and middle-income countries. Health Policy Plan. 2014;29(Suppl. 2):ii29–39.
3. Rapport F, Braithwaite J. Are we on the cusp of a fourth research paradigm? Predicting the future for a new approach to methods-use in medical and health services research. BMC Med Res Methodol. 2018;18(1):1–7.
4. Mack N. Qualitative research methods: a data collector's field guide. 2005.
5. UNICEF, WHO. Framework for operations and implementation research in health and disease control programs. 2008.
6. Bauer MS, Damschroder L, Hagedorn H, Smith J, Kilbourne AM. An introduction to implementation science for the non-specialist. BMC Psychol. 2015;3(1):1–12.
7. Damschroder LJ, Aron DC, Keith RE, Kirsh SR, Alexander JA, Lowery JC. Fostering implementation of health services research findings into practice: a consolidated framework for advancing implementation science. Implement Sci. 2009;4(1):1–15.
8. Organization WH. Everybody's business: strengthening health systems to improve health outcomes: WHO's framework for action. Geneva: WHO; 2007. p. 2017.
9. Beaumier G, Wernli D. Systems analysis. Key concepts in research methods; 2021. p. 277–81.
10. Capra F, Luisi PL. The systems view of life: a unifying vision. Cambridge University Press; 2014.
11. Akrich M, Callon M, Latour B. Sociologie de la traduction: textes fondateurs. Paris: Les presses de l'école des mines; 2006. p. 303.
12. Wernli D, Tanner M, Kickbusch I, Escher G, Paccaud F, Flahault A. Moving global health forward in academic institutions. J Glob Health. 2016;6(1):010409.
13. Taylor SJ, Bogdan R, DeVault M. Introduction to qualitative research methods: a guidebook and resource. John Wiley & Sons; 2015.
14. Pawson R, Tilley N. Realist evaluation 2014.

GRADE: A Transparent Approach for Evidence-Based Recommendations and Decisions in Health

84

Holger J. Schünemann and Marge Reinap

Abstract

Trustworthy evidence syntheses using systematic review methodology are essential to make trustworthy decisions. To assess the certainty of a body of evidence included in a systematic review, the Grading of Recommendations Assessment, Development and Evaluation (GRADE) working group has developed an approach that is used by over 110 organizations, including the World Health Organization and the Cochrane Collaboration. GRADE provides operational definitions and instructions to rate the certainty of the evidence for each outcome in a review as high, moderate, low, or very low for the effects of interventions, prognostic estimates, values and preferences, test accuracy, resource utilization and other health questions. The assessment includes assessing the possible impact of risk of bias, imprecision, inconsistency, indirectness, and publication bias, the magnitude of effects, dose-response relations and residual plausible bias on effects or associations. Summary statistical information and assessments of certainty are presented in GRADE evidence summary tables, which are supported by GRADE's official GRADEpro software tool. The evidence summary tables feed into the GRADE Evidence to Decision frameworks which allow creating bridges across health decision-making disciplines and support transparency and trust when making recommendations and informing health policy.

Keywords

GRADE · Guidelines · Recommendations · Systematic reviews · Evidence

H. J. Schünemann (✉)
Department of Health Research Methods, Evidence, and Impact, McMaster University, Hamilton, ON, Canada

Department of Medicine, McMaster University, Hamilton, ON, Canada

Department of Biomedical Sciences, Humanitas University, Milan, Italy
e-mail: schuneh@mcmaster.ca

M. Reinap
Division of Country Health Policies and Systems, WHO Regional Office for Europe, Copenhagen, Denmark
e-mail: reinapm@who.int

84.1 Introduction

Decisions in global health should be based on the best available evidence to ensure the biggest impact within the limited resources. Decision-makers should make the judgments based on that evidence as well as the factors (criteria), that were considered in decision-making, transparent.

M. C. B. Raviglione et al. (eds.), *Global Health Essentials*, Sustainable Development Goals Series,
https://doi.org/10.1007/978-3-031-33851-9_84

Evidence to Decision (EtD) frameworks support such efforts by helping groups of people to move from evidence to decisions [1]. EtDs provide a basis for structured and comprehensive decision-making deliberation through presenting transparently the research evidence building on systematic reviews [2, 3] in a well-structured and systematized way covering a range of key criteria important for decision-making, such as benefits and harms, feasibility and acceptability, resources required. Decision-making based on EtDs facilitates the communication, but also revision of decisions when conditions change or new evidence becomes available. EtD frameworks have been used to formulate 1000's of recommendations, mostly in guidelines, which are systematically developed evidence-based statements that assist providers, patients, policy makers, and other stakeholders to make informed health systems, global health, and public health decisions [4].

The Grading of Recommendations, Assessment, Development and Evaluation (GRADE) working group (www.gradeworkinggroup.org), a collaboration of over 1000 scientists, epidemiologists, clinical and public health specialists, and people with other backgrounds, have developed widely used EtD frameworks for public health and health system decisions to support global health. The approach to EtDs advanced by GRADE working group (simply GRADE) is based on rating the certainty of evidence, an essential step in evidence-based decision-making[1]and is considered the gold-standard in developing recommendations. It is used by over 110 organizations, including the World Health Organization (WHO) and the Cochrane Collaboration in guiding global and national decision-making in health. GRADE is applicable to different types of evidence, including evidence about intervention effects (including multiple treatment comparisons), test accuracy, prognosis, resources, and values and preferences of key stakeholders, including the end users.

EtD frameworks can create bridges across health decision-makers by linkage through the criteria that are used by different actors in the health care space aiming to avoid conflicting decisions in health system and for ensuring optimal resource use [5].

In summary, structured decision-making process decisions are informed by interpretation of evidence. Expert opinion, defined as a combination of an interpretation and judgments based on this interpretation of relevant data ideally compiled through systematic research, is of crucial importance for decisions. Decision-makers should make the data and research evidence used and their interpretation fully transparent. GRADE's EtDs and systematic reviews play an important role in this context. This chapter provides a brief introduction and overview of GRADE.

84.2 The Role of Systematic Reviews and GRADE in Decision-Making

Systematic reviews increase trustworthiness of decisions by ensuring that all members of a panel consider the same, comprehensively collected and rigorously assessed body of evidence. Systematically reviewed bodies of evidence are relevant for all aspects that influence the direction of a decisions and how confident one can be in it. Systematic reviews require an assessment of the quality or certainty that one can place in the summarized evidence using GRADE.

GRADE defines the certainty of the whole body of evidence as the "extent to which one can be confident that an estimate of the effect or association is correct or, more specifically, is beyond a threshold or within a specific range [6]." In the context of decisions, the certainty of the evidence reflects the confidence that the estimates of an effect are adequate to support a particular decision. GRADE uses the terms certainty of the

[1]In policy making, the term evidence-informed is often used but this is based on an understanding that evidence is one of many different types of factors informing a decision, which have been explicitly included into an EtD, including the context, feasibility, acceptability, and so on and are underpinned in evidence. Thus, we use the term evidence-based throughout emphasizing that evidence should be at the forefront of making decisions, regardless of context, by using rigorous methods to inform the context.

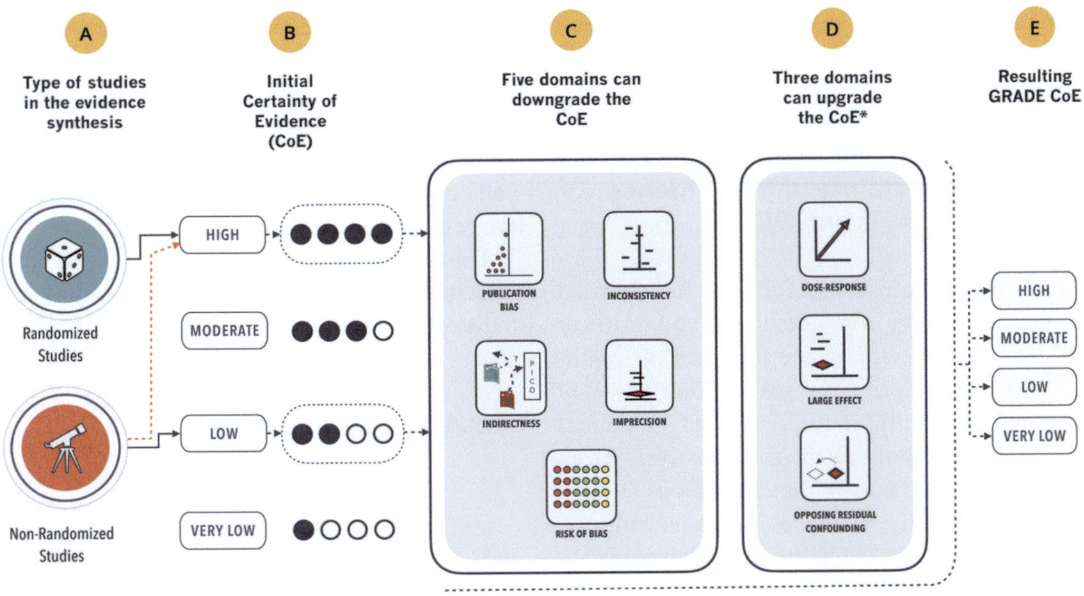

Fig. 84.1 (Designed by Carlos Cuello-Garcia). GRADE approach to rating the certainty of evidence of intervention effects

evidence, quality of the evidence, strength of the evidence, and confidence in estimates interchangeably but the preferred term is certainty of the evidence. Certainty of the evidence is one of several "criteria" used for decision-making, including grading the strength and direction of a recommendation or decision in EtD frameworks [1]. Figure 84.1 presents the detailed domains in GRADE's approach to assessing the certainty of evidence.

84.3 The Certainty of the Evidence, Quality of the Evidence, or Strength of the Evidence

GRADE categorizes the certainty of the evidence as *high*, *moderate*, *low*, or *very low* (see Fig. 84.1). These certainty levels apply to the body of evidence assessed for each key question, not to individual studies. However, an assessment of the risk of bias is needed for each individual study in order to assess the certainty of the evidence. This assessment can lead to lowering or increasing the certainty of the evidence.

84.3.1 Evidence on the Effects of Interventions

For interventions [7] the starting point for rating the certainty of evidence is the study design, broadly categorized into two types:

- Randomized controlled trials (RCTs).
- Non-randomized studies (NRS) or observational studies (including but not limited to cohort studies, and case-control studies, cross-sectional studies, case series, and case reports).

Although RCTs are the preferred source of evidence to assess interventions, in many instances guideline developers must rely on information from NRS, in particular to evaluate potential harms and other EtD criteria talked about earlier. Relevant data can be obtained from both RCTs and NRS, with each type of evidence complementing the other, including both qualitative and quantitative evidence [7]. In GRADE, a body of evidence from RCTs begins with a high-certainty rating while a body of evidence from NRS begins with a low-certainty rating. The lower rating with NRS is the result of the potential bias induced by the lack of randomization (i.e., confounding and selection bias).

84.3.2 Five Domains Can Lower the Certainty of the Evidence from RCTs and NRS

These initial ratings are followed by detailed ratings across the five domains that can lower the certainty. Firstly, in the presence of limitations in study design and execution or *risk of bias* [8]. Secondly, if the results of individual studies contributing to the meta-analysis of an outcome are statistically heterogeneous *(inconsistency)*. Thirdly, if the evidence is indirect, *Indirectness* arises when the identified evidence differs with respect to at least one of the population, intervention, comparator, outcome (PICO) elements relative to the target question formulated by the decision-making panel, such as guideline development group or the systematic reviewers. Fourthly, due to *imprecision*—if the results are imprecise, such as the body of evidence includes few participants and few events, with wide confidence intervals around the estimate of the effect. And finally, the presence of *publication bias*—the systematic deviation of the effect estimated in a systematic review from the underlying true effect due to the selective publication of studies.

The ratings in systematic reviews are conducted initially on a "per outcome" level [8]. This requires detailed knowledge of the individual studies included in the body of evidence. For details, the readers are referred to the online GRADE Handbook and the cited publications.

84.3.3 Three Factors Can Increase the Certainty of the Evidence of NRS

If, and only if, there are no further limitations, i.e., there is no reason for downgrading the quality of a body of evidence from NRS, then upgrading the certainty of the evidence may be possible, within the following three domains [8].

Firstly, the presence of a dose-response gradient increasing the confidence in the findings of NRS, and thereby increase the certainty of the evidence. Secondly, if plausible, but not accounted for residual confounders or biases in a well conducted NRS would result in an underestimate of an observed treatment effect.

Thirdly, if a large or very large effect is observed, this will generally increase confidence in the results [8].

84.3.4 GRADE Evidence Profiles and Summary of Findings Tables: Summaries of Evidence

GRADE Evidence Profiles include the detailed assessment of the quality or certainty of the evidence for each outcome [8]. Figure 84.2 shows an example from a clinical practice guideline of the use of masks for COVID-19 [9]. The effects of the intervention are summarized both in relative terms and as absolute risk differences. The main reason for a certainty assessment or other noteworthy points is documented in explanatory footnotes that constitute an essential part of GRADE tables [10]. The Summary of Findings (SoF) table includes an assessment of the quality of evidence for each outcome but not the detailed judgments on which that assessment is based. SoF tables are intended for a broader audience, for example, users of guidelines: they provide a concise summary of the key information underlying a recommendation.

84.3.5 How Is the Overall Certainty of the Evidence for a Decision or Recommendation Determined?

Those making decisions should assess all the information from the systematic review(s) presented in GRADE Evidence Profiles and SoF tables. Panels then determine the overall certainty of the evidence across all the critical outcomes for a recommendation. Because certainty of the

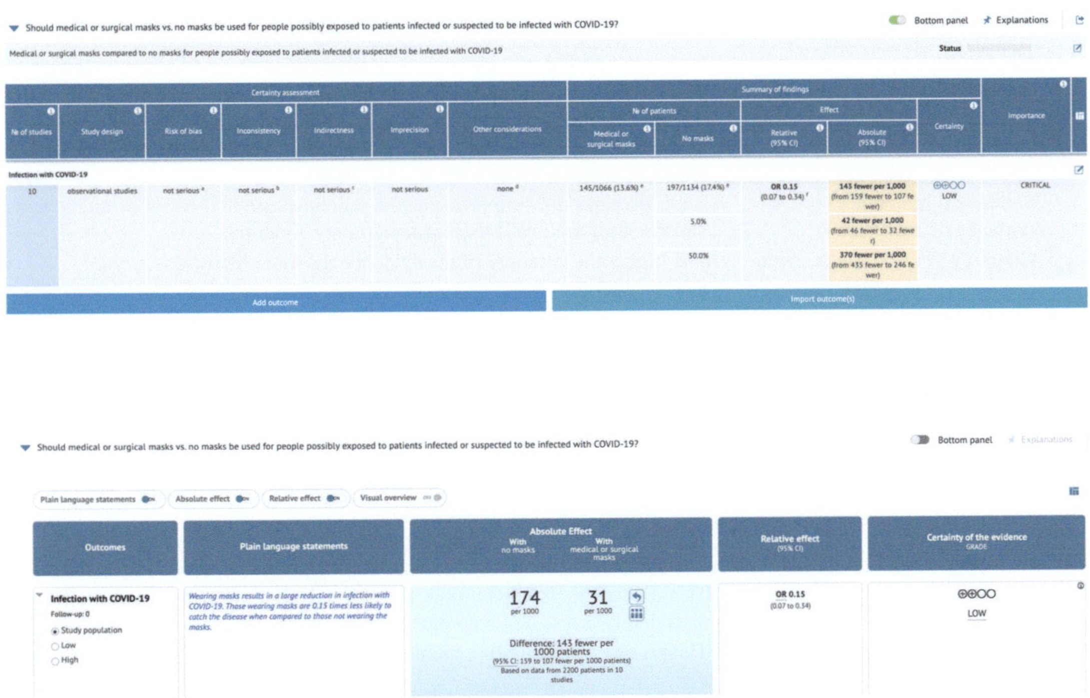

Fig. 84.2 An evidence profile and summary of findings table showing one outcome [9]

evidence is rated separately for each outcome, the certainty usually differs across outcomes reflecting the state of the evidence. The overall certainty of the recommendation is not higher than the lowest certainty for any outcome that is critical for a decision.

84.4 Developing Recommendations and Making Decisions Based on Evidence

The EtD framework consists of three sections: the PICO questions, summaries of the evidence, and the conclusions [1]. The GRADE criteria that determine the direction and strength of the recommendation and a description of how they influence the recommendation are summarized in Table 84.1. This emphasizes that for many of the criteria NRS will provide critical evidence, e.g., for prognostic and baseline risk questions, on values and on economic and feasibility related evidence, although experimental studies with credible designs should be used as much as possible.

The strength of a recommendation reflects the confidence of a guideline development group in the balance of the desirable and undesirable consequences of implementing a recommendation:

- *Strong*: the guideline group is confident that the desirable effects outweigh any undesirable consequences.
- *Conditional or weak*: there is considerable uncertainty about the balance of desirable and undesirable effects.

Strong recommendations are not very common: those making recommendations are often dealing with low or very low-certainty evidence and therefore should be reluctant to make strong recommendations [11]. The EtD framework documents not only the evidence and the judgments leading to a recommendation, but also the justifications for the direction and strength of the recommendation, and the process. Considerations on subgroups of people, implementation of the

Table 84.1 Criteria that influence the strength and direction in the GRADE evidence to decision frameworks

Criteria	How the criterion influences the direction and strength of a recommendation
1. Problem	The judgment about the problem is determined by the importance and frequency of the health care issue that is addressed (burden of disease, prevalence, cost or baseline risk). If the problem is of great importance a strong recommendation may be more likely
2. Values and preferences or the importance of outcomes	This describes how important health outcomes are to those affected, how variable they are and if there is uncertainty about this
3. Certainty of the evidence about the health benefits and harm	The higher the certainty of the evidence the more likely is a strong recommendation
4. Health benefits and harms and burden and their balance	This requires an evaluation of the absolute effects of both the benefits and harms and their importance including the judgment about criterion 2. The greater the net benefit or net harm the more likely is a strong recommendation for or against the option
5. Resource implications	This describes how resource intense an option is if it is cost-effective and if there is incremental benefit. The more advantageous or clearly disadvantageous these resource implications are the more likely is a strong recommendation
6. Equity	The greater the likelihood to reduce inequities or increase equity and the more accessible an option is, the more likely is a strong recommendation
7. Acceptability	The greater the acceptability of an option to all or most stakeholders, the more likely is a strong recommendation
8. Feasibility	The greater the feasibility, the more likely is a strong recommendation

recommendation, evaluation, and monitoring gaps may also be covered.

The systematic assessment of the certainty of the evidence in GRADE helps reviewers to identify and report on important gaps in the evidence base. Table 84.2 illustrates how review authors may interpret a body of evidence and draw conclusions about the need for future research. The GRADE process from creating a (interactive) SoF table to interactive EtD frameworks and full guidelines is facilitated by the GRADEpro software (www.gradepro.org).

84.5 Outlook

The strength of the GRADE approach rests in the structured framework for the assessment of evidence independent of the actual intervention or question, and the requirement for explicit processes and transparent judgments. This provides a good basis for increasing trust in decision-making and cross-utilization of evidence products between different decision-making streams to reduce conflicting decisions and wasted resources. GRADE has been applied to a wide range of health care interventions, from clinical to public health and health policy questions including in global health decisions [12]. The ease of applying the GRADE approach will vary according to the type of evidence being assessed, the circumstances in which GRADE cannot be usefully applied are rare. GRADE has also been used for questions about diagnostical tests, prognosis, resource use, values, and preferences. GRADE, as any approach in science, is not perfect and will evolve in the light of future research [13].

Detailed information on GRADE is available through the following resources:

- GRADE working group: http://www.gradeworkinggroup.org
- GRADE profiler software (GRADEpro) and GRADE apps in the GRADEpro Guideline Development Tool (GDT): http://www.gradepro.org (includes a detailed handbook on GRADE)
- GRADE online training modules: http://heigrade.mcmaster.ca
- GRADE training resource compilation by Cochrane: https://training.cochrane.org/grade-approach

Table 84.2 Interpretation of the certainty of a body of evidence for both research and practice, according to individual GRADE domains

By outcome	Implications for research	Examples	Implications for practice
Risk of bias	Need for methodologically better designed and executed studies	All studies suffered from lack of blinding of outcome assessors. Trials of this type are required	The estimates of effect may be biased because of a lack of blinding
Inconsistency	Unexplained inconsistency: Need for individual participant data meta-analysis (IPDMA) to explore subgroup effects; need for studies in relevant subgroups	Studies in patients with small cell lung cancer are needed to understand if the effects differ from those in patients with pancreatic cancer	Unexplained inconsistency: Consider and interpret overall effect estimates as for the certainty of a body of evidence Explained inconsistency (if results are presented in strata): Consider and interpret effects estimates by subgroup
Indirectness	Need for studies that more directly address the PICO question of interest	Studies in patients with early cancer are needed because the evidence is from studies with advanced cancer	It is uncertain if the results directly apply to the patients or the way that the intervention is applied in your setting
Imprecision	Need for more studies with more participants to reach optimal information size	Studies with approximately 200 more events in the treatment and control group are required	Same as for certainty of a body of evidence
Publication bias	Need to investigate and identify unpublished data; large studies might help resolve this issue		Same as for certainty of a body of evidence
Large effects	No implications	No implications	The effect is large in the populations that were included in the studies. The effect is going to be in the vicinity of the observed effect
Dose effects	No implications	No implications	The greater the reduction in the exposure the larger is the expected benefit (harm)
Opposing bias and confounding	Studies controlling for the residual bias and confounding may be needed to better estimate the effects	Studies controlling for following possible confounders may be required smoking, degree of education	The effect could be even larger than the one that is observed in the studies presented here

Acknowledgments This work benefitted from the many contributions of members of the GRADE working group to developing GRADE and its official tools.

Conflict of Interest HJS is the co-chair of the GRADE Working Group. The author (MR) affiliated with the World Health Organization (WHO) is alone responsible for the views expressed in this publication and they do not necessarily represent the decisions or policies of the WHO.

References

1. Alonso-Coello P, Oxman AD, Moberg J, et al. GRADE Evidence to Decision (EtD) frameworks: a systematic and transparent approach to making well informed healthcare choices. 2: Clinical practice guidelines. BMJ. 2016;353:i2089.
2. Oxman AD, Schunemann HJ, Fretheim A. Improving the use of research evidence in guideline development: 8. Synthesis and presentation of evidence. Health Res Policy Syst. 2006;4:20.

3. Graham R, Mancher M, Miller Wolman D, Greenfield S, Steinberg E. Clinical practice guidelines we can trust. Washington DC: The National Academy of Sciences; 2011.
4. Moberg J, Oxman AD, Rosenbaum S, et al. The GRADE evidence to decision (EtD) framework for health system and public health decisions. Health Res Policy Syst. 2018;16(1):45.
5. Schunemann HJ, Reinap M, Piggott T, et al. The ecosystem of health decision making: from fragmentation to synergy. Lancet Public Health. 2022;7(4):e378–90.
6. Schunemann HJ. Interpreting GRADE's levels of certainty or quality of the evidence: GRADE for statisticians, considering review information size or less emphasis on imprecision? J Clin Epidemiol. 2016;75:6–15.
7. Schunemann HJ, Tugwell P, Reeves BC, et al. Non-randomized studies as a source of complementary, sequential or replacement evidence for randomized controlled trials in systematic reviews on the effects of interventions. Res Synth Methods. 2013;4(1):49–62.
8. Zhang Y, Akl EA, Schunemann HJ. Using systematic reviews in guideline development: the GRADE approach. Res Synth Methods. 2018;10:312.
9. Chu DK, Akl EA, Duda S, et al. Physical distancing, face masks, and eye protection to prevent person-to-person transmission of SARS-CoV-2 and COVID-19: a systematic review and meta-analysis. Lancet. 2020;395(10242):1973–87.
10. Santesso N, Carrasco-Labra A, Langendam M, et al. Improving GRADE evidence tables part 3: detailed guidance for explanatory footnotes supports creating and understanding GRADE certainty in the evidence judgments. J Clin Epidemiol. 2016;74:28–39.
11. Neumann I, Santesso N, Akl EA, et al. A guide for health professionals to interpret and use recommendations in guidelines developed with the GRADE approach. J Clin Epidemiol. 2016;72:45–55.
12. Akl EA, Kennedy C, Konda K, et al. Using GRADE methodology for the development of public health guidelines for the prevention and treatment of HIV and other STIs among men who have sex with men and transgender people. BMC Public Health. 2012;12:386.
13. Norris SL, Bero L. GRADE methods for guideline development: time to evolve? Ann Intern Med. 2016;165(11):810–1.

85 Methods in Surveillance and Monitoring and Evaluation

Marcos A. Espinal and Prabhjot Singh

Abstract

Public health surveillance involves collection and analysis of health-related data. It could be indicator-based or event-based. The latter involves monitoring of formal sources like newspapers or informal-like social media for health-related information; it has the potential to detect outbreaks earlier. Indicator-based surveillance could be established using unconfirmed disease syndromes, like fever, or diseases confirmed using laboratory diagnosis. It could be disease-specific or integrate information for multiple diseases. It may have information transmitted passively or require actively looking for health-related information. Demographic surveillance uses census or civil registration of vital events like births and deaths as a source of information. Health and demographic surveillance system sites in some countries of the Global South offer an in-depth understanding of changes in population and the causes thereof. Monitoring and evaluation of public health programmes provide information about how well the programme is functioning and what interventions are having the most impact.

Keywords

Indicator-based surveillance · Disease-based surveillance · Event-based surveillance · Demographic surveillance · Monitoring and evaluation

85.1 Introduction and Background

Implementation of health systems requires information. Information about types of diseases prevalent within a population, their magnitude and trends would help in assessing current and near future needs; like increasing fever cases could be due to an outbreak of dengue which would require investigation of cases and mosquito control. The demographic structure of population and long-term trends therein would help projecting future needs. A very rapid increase in proportion of people in older age groups, for instance, would require scaling up of geriatric health services.

M. A. Espinal (✉)
Pan American Health Organization, Washington, DC, USA
e-mail: espinalm@paho.org

P. Singh
Barbados and the Eastern Caribbean Countries, Pan American Health Organization, Bridgetown, Barbados
e-mail: singhpra@paho.org

M. C. B. Raviglione et al. (eds.), *Global Health Essentials*, Sustainable Development Goals Series,
https://doi.org/10.1007/978-3-031-33851-9_85

85.2 Public Health Surveillance

The World Health Organization defines public health surveillance as 'continuous, systematic collection, analysis and interpretation of health-related data'. The sharing of information about the number of cases of a particular disease seen in a health centre and its analysis to ascertain whether it is normal to see that number or if it represents an outbreak is the core of public health surveillance. Based on the source of information, traditional and structured-like health centres or unstructured like news reports, public health surveillance is called indicator-based or event-based, respectively.

85.2.1 Indicator-Based Surveillance

Indicator-based surveillance includes traditional methods of reporting diseases to government health personnel from hospitals, health centres or clinics, usually in a structured and standardized manner. The following are various strategies used within indicator-based surveillance.

85.2.1.1 Syndromic Surveillance

Syndromic surveillance was developed for detecting and responding to bioterrorism attacks and has been widely adopted as an early warning system in public health. Data is collected from health centres on illnesses like fever, fever with rash or gastroenteritis. Any increase in cases of an illness over a predetermined threshold (or a threshold calculated using seasonal variations in previous years) is considered as an alert and precursor for intervention. Other than illnesses, surrogates like school absenteeism or over the counter drug use have also been used. The objective is to identify illness clusters early or earlier than traditional methods of surveillance and this is very useful in resource limited settings where the health staff are limited or overburdened. But, since symptoms like fever and not the actual disease is being followed up, an investigation is still required to identify the underlying cause. Often, this could require a laboratory diagnosis which may not be feasible in resource limited settings or in rural areas.

85.2.1.2 Laboratory-Based Surveillance

Laboratory-based surveillance focuses on definitive diagnosis of diseases before data is analysed. While this has the advantage that all episodes included are certainly due to the disease under surveillance, some diagnosis techniques could be difficult to implement in resource limited settings. COVID-19 confirmed cases required reverse transcriptase polymerase chain reaction (rt-PCR) which wasn't available at the start of pandemic in most laboratories even in developed countries. In early days of the pandemic, sometimes in resource limited countries samples had to be sent outside the country, often delaying the diagnosis by days as also the response. Additionally, the accuracy of a diagnosis technique varies and even the most accurate techniques will miss or misclassify some disease cases (Box 85.1). When several diseases must be checked against in one patient, one test would be required for each one of them leading to delay in getting results, increased cost, and time the laboratory personnel will take. Progress is being made in developing tests, like multiplex platforms, that would test for multiple diseases from one sample in a single test, thereby alleviating the need for individual tests in most situations.

Box 85.1

HIV tests are accurate, but their performance varies by when a test is conducted as also what a test is looking for. Tests can look for HIV RNA, HIV antigen (p24) or antibodies to HIV. Nucleic acid tests (NAT) detect HIV RNA. The fourth-generation rapid tests that detect both HIV antigen and antibodies to the virus have a sensitivity and specificity higher than 99.5%. Sensitivity is the probability that a person with disease will receive a correct test result, i.e. positive, while specificity is the probability that a person without disease will receive a correct test result, i.e. negative. However, HIV RNA become detectable by NAT after 10 days of infection. It takes another 4–10 days for the HIV antigen to reach levels detectable by fourth generation rapid tests. But the antigen is present for a short window as antibodies are formed against it. These antibodies are detectable 3–5 days after the antigen appears, or 10–13 days after the HIV RNA appears. Thus, even with highly sensitive and specific diagnosis tools, the time at which a test is done since HIV infection would also determine the accuracy of the diagnosis result.

85.2.2 Disease-Specific and Integrated Disease Surveillance

Disease-specific surveillance is a completely vertical system. Herein comprehensive information including number of cases of a single disease by age and sex, people tested, or even a line list of each confirmed case is shared regularly. This has helped resource limited countries focus efforts on major problems like tuberculosis or malaria. However, resources pooled in for disease-specific surveillance have limited benefits for the broader health surveillance or population health. In integrated disease surveillance, information about predetermined set of diseases is shared regularly from the health centre onwards. The information shared is common for all diseases, like number of confirmed cases. Advancements in multiplex platforms would further aid integrated surveillance right from the laboratory. While useful to detect major trends and outbreaks, integrated surveillance may not provide adequate information needed for a response, like risk profile of patients, probable place of occurrence or associated factors, all of which would need details of each patient.

85.2.2.1 Special Surveys

When routine surveillance is not able to capture the true magnitude of a disease, or information is required which isn't captured by it, for e.g. lifestyle risk factors in otherwise healthy individuals, surveys may need to be conducted. It could be based on a questionnaire specific to a disease or could gather information about multiple diseases or risk factors. The Behavioural Risk Factor Surveillance System (BRFSS) is a telephone-based survey in USA that has been used to monitor seat belt use. Surveys, however, are costly and logistically difficult to do very frequently, often limiting their use.

85.2.2.2 Active and Passive Surveillance

When sick, a patient may seek care at a health centre, polyclinic or hospital, be it private or public. Information so generated and reported passively to health authorities is considered as passive surveillance. This forms the backbone of surveillance in most countries, owing to its simplicity and lower costs once established. However, the quality and type of information depend upon the health centres reporting correctly on all items.

On the other hand, health staff may actively seek information from a health centre or go house to house to look for those who are sick, or test all those who have been in contact with a known case of disease. Such information forms part of active surveillance. The quality of information and its completeness is higher in active surveillance, but the extra cost—financial and in time—of actively seeking information make it difficult to implement and maintain.

85.2.3 Event-Based Surveillance

The International Health Regulations require countries to have "the capacity to detect, assess, notify and report events." A disease itself or a situation that could lead to potential disease is an event. Event-based surveillance is the organized and rapid capture of information about events that are a potential risk to public health. This information could be news reports, rumours and other ad-hoc reports transmitted through established formal channels or informal channels like news channels or social media. Event-based surveillance can potentially detect outbreaks. Table 85.1 presents the advantages of this strategy compared to others.

85.2.4 Public Health Surveillance and Digitalization

As if the adoption of digital tools was not fast enough, the COVID-19 pandemic and associated infection prevention strategies have led to a massive increase in the adoption of digitalization in public health surveillance. The area is still in its infancy and is quite wide applying both to the adoption of digital tools in public health surveillance and the use of digital information for public health surveillance. The move towards reporting via smartphones, automation of data consolidation, cleaning, analytics and reporting, interoperability between hitherto siloed databases has massively increased the efficiency of public health surveillance. On the other hand, increased trend of use of social media, search engines and associated digital history has provided other avenues to infer trends in diseases and risk factors. The COVID-19 Mobility Reports produced by Google® and Apple® provided an instant tool for public health practitioners to study adherence to stay at home and quarantine orders and their impact at the start of the pandemic.

Table 85.1 Advantages and disadvantages of surveillance strategies

Surveillance type	Advantages	Disadvantages
Indicator-based surveillance		
• Syndromic	Easy to implement	Further investigation is required Confirmation of diagnosis required in some cases
• Lab-based	Certainty of cause of increase or outbreaks	Could be resource intensive Certainty depends on diagnosis technique
• Disease specific	Provides highly specific and relevant information	Resource intensive Doesn't add to surveillance of other diseases
• Integrated	Information on most important diseases Optimal use of resources	Additional disease-specific information may still be needed
• Special surveys	Higher coverage, especially of populations not traditionally included Surveillance of risk factors is possible	Costly Variance in methodology over time could make surveys incomparable
• Passive	Easier to maintain once established Allows estimation of trends, disease burdens, risk factors	Quality of data depends on health centres Complete reporting from all health centres is difficult to maintain
• Active	Higher quality of information Almost complete records Useful for specific analyses	Costly to implement or maintain
• Event-based surveillance	Allows inclusion of non-traditional and informal sources Possible detection of outbreaks by unknown diseases	Verification of information is required

85.3 Demographic Surveillance Strategies

85.3.1 Census

"The total process of collecting, compiling, analysing, and publishing or otherwise disseminating demographic, economic and social data pertaining to all persons in a country or in a well-delineated part of a country at a specified time" is defined as census by the United Nations. Thus, a census is more than just a simple headcount done every 10 or so years in a country. It provides information down to the lowest unit of administration, something that surveys cannot provide. Although the cost of asking for additional demographic and other information is marginal, the length of census forms could become long and cumbersome leading to lower quality of data. Given the size and complexity of a census, quality control efforts are limited at best. In an ever more globalized world, accelerated internal and external migration has decreased the usefulness of a decennial census. Some developed countries like Sweden and Norway have stopped collecting population data by census altogether and being replaced with population registers among other tools.

85.3.2 Civil Registration and Vital Statistics

United Nations defined vital statistics to constitute "life and death of individuals, as well as their family and civil status." Further, civil registration and vital statistics system (CRVS) is defined as the "continuous, permanent, compulsory and universal recording of the occurrence and characteristics of vital events pertaining to the population, as provided through decree or regulation in accordance with the legal requirements in each country". Enacted laws require each birth and death, be it within a hospital and health centre or outside it, to be registered. CRVS helps in updating intercensal population estimates while analysis of cause of deaths could provide trends that would need intervention. The rising number of deaths due to opioids in USA, analysis partly based on National Vital Statistics System mortality data, helped identify the epidemic of opioid overdose and its relation to prescribing practices. In resource limited countries, not all births and deaths happen at a health institution or are reported to local health authorities, which limits the use of CRVS.

85.3.3 Health and Demographic Surveillance System

The Health and Demographic Surveillance System (HDSS) refers to a specific longitudinal surveillance system that originated in 1960s. In countries where a proportion of births and deaths may happen outside of the health centres, CRVS will not capture demographic trends well. HDSS sites were established in mostly resource limited countries, wherein the total population of a specific defined area would be followed up more intensely than the rest of the population. Changes in population due to births, deaths and migration into or out of the HDSS site are documented continuously through resident enumerators. This is complemented with ongoing retrospective surveys done in all households of the site. An INDEPTH network has been created and as of 2022, 47 HDSS sites were part of this. This allows collecting standardized data across HDSS sites located in different countries which helps in comparison.

85.4 Monitoring and Evaluation

Monitoring and evaluation (M&E) are the techniques used to assess how well a health programme is achieving its goals. While *monitoring* refers to the ongoing assessment of progress and is usually conducted by internal teams, *evaluation* involves a systematic review of the progress conducted or the impact of the programme at set intervals, say once every 5 years or at the end of a programme, and done usually by an external team. Monitoring focuses on if things are being done correctly, while evaluation assesses if correct things were done. Eventually M&E helps improve the health of a population by improving the efficiency and efficacy of a public health programme.

The adoption of Millennium Development Goals (MDGs) and Sustainable Development Goals has led to internalization of M&E in all aspects of governance, especially health sector. MDG-3 focussed on decreasing the burden of HIV/AIDS, tuberculosis and malaria. In malaria, distribution of bednets was the bedrock of preventing the disease. Monitoring tools used provided the information on how efficient bed net distribution campaigns were, challenges in distribution and subsequent use by the population. Evaluation provided evidence that mass distribution of bednets was a correct strategy and led to decline in deaths due to malaria in children.

Indicators developed at the start of a programme guide the M&E process. These could be input, output, outcome or impact indicators. Input indicators measure what has been put in, like the number of bednets purchased. Output indicators measure the effort put into a programme, like number of bednets distributed. Outcome indicators assess the effectiveness of the programme, like the percentage of population of a village that received a bednet. Impact indicators would measure the actual change in the disease, like the decline in deaths before and after the bednet distribution. Established at the start of a programme, indicators and their targets provide clarity for health personnel on how performance will be measured and guidance in course correction.

85.5 Conclusions

Various strategies of public health surveillance exist, and their use in a context depends on available resources, both financial and human. The lack of trained human resources has been the bane in large resource limited countries and exacerbated in small island developing states. The use of digital tools may increase the efficiency of public health, resolving the paucity of resources to some extent. Censuses are still the backbone of demographic data for most countries, but increasing global migration is becoming challenging to factor in. Robust CRVS development requires legal framework and compliance by the population.

Suggested Reading

Centers for Disease Control and Prevention and Association of Public Health Laboratories. Laboratory testing for the diagnosis of HIV infection: updated recommendations. https://doi.org/10.15620/cdc.23447. Published 27 Jun 2014. Accessed May 2022.

Coleman D. The twilight of the census. Popul Dev Rev. 2013;38:334–51. https://doi.org/10.1111/j.1728-4457.2013.00568.x.

Henning KJ. What is syndromic surveillance? MMWR. 2004;53S:5–11.

Hossein Abad ZS, Kline A, Sultana M, et al. Digital public health surveillance: a systematic scoping review. NPJ Digit Med. 2021;4(1):1–13. https://doi.org/10.1038/s41746-021-00407-6.

Kaneko S, K'opiyo J, Kiche I, Wanyua S, Goto K, Tanaka J, et al. Health and demographic surveillance system in the Western and coastal areas of Kenya: an infrastructure for epidemiologic studies in Africa. J Epidemiol. 2012;22(3):276–85. https://doi.org/10.2188/jea.je20110078.

Lankester T. Monitoring and evaluating the health programme. In: Lankester T, Grills N, editors. Setting up community health Programmes in low and middle income countries. 4th ed. Oxford University Press; 2019.

Lindblade KA, Eisele TP, Gimnig JE, Alaii JA, Odhiambo F, ter Kuile OF, et al. Sustainability of reductions in malaria transmission and infant mortality in western Kenya with use of insecticide-treated bednets: 4 to 6 years of follow-up. JAMA. 2004;291(21):2571–80. https://doi.org/10.1001/jama.291.21.2571.

McKee M, van Schalkwyk MCI, Stuckler D. The second information revolution: digitalization brings opportunities and concerns for public health. Eur J Pub Health. 2019;29(S3):3–6. https://doi.org/10.1093/eurpub/ckz160.

Mirza N, Reynolds TL, Coletta M, Suda K, Soyiri I, Markle A, et al. Steps to a sustainable public health surveillance enterprise. A commentary from the international society for disease surveillance. OJPHI. 2013;5(2):210. https://ojphi.org/ojs/index.php/ojphi/article/view/4703.

Nsubuga P, White ME, Thacker SB, et al. Public health surveillance: a tool for targeting and monitoring interventions. In: Jamison DT, Breman JG, Measham AR, et al., editors. Disease control priorities in developing countries. 2nd ed. Washington (DC): The International Bank for Reconstruction and Development/the World Bank; 2006. Chapter 53. https://www.ncbi.nlm.nih.gov/books/NBK11770/ co-published by Oxford university press, N Y.

Porta M, editor. A dictionary of epidemiology. Oxford university press; 2008.

Rolle-Lake L, Robbins E. Behavioral risk factor surveillance system. StatPearls, StatPearls Publishing; 2022.

Teutsch SM, Churchill RE, editors. Principles and practice of public health surveillance. USA: Oxford University Press; 2000.

Thacker SB, Berkelman RL. Public health surveillance in the United States. Epidemiol Rev. 1988;10(1):164–90. https://doi.org/10.1093/oxfordjournals.epirev.a036021.

United Nations. Definition, concepts and uses of vital statistics. In: Principles and recommendations for a vital statistics system; 2014. https://doi.org/10.18356/25930282-en.

World Health Organization. Surveillance in emergencies. Emergencies, World Health Organization; 2022. www.who.int/emergencies/surveillance. Accessed 1 Jun 2022

Yilmazkuday H. Stay-at-home works to fight against COVID-19: international evidence from Google mobility data. J Hum Behav Soc Environ. 2021;31(1–4):210–20. https://doi.org/10.1080/10911359.2020.1845903.

Economics of Global Health

86

Gerard Abou Jaoude, Neha Batura, Ana Correa, Hassan Haghparast-Bidgoli, Rolando Leiva Granados, Tom Palmer, Stavros Poupakis, Francesco Salustri, and Jolene Skordis

Abstract

Population health and economic development are directly dependent on each other, as good health facilitates productivity and higher incomes enable better nutrition and care seeking. The design of health systems financing can impact the distribution of economic gains and health risks in a population. Further, the human and financial resources available for health provision are limited and some priority setting will be inevitable. After describing the relationship between population health and economic development, this chapter evaluates the main mechanisms for health systems financing and considers the potentially impoverishing effect of health spending in many contexts. Finally, the efficiency of systems is considered, with a focus on incentivising health workers through appropriate payment systems, reducing waste and selecting the highest priority health interventions.

Keywords

Economic development · Health financing system · Health expenditure · Health systems · Disease burden

86.1 Introduction

This chapter explores the economics of health at a time when health spending comprises 9.8% of gross domestic product (GDP) globally, according to the World Bank. Health spending is expected to increase further as populations age and the prevalence of non-communicable diseases rise, while infectious diseases remain common. After describing the relationship between population health and economic development, this chapter evaluates the main mechanisms for health systems financing and considers the potentially impoverishing effect of health spending in many contexts. Finally, the efficiency of systems is considered, with a focus on incentivising health workers through appropriate payment systems, reducing waste and selecting the highest priority health interventions.

G. Abou Jaoude · N. Batura · A. Correa · H. Haghparast-Bidgoli · R. Leiva Granados · T. Palmer · S. Poupakis · J. Skordis (✉)
University College London, London, UK
e-mail: gerard.jaoude.15@ucl.ac.uk; n.batura@ucl.ac.uk; a.correa@ucl.ac.uk; h.haghparast-bidgoli@ucl.ac.uk; rolando.granados.19@ucl.ac.uk; t.palmer@ucl.ac.uk; s.poupakis@ucl.ac.uk; j.skordis@ucl.ac.uk

F. Salustri
University College London, London, UK

Roma Tre University, Rome, Italy
e-mail: f.salustri@ucl.ac.uk

M. C. B. Raviglione et al. (eds.), *Global Health Essentials*, Sustainable Development Goals Series,
https://doi.org/10.1007/978-3-031-33851-9_86

86.2 The Relationship Between Population Health and Economic Development

There is a well-established relationship between population health and economic development. In the 1970s, the Preston curve described the positive relationship between life-expectancy and GDP per capita [1]. This relationship is supported theoretically in two ways. Firstly, rising income improves nutrition and public health infrastructure, which have a direct effect on health. Secondly, health is a component of human capital, an input to economic development through higher productivity [2].

In 2001, the World Health Organization's (WHO) Commission on Macroeconomics and Health comprehensively demonstrated how health was a central input to economic development and poverty reduction, while being a priority in its own right. The Commission estimated that eight million lives could be saved from infectious diseases and nutritional deficiencies, which translated then into a direct economic benefit of $186 billion per year. Additionally, that economic dividend would accelerate economic growth, interrupt the medical poverty trap and add '*billions of dollars more per year through increased per capita incomes*' [3].

Globally, health expenditure has increased over the last decade, with the trend looking set to continue. Donor investment in health also accelerated in the early part of this century, but efforts to increase and co-ordinate donor funding have since foundered and aid to the health sector was in steady decline before the COVID-19 pandemic. Supporting health systems to support development remains a high priority challenge, although investment will be likely be challenged by a volatile and contracting economic climate globally.

86.3 Health Financing Systems: The Role of Health Insurance and Incentives of Provider Payments

While health funding can be collected before or at the point of use, populations always ultimately finance services [4]. Health financing systems therefore perform three main functions: (1) revenue collection, (2) fund and risk pooling, and (3) purchasing services/paying health providers [5]. In practice, this means deciding who pays, how much, and when. Health financing systems can perform these functions through various mechanisms, each with its advantages and shortfalls (Table 86.1). Direct and indirect taxes, health insurance premiums, and donor funding are all types of revenue collected before health services are used. Funds can be pooled together and used to purchase health services on behalf of individuals entitled to a given pool. Typically, bigger funding pools have more diverse health risks and are most efficient [5]. It is thus increasingly recognised that single or integrated pools, which are primarily general tax-funded and cover entire populations, are required for progress toward universal health coverage [5, 6].

The way in which health care providers are paid affects the type and quantity of services provided. Health workers can be incentivised to work longer and provide higher quality, cost-effective services. Table 86.2 presents the common provider payment mechanisms and the incentives each one creates. No one payment method is most effective. Payment mechanisms need to consider the context and balance positive and negative incentives against the cost of administration. Some studies show that a combination of mechanisms may be most effective [16].

Table 86.1 An overview of health financing systems and consequences

Mechanism	Implications on pooling function	Fair financing	Universal health coverage	Ease of operation	Financial sustainability
Tax-based (e.g., *United Kingdom)*	+ Large, national pool is possible + Pooling of funds and risk spreading across time and individuals/households	+ Can be funded through progressive taxation where the rich cross-subsidise the poor [6] – Certain taxes (e.g. VAT) can be regressive and disproportionately burden poorer populations	+ Can ensure everyone is able to access publicly funded services for free at the point of use [7] – Only a limited set of services can be offered when relying solely on taxation in lower income settings with a small tax base [8]	– Costly to set up – Requires substantial government capacity to effectively collect, manage and spend taxes – Challenging to collect certain taxes, for example income tax, in settings with high levels of informal labour or unemployment [6] –Requires expertise from the government to identify the needs of the population and purchase an appropriate package of health services	+ Can be sustainable and can mobilise additional funding in several ways, such as spending more on health as a percentage of GDP or introducing new taxes + Can be used to invest in public health and prevention which can lower costs over time – Requires substantial priority setting and a limited set of publicly financed services to be sustainable in lower income settings where tax-bases limited [8] – Susceptible to changes in government and their commitment to health [7]

(continued)

Table 86.1 (continued)

Mechanism	Implications on pooling function	Fair financing	Universal health coverage	Ease of operation	Financial sustainability
Social health insurance (e.g., France)	+ Large pools + Pooling of funds and risk spreading across time and individuals/households – Can create segmented pools of employed, informally employed and unemployed individuals[6]	+ Can be progressive, especially when there is a large pool enabling cross-subsidisation of the poor by the rich [9] – Can result in separate pools without cross-subsidisation between rich and poor [6]	+ Can ensure health service provision that is subsidised or free at the point of use for those entitled [7] – Not all population groups may be entitled to the same services and patient pathways when there is more than one pool	– Costly to set-up – Requires actuarial expertise – Reimbursement procedures, provider purchasing and negotiation of tariffs/fees can be challenging to implement effectively [10]	+ Funding is less susceptible to changes in government and their commitment to health compared with tax-based mechanisms. [7] – Effective priority setting and purchasing agreements are required to prevent escalating costs of services –Balancing population needs and the sustainability of pooled resources might be difficult, especially for the smallest schemes when there is more than one pool
Community-based health insurance (e.g., Rwanda)	+ Pooling of funds and risk spreading across time and individuals/households – Many small/fragmented pools of individuals/ households with similar risk profiles and from similar communities [11]	– There is usually little scope for cross-subsidisation between rich and poor as members are often from the same community [11]	+ Can help improve access to services – Not all population groups may be entitled to the same services and patient pathways—with differences in quality of care [11] + Can provide financial protection if fees are based on socioeconomic status rather than on a flat rate [12]	– Requires actuarial expertise, especially larger funds	– Challenging to ensure sufficient contributions and funds to cover included services if the pool is not big enough [12] – Often actuarial expertise is lacking to ensure financial feasibility and sustainability of the schemes [11]

Private health insurance (e.g., *universally private such as Switzerland and Netherlands; and mostly private insurance such as the United States)*	+ Pooling of funds and risk across time and across individuals/households – Relying solely on private health insurance results in fragmented pools + – Individuals are the purchasers of their own health care. Restricted to what is covered by their private insurance, they can decide which services to purchase and from which providers [7]	– Private health insurance in fragmented financing systems is typically regressive. Poorer populations have lower access to costlier services [13] + Can be progressive in contexts with compulsory contributions to large funding pools (e.g. Switzerland). Richer populations pay into large public pools but do not use the services [7]	+ Can complement/supplement publicly subsidised services free at the point of use [7] – Private health insurance in fragmented financing systems can lead to lower access to health services, especially among the poorest. Relying solely on private health insurance can result in populations, especially poorer and unhealthier groups, being excluded from schemes based on higher risk of illness or high costs [7] – Curative driven care, little to no emphasis on public health and prevention	– Requires actuarial expertise and is costly to operate [7] – Requires some expertise from the individuals to know what services are covered and at what rates they will be reimbursed by their insurance schemes	– Costlier to operate due to smaller pools and higher technical and administration costs relative to the size of the pool [7]
User fees (e.g., *Mali, co-payments)*	– No pooling across households and no spreading of risk over time +–Individuals are the purchasers. They purchase only the services they can afford with their income or personal savings	– No cross-subsidisation of rich and poor – Disproportionately burdens poorer populations and can lead to medical impoverishment [5]	+ Can in some circumstances mitigate excess demand and ensure the availability of certain services [7] – Often deters service usage, especially among poorer populations [14]	+ Comparatively easy to operate depending on the amount and type of exemptions – Can be difficult to regulate	Payments may cause individuals/households to experience catastrophic payments that can lead to financial instability and impoverishment

(continued)

Table 86.1 (continued)

Mechanism	Implications on pooling function	Fair financing	Universal health coverage	Ease of operation	Financial sustainability
Medical savings account (e.g., *Singapore*)	– Can prevent the displacement of necessary consumption due to healthcare costs + – No pooling across households but spreads risk over time. + – Individuals are the purchasers. They purchase the services they can afford with their Medical Savings Account (MSA). However, they might be allowed to use their MSA to pay only for a set of approved services [15]	– There is usually little scope for cross-subsidisation between rich and poor	+ Compared to user fees, it can help to spread risk over time – Compared to tax based or social health insurance, can deter service usage of expensive medical procedures – Medical savings are usually linked to individual income. Therefore, low-income individuals may deplete their accounts when purchasing high-cost medical services	–Requires some expertise from the individuals to know which services can be paid for using their MSA	–Individuals can deplete their accounts quickly if they experience high-cost medical procedures –Individuals may experience catastrophic payments, which can lead to financial instability and impoverishment
Donor funding (e.g., *Ethiopia*)	– Donor funding often cannot be pooled with other public funds	+ Donor funding often targets pro-poor health and public health services	+ Can supplement government budgets and support the provision of essential services free at the point of use – Can result in fragmented health systems with separate patient pathways depending on whether services are donor funded or not	– Government absorptive capacity, the extent to which recipient governments can effectively spend financial resources, is essential for donor funding to have an impact	– Can displace government funding and create fragmentation of funding for different services – Donor funding can fluctuate between funding cycles (e.g. 3–5 years) and reduces as a recipient country's GDP increases – Replacement of donor funding with government funding is often slower than the withdrawal of donor funds

Table 86.2 Common provider payment mechanisms and incentives[a]

Payment mechanism	Definition	Incentives for provider
Fee for service (FFS)	Provider is reimbursed (retrospectively) for each individual service deliver	Increase the number of services, including beyond what is necessary (leads to oversupply or supplier induced demand), reduce inputs per service (improve technical efficiency)
Capitation	Provider receive a fixed payment per each registered individual for a fixed period of time to provide an agreed package of services	Attract more enrollees, undersupply services, decrease inputs (may improve efficiency), provide less expensive interventions and increase referrals to next level, attempt to select healthier (less costly) enrollees (called 'cream skimming' behaviour)
Salary	Provider, usually employed by an institution, receive a fixed salary every month	No incentive to improve efficiency, quality of life or oversupply
Pay for performance (performance-based payment)	Provider is paid on the basis of achieving certain performance thresholds	Increase provision of the targeted services, overreport provision of targeted services ('gaming' behaviour)
Line-item budget	Providers (mainly hospitals) receive prospectively a given amount of money to spend on specific inputs or line items (e.g. staff, medicine, food etc.). Budget generally decided based on the previous years' budget. Spending the budget is not flexible	Undersupply services, increase referrals (in particular, complex patients), spend remaining budget by the end of the budget year. No incentive to improve quality of care and efficiency
Global budget	Providers (mainly hospitals) receive prospectively a lump sum payment to spend, flexibly, to deliver a specified package of services over a period of time (usually a year)	Undersupply services, increase referrals, decrease inputs (may improve efficiency)
Per diem	Provider (mainly hospital) is paid a fixed amount to provide given services per day	Increase the number of inpatient days or lengths of hospital stay; reduce inputs per inpatient day (may improve the efficiency)
Case-based (e.g. diagnosis-related groups-DRGs)	Health care provider (mainly hospital) is paid a flat amount per case such as for each diagnosis, admission, or discharge	Increase admissions (may leads to oversupply); reduce inputs per case (may improve efficiency); admit less severe cases ('cream skimming')

[a] Sources: Adapted from [16, 17, 18]

86.4 Impoverishing Effects of Health Expenditure

In the absence of prepayment mechanisms such as taxes or insurance, patients pay providers at the point of use. These payments are also known as out-of-pocket payments (OOPs) and can deter service usage [14], especially among the poor and for preventive services. OOPs include deductibles, co-payments for consultation fees or medication and any other costs that are not pre-paid before the point of use of a service [19]. Prices charged by healthcare providers often do not consider an individual's ability to pay. This financing mechanism reduces or eliminates risk pooling, and the highest cost burden tends to fall on the poor, children or the elderly [20]. Two main indicators are used to estimate the financial burden caused by OOPs: (a) catastrophic health expenditure, and (b) health impoverishment.

Catastrophic health expenditure measures whether OOPs exceed a threshold of a household's income or non-food consumption (e.g. 10% or 40%) [21]. This aims to estimate whether OOPs displace other necessary consumption. Health impoverishment measures if OOPs drive vulnerable households into poverty or deepen poverty among the poor [22]. This is known as a medical poverty trap, which can have severe consequences such as delayed care seeking leading to more severe or untreated illnesses, and inappropriate or irrational drug use leading to drug resistance. This results in further health deterioration and higher health costs [20]. To avoid or alleviate large financial burdens, the WHO recommends that:

- Population coverage be extended through public prepayment mechanisms;
- The poor and disadvantaged are protected through exemptions;
- Designing an essential benefits package for all (horizontal programme); and
- Deciding the level of cost sharing by the patients [23].

86.5 How to Reduce Waste in Health Systems

Countries have limited resources and must avoid ineffective spending. An estimated one-fifth of Organisation for Economic Co-operation and Development (OECD) health expenditure [24] and 20–40% of health expenditure globally [5] does not contribute to improved health outcomes.

Wasteful spending is mainly caused by technical and allocative inefficiencies, but also corruption and fraud [5]. Examples of technical inefficiencies include underuse of generic drugs, use of ineffective and low-quality drugs, inappropriate staff mix or poor incentive/payment mechanisms. Allocative inefficiency is caused by an inefficient mix of interventions [5, 25]. Health Technology Assessment, where cost-effectiveness estimates for different interventions are compared, informs allocative efficiency. Health economics can also inform the design of payment mechanisms that aim to align individual and health system incentives by rewarding waste-averting decisions [26]. However, health economics alone cannot address the forms of waste that require institutional or legislative reform.

86.6 Using Burden of Disease for Priority Setting

Given limited resources, countries must find the most effective interventions to tackle the most pressing health needs. This is known as priority setting [27]. There is no standardised method for setting priorities but most use burden of disease to understand the greatest need [28]. Burden of disease can be measured in different ways including years of life lost, healthy years of life lost, quality adjusted life years (QALYs), or disability-adjusted life years (DALYs) [29].

Burden of disease can aid priority setting by identifying the regions or populations suffering the highest burden [28]. Similarly, it can help monitor progress and re-organise priorities if the burden increases in previously neglected areas.

Investing resources in the areas with the highest burden of disease does not, however, guarantee that the most cost-effective interventions will be used [30]. Additionally, burden of disease is a population-level aggregate measure that cannot identify the worst-off, who are generally defined in terms of non-health dimensions such as gender or socio-economic status [28]. The risk of introducing allocatively inefficient interventions or exacerbating health inequity must always be considered.

86.7 Conclusion

Despite the high priority given to health within global development goals, prevailing economic conditions are likely to challenge investment in this critical area. Economic tools are needed to ensure financing mechanisms spread risk through large risk pools, healthcare workers are incentivised appropriately, and that allocative and technical efficiency are maximised within systems. Priority setting is a complex process that should incorporate insights from evidence-based medicine, cost-effectiveness analyses and equity considerations [28, 31].

References

1. Preston SH. The changing relation between mortality and level of economic development. Popul Stud. 1975;29(2):231–48.
2. Smith JP. Healthy bodies and thick wallets: the dual relation between health and economic status. J Econ Perspect. 1999;13(2):145–66.
3. World Health Organization. Macroeconomics and health: investing in health for economic development: executive summary/report of the commission on macroeconomics and health. In: Macroeconomics and health: investing in health for economic development: executive summary/report of the Commission on Macroeconomics and Health; 2001.
4. Kutzin J. A descriptive framework for country-level analysis of health care financing arrangements. Health Policy. 2001;56(3):171–204.
5. World Health Organization. The world health report: health systems financing: the path to universal coverage. World Health Organization; 2010.
6. Yazbeck AS, Savedoff WD, Hsiao WC, Kutzin J, Soucat A, Tandon A, Chi-Man Yip W, et al. The case against labor-tax-financed social health insurance for low-and low-middle-income countries: a summary of recent research into labor-tax financing of social health insurance in low-and low-middle-income countries. Health Aff. 2020;39(5):892–7.
7. The King's Fund (2017). How health care is funded.. Retrieved from https://www.kingsfund.org.uk/publications/how-health-care-is-funded.
8. Watkins DA, Qi J, Kawakatsu Y, Pickersgill SJ, Horton SE, Jamison DT. Resource requirements for essential universal health coverage: a modelling study based on findings from disease control priorities. Lancet Glob Health. 2020;8(6):e829–39.
9. Smith P, Witter S. Risk pooling in health care financing: the implications for health system performance. Washington: The World Bank; 2004.
10. Wagstaff A. Social health insurance reexamined. Health Econ. 2010;19(5):503–17.
11. Carrin G, Waelkens MP, Criel B. Community-based health insurance in developing countries: a study of its contribution to the performance of health financing systems. Tropical Med Int Health. 2005;10(8):799–811.
12. Ekman B. Community-based health insurance in low-income countries: a systematic review of the evidence. Health Policy Plan. 2004;19(5):249–70.
13. Doorslaer EV, Wagstaff A, Rutten F. Equity in the finance and delivery of health care: an international perspective. Oxford University Press; 1992.
14. Lagarde M, Palmer N. The impact of user fees on access to health services in low-and middle-income countries. Cochrane Database Syst Rev. 2011;2011(4):CD009094.
15. Tan CC, Lam CS, Matchar DB, Zee YK, Wong JE. Singapore's health-care system: key features, challenges, and shifts. Lancet. 2021;398(10305):1091–104.
16. Cashin C. Assessing health provider payment systems: A practical guide for countries working toward universal health coverage. Washington, DC: Joint Learning Network for Universal Health Coverage; 2015.
17. Langenbrunner J, Cashin C, O'Dougherty S, World Bank. Designing and implementing health care provider payment systems: how-to manuals. Washington, D.C.: World Bank; 2009.
18. Guinness L, Wiseman V. Introduction to heath economics. Second ed. Open University Press; 2011.
19. McPake B, Normand C, Smith S, Nolan A. Tax and social health insurance mechanisms. In: McPake B, Normand C, Smith S, Nolan A, editors. Health economics: an international perspective. London: Routledge; 2020.
20. Whitehead M, Dahlgren G, Evans T. Equity and health sector reforms: can low-income countries escape the medical poverty trap? Lancet. 2001;358(9284):833–6.
21. Wagstaff A, Flores G, Hsu J, Smitz M-F, Chepynoga K, Buisman LR, Eozenou P, et al. Progress on catastrophic health spending in 133 countries: a retro-

spective observational study. Lancet Glob Health. 2018a;6(2):e169–79.
22. Wagstaff A, Flores G, Smitz M-F, Hsu J, Chepynoga K, Eozenou P. Progress on impoverishing health spending in 122 countries: a retrospective observational study. Lancet Glob Health. 2018b;6(2):e180–92.
23. World Health Organization. (2005). Designing health financing systems to reduce catastrophic health expenditure.. Retrieved from.
24. Organization for Economic Co-operation and Development. Tackling wasteful spending on health; 2017.
25. Cylus J, Papanicolas I, Smith PC. A framework for thinking about health system efficiency. In: Health system efficiency, vol. 1. Copenhagen (Denmark): European Observatory on Health Systems and Policies; 2016.
26. Luft HS. Economic incentives to promote innovation in healthcare delivery. Clin Orthop Relat Res. 2009;467(10):2497–505.
27. Shiell A, Donaldson C, Mitton C, Currie G. Health economic evaluation. J Epidemiol Community Health. 2002;56(2):85.
28. Ottersen T, Norheim OF. The uses of burden-of-disease data for priority setting. In: Measuring the global burden of disease: philosophical dimensions; 2020. p. 293.
29. Murray CJ, Lopez AD. Measuring the global burden of disease. N Engl J Med. 2013;369(5):448–57.
30. Mooney G, Wiseman V. Burden of disease and priority setting. Health Econ. 2000;9(5):369–72.
31. Baltussen R, Niessen L. Priority setting of health interventions: the need for multi-criteria decision analysis. Cost Eff Resour Alloc. 2006;4(1):1–9.

87 Priority Setting: How to Increase Value for Money in Health Investments

Javier Guzman

Abstract

Priority setting is a critical tool to support donors and governments in maximizing the "value for money" of health spending; ensuring access to safe, effective, quality assured, and affordable medicines and vaccines; and ultimately achieving universal health coverage. Low- and middle-income countries often utilize priority setting in the face of growing health needs and resource constraints in order to shift from aspirational and implicit approaches where all health technologies and services are covered to explicit packages, which specify what services and products are provided to whom and at what price. The priority setting process requires adequate structures and institutional arrangements, should be underpinned by clear governing principles, and should follow a set of systematic steps. If done properly, decisions will be more effective, legitimate, and accepted, likely leading to more sustainable health systems and better health outcomes.

Keywords

Priority setting · Universal health coverage · Cost-effectiveness · Health benefit package · Decision-making

J. Guzman (✉)
Center for Global Development, Washington, DC, USA
e-mail: jguzman@cgdev.org

87.1 Introduction

Medicines, vaccines, procedures, and other health technologies are essential to prevent, diagnose, and treat disease and improve quality of life. Due to their importance, equitable access to them is a global priority embedded in the Sustainable Development Goals (SGDs). In particular, Target 3.8.1 explicitly talks about achieving universal health coverage (UHC), including access to safe, effective, quality assured, and affordable essential medicines and vaccines for all.

Despite this laudable aspiration and the progress made before the COVID-19 pandemic—the UHC Service Coverage Index, which measures progress against target 3.8.1, increased from an average of 45/100 in 2000 to 66/100 in 2017 [1], health systems in low- and middle-income countries (LMICs), face a critical challenge. How to address growing health needs and allocate resources within the constraint of limited funding. Donors and governments must decide what investments will secure for society the greatest "value for money." They must decide what health technologies and services are provided to whom using public funds,, and at what price. This process of selecting among different options for addressing the most important health needs, given limited resources is referred to as "priority setting" [2].

M. C. B. Raviglione et al. (eds.), *Global Health Essentials*, Sustainable Development Goals Series,
https://doi.org/10.1007/978-3-031-33851-9_87

This chapter outlines where priority setting takes place, the principles that should govern the process, and the steps and methods that should be followed at the national level for priority setting to be successful.

87.2 Where Does Priority Setting Take Place?

Funders at all levels (e.g., global, national, subnational) make decisions on their priorities either by action or inaction. Donors, for example, might decide to prioritize a disease (e.g., HIV), an institution (e.g., Gavi, The Vaccine Alliance), or a population (e.g., children under 5 years of age). At the national level, LMIC governments tend to start with implicit rationing approaches. For example, countries might guarantee "all necessary services and products" on paper while, in reality, the treatments patients actually receive are severely restricted by budget size, lack of infrastructure, scarce human resources, and other constraints [3].

As LMICs move toward UHC with the goal of expanding priority services, including more people, and reducing out-of-pocket payments, they start moving toward explicit approaches including defining a health benefit package (HBP)—an explicit list of health services to be provided using public funds. Then, as processes mature, countries often move to making only incremental adjustments to their HBP, usually adding or excluding single interventions. This is not a linear process, and countries often move from implicit approaches to incremental adjustments, or from an explicit HBP to implicit rationing approaches. Since LMICs spend a high proportion of their health budgets on health technologies—the World Health Organization estimates that LMICs spend between 20 and 60% of their health budgets on medicines [4]-, explicit priority setting often focuses on health technologies there.

87.3 Governing Principles

Any priority setting process must be embedded in appropriate legal frameworks with clear overarching governing principles and institutional arrangements. Governments must also ensure adequate financing, sufficient expertise, and reasonable timeframes for priority setting to be successful. Different authors have recommended several principles to guide priority setting [5–7]. Overall, the process must be:

- *Based on national values, translated into clear policy goals and decision criteria*: values and goals might include health improvement, fair distribution of health outcomes, solidarity, or fair financial risk protection. Values and goals should be translated into decision criteria such as burden of disease, cost and effectiveness of the intervention, and equity and priority to the worse off, among others.
- *Transparent*: citizens and stakeholders should have access to the information they need to understand the process and its results. Anyone should be able to look at and understand what is covered and how and why decisions were made.
- *Participatory*: all interested parties should be systematically involved in the different stages of the priority setting process and should be actively engaged, exchanging views on argumentation and evidence. Potential conflicts of interests should be managed to reduce the potential for undue influence.
- *Evidenced-based and data driven*: decisions should be informed by data on each of the selected decision criteria. Established methodologies, such as health technology assessment, offer a systematic approach to measure the medical, economic, social, and ethical issues related to the use of a health technology [8].
- *Consistent*: the process should be stable, should follow explicit rules, and should not

change arbitrarily or every time leadership changes.

- *Implementable*: the final list of services to be provided should be costed, based on realistic projections of current and future utilization. Decisions should also be linked to adequate policies to ensure that resources (e.g., financial, human) required for these services to be delivered are guaranteed.

Implementing these principles will increase legitimacy, rigor, fairness, and will improve the quality of decision-making. This will make the process and its decisions more likely to be sustainable.

87.4 Stages of the Priority Setting Process

Several stages should be followed for adequately implementing priority setting process [9, 10] - see Fig. 87.1. These steps are not always linear, and decision-makers often incorporate the elements outlined in each step differently.

Establishing governance and institutional arrangements: involves setting up adequate structures and operationalizing the governing principles described in the previous section.

Identifying goals and defining decision criteria: decision-makers clearly state the intended impact of the process as well as the decision criteria that will be used. They should reach these conclusions following a transparent and participatory approach.

Choosing shape and scoping technologies for assessment: decision-makers determine the structure of the HBP, the level of detail it will include and the scope of the exercise (e.g., whole package review vs incremental process). Consequently, and in a participatory manner, they identify health technologies for evaluation.

Evaluating: different methods are used to assess identified health technologies against the decision criteria that have been established. Cost-effectiveness analysis, for example, provides information on incremental costs and incremental health benefits, usually measured in terms of expected health gain (see illustration in Fig. 87.2). Budget impact analysis quantifies the potential financial and fiscal impact of adopting and/or increasing coverage to a technology. Adaptive approaches are often used.

> If the costs and benefits of two interventions are compared, four possible outcomes exist. Two of those don't present any difficulty for decision-making (no-brainers) but two require decision-makers to determine their willingness to pay (i.e., how much money they are willing to pay for an additional unit of health value?)

- *Appraising the evidence*: an advisory committee normally reviews the evidence gathered as part of the evaluation and makes recommen-

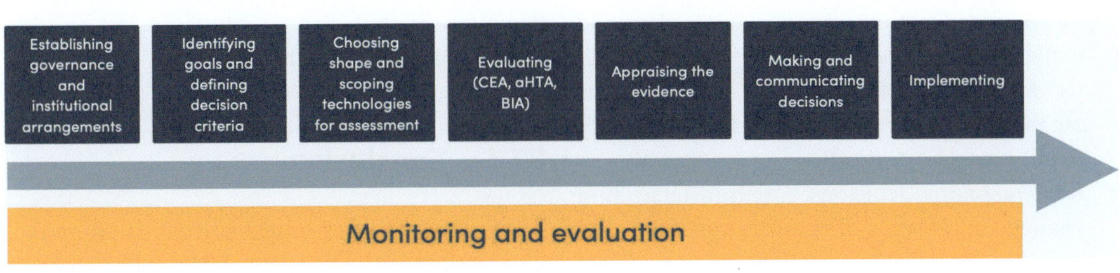

Fig. 87.1 Steps to implement priority setting processes

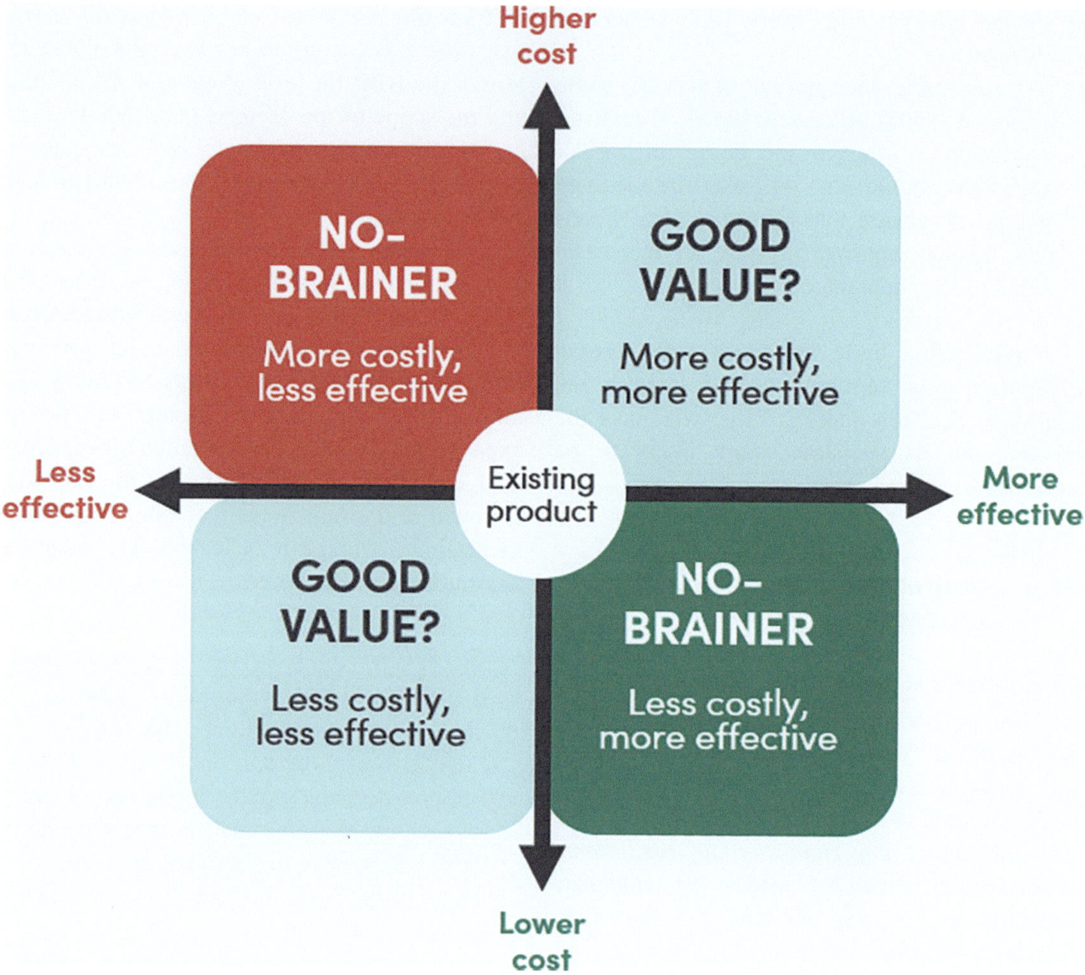

Fig. 87.2 Cost-effectiveness plane

dations to finance or not to finance with public funding.

- *Making and communicating decisions*: decision-making body assesses the recommendations from the appraisal committee and makes the final decision to include a health technology in public budgets. These decisions are then communicated clearly and effectively to all relevant actors, allowing for appeals.
- *Implementing*: decisions are translated into changes in resource allocation, coverage, and use, through different mechanisms (e.g., fiscal transfers, reimbursements, product procurement). Securing quality in the delivery of those interventions and products is essential.

It is important that the process and its implementation are systematically measured, both to guarantee compliance and improve performance but also to identify shortcomings and update decisions made based on new evidence and lessons from implementation.

87.5 Conclusion

Explicit, evidenced-based priority setting is a cornerstone to achieving UHC. The process requires adequate structures and institutional arrangements, should be underpinned by clear governing principles, and should follow a set of systematic steps. It implies moving from aspirational and implicit approaches where everything is covered in theory to explicit packages, which specify what services and products are provided to whom and at what price. If done properly, decisions will be more effective, legitimate, and accepted. This will increase sustainability and likely lead to better health.

References

1. United Nations. The sustainable development goals report. 2021. https://unstats.un.org/sdgs/report/2021/The-Sustainable-Development-Goals-Report-2021.pdf.
2. Terwindt F, Rajan D, Soucat A. Chapter 4. Priority setting for national health policies, strategies and plans. In: Schmets G, Rajan D, Kadandale S, editors. Strategizing national health in the 21st century: a handbook. Geneva: World Health Organization; 2016.
3. Glassman A, Chalkidou K. And the priority-setting institutions for Global Health working group. Priority-setting in health: building institutions for smarter public spending. Washington, DC: Center for Global Development; 2012. http://www.cgdev.org/sites/default/files/1426240_file_priority_setting_global_health_FINAL_0.pdf. Accessed 14 October 2015.
4. World Health Organization. Access to Medicines and Vaccines. Report by the Director General. A72/17. Geneva. 2019. https://apps.who.int/gb/ebwha/pdf_files/WHA72/A72_17-en.pdf.
5. World Health Organization. Principles of health benefit packages. Geneva: World Health Organization; 2021. https://www.who.int/publications/i/item/9789240020689.
6. Norheim OF, Baltussen R, Johri M, et al. Guidance on priority setting in health care (GPS-health): the inclusion of equity criteria not captured by cost-effectiveness analysis. Cost Eff Resour Alloc. 2014;12:18. https://doi.org/10.1186/1478-7547-12-18.
7. Giedion U, Guzman J. Defining the rules of the game: good governance principles for the design and revision of the health benefits package. In: Glassman A, Giedion U, Smith P, editors. What's in, what's out: designing benefits for Universal Health Coverage. Washington DC: Center for Global Development; 2017.
8. Bertram M, Dhaene G, Tan-Torres Edejer T, editors. Institutionalizing health technology assessment mechanisms: a how to guide. Geneva: World Health Organization; 2021.
9. Glassman A, Giedion U, Smith P. What's in, What's out: designing benefits for universal health coverage. Washington DC: Center for Global Development; 2017.
10. Oortwijn W, Jansen M, Baltussen R. Evidence-informed deliberative processes for health benefit package design – Part II: A practical guide. Int J Health Policy Manag. 2021;11(10):2327–36. https://doi.org/10.34172/ijhpm.2021.159.

Principles of Global Health Project Management

88

Federico Lega and Elena Maggioni

Abstract

Global Health programs and projects require robust project management as they are often extremely complex due to their technical contents, sensitive issues addressed, political and social environment where they take place, multi-stakeholders expectations and interests, timing, and funding. Therefore, mastering the project management cycle, adopting the right tools, and playing at its best the role of project manager are of paramount importance for organizations and institutions involved in Global Health. The chapter provides the principles and foundations that should inform the way project management is developed and the role of the manager played.

Keywords

Project management · Project planning · Project cycle management · Logical framework approach · Global health projects

F. Lega (✉)
Department of Biomedical Sciences for Health and Acting Director of the Research Center in Health Administration (HEAD), University of Milan, Milan, Italy
e-mail: federico.lega@unimi.it

E. Maggioni
Research Center in Health Administration (HEAD), University of Milan, Milan, Italy
e-mail: elena.maggioni@unimi.it

88.1 Why Project Management Is Key in Global Health

International institutions, supranational agencies, and non-governmental organizations working in the Global Health environment (hereafter Global Health Organizations—GHOs) deliver their "services" often through ad hoc projects.

In this perspective, a fundamental role played by their front-line staff is that of project manager.

Building and delivering a project concerning Global Health issues generate several challenges, as it often involves—just to say a few—multiple stakeholders, institutional (e.g., formal, bureaucratic, ambiguous, ceremonial) procedures, complex accountability systems, and difficult and uncertain sustainability. Last but not least, Global Health programs run by GHOs are usually a bundle of several different projects, a situation that increases the importance of good coordination and governance of the full spectrum of projects as they often impact on same targets, stakeholders, outcomes and have cross-effects on social/economic/cultural dynamics.

Further, GHOs operate in a highly competitive context when one looks at sources of funding and have the need to plan and organize their projects to manage them efficiently and improve the attractiveness of proposals/request for financial support to potential funders/donors.

M. C. B. Raviglione et al. (eds.), *Global Health Essentials*, Sustainable Development Goals Series,
https://doi.org/10.1007/978-3-031-33851-9_88

Therefore, sound project management is a key "management" competence much seek after by GHOs, a core focus in their recruitment policy and without doubt one of the scarcest professional expertise available on the market. This chapter will frame and outline the foundations of the cycle of project management that could be used as a reference.

Project management, or management by project, can be defined as the application of knowledge, professional and personal skills, methods, techniques, and tools to the activities of a project to meet its requirements. Project management is considered successful when allows achieving the project's objectives on time, within the budgeted costs, with the desired level of performance, and with the satisfaction of end users and all stakeholders [1]. By "project" we usually mean a group of activities to produce a specific goal in a fixed time frame for a specific target (e.g., group or cluster of people, single organization); while a "program" is a series of projects whose objectives together contribute to a greater objective beneficial for a "greater" target, like a country, a sector, the government, or a whole population [2].

The frameworks and reflections presented throughout this chapter are suitable for both, though we'll refer just to project from now on.

88.2 The Project Management Cycle [2]

Projects are planned and carried out following a predetermined sequence of actions that defines its management cycle. Hence, the project cycle provides "structure" to ensure a clear and linear identification of activities that need to be organized and supervised by the project manager during the lifetime of the project itself (Fig. 88.1). While the duration and importance of each phase may vary for different projects, the framework presents some essential characteristics: key decisions, required information, and responsibilities are defined at each phase; the phases in the cycle are strictly progressive and stakeholders should be involved in the process as much as possible.

These stages can be summarized as follows:

1. *Programming*. The output of this phase is a multi-annual document that identifies problems, constraints, and opportunities that should or could be faced with the project. A specific strategic document can be developed in this phase stating the reasons for the project, the key players to be involved, the time frame, and the expected impact. This document can be the starting point for the development of the next steps of a full business plan for the project, which will be required to obtain institutional and financial support from the key stakeholders/donors. An example of contents that should be included in this strategic document is the template designed by European Commission for project proposals (Box 88.1). A description of the background of the project is usually the starting point for any PjM's plan. Project managers must develop analyses to describe the sector/context and identify problems or opportunities connected to the projects, also through a specific stakeholders' analysis. Therefore, the template includes a detailed description of the project's aims (objectives, targets to be achieved and strategic priorities), its operations and timing (estimated costs, timetable, monitoring, and evaluation), features and impacts (technologies used, socio-cultural aspects, gender equality, environmental protection), and sustainability (financial and economic viability). This programming process includes the major elements developed through the Logical Framework Approach (LFA or Logframe Approach) explained in Box 88.2.
2. *Identification*. Analysis of the stakeholders and of target groups, beneficiaries (e.g., women, socio-economic groups), and situations that could be faced. Thus, the expected outcome is a pre-feasibility analysis, outlining different options to reach the identified objectives and suggesting the one(s) to be further studied during the appraisal phase, examining the coherence between the project and the objectives defined.
3. *Appraisal*. Preparatory studies that include technical, contractual, and financial aspects of

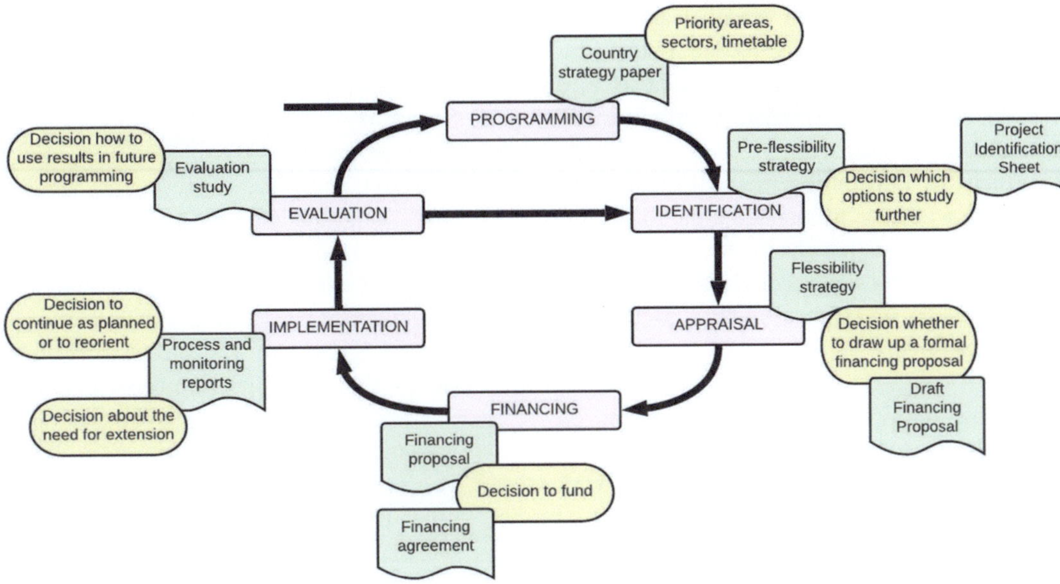

Fig. 88.1 Steps in the project cycle management

the projects focused on the feasibility, sustainability, and quality of the suggested intervention. This phase allows an *"ex-ante"* evaluation of an ongoing or completed project through cost-effective analysis. The Logframe framework should be completed at the end of the appraisal phase.

4. *Financing*. Entities and governments examine proposals on whether to fund the project. Hence, during this phase, a final version of the financing proposal needs to be drafted and assessed, also including the analysis carried out during the previous stages such as stakeholder analysis, target/beneficiaries' identification, project description, and so on.
5. *Implementation*. This phase is usually characterized by meetings finalized to the contract signature for studies, technical assistance, works, or supplies. This stage also includes monitoring and reporting activities to enable adjustment to change circumstances. Execution is the focus of the project management activity and respect of timing and goals become the key objectives.
6. *Evaluation*. The evaluation of the project must consider both the project as a whole and the results per specific target (i.e., country/region) or stakeholder. An evaluation can be done during implementation ("mid-term"), at its end ("final evaluation"), or afterward ("ex-post evaluation"), either to help steer the project or to draw lessons for future projects and programming.

88.3 Some Remarks on Project Managers

Project management requires the designation of a project manager who supervises all the above steps and ensures the right implementation and execution of activities designed for each phase of the project. The project manager usually leads a team, the project team, which is a time-limited continuing work unit producing one-time outputs. The Project Manager (PjM) should have hierarchical authority over members of the team, which are selected from different organizational units or recruited ad hoc for the project, and permanently assigned to the team for all its duration. If the PjM has not full (or at least partial) hierarchical authority then his/her work becomes more complex as the source of "power" becomes his/her capacity to be influential over the group members, building even a stronger leadership than what it would be usually needed. In this situation, it would be advisable to appoint as PjM someone with strong expertise, credibility, and informal recognition.

Further, the PjM during the project management cycle will have to manage a parallel cycle defined by the steps that characterize the dynamics of the team. It is well recognized in the literature that teams will (most likely) go through stages such as [3]:

- Forming, during which the team agrees on goals, begins to know each other, and acknowledge challenges and opportunities in the work to come.
- Storming, the second stage of team development, where the group starts to sort itself out and gain each other's trust to generate the team's own identity. Conflict may arise between team members as power and status are assigned, working styles emerge, priorities differ. Here the PjM must establish quickly his/her leadership.
- Norming, when rules, roles and expected behaviors are agreed and the team starts to cooperate in an efficient and effective mode.
- Performing, when the team works as a unity and decision-making processes are well structured, roles are recognized and respected, focus on achieving goals.
- Adjourning (or mourning) is the time for celebrating successes and manage properly the breaking up of the team.

The role of the PjM is then of paramount importance both for the identification of tools and models that best fit the need of project management of the specific program/project and for the supervision of the group's dynamics that ultimately could determine the success or failure.

Box 88.1 Template for Project Planning Proposed by European Commission

1. **Summary**
2. **Background:** Overall EC and Government policy objectives, and links with the Commission's country programme or strategy, the commitment of Government to overarching policy objectives of the EC such as respect of human rights
3. **Sectoral and problem analysis**, including stakeholder analysis and their potentials
4. **Project/programme description,** objectives, and the strategy to attain them
   - Including lessons from past experience, and linkage with other donors' activities
   - Description of the intervention (objectives, and strategy to reach them, including Project Purpose, Results and Activities and main indicators)
5. **Assumptions, risks**
6. **Implementation arrangements**
   - Physical and non-physical means
   - Organisation and implementation procedures
   - Timetable (work plan)
   - Estimated cost and financing plan
   - Special conditions and accompanying measures by Government/partners
   - Monitoring and Evaluation
7. **Quality factors**
   - Participation and ownership by beneficiaries
   - Policy support

- Appropriate technology
- Socio-cultural aspects
- Gender equality
- Environmental protection
- Institutional and management capacities
- Financial and economic viability

Annex: Logframe (completed or outline, depending on the phase)

Box 88.2 Logical Framework Matrix [4]

A logical framework matrix (or Logframe) is the output of a program design process where program/project activities are listed and linked with immediate outputs and final outcomes and goal. Logframe helps to identify and analyze the contingent situation (and connected risks/opportunities) to better design the activities that should be undertaken to manage and monitor the implementation of the program/project. Here below is provided a template for a Logframe. It is important to underline that to complete the analysis, it is necessary also to include specific inputs on expectations of stakeholders/beneficiaries of the program/project and situational analysis of the political/social/institutional contexts that might impose constraints and priorities on project timing and development.

Logical framework (Logframe) template

	Project summary	Indicators	Means of verification	Risks/assumptions
Goal				
Outcomes				
Outputs				
Activities				

References

1. Dal Maso M, Mastrofini E, Rambaldi E. Capitolo 3–Gli elementi di conoscenza della certificazione ISIPM. In: I. I. Management, editor. Guida alla certificazione base di project management in sanità. Milano: FrancoAngeli Srl; 2009. p. 28–31.
2. European Commission—EuropAid Co-operation Office. Project cycle management—handbook. Freiburg, Germany: PARTICIP GmbH; 2022.
3. Tuckman, B., & Jensen, M. (1977). Stages of small-group development revisited (Vols. 2(4)). Group & Organization Studies.
4. Bording Collins K. What is a logframe? Washington DC: American University; 2021. https://programs.online.american.edu/online-graduate-certificates/project-monitoring/resources/what-is-a-logframe.

Correction to: Global Oral Health

Sante Leandro Baldi, Gemma Bridge,
and Richard G. Watt

Correction to:
Chapter 32 in: M. C. B. Raviglione et al. (eds.), *Global Health Essentials*, Sustainable Development Goals Series,
https://doi.org/10.1007/978-3-031-33851-9_32

The original version of Chapter 32 was inadvertently published with incorrect affiliation of Richard G. Watt. The affiliation has been corrected as follows:

Department of Epidemiology and Public Health, University College London, WHO Collaborating Center for Oral Health Inequalities and Public Health, London. r.watt@ucl.ac.uk

The updated version of this chapter can be found at https://doi.org/10.1007/978-3-031-33851-9_32

M. C. B. Raviglione et al. (eds.), *Global Health Essentials*, Sustainable Development Goals Series,
https://doi.org/10.1007/978-3-031-33851-9_89

MIX
Papier aus verantwortungsvollen Quellen
Paper from responsible sources
FSC® C105338

If you have any concerns about our products,
you can contact us on
ProductSafety@springernature.com

In case Publisher is established outside the EU,
the EU authorized representative is:
Springer Nature Customer Service Center GmbH
Europaplatz 3, 69115 Heidelberg, Germany

Printed by Libri Plureos GmbH
in Hamburg, Germany